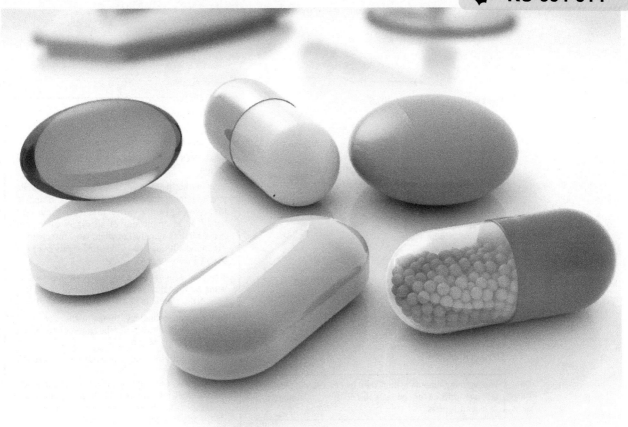

BMJ Research Methods and Reporting:

Reporting Research

Edited by
Professor Adrian Hunnisett

BPP
UNIVERSITY
SCHOOL OF HEALTH

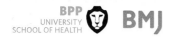

First edition February 2016

ISBN 9781 4727 4557 6
eISBN 9781 4727 4564 4
eISBN 9781 4727 4571 2

British Library Cataloguing-in-Publication Data
A catalogue record for this book is available
from the British Library

Published by
BPP Learning Media Ltd
BPP House, Aldine Place
London W12 8AA

www.bpp.com/health

Printed in the United Kingdom by
CPI Antony Rowe

Bumper's Farm,
Chippenham,
Wiltshire
SN14 6LH

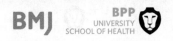

About the publisher

BPP Learning Media is dedicated to supporting aspiring professionals with top quality learning material. BPP Learning Media's commitment to success is shown by our record of quality, innovation and market leadership in paper-based and e-learning materials. BPP Learning Media's study materials are written by professionally-qualified specialists who know from personal experience the importance of top quality materials for success.

About The BMJ

The BMJ (formerly the British Medical Journal) in print has a long history and has been published without interruption since 1840. The BMJ's vision is to be the world's most influential and widely read medical journal. Our mission is to lead the debate on health and to engage, inform, and stimulate doctors, researchers, and other health professionals in ways that will improve outcomes for patients. We aim to help doctors to make better decisions. BMJ, the company, advances healthcare worldwide by sharing knowledge and expertise to improve experiences, outcomes and value.

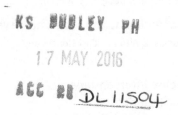

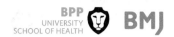

Contents

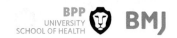

About the author

Professor Adrian Hunnisett is a biomedical scientist specialising in clinical biochemistry and haematology. He completed initial BMS training at Gloucester Royal Hospital and then graduated from Oxford Brookes University, completing research training in Oxford and London. He has worked in a variety of roles within the NHS and private medical sectors, most recently as Head of Clinical R&D at Southampton General Hospital. He is now Professor of Evidence-Based Healthcare at BPP University.

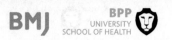

Introduction to Research Methods and Reporting series

As a healthcare worker, you are working in an "evidence-based" or "evidence-informed" professional environment whatever your professional discipline, whether you are doctors, nurses, physiotherapists, occupational therapist or part of the emerging plethora of allied professions. The evidence you use, the research base, is being generated constantly and that is impacting on clinical practice at all levels. The information you all learned in your clinical training has rapidly, and inevitably, become outdated. As a result there is a clear need to understand the principles of research and research methods to help you make decisions about the mass of new knowledge and integrating it into your practice whilst discontinuing the "old traditions".

Over recent years, the teaching of clinical research methods, research practice and the evaluation of clinical evidence has become a core addition to undergraduate and postgraduate curricula across all healthcare disciplines. In addition, many clinical journals have articles and sections concentrating on continuing education providing tools for reading and critiquing the vast amount of emerging research. Such material is considered so important in the development of evidence-based practice that they may attract credits toward the CPD portfolios required by many of the professional registration bodies today.

The BMJ Research Methods & Reporting books bring together a collection of review articles first published in the British Medical Journal. They are not designed to replace the basic knowledge of research methods and evaluation, but rather to answer some of the key questions that researchers at all levels ask along with updates in the reporting structures and regulations for articles in the medical press. Each of the articles is written by acknowledged experts in their fields and they offer a broad update on many aspects of research, research methodology and guidelines for undertaking and reporting research. They are written in a user-friendly way that is easy to follow and understand by the non-specialist. In addition, each article is fully referenced with links to further information and evidence to support the statements made in the article. The collections are aimed at non-specialist doctors, general practitioners, research nurses and healthcare practitioners. They can also be used by individuals who may be preparing for any postgraduate examinations that have a research element.

There are two separate volumes, each concentrating on a different aspect of the research process. The first volume examines some key messages about the basics of research along with up to date articles on statistical approaches, methods and interpretation. The topics covered concentrate on subjects such as confidence intervals, p values, sample size calculations, use of patient reported outcome measures, conundrums in the application of RCT and more complex statistical analysis. It also highlights implementation research and prognostic research. The second is more specific with articles on the reporting requirements for research. It examines guidelines such as CONSORT, SPIRIT, GPP2, PRISMA and the IDEAL framework for surgical innovation. It also gives some guidance on economic evaluations, policy and service interventions and publication guidelines, as well as providing useful tips on preparing data for publication.

Each book is a stand-alone volume, but together they will give the reader a comprehensive overview of the commoner research issues and guidelines.

Adrian Hunnisett (November 2015).

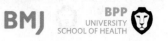

CONSORT 2010 Explanation and Elaboration: updated guidelines for reporting parallel group randomised trials

David Moher, senior scientist[1], Sally Hopewell, senior research fellow[2], Kenneth F Schulz, distinguished scientist and vice president[3], Victor Montori, professor of medicine[4], Peter C Gøtzsche, director[5], P J Devereaux, clinical scholar[6], Diana Elbourne, professor of health care evaluation[7], Matthias Egger, head of department and professor of epidemiology and public health[8], Douglas G Altman, professor[2]

[1]Ottawa Methods Centre, Clinical Epidemiology Program, Ottawa Hospital Research Institute, Ottawa Hospital, Ottawa, Ontario, Canada, K1H 8L6

[2]Centre for Statistics in Medicine, University of Oxford, Wolfson College, Oxford

[3]Family Health International, Research Triangle Park, NC 27709, USA

[4]UK Knowledge and Encounter Research Unit, Mayo Clinic, Rochester, MN, USA

[5]The Nordic Cochrane Centre, Rigshospitalet, Blegdamsvej 9, Copenhagen, Denmark

[6]McMaster University Health Sciences Centre, Hamilton, Canada

[7]Medical Statistics Unit, London School of Hygiene and Tropical Medicine, London

[8]Institute of Social and Preventive Medicine (ISPM), University of Bern, Switzerland

Correspondence to: D Moher
dmoher@ohri.ca

Cite this as: BMJ 2010;340:c869

DOI: 10.1136/bmj.c869

http://www.bmj.com/content/340/bmj.c869

"The whole of medicine depends on the transparent reporting of clinical trials."[1]

Well designed and properly executed randomised controlled trials (RCTs) provide the most reliable evidence on the efficacy of healthcare interventions, but trials with inadequate methods are associated with bias, especially exaggerated treatment effects.[2][3][4][5] Biased results from poorly designed and reported trials can mislead decision making in health care at all levels, from treatment decisions for a patient to formulation of national public health policies.

Critical appraisal of the quality of clinical trials is possible only if the design, conduct, and analysis of RCTs are thoroughly and accurately described in the report. Far from being transparent, the reporting of RCTs is often incomplete,[6][7][8][9] compounding problems arising from poor methodology.[10][11][12][13][14][15]

Incomplete and inaccurate reporting

Many reviews have documented deficiencies in reports of clinical trials. For example, information on the method used in a trial to assign participants to comparison groups was reported in only 21% of 519 trial reports indexed in PubMed in 2000,[16] and only 34% of 616 reports indexed in 2006.[17] Similarly, only 45% of trial reports indexed in PubMed in 2000[16] and 53% in 2006[17] defined a primary end point, and only 27% in 2000 and 45% in 2006 reported a sample size calculation. Reporting is not only often incomplete but also sometimes inaccurate. Of 119 reports stating that all participants were included in the analysis in the groups to which they were originally assigned (intention-to-treat analysis), 15 (13%) excluded patients or did not analyse all patients as allocated.[18] Many other reviews have found that inadequate reporting is common in specialty journals[16][19] and journals published in languages other than English.[20][21]

Proper randomisation reduces selection bias at trial entry and is the crucial component of high quality RCTs.[22] Successful randomisation hinges on two steps: generation of an unpredictable allocation sequence and concealment of this sequence from the investigators enrolling participants (see box 1).[2][23]

Unfortunately, despite that central role, reporting of the methods used for allocation of participants to interventions is also generally inadequate. For example, 5% of 206 reports of supposed RCTs in obstetrics and gynaecology journals described studies that were not truly randomised.[23] This estimate is conservative, as most reports do not at present provide adequate information about the method of allocation.[20][23][30][31][32][33]

ABSTRACT

Overwhelming evidence shows the quality of reporting of randomised controlled trials (RCTs) is not optimal. Without transparent reporting, readers cannot judge the reliability and validity of trial findings nor extract information for systematic reviews. Recent methodological analyses indicate that inadequate reporting and design are associated with biased estimates of treatment effects. Such systematic error is seriously damaging to RCTs, which are considered the gold standard for evaluating interventions because of their ability to minimise or avoid bias.

A group of scientists and editors developed the CONSORT (Consolidated Standards of Reporting Trials) statement to improve the quality of reporting of RCTs. It was first published in 1996 and updated in 2001. The statement consists of a checklist and flow diagram that authors can use for reporting an RCT. Many leading medical journals and major international editorial groups have endorsed the CONSORT statement. The statement facilitates critical appraisal and interpretation of RCTs.

During the 2001 CONSORT revision, it became clear that explanation and elaboration of the principles underlying the CONSORT statement would help investigators and others to write or appraise trial reports. A CONSORT explanation and elaboration article was published in 2001 alongside the 2001 version of the CONSORT statement.

After an expert meeting in January 2007, the CONSORT statement has been further revised and is published as the CONSORT 2010 Statement. This update improves the wording and clarity of the previous checklist and incorporates recommendations related to topics that have only recently received recognition, such as selective outcome reporting bias.

This explanatory and elaboration document—intended to enhance the use, understanding, and dissemination of the CONSORT statement—has also been extensively revised. It presents the meaning and rationale for each new and updated checklist item providing examples of good reporting and, where possible, references to relevant empirical studies. Several examples of flow diagrams are included.

The CONSORT 2010 Statement, this revised explanatory and elaboration document, and the associated website (www.consort-statement.org) should be helpful resources to improve reporting of randomised trials.

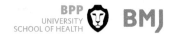

Improving the reporting of RCTs: the CONSORT statement

DerSimonian and colleagues suggested that "editors could greatly improve the reporting of clinical trials by providing authors with a list of items that they expected to be strictly reported."[34] Early in the 1990s, two groups of journal editors, trialists, and methodologists independently published recommendations on the reporting of trials.[35] [36] In a subsequent editorial, Rennie urged the two groups to meet and develop a common set of recommendations [37]; the outcome was the CONSORT statement (Consolidated Standards of Reporting Trials).[38]

The CONSORT statement (or simply CONSORT) comprises a checklist of essential items that should be included in reports of RCTs and a diagram for documenting the flow of participants through a trial. It is aimed at primary reports of RCTs with two group, parallel designs. Most of CONSORT is also relevant to a wider class of trial designs, such as non-inferiority, equivalence, factorial, cluster, and crossover trials. Extensions to the CONSORT checklist for reporting trials with some of these designs have been published,[39] [40] [41] as have those for reporting certain types of data (harms [42]), types of interventions (non-pharmacological treatments [43], herbal interventions[44]), and abstracts.[45]

The objective of CONSORT is to provide guidance to authors about how to improve the reporting of their trials. Trial reports need be clear, complete, and transparent. Readers, peer reviewers, and editors can also use CONSORT to help them critically appraise and interpret reports of RCTs. However, CONSORT was not meant to be used as a quality assessment instrument. Rather, the content of CONSORT focuses on items related to the internal and external validity of trials. Many items not explicitly mentioned in CONSORT should also be included in a report, such as information about approval by an ethics committee, obtaining informed consent from participants, and, where relevant, existence of a data safety and monitoring committee. In addition, any other aspects of a trial that are mentioned should be properly reported, such as information pertinent to cost effectiveness analysis.[46] [47] [48]

Since its publication in 1996, CONSORT has been supported by more than 400 journals (www.consort-statement.org) and several editorial groups, such as the International Committee of Medical Journal Editors.[49] The introduction of CONSORT within journals is associated with improved quality of reports of RCTs.[17] [50] [51] However, CONSORT is an ongoing initiative, and the CONSORT statement is revised periodically.[3] CONSORT was last revised nine years ago, in 2001.[52] [53] [54] Since then the evidence base to inform CONSORT has grown considerably; empirical data have highlighted new concerns regarding the reporting of RCTs, such as selective outcome reporting.[55] [56] [57] A CONSORT Group meeting was therefore convened in January 2007, in Canada, to revise the 2001 CONSORT statement and its accompanying explanation and elaboration document. The revised checklist is shown in table 1 and the flow diagram, not revised, in fig 1.[52] [53] [54]

The CONSORT 2010 Statement: explanation and elaboration

During the 2001 CONSORT revision, it became clear that explanation and elaboration of the principles underlying the CONSORT statement would help investigators and others to write or appraise trial reports. The CONSORT explanation and elaboration article[58] was published in 2001 alongside the 2001 version of the CONSORT statement. It discussed the rationale and scientific background for each item and provided published examples of good reporting. The rationale for revising that article is similar to that for revising the statement, described above. We briefly describe below the main additions and deletions to this version of the explanation and elaboration article.

The CONSORT 2010 Explanation and Elaboration: changes

We have made several substantive and some cosmetic changes to this version of the CONSORT explanatory document (full details are highlighted in the 2010 version of the CONSORT statement[59]). Some reflect changes to the CONSORT checklist; there are three new checklist items in the CONSORT 2010 checklist—such as item 24, which asks authors to report where their trial protocol can be accessed. We have also updated some existing explanations, including adding more recent references to methodological evidence, and used some better examples. We have removed the glossary, which is now available on the CONSORT website (www.consort-statement.org). Where possible, we describe the findings of relevant empirical studies. Many excellent books on clinical trials offer fuller discussion of methodological issues.[60] [61] [62] Finally, for convenience, we sometimes refer to "treatments" and "patients," although we recognise that not all interventions evaluated in RCTs are treatments and not all participants are patients.

BOX 1 TREATMENT ALLOCATION. WHAT'S SO SPECIAL ABOUT RANDOMISATION?

The method used to assign interventions to trial participants is a crucial aspect of clinical trial design. Random assignment is the preferred method; it has been successfully used regularly in trials for more than 50 years.[24] Randomisation has three major advantages.[25] First, when properly implemented, it eliminates selection bias, balancing both known and unknown prognostic factors, in the assignment of treatments. Without randomisation, treatment comparisons may be prejudiced, whether consciously or not, by selection of participants of a particular kind to receive a particular treatment. Second, random assignment permits the use of probability theory to express the likelihood that any difference in outcome between intervention groups merely reflects chance.[26] Third, random allocation, in some situations, facilitates blinding the identity of treatments to the investigators, participants, and evaluators, possibly by use of a placebo, which reduces bias after assignment of treatments.[27] Of these three advantages, reducing selection bias at trial entry is usually the most important.[28]

Successful randomisation in practice depends on two interrelated aspects—adequate generation of an unpredictable allocation sequence and concealment of that sequence until assignment occurs.[2] [23] A key issue is whether the schedule is known or predictable by the people involved in allocating participants to the comparison groups.[29] The treatment allocation system should thus be set up so that the person enrolling participants does not know in advance which treatment the next person will get, a process termed allocation concealment.[2] [23] Proper allocation concealment shields knowledge of forthcoming assignments, whereas proper random sequences prevent correct anticipation of future assignments based on knowledge of past assignments.

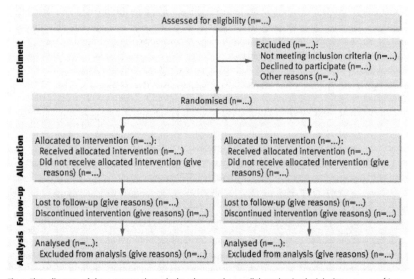

Fig 1 Flow diagram of the progress through the phases of a parallel randomised trial of two groups (that is, enrolment, intervention allocation, follow-up, and data analysis)[52] [53] [54]

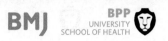

Table 1 CONSORT 2010 checklist of information to include when reporting a randomised trial*

Section/Topic	Item No	Checklist item	Reported on page No
Title and abstract			
	1a	Identification as a randomised trial in the title	
	1b	Structured summary of trial design, methods, results, and conclusions (for specific guidance see CONSORT for abstracts[45 65])	
Introduction			
Background and objectives	2a	Scientific background and explanation of rationale	
	2b	Specific objectives or hypotheses	
Methods			
Trial design	3a	Description of trial design (such as parallel, factorial) including allocation ratio	
	3b	Important changes to methods after trial commencement (such as eligibility criteria), with reasons	
Participants	4a	Eligibility criteria for participants	
	4b	Settings and locations where the data were collected	
Interventions	5	The interventions for each group with sufficient details to allow replication, including how and when they were actually administered	
Outcomes	6a	Completely defined pre-specified primary and secondary outcome measures, including how and when they were assessed	
	6b	Any changes to trial outcomes after the trial commenced, with reasons	
Sample size	7a	How sample size was determined	
	7b	When applicable, explanation of any interim analyses and stopping guidelines	
Randomisation:			
Sequence generation	8a	Method used to generate the random allocation sequence	
	8b	Type of randomisation; details of any restriction (such as blocking and block size)	
Allocation concealment mechanism	9	Mechanism used to implement the random allocation sequence (such as sequentially numbered containers), describing any steps taken to conceal the sequence until interventions were assigned	
Implementation	10	Who generated the random allocation sequence, who enrolled participants, and who assigned participants to interventions	
Blinding	11a	If done, who was blinded after assignment to interventions (for example, participants, care providers, those assessing outcomes) and how	
	11b	If relevant, description of the similarity of interventions	
Statistical methods	12a	Statistical methods used to compare groups for primary and secondary outcomes	
	12b	Methods for additional analyses, such as subgroup analyses and adjusted analyses	
Results			
Participant flow (a diagram is strongly recommended)	13a	For each group, the numbers of participants who were randomly assigned, received intended treatment, and were analysed for the primary outcome	
	13b	For each group, losses and exclusions after randomisation, together with reasons	
Recruitment	14a	Dates defining the periods of recruitment and follow-up	
	14b	Why the trial ended or was stopped	
Baseline data	15	A table showing baseline demographic and clinical characteristics for each group	
Numbers analysed	16	For each group, number of participants (denominator) included in each analysis and whether the analysis was by original assigned groups	
Outcomes and estimation	17a	For each primary and secondary outcome, results for each group, and the estimated effect size and its precision (such as 95% confidence interval)	
	17b	For binary outcomes, presentation of both absolute and relative effect sizes is recommended	
Ancillary analyses	18	Results of any other analyses performed, including subgroup analyses and adjusted analyses, distinguishing pre-specified from exploratory	
Harms	19	All important harms or unintended effects in each group (for specific guidance see CONSORT for harms[42])	
Discussion			
Limitations	20	Trial limitations, addressing sources of potential bias, imprecision, and, if relevant, multiplicity of analyses	
Generalisability	21	Generalisability (external validity, applicability) of the trial findings	
Interpretation	22	Interpretation consistent with results, balancing benefits and harms, and considering other relevant evidence	
Other information			
Registration	23	Registration number and name of trial registry	
Protocol	24	Where the full trial protocol can be accessed, if available	
Funding	25	Sources of funding and other support (such as supply of drugs), role of funders	

*We strongly recommend reading this statement in conjunction with the CONSORT 2010 Explanation and Elaboration for important clarifications on all the items. If relevant, we also recommend reading CONSORT extensions for cluster randomised trials,[40] non-inferiority and equivalence trials,[39] non-pharmacological treatments,[43] herbal interventions,[44] and pragmatic trials.[41] Additional extensions are forthcoming: for those and for up to date references relevant to this checklist, see www.consort-statement.org.

Checklist items
Title and abstract
Item 1a. Identification as a randomised trial in the title.

Example—"Smoking reduction with oral nicotine inhalers: double blind, randomised clinical trial of efficacy and safety."[63]

Explanation—The ability to identify a report of a randomised trial in an electronic database depends to a large extent on how it was indexed. Indexers may not classify a report as a randomised trial if the authors do not explicitly report this information.[64] To help ensure that a study is appropriately indexed and easily identified, authors should use the word "randomised" in the title to indicate that the participants were randomly assigned to their comparison groups.

Item 1b. Structured summary of trial design, methods, results, and conclusions
For specific guidance see CONSORT for abstracts.[45 65]

Explanation—Clear, transparent, and sufficiently detailed abstracts are important because readers often base their assessment of a trial on such information. Some readers use an abstract as a screening tool to decide whether to read the full article. However, as not all trials are freely available and some health professionals do not have access to the full trial reports, healthcare decisions are sometimes made on the basis of abstracts of randomised trials.[66]

A journal abstract should contain sufficient information about a trial to serve as an accurate record of its conduct and findings, providing optimal information about the trial within the space constraints and format of a journal. A properly constructed and written abstract helps individuals to assess quickly the relevance of the findings and aids the retrieval of relevant reports from electronic databases.[67] The abstract should accurately reflect what is included in the full journal article and should not include information that does not appear in the body of the paper. Studies comparing the accuracy of information reported in a journal abstract with that reported in the text of the full publication have found claims that are inconsistent with, or missing from, the body of the full article.[68 69 70 71] Conversely, omitting important harms from the abstract could seriously mislead someone's interpretation of the trial findings.[42 72]

A recent extension to the CONSORT statement provides a list of essential items that authors should include when reporting the main results of a randomised trial in a journal (or conference) abstract (see table 2).[45] We strongly recommend the use of structured abstracts for reporting randomised trials. They provide readers with information about the trial under a series of headings pertaining to the design, conduct, analysis, and interpretation.[73] Some studies have found that structured abstracts are of higher quality than the more traditional descriptive abstracts[74 75] and that they allow readers to find information more easily.[76] We recognise that many journals have developed their own structure and word limit for reporting abstracts. It is not our intention to suggest changes to these formats, but to recommend what information should be reported.

Introduction

Item 2a. Scientific background and explanation of rationale
Example—"Surgery is the treatment of choice for patients with disease stage I and II non-small cell lung cancer (NSCLC) ... An NSCLC meta-analysis combined the results from eight randomised trials of surgery versus surgery plus adjuvant

cisplatin-based chemotherapy and showed a small, but not significant (p=0.08), absolute survival benefit of around 5% at 5 years (from 50% to 55%). At the time the current trial was designed (mid-1990s), adjuvant chemotherapy had not become standard clinical practice ... The clinical rationale for neo-adjuvant chemotherapy is three-fold: regression of the primary cancer could be achieved thereby facilitating and simplifying or reducing subsequent surgery; undetected micro-metastases could be dealt with at the start of treatment; and there might be inhibition of the putative stimulus to residual cancer by growth factors released by surgery and by subsequent wound healing ... The current trial was therefore set up to compare, in patients with resectable NSCLC, surgery alone versus three cycles of platinum-based chemotherapy followed by surgery in terms of overall survival, quality of life, pathological staging, resectability rates, extent of surgery, and time to and site of relapse."[77]

Explanation—Typically, the introduction consists of free flowing text, in which authors explain the scientific background and rationale for their trial, and its general outline. It may also be appropriate to include here the objectives of the trial (see item 2b).The rationale may be explanatory (for example, to assess the possible influence of a drug on renal function) or pragmatic (for example, to guide practice by comparing the benefits and harms of two treatments). Authors should report any evidence of the benefits and harms of active interventions included in a trial and should suggest a plausible explanation for how the interventions might work, if this is not obvious.[78]

The Declaration of Helsinki states that biomedical research involving people should be based on a thorough knowledge of the scientific literature.[79] That is, it is unethical to expose humans unnecessarily to the risks of research. Some clinical trials have been shown to have been unnecessary because the question they addressed had been or could have been answered by a systematic review of the existing literature.[80 81] Thus, the need for a new trial should be justified in the introduction. Ideally, it should include a reference to a systematic review of previous similar trials or a note of the absence of such trials.[82]

Item 2b. Specific objectives or hypotheses
Example—"In the current study we tested the hypothesis that a policy of active management of nulliparous labour would: 1. reduce the rate of caesarean section, 2. reduce the rate of prolonged labour; 3. not influence maternal satisfaction with the birth experience."[83]

Explanation—Objectives are the questions that the trial was designed to answer. They often relate to the efficacy of a particular therapeutic or preventive intervention. Hypotheses are pre-specified questions being tested to help meet the objectives. Hypotheses are more specific than objectives and are amenable to explicit statistical evaluation. In practice, objectives and hypotheses are not always easily differentiated. Most reports of RCTs provide adequate information about trial objectives and hypotheses.[84]

Methods

Item 3a. Description of trial design (such as parallel, factorial) including allocation ratio

Example—"This was a multicenter, stratified (6 to 11 years and 12 to 17 years of age, with imbalanced randomisation [2:1]), double-blind, placebo-controlled, parallel-group study conducted in the United States (41 sites)."[85]

Explanation—The word "design" is often used to refer to all aspects of how a trial is set up, but it also has a narrower

Table 2   Items to include when reporting a randomised trial in a journal abstract

Item	Description
Authors	Contact details for the corresponding author
Trial design	Description of the trial design (such as parallel, cluster, non-inferiority)
Methods:	
Participants	Eligibility criteria for participants and the settings where the data were collected
Interventions	Interventions intended for each group
Objective	Specific objective or hypothesis
Outcome	Clearly defined primary outcome for this report
Randomisation	How participants were allocated to interventions
Blinding (masking)	Whether participants, care givers, and those assessing the outcomes were blinded to group assignment
Results:	
Numbers randomised	Number of participants randomised to each group
Recruitment	Trial status
Numbers analysed	Number of participants analysed in each group
Outcome	For the primary outcome, a result for each group and the estimated effect size and its precision
Harms	Important adverse events or side effects
Conclusions	General interpretation of the results
Trial registration	Registration number and name of trial register
Funding	Source of funding

interpretation. Many specific aspects of the broader trial design, including details of randomisation and blinding, are addressed elsewhere in the CONSORT checklist. Here we seek information on the type of trial, such as parallel group or factorial, and the conceptual framework, such as superiority or non-inferiority, and other related issues not addressed elsewhere in the checklist.

The CONSORT statement focuses mainly on trials with participants individually randomised to one of two "parallel" groups. In fact, little more than half of published trials have such a design.[16] The main alternative designs are multi-arm parallel, crossover, cluster,[40] and factorial designs. Also, most trials are set to identify the superiority of a new intervention, if it exists, but others are designed to assess non-inferiority or equivalence.[39] It is important that researchers clearly describe these aspects of their trial, including the unit of randomisation (such as patient, GP practice, lesion). It is desirable also to include these details in the abstract (see item 1b).

If a less common design is employed, authors are encouraged to explain their choice, especially as such designs may imply the need for a larger sample size or more complex analysis and interpretation.

Although most trials use equal randomisation (such as 1:1 for two groups), it is helpful to provide the allocation ratio explicitly. For drug trials, specifying the phase of the trial (I-IV) may also be relevant.

Item 3b. Important changes to methods after trial commencement (such as eligibility criteria), with reasons
Example—"Patients were randomly assigned to one of six parallel groups, initially in 1:1:1:1:1:1 ratio, to receive either one of five otamixaban … regimens … or an active control of unfractionated heparin … an independent Data Monitoring Committee reviewed unblinded data for patient safety; no interim analyses for efficacy or futility were done. During the trial, this committee recommended that the group receiving the lowest dose of otamixaban (0·035 mg/kg/h) be discontinued because of clinical evidence of inadequate anticoagulation. The protocol was immediately amended in accordance with that recommendation, and participants were subsequently randomly assigned in 2:2:2:2:1 ratio to the remaining otamixaban and control groups, respectively."[86]

Explanation—A few trials may start without any fixed plan (that is, are entirely exploratory), but the most will have a protocol that specifies in great detail how the trial will be conducted. There may be deviations from the original protocol, as it is impossible to predict every possible change in circumstances during the course of a trial. Some trials will therefore have important changes to the methods after trial commencement.

Changes could be due to external information becoming available from other studies, or internal financial difficulties, or could be due to a disappointing recruitment rate. Such protocol changes should be made without breaking the blinding on the accumulating data on participants' outcomes. In some trials, an independent data monitoring committee will have as part of its remit the possibility of recommending protocol changes based on seeing unblinded data. Such changes might affect the study methods (such as changes to treatment regimens, eligibility criteria, randomisation ratio, or duration of follow-up) or trial conduct (such as dropping a centre with poor data quality).[87]

Some trials are set up with a formal "adaptive" design. There is no universally accepted definition of these designs, but a working definition might be "a multistage study design that uses accumulating data to decide how to modify aspects of the study without undermining the validity and integrity of the trial."[88] The modifications are usually to the sample sizes and the number of treatment arms and can lead to decisions being made more quickly and with more efficient use of resources. There are, however, important ethical, statistical, and practical issues in considering such a design.[89] [90]

Whether the modifications are explicitly part of the trial design or in response to changing circumstances, it is essential that they are fully reported to help the reader interpret the results. Changes from protocols are not currently well reported. A review of comparisons with protocols showed that about half of journal articles describing RCTs had an unexplained discrepancy in the primary outcomes.[57] Frequent unexplained discrepancies have also been observed for details of randomisation, blinding,[91] and statistical analyses.[92]

Item 4a. Eligibility criteria for participants
Example—"Eligible participants were all adults aged 18 or over with HIV who met the eligibility criteria for antiretroviral therapy according to the Malawian national HIV treatment guidelines (WHO clinical stage III or IV or any WHO stage with a CD4 count <250/mm³) and who were starting treatment with a BMI <18.5. Exclusion criteria were pregnancy and lactation or participation in another supplementary feeding programme."[93]

Explanation—A comprehensive description of the eligibility criteria used to select the trial participants is needed to help readers interpret the study. In particular, a clear understanding of these criteria is one of several elements required to judge to whom the results of a trial apply—that is, the trial's generalisability (applicability) and relevance to clinical or public health practice (see item 21).[94] A description of the method of recruitment, such as by referral or self selection (for example, through advertisements), is also important in this context. Because they are applied before randomisation, eligibility criteria do not affect the internal validity of a trial, but they are central to its external validity.

Typical and widely accepted selection criteria relate to the nature and stage of the disease being studied, the exclusion of persons thought to be particularly vulnerable to harm from the study intervention, and to issues required to ensure that the study satisfies legal and ethical norms. Informed consent by study participants, for example, is typically required in intervention studies. The common distinction between inclusion and exclusion criteria is unnecessary; the same criterion can be phrased to include or exclude participants.[95]

Despite their importance, eligibility criteria are often not reported adequately. For example, eight published trials leading to clinical alerts by the National Institutes of Health specified an average of 31 eligibility criteria in their protocols, but only 63% of the criteria were mentioned in the journal articles, and only 19% were mentioned in the clinical alerts.[96] Similar deficiencies were found for HIV clinical trials.[97] Among 364 reports of RCTs in surgery, 25% did not specify any eligibility criteria.[98]

Item 4b. Settings and locations where the data were collected
Example—"The study took place at the antiretroviral therapy clinic of Queen Elizabeth Central Hospital in Blantyre, Malawi, from January 2006 to April 2007. Blantyre is the

major commercial city of Malawi, with a population of 1 000 000 and an estimated HIV prevalence of 27% in adults in 2004."[93]

Explanation—Along with the eligibility criteria for participants (see item 4a) and the description of the interventions (see item 5), information on the settings and locations is crucial to judge the applicability and generalisability of a trial. Were participants recruited from primary, secondary, or tertiary health care or from the community? Healthcare institutions vary greatly in their organisation, experience, and resources and the baseline risk for the condition under investigation. Other aspects of the setting (including the social, economic, and cultural environment and the climate) may also affect a study's external validity.

Authors should report the number and type of settings and describe the care providers involved. They should report the locations in which the study was carried out, including the country, city if applicable, and immediate environment (for example, community, office practice, hospital clinic, or inpatient unit). In particular, it should be clear whether the trial was carried out in one or several centres ("multicentre trials"). This description should provide enough information so that readers can judge whether the results of the trial could be relevant to their own setting. The environment in which the trial is conducted may differ considerably from the setting in which the trial's results are later used to guide practice and policy.[94 99] Authors should also report any other information about the settings and locations that could have influenced the observed results, such as problems with transportation that might have affected patient participation or delays in administering interventions.

Item 5. The interventions for each group with sufficient details to allow replication, including how and when they were actually administered

Examples—"In POISE, patients received the first dose of the study drug (ie, oral extended-release metoprolol 100 mg or matching placebo) 2-4 h before surgery. Study drug administration required a heart rate of 50 bpm or more and a systolic blood pressure of 100 mm Hg or greater; these haemodynamics were checked before each administration. If, at any time during the first 6 h after surgery, heart rate was 80 bpm or more and systolic blood pressure was 100 mm Hg or higher, patients received their first postoperative dose (extended-release metoprolol 100 mg or matched placebo) orally. If the study drug was not given during the first 6 h, patients received their first postoperative dose at 6 h after surgery. 12 h after the first postoperative dose, patients started taking oral extended-release metoprolol 200 mg or placebo every day for 30 days. If a patient's heart rate was consistently below 45 bpm or their systolic blood pressure dropped below 100 mm Hg, study drug was withheld until their heart rate or systolic blood pressure recovered; the study drug was then restarted at 100 mg once daily. Patients whose heart rate was consistently 45-49 bpm and systolic blood pressure exceeded 100 mm Hg delayed taking the study drug for 12 h."[100]

"Patients were randomly assigned to receive a custom-made neoprene splint to be worn at night or to usual care. The splint was a rigid rest orthosis recommended for use only at night. It covered the base of the thumb and the thenar eminence but not the wrist (Figure 1). Splints were made by 3 trained occupational therapists, who adjusted the splint for each patient so that the first web could be opened and the thumb placed in opposition with the first long finger. Patients were encouraged to contact the occupational therapist if they felt that the splint needed adjustment, pain increased while wearing the splint, or they had adverse effects (such as skin erosion). Because no treatment can be considered the gold standard in this situation, patients in the control and intervention groups received usual care at the discretion of their physician (general practitioner or rheumatologist). We decided not to use a placebo because, to our knowledge, no placebo for splinting has achieved successful blinding of patients, as recommended."[101]

Explanation—Authors should describe each intervention thoroughly, including control interventions. The description should allow a clinician wanting to use the intervention to know exactly how to administer the intervention that was evaluated in the trial.[102] For a drug intervention, information would include the drug name, dose, method of administration (such as oral, intravenous), timing and duration of administration, conditions under which interventions are withheld, and titration regimen if applicable. If the control group is to receive "usual care" it is important to describe thoroughly what that constitutes. If the control group or intervention group is to receive a combination of interventions the authors should provide a thorough description of each intervention, an explanation of the order in which the combination of interventions are introduced or withdrawn, and the triggers for their introduction if applicable.

Specific extensions of the CONSORT statement address the reporting of non-pharmacologic and herbal interventions and their particular reporting requirements (such as expertise, details of how the interventions were standardised).[43 44] We recommend readers consult the statements for non-pharmacologic and herbal interventions as appropriate.

Item 6a. Completely defined pre-specified primary and secondary outcome measures, including how and when they were assessed

Example—"The primary endpoint with respect to efficacy in psoriasis was the proportion of patients achieving a 75% improvement in psoriasis activity from baseline to 12 weeks as measured by the PASI [psoriasis area and severity index] Additional analyses were done on the percentage change in PASI scores and improvement in target psoriasis lesions."[103]

Explanation—All RCTs assess response variables, or outcomes (end points), for which the groups are compared. Most trials have several outcomes, some of which are of more interest than others. The primary outcome measure is the pre-specified outcome considered to be of greatest importance to relevant stakeholders (such a patients, policy makers, clinicians, funders) and is usually the one used in the sample size calculation (see item 7). Some trials may have more than one primary outcome. Having several primary outcomes, however, incurs the problems of interpretation associated with multiplicity of analyses (see items 18 and 20) and is not recommended. Primary outcomes should be explicitly indicated as such in the report of an RCT. Other outcomes of interest are secondary outcomes (additional outcomes). There may be several secondary outcomes, which often include unanticipated or unintended effects of the intervention (see item 19), although harms should always be viewed as important whether they are labelled primary or secondary.

All outcome measures, whether primary or secondary, should be identified and completely defined. The principle here is that the information provided should be sufficient to allow others to use the same outcomes.[102] When outcomes are assessed at several time points after randomisation, authors should also indicate the pre-specified time point of primary interest. For many non-pharmacological interventions it is helpful to specify who assessed outcomes (for example, if special skills are required to do so) and how many assessors there were.[43]

Where available and appropriate, the use of previously developed and validated scales or consensus guidelines should be reported,[104] [105] both to enhance quality of measurement and to assist in comparison with similar studies.[106] For example, assessment of quality of life is likely to be improved by using a validated instrument.[107] Authors should indicate the provenance and properties of scales.

More than 70 outcomes were used in 196 RCTs of non-steroidal anti-inflammatory drugs for rheumatoid arthritis,[108] and 640 different instruments had been used in 2000 trials in schizophrenia, of which 369 had been used only once.[33] Investigation of 149 of those 2000 trials showed that unpublished scales were a source of bias. In non-pharmacological trials, a third of the claims of treatment superiority based on unpublished scales would not have been made if a published scale had been used.[109] Similar data have been reported elsewhere.[110] [111] Only 45% of a cohort of 519 RCTs published in 2000 specified the primary outcome[16]; this compares with 53% for a similar cohort of 614 RCTs published in 2006.[17]

Item 6b. Any changes to trial outcomes after the trial commenced, with reasons

Example—"The original primary endpoint was all-cause mortality, but, during a masked analysis, the data and safety monitoring board noted that overall mortality was lower than had been predicted and that the study could not be completed with the sample size and power originally planned. The steering committee therefore decided to adopt co-primary endpoints of all-cause mortality (the original primary endpoint), together with all-cause mortality or cardiovascular hospital admissions (the first prespecified secondary endpoint)."[112]

Explanation—There are many reasons for departures from the initial study protocol (see item 24). Authors should report all major changes to the protocol, including unplanned changes to eligibility criteria, interventions, examinations, data collection, methods of analysis, and outcomes. Such information is not always reported.

As indicated earlier (see item 6a), most trials record multiple outcomes, with the risk that results will be reported for only a selected subset (see item 17). Pre-specification and reporting of primary and secondary outcomes (see item 6a) should remove such a risk. In some trials, however, circumstances require a change in the way an outcome is assessed or even, as in the example above, a switch to a different outcome. For example, there may be external evidence from other trials or systematic reviews suggesting the end point might not be appropriate, or recruitment or the overall event rate in the trial may be lower than expected.[112] Changing an end point based on unblinded data is much more problematic, although it may be specified in the context of an adaptive trial design.[88] Authors should identify and explain any such changes. Likewise, any changes after the trial began of the designation of outcomes as primary or secondary should be reported and explained.

A comparison of protocols and publications of 102 randomised trials found that 62% of trials reports had at least one primary outcome that was changed, introduced, or omitted compared with the protocol.[55] Primary outcomes also differed between protocols and publications for 40%

of a cohort of 48 trials funded by the Canadian Institutes of Health Research.[113] Not one of the subsequent 150 trial reports mentioned, let alone explained, changes from the protocol. Similar results from other studies have been reported recently in a systematic review of empirical studies examining outcome reporting bias.[57]

Item 7a. How sample size was determined

Examples—"To detect a reduction in PHS (postoperative hospital stay) of 3 days (SD 5 days), which is in agreement with the study of Lobo et al[17] with a two-sided 5% significance level and a power of 80%, a sample size of 50 patients per group was necessary, given an anticipated dropout rate of 10%. To recruit this number of patients a 12-month inclusion period was anticipated."[114]

"Based on an expected incidence of the primary composite endpoint of 11% at 2.25 years in the placebo group, we calculated that we would need 950 primary endpoint events and a sample size of 9650 patients to give 90% power to detect a significant difference between ivabradine and placebo, corresponding to a 19% reduction of relative risk (with a two-sided type 1 error of 5%). We initially designed an event-driven trial, and planned to stop when 950 primary endpoint events had occurred. However, the incidence of the primary endpoint was higher than predicted, perhaps because of baseline characteristics of the recruited patients, who had higher risk than expected (e.g., lower proportion of NYHA class I and higher rates of diabetes and hypertension). We calculated that when 950 primary endpoint events had occurred, the most recently included patients would only have been treated for about 3 months. Therefore, in January 2007, the executive committee decided to change the study from being event-driven to time-driven, and to continue the study until the patients who were randomised last had been followed up for 12 months. This change did not alter the planned study duration of 3 years."[115]

Explanation—For scientific and ethical reasons, the sample size for a trial needs to be planned carefully, with a balance between medical and statistical considerations. Ideally, a study should be large enough to have a high probability (power) of detecting as statistically significant a clinically important difference of a given size if such a difference exists. The size of effect deemed important is inversely related to the sample size necessary to detect it; that is, large samples are necessary to detect small differences. Elements of the sample size calculation are (1) the estimated outcomes in each group (which implies the clinically important target difference between the intervention groups); (2) the α (type I) error level; (3) the statistical power (or the β (type II) error level); and (4), for continuous outcomes, the standard deviation of the measurements.[116] The interplay of these elements and their reporting will differ for cluster trials[40] and non-inferiority and equivalence trials.[39]

Authors should indicate how the sample size was determined. If a formal power calculation was used, the authors should identify the primary outcome on which the calculation was based (see item 6a), all the quantities used in the calculation, and the resulting target sample size per study group. It is preferable to quote the expected result in the control group and the difference between the groups one would not like to overlook. Alternatively, authors could present the percentage with the event or mean for each group used in their calculations. Details should be given of any allowance made for attrition or non-compliance during the study.

Some methodologists have written that so called underpowered trials may be acceptable because they could ultimately be combined in a systematic review and meta-analysis,[117] [118] [119] and because some information is better than no information. Of note, important caveats apply—such as the trial should be unbiased, reported properly, and published irrespective of the results, thereby becoming available for meta-analysis.[118] On the other hand, many medical researchers worry that underpowered trials with indeterminate results will remain unpublished and insist that all trials should individually have "sufficient power." This debate will continue, and members of the CONSORT Group have varying views. Critically however, the debate and those views are immaterial to reporting a trial. Whatever the power of a trial, authors need to properly report their intended size with all their methods and assumptions.[118] That transparently reveals the power of the trial to readers and gives them a measure by which to assess whether the trial attained its planned size.

In some trials, interim analyses are used to help decide whether to stop early or to continue recruiting sometimes beyond the planned trial end (see item 7b). If the actual sample size differed from the originally intended sample size for some other reason (for example, because of poor recruitment or revision of the target sample size), the explanation should be given.

Reports of studies with small samples frequently include the erroneous conclusion that the intervention groups do not differ, when in fact too few patients were studied to make such a claim.[120] Reviews of published trials have consistently found that a high proportion of trials have low power to detect clinically meaningful treatment effects.[121] [122] [123] In reality, small but clinically meaningful true differences are much more likely than large differences to exist, but large trials are required to detect them.[124]

In general, the reported sample sizes in trials seem small. The median sample size was 54 patients in 196 trials in arthritis,[108] 46 patients in 73 trials in dermatology,[8] and 65 patients in 2000 trials in schizophrenia.[33] These small sample sizes are consistent with those of a study of 519 trials indexed in PubMed in December 2000[16] and a similar cohort of trials (n=616) indexed in PubMed in 2006,[17] where the median number of patients recruited for parallel group trials was 80 across both years. Moreover, many reviews have found that few authors report how they determined the sample size.[8] [14] [32] [33] [123]

There is little merit in a post hoc calculation of statistical power using the results of a trial; the power is then appropriately indicated by confidence intervals (see item 17).[125]

Item 7b. When applicable, explanation of any interim analyses and stopping guidelines

Examples—"Two interim analyses were performed during the trial. The levels of significance maintained an overall P value of 0.05 and were calculated according to the O'Brien-Fleming stopping boundaries. This final analysis used a Z score of 1.985 with an associated P value of 0.0471."[126]

"An independent data and safety monitoring board periodically reviewed the efficacy and safety data. Stopping rules were based on modified Haybittle-Peto boundaries of 4 SD in the first half of the study and 3 SD in the second half for efficacy data, and 3 SD in the first half of the study and 2 SD in the second half for safety data. Two formal interim analyses of efficacy were performed when 50% and 75% of the expected number of primary events had accrued; no correction of the reported P value for these interim tests was performed."[127]

Explanation—Many trials recruit participants over a long period. If an intervention is working particularly well or badly, the study may need to be ended early for ethical reasons. This concern can be addressed by examining results as the data accumulate, preferably by an independent data monitoring committee. However, performing multiple statistical examinations of accumulating data without appropriate correction can lead to erroneous results and interpretations.[128] If the accumulating data from a trial are examined at five interim analyses that use a P value of 0.05, the overall false positive rate is nearer to 19% than to the nominal 5%.

Several group sequential statistical methods are available to adjust for multiple analyses,[129] [130] [131] and their use should be pre-specified in the trial protocol. With these methods, data are compared at each interim analysis, and a P value less than the critical value specified by the group sequential method indicates statistical significance. Some trialists use group sequential methods as an aid to decision making,[132] whereas others treat them as a formal stopping rule (with the intention that the trial will cease if the observed P value is smaller than the critical value).

Authors should report whether they or a data monitoring committee took multiple "looks" at the data and, if so, how many there were, what triggered them, the statistical methods used (including any formal stopping rule), and whether they were planned before the start of the trial, before the data monitoring committee saw any interim data by allocation, or some time thereafter. This information is often not included in published trial reports,[133] even in trials that report stopping earlier than planned.[134]

Item 8a. Method used to generate the random allocation sequence

Examples—"Independent pharmacists dispensed either active or placebo inhalers according to a computer generated randomisation list."[63]

"For allocation of the participants, a computer-generated list of random numbers was used."[135]

Explanation—Participants should be assigned to comparison groups in the trial on the basis of a chance (random) process characterised by unpredictability (see box 1). Authors should provide sufficient information that the reader can assess the methods used to generate the random allocation sequence and the likelihood of bias in group assignment. It is important that information on the process of randomisation is included in the body of the main article and not as a separate supplementary file; where it can be missed by the reader.

The term "random" has a precise technical meaning. With random allocation, each participant has a known probability of receiving each intervention before one is assigned, but the assigned intervention is determined by a chance process and cannot be predicted. However, "random" is often used inappropriately in the literature to describe trials in which non-random, deterministic allocation methods were used, such as alternation, hospital numbers, or date of birth. When investigators use such non-random methods, they should describe them precisely and should not use the term "random" or any variation of it. Even the term "quasi-random" is unacceptable for describing such trials. Trials based on non-random methods generally yield biased

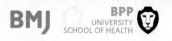

results.[2] [3] [4] [136] Bias presumably arises from the inability to conceal these allocation systems adequately (see item 9).

Many methods of sequence generation are adequate. However, readers cannot judge adequacy from such terms as "random allocation," "randomisation," or "random" without further elaboration. Authors should specify the method of sequence generation, such as a random-number table or a computerised random number generator. The sequence may be generated by the process of minimisation, a non-random but generally acceptable method (see box 2).

In some trials, participants are intentionally allocated in unequal numbers to each intervention: for example, to gain more experience with a new procedure or to limit costs of the trial. In such cases, authors should report the randomisation ratio (for example, 2:1 or two treatment participants per each control participant) (see item 3a).

In a representative sample of PubMed indexed trials in 2000, only 21% reported an adequate approach to random sequence generation[16]; this increased to 34% for a similar cohort of PubMed indexed trials in 2006.[17] In more than 90% of these cases, researchers used a random number generator on a computer or a random number table.

Item 8b. Type of randomisation; details of any restriction (such as blocking and block size)

Examples—"Randomization sequence was created using Stata 9.0 (StataCorp, College Station, TX) statistical software and was stratified by center with a 1:1 allocation using random block sizes of 2, 4, and 6."[137]

"Participants were randomly assigned following simple randomization procedures (computerized random numbers) to 1 of 2 treatment groups."[138]

Explanation—In trials of several hundred participants or more simple randomisation can usually be trusted to generate similar numbers in the two trial groups[139] and to generate groups that are roughly comparable in terms of known and unknown prognostic variables.[140] For smaller trials (see item 7a)—and even for trials that are not intended to be small, as they may stop before reaching their target size—some restricted randomisation (procedures to help achieve balance between groups in size or characteristics) may be useful (see box 2).

It is important to indicate whether no restriction was used, by stating such or by stating that "simple randomisation" was done. Otherwise, the methods used to restrict the randomisation, along with the method used for random selection, should be specified. For block randomisation, authors should provide details on how the blocks were generated (for example, by using a permuted block design with a computer random number generator), the block size or sizes, and whether the block size was fixed or randomly varied. If the trialists became aware of the block size(s), that information should also be reported as such knowledge could lead to code breaking. Authors should specify whether stratification was used, and if so, which factors were involved (such as recruitment site, sex, disease stage), the categorisation cut-off values within strata, and the method used for restriction. Although stratification is a useful technique, especially for smaller trials, it is complicated to implement and may be impossible if many stratifying factors are used. If minimisation (see box 2) was used, it should be explicitly identified, as should the variables incorporated into the scheme. If used, a random element should be indicated.

Only 9% of 206 reports of trials in specialty journals[23] and 39% of 80 trials in general medical journals reported use of stratification.[32] In each case, only about half of the reports mentioned the use of restricted randomisation.

BOX 2 RANDOMISATION AND MINIMISATION

- **Simple randomisation—**Pure randomisation based on a single allocation ratio is known as simple randomisation. Simple randomisation with a 1:1 allocation ratio is analogous to a coin toss, although we do not advocate coin tossing for randomisation in an RCT. "Simple" is somewhat of a misnomer. While other randomisation schemes sound complex and more sophisticated, in reality, simple randomisation is elegantly sophisticated in that it is more unpredictable and surpasses the bias prevention levels of all other alternatives.

- **Restricted randomisation—**Any randomised approach that is not simple randomisation. Blocked randomisation is the most common form. Other means of restricted randomisation include replacement, biased coin, and urn randomisation, although these are used much less frequently.[141]

- **Blocked randomisation—**Blocking is used to ensure that comparison groups will be generated according to a predetermined ratio, usually 1:1 or groups of approximately the same size. Blocking can be used to ensure close balance of the numbers in each group at any time during the trial. For every block of eight participants, for example, four would be allocated to each arm of the trial.[142] Improved balance comes at the cost of reducing the unpredictability of the sequence. Although the order of interventions varies randomly within each block, a person running the trial could deduce some of the next treatment allocations if he or she knew the block size.[143] Blinding the interventions, using larger block sizes, and randomly varying the block size can ameliorate this problem.

- **Stratified randomisation—**Stratification is used to ensure good balance of participant characteristics in each group. By chance, particularly in small trials, study groups may not be well matched for baseline characteristics, such as age and stage of disease. This weakens the trial's credibility.[144] Such imbalances can be avoided without sacrificing the advantages of randomisation. Stratification ensures that the numbers of participants receiving each intervention are closely balanced within each stratum. Stratified randomisation is achieved by performing a separate randomisation procedure within each of two or more subsets of participants (for example, those defining each study centre, age, or disease severity). Stratification by centre is common in multicentre trials. Stratification requires some form of restriction (such as blocking within strata). Stratification without blocking is ineffective.

- **Minimisation—**Minimisation ensures balance between intervention groups for several selected patient factors (such as age).[22] [60] The first patient is truly randomly allocated; for each subsequent participant, the treatment allocation that minimises the imbalance on the selected factors between groups at that time is identified. That allocation may then be used, or a choice may be made at random with a heavy weighting in favour of the intervention that would minimise imbalance (for example, with a probability of 0.8). The use of a random component is generally preferable. Minimisation has the advantage of making small groups closely similar in terms of participant characteristics at all stages of the trial. Minimisation offers the only acceptable alternative to randomisation, and some have argued that it is superior.[145] On the other hand, minimisation lacks the theoretical basis for eliminating bias on all known and unknown factors. Nevertheless, in general, trials that use minimisation are considered methodologically equivalent to randomised trials, even when a random element is not incorporated.

However, these studies and that of Adetugbo and Williams[8] found that the sizes of the treatment groups in many trials were the same or quite similar, yet blocking or stratification had not been mentioned. One possible explanation for the close balance in numbers is underreporting of the use of restricted randomisation.

Item 9. Mechanism used to implement the random allocation sequence (such as sequentially numbered containers), describing any steps taken to conceal the sequence until interventions were assigned

Examples—"The doxycycline and placebo were in capsule form and identical in appearance. They were prepacked in bottles and consecutively numbered for each woman according to the randomisation schedule. Each woman was assigned an order number and received the capsules in the corresponding prepacked bottle."[146]

"The allocation sequence was concealed from the researcher (JR) enrolling and assessing participants in sequentially numbered, opaque, sealed and stapled envelopes. Aluminium foil inside the envelope was used to render the envelope impermeable to intense light. To prevent subversion of the allocation sequence, the name and date of birth of the participant was written on the envelope and a video tape made of the sealed envelope with participant details visible. Carbon paper inside the envelope transferred the information onto the allocation card inside the envelope and a second researcher (CC) later viewed video tapes to ensure envelopes were still sealed when participants' names were written on them. Corresponding envelopes were opened only after the enrolled participants completed all baseline assessments and it was time to allocate the intervention."[147]

Explanation—Item 8a discussed generation of an unpredictable sequence of assignments. Of considerable importance is how this sequence is applied when participants are enrolled into the trial (see box 1). A generated allocation schedule should be implemented by using allocation concealment,[23] a critical mechanism that prevents foreknowledge of treatment assignment and thus shields those who enroll participants from being influenced by this knowledge. The decision to accept or reject a participant should be made, and informed consent should be obtained from the participant, in ignorance of the next assignment in the sequence.[148]

The allocation concealment should not be confused with blinding (see item 11). Allocation concealment seeks to prevent selection bias, protects the assignment sequence until allocation, and can always be successfully implemented.[2] In contrast, blinding seeks to prevent performance and ascertainment bias, protects the sequence after allocation, and cannot always be implemented.[23] Without adequate allocation concealment, however, even random, unpredictable assignment sequences can be subverted.[2][149]

Centralised or "third-party" assignment is especially desirable. Many good allocation concealment mechanisms incorporate external involvement. Use of a pharmacy or central telephone randomisation system are two common techniques. Automated assignment systems are likely to become more common.[150] When external involvement is not feasible, an excellent method of allocation concealment is the use of numbered containers. The interventions (often drugs) are sealed in sequentially numbered identical containers according to the allocation sequence.[151] Enclosing assignments in sequentially numbered, opaque, sealed envelopes can be a good allocation concealment mechanism if it is developed and monitored diligently. This method can be corrupted, however, particularly if it is poorly executed. Investigators should ensure that the envelopes are opaque when held to the light, and opened sequentially and only after the participant's name and other details are written on the appropriate envelope.[143]

A number of methodological studies provide empirical evidence to support these precautions.[152][153] Trials in which the allocation sequence had been inadequately or unclearly concealed yielded larger estimates of treatment effects than did trials in which authors reported adequate allocation concealment. These findings provide strong empirical evidence that inadequate allocation concealment contributes to bias in estimating treatment effects.

Despite the importance of the mechanism of allocation concealment, published reports often omit such details. The mechanism used to allocate interventions was omitted in reports of 89% of trials in rheumatoid arthritis,[108] 48% of trials in obstetrics and gynaecology journals,[23] and 44% of trials in general medical journals.[32] In a more broadly representative sample of all randomised trials indexed on PubMed, only 18% reported any allocation concealment mechanism, but some of those reported mechanisms were inadequate.[16]

Item 10. Who generated the allocation sequence, who enrolled participants, and who assigned participants to interventions

Examples—"Determination of whether a patient would be treated by streptomycin and bed-rest (S case) or by bed-rest alone (C case) was made by reference to a statistical series based on random sampling numbers drawn up for each sex at each centre by Professor Bradford Hill; the details of the series were unknown to any of the investigators or to the co-ordinator … After acceptance of a patient by the panel, and before admission to the streptomycin centre, the appropriate numbered envelope was opened at the central office; the card inside told if the patient was to be an S or a C case, and this information was then given to the medical officer of the centre."[24]

"Details of the allocated group were given on coloured cards contained in sequentially numbered, opaque, sealed envelopes. These were prepared at the NPEU and kept in an agreed location on each ward. Randomisation took place at the end of the 2nd stage of labour when the midwife considered a vaginal birth was imminent. To enter a women into the study, the midwife opened the next consecutively numbered envelope."[154]

"Block randomisation was by a computer generated random number list prepared by an investigator with no clinical involvement in the trial. We stratified by admission for an oncology related procedure. After the research nurse had obtained the patient's consent, she telephoned a contact who was independent of the recruitment process for allocation consignment."[155]

Explanation—As noted in item 9, concealment of the allocated intervention at the time of enrolment is especially important. Thus, in addition to knowing the methods used, it is also important to understand how the random sequence was implemented—specifically, who generated the allocation sequence, who enrolled participants, and who assigned participants to trial groups.

The process of randomising participants into a trial has three different steps: sequence generation, allocation

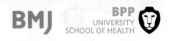

concealment, and implementation (see box 3). Although the same people may carry out more than one process under each heading, investigators should strive for complete separation of the people involved with generation and allocation concealment from the people involved in the implementation of assignments. Thus, if someone is involved in the sequence generation or allocation concealment steps, ideally they should not be involved in the implementation step.

Even with flawless sequence generation and allocation concealment, failure to separate creation and concealment of the allocation sequence from assignment to study group may introduce bias. For example, the person who generated an allocation sequence could retain a copy and consult it when interviewing potential participants for a trial. Thus, that person could bias the enrolment or assignment process, regardless of the unpredictability of the assignment sequence. Investigators must then ensure that the assignment schedule is unpredictable and locked away (such as in a safe deposit box in a building rather inaccessible to the enrolment location) from even the person who generated it. The report of the trial should specify where the investigators stored the allocation list.

BOX 3 STEPS IN A TYPICAL RANDOMISATION PROCESS

Sequence generation
- Generate allocation sequence by some random procedure

Allocation concealment
- Develop allocation concealment mechanism (such as numbered, identical bottles or sequentially numbered, sealed, opaque envelopes)
- Prepare the allocation concealment mechanism using the allocation sequence from the sequence generation step

Implementation
- Enrol participants:
- Assess eligibility
- Discuss the trial
- Obtain informed consent
- Enrol participant in trial
- Ascertain intervention assignment (such as opening next envelope)
- Administer intervention

BOX 4 BLINDING TERMINOLOGY

In order for a technical term to have utility it must have consistency in its use and interpretation. Authors of trials commonly use the term "double blind" and, less commonly, the terms "single blind"or "triple blind." A problem with this lexicon is that there is great variability in clinician interpretations and epidemiological textbook definitions of these terms.[169] Moreover, a study of 200 RCTs reported as double blind found 18 different combinations of groups actually blinded when the authors of these trials were surveyed, and about one in every five of these trials—reported as double blind—did not blind participants, healthcare providers, or data collectors.[170] This research shows that terms are ambiguous and, as such, authors and editors should abandon their use. Authors should instead explicitly report the blinding status of the people involved for whom blinding may influence the validity of a trial.

Healthcare providers include all personnel (for example, physicians, chiropractors, physiotherapists, nurses) who care for the participants during the trial. Data collectors are the individuals who collect data on the trial outcomes. Outcome adjudicators are the individuals who determine whether a participant did experience the outcomes of interest.

Some researchers have also advocated blinding and reporting the blinding status of the data monitoring committee and the manuscript writers.[160] Blinding of these groups is uncommon, and the value of blinding them is debated.[171]

Sometimes one group of individuals (such as the healthcare providers) are the same individuals fulfilling another role in a trial (such as data collectors). Even if this is the case, the authors should explicitly state the blinding status of these groups to allow readers to judge the validity of the trial.

Item 11a. If done, who was blinded after assignment to interventions (for example, participants, care providers, those assessing outcomes) and how

Examples—"Whereas patients and physicians allocated to the intervention group were aware of the allocated arm, outcome assessors and data analysts were kept blinded to the allocation."[156]

"Blinding and equipoise were strictly maintained by emphasising to intervention staff and participants that each diet adheres to healthy principles, and each is advocated by certain experts to be superior for long-term weight-loss. Except for the interventionists (dieticians and behavioural psychologists), investigators and staff were kept blind to diet assignment of the participants. The trial adhered to established procedures to maintain separation between staff that take outcome measurements and staff that deliver the intervention. Staff members who obtained outcome measurements were not informed of the diet group assignment. Intervention staff, dieticians and behavioural psychologists who delivered the intervention did not take outcome measurements. All investigators, staff, and participants were kept masked to outcome measurements and trial results."[157]

Explanation—The term "blinding" or "masking" refers to withholding information about the assigned interventions from people involved in the trial who may potentially be influenced by this knowledge. Blinding is an important safeguard against bias, particularly when assessing subjective outcomes.[153]

Benjamin Franklin has been credited as being the first to use blinding in a scientific experiment.[158] He blindfolded participants so they would not know when he was applying mesmerism (a popular "healing fluid" of the 18th century) and in so doing showed that mesmerism was a sham. Based on this experiment, the scientific community recognised the power of blinding to reduce bias, and it has remained a commonly used strategy in scientific experiments.

Box 4, on blinding terminology, defines the groups of individuals (that is, participants, healthcare providers, data collectors, outcome adjudicators, and data analysts) who can potentially introduce bias into a trial through knowledge of the treatment assignments. Participants may respond differently if they are aware of their treatment assignment (such as responding more favourably when they receive the new treatment).[153] Lack of blinding may also influence compliance with the intervention, use of co-interventions, and risk of dropping out of the trial.

Unblinded healthcare providers may introduce similar biases, and unblinded data collectors may differentially assess outcomes (such as frequency or timing), repeat measurements of abnormal findings, or provide encouragement during performance testing. Unblinded outcome adjudicators may differentially assess subjective outcomes, and unblinded data analysts may introduce bias through the choice of analytical strategies, such as the selection of favourable time points or outcomes, and by decisions to remove patients from the analyses. These biases have been well documented.[71] [153] [159] [160] [161] [162]

Blinding, unlike allocation concealment (see item 10), may not always be appropriate or possible. An example is a trial comparing levels of pain associated with sampling blood from the ear or thumb.[163] Blinding is particularly important when outcome measures involve some subjectivity, such as assessment of pain. Blinding of data collectors and outcome adjudicators is unlikely to matter for objective outcomes, such as death from any cause. Even then, however, lack of participant or healthcare provider blinding can lead to other problems, such as differential attrition.[164] In certain trials, especially surgical trials, blinding of participants and surgeons is often difficult or impossible, but blinding of data collectors and outcome adjudicators is often achievable. For example, lesions can be photographed before and after treatment and assessed by an external observer.[165] Regardless of whether blinding is possible, authors can and should always state who was blinded (that is, participants, healthcare providers, data collectors, and outcome adjudicators).

Unfortunately, authors often do not report whether blinding was used.[166] For example, reports of 51% of 506 trials in cystic fibrosis,[167] 33% of 196 trials in rheumatoid arthritis,[108] and 38% of 68 trials in dermatology[8] did not state whether blinding was used. Until authors of trials improve their reporting of blinding, readers will have difficulty in judging the validity of the trials that they may wish to use to guide their clinical practice.

The term masking is sometimes used in preference to blinding to avoid confusion with the medical condition of being without sight. However, "blinding" in its methodological sense seems to be understood worldwide and is acceptable for reporting clinical trials.[165] [168]

Item 11b. If relevant, description of the similarity of interventions

Example—"Jamieson Laboratories Inc provided 500-mg immediate release niacin in a white, oblong, bisect caplet. We independently confirmed caplet content using high performance liquid chromatography … The placebo was matched to the study drug for taste, color, and size, and contained microcrystalline cellulose, silicon dioxide, dicalcium phosphate, magnesium stearate, and stearic acid."[172]

Explanation—Just as we seek evidence of concealment to assure us that assignment was truly random, we seek evidence of the method of blinding. In trials with blinding of participants or healthcare providers, authors should state the similarity of the characteristics of the interventions (such as appearance, taste, smell, and method of administration).[35] [173]

Some people have advocated testing for blinding by asking participants or healthcare providers at the end of a trial whether they think the participant received the experimental or control intervention.[174] Because participants and healthcare providers will usually know whether the participant has experienced the primary outcome, this makes it difficult to determine if their responses reflect failure of blinding or accurate assumptions about the efficacy of the intervention.[175] Given the uncertainty this type of information provides, we have removed advocating reporting this type of testing for blinding from the CONSORT 2010 Statement. We do, however, advocate that the authors report any known compromises in blinding. For example, authors should report if it was necessary to unblind any participants at any point during the conduct of a trial.

Item 12a. Statistical methods used to compare groups for primary and secondary outcomes

Example—"The primary endpoint was change in bodyweight during the 20 weeks of the study in the intention-to-treat population … Secondary efficacy endpoints included change in waist circumference, systolic and diastolic blood pressure, prevalence of metabolic syndrome … We used an analysis of covariance (ANCOVA) for the primary endpoint and for secondary endpoints waist circumference, blood pressure, and patient-reported outcome scores; this was supplemented by a repeated measures analysis. The ANCOVA model included treatment, country, and sex as fixed effects, and bodyweight at randomisation as covariate. We aimed to assess whether data provided evidence of superiority of each liraglutide dose to placebo (primary objective) and to orlistat (secondary objective)."[176]

Explanation—Data can be analysed in many ways, some of which may not be strictly appropriate in a particular situation. It is essential to specify which statistical procedure was used for each analysis, and further clarification may be necessary in the results section of the report. The principle to follow is to, "Describe statistical methods with enough detail to enable a knowledgeable reader with access to the original data to verify the reported results" (www.icmje.org). It is also important to describe details of the statistical analysis such as intention-to-treat analysis (see box 6).

Almost all methods of analysis yield an estimate of the treatment effect, which is a contrast between the outcomes in the comparison groups. Authors should accompany this by a confidence interval for the estimated effect, which indicates a central range of uncertainty for the true treatment effect. The confidence interval may be interpreted as the range of values for the treatment effect that is compatible with the observed data. It is customary to present a 95% confidence interval, which gives the range expected to include the true value in 95 of 100 similar studies.

Study findings can also be assessed in terms of their statistical significance. The P value represents the probability that the observed data (or a more extreme result) could have arisen by chance when the interventions did not truly differ. Actual P values (for example, P=0.003) are strongly preferable to imprecise threshold reports such as P<0.05.[48] [177]

Standard methods of analysis assume that the data are "independent." For controlled trials, this usually means that there is one observation per participant. Treating multiple observations from one participant as independent data is a serious error; such data are produced when outcomes can be measured on different parts of the body, as in dentistry or rheumatology. Data analysis should be based on counting each participant once[178] [179] or should be done by using more complex statistical procedures.[180] Incorrect analysis of multiple observations per individual was seen in 123 (63%) of 196 trials in rheumatoid arthritis.[108]

Item 12b. Methods for additional analyses, such as subgroup analyses and adjusted analyses

Examples—"Proportions of patients responding were compared between treatment groups with the Mantel-Haenszel χ^2 test, adjusted for the stratification variable, methotrexate use."[103]

"Pre-specified subgroup analyses according to antioxidant treatment assignment(s), presence or absence of prior CVD, dietary folic acid intake, smoking, diabetes, aspirin, hormone therapy, and multivitamin use were performed using stratified Cox proportional hazards models. These analyses used baseline exposure assessments and were restricted to participants with nonmissing subgroup data at baseline."[181]

Explanation—As is the case for primary analyses, the method of subgroup analysis should be clearly specified. The strongest analyses are those that look for evidence of a difference in treatment effect in complementary subgroups (for example, older and younger participants), a comparison

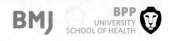

known as a test of interaction.[182] [183] A common but misleading approach is to compare P values for separate analyses of the treatment effect in each group. It is incorrect to infer a subgroup effect (interaction) from one significant and one non-significant P value.[184] Such inferences have a high false positive rate.

Because of the high risk for spurious findings, subgroup analyses are often discouraged.[14] [185] Post hoc subgroup comparisons (analyses done after looking at the data) are especially likely not to be confirmed by further studies. Such analyses do not have great credibility.

In some studies, imbalances in participant characteristics are adjusted for by using some form of multiple regression analysis. Although the need for adjustment is much less in RCTs than in epidemiological studies, an adjusted analysis may be sensible, especially if one or more variables is thought to be prognostic.[186] Ideally, adjusted analyses should be specified in the study protocol (see item 24). For example, adjustment is often recommended for any stratification variables (see item 8b) on the principle that the analysis strategy should follow the design. In RCTs, the decision to adjust should not be determined by whether baseline differences are statistically significant (see item 16).[183] [187] The rationale for any adjusted analyses and the statistical methods used should be specified.

Authors should clarify the choice of variables that were adjusted for, indicate how continuous variables were handled, and specify whether the analysis was planned or suggested by the data.[188] Reviews of published studies show that reporting of adjusted analyses is inadequate with regard to all of these aspects.[188] [189] [190] [191]

BOX 5 EARLY STOPPING

RCTs can end when they reach their sample size goal, their event count goal, their length of follow-up goal, or when they reach their scheduled date of closure. In these situations the trial will stop in a manner independent of its results, and stopping is unlikely to introduce bias in the results. Alternatively, RCTs can stop earlier than planned because of the result of an interim analysis showing larger than expected benefit or harm on the experimental intervention. Also RCTs can stop earlier than planned when investigators find evidence of no important difference between experimental and control interventions (that is, stopping for futility). In addition, trials may stop early because the trial becomes unviable: funding vanishes, researchers cannot access eligible patients or study interventions, or the results of other studies make the research question irrelevant.

Full reporting of why a trial ended is important for evidence based decision making (see item 14b). Researchers examining why 143 trials stopped early for benefit found that many failed to report key methodological information regarding how the decision to stop was reached—the planned sample size (n=28), interim analysis after which the trial was stopped (n=45), or whether a stopping rule informed the decision (n=48).[134] Item 7b of the checklist requires the reporting of timing of interim analyses, what triggered them, how many took place, whether these were planned or ad hoc, and whether there were statistical guidelines and stopping rules in place a priori. Furthermore, it is helpful to know whether an independent data monitoring committee participated in the analyses (and who composed it, with particular attention to the role of the funding source) and who made the decision to stop. Often the data safety and monitoring committee makes recommendations and the funders (sponsors) or the investigators make the decision to stop.

Trials that stop early for reasons apparently independent of trial findings, and trials that reach their planned termination, are unlikely to introduce bias by stopping.[207] In these cases, the authors should report whether interim analyses took place and whether these results were available to the funder.

The push for trials that change the intervention in response to interim results, thus enabling a faster evaluation of promising interventions for rapidly evolving and fatal conditions, will require even more careful reporting of the process and decision to stop trials early.[208]

BOX 6 INTENTION-TO-TREAT ANALYSIS

The special strength of the RCT is the avoidance of bias when allocating interventions to trial participants (see box 1). That strength allows strong inferences about cause and effect that are not justified with other study designs. In order to preserve fully the huge benefit of randomisation we should include all randomised participants in the analysis, all retained in the group to which they were allocated. Those two conditions define an "intention-to-treat" analysis, which is widely recommended as the preferred analysis strategy.[18] [223] Intention-to-treat analysis corresponds to analysing the groups exactly as randomised. Strict intention-to-treat analysis is often hard to achieve for two main reasons—missing outcomes for some participants and non-adherence to the trial protocol.

Missing outcomes

Many trialists exclude patients without an observed outcome. Often this is reasonable, but once any randomised participants are excluded the analysis is not strictly an intention-to-treat analysis. Indeed, most randomised trials have some missing observations. Trialists effectively must choose between omitting the participants without final outcome data or imputing their missing outcome data.[225] A "complete case" (or "available case") analysis includes only those whose outcome is known. While a few missing outcomes will not cause a problem, in half of trials more than 10% of randomised patients may have missing outcomes.[226] This common approach will lose power by reducing the sample size, and bias may well be introduced if being lost to follow-up is related to a patient's response to treatment. There should be concern when the frequency or the causes of dropping out differ between the intervention groups.

Participants with missing outcomes can be included in the analysis only if their outcomes are imputed (that is, their outcomes are estimated from other information that was collected). Imputation of the missing data allows the analysis to conform to intention-to-treat analysis but requires strong assumptions, which may be hard to justify.[227] Simple imputation methods are appealing, but their use may be inadvisable. In particular, a widely used method is "last observation carried forward" in which missing final values of the outcome variable are replaced by the last known value before the participant was lost to follow up. This is appealing through its simplicity, but the method may introduce bias,[228] and no allowance is made for the uncertainty of imputation.[229] Many authors have severely criticised last observation carried forward.[229] [230] [231]

Non-adherence to the protocol

A separate issue is that the trial protocol may not have been followed fully for some trial participants. Common examples are participants who did not meet the inclusion criteria (such as wrong diagnosis, too young), received a proscribed co-intervention, did not take all the intended treatment, or received a different treatment or no intervention. The simple way to deal with any protocol deviations is to ignore them: all participants can be included in the analysis regardless of adherence to the protocol, and this is the intention-to-treat approach. Thus, exclusion of any participants for such reasons is incompatible with intention-to-treat analysis.

The term "modified intention-to-treat" is quite widely used to describe an analysis that excludes participants who did not adequately adhere to the protocol, in particular those who did not receive a defined minimum amount of the intervention.[232] An alternative term is "per protocol." Though a per protocol analysis may be appropriate in some settings, it should be properly labelled as a non-randomised, observational comparison. Any exclusion of patients from the analysis compromises the randomisation and may lead to bias in the results.

Like "intention-to-treat," none of these other labels reliably clarifies exactly which patients were included. Thus, in the CONSORT checklist we have dropped the specific request for intention-to-treat analysis in favour of a clear description of exactly who was included in each analysis.

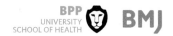

Results

Item 13. Participant flow (a diagram is strongly recommended) Item 13a. For each group, the numbers of participants who were randomly assigned, received intended treatment, and were analysed for the primary outcome

Examples—See figs 2 and 3.

Explanation—The design and conduct of some RCTs is straightforward, and the flow of participants, particularly were there are no losses to follow-up or exclusions, through each phase of the study can be described adequately in a few sentences. In more complex studies, it may be difficult for readers to discern whether and why some participants did not receive the treatment as allocated, were lost to follow-up, or were excluded from the analysis.[51] This information is crucial for several reasons. Participants who were excluded after allocation are unlikely to be representative of all participants in the study. For example, patients may not be available for follow-up evaluation because they experienced an acute exacerbation of their illness or harms of treatment.[22][192]

Attrition as a result of loss to follow up, which is often unavoidable, needs to be distinguished from investigator-determined exclusion for such reasons as ineligibility, withdrawal from treatment, and poor adherence to the trial protocol. Erroneous conclusions can be reached if participants are excluded from analysis, and imbalances in such omissions between groups may be especially indicative of bias.[192][193][194] Information about whether the investigators included in the analysis all participants who underwent randomisation, in the groups to which they were originally allocated (intention-to-treat analysis (see item 16 and box 6)), is therefore of particular importance. Knowing the number of participants who did not receive the intervention as allocated or did not complete treatment permits the reader to assess to what extent the estimated efficacy of therapy might be underestimated in comparison with ideal circumstances.

If available, the number of people assessed for eligibility should also be reported. Although this number is relevant to external validity only and is arguably less important than the other counts,[195] it is a useful indicator of whether trial participants were likely to be representative of all eligible participants.

A review of RCTs published in five leading general and internal medicine journals in 1998 found that reporting of the flow of participants was often incomplete, particularly with regard to the number of participants receiving the allocated intervention and the number lost to follow-up.[51] Even information as basic as the number of participants who underwent randomisation and the number excluded from analyses was not available in up to 20% of articles.[51] Reporting was considerably more thorough in articles that included a diagram of the flow of participants through a trial, as recommended by CONSORT. This study informed the design of the revised flow diagram in the revised CONSORT statement.[52][53][54] The suggested template is shown in fig 1, and the counts required are described in detail in table 3.

Some information, such as the number of individuals assessed for eligibility, may not always be known,[14] and, depending on the nature of a trial, some counts may be more relevant than others. It will sometimes be useful or necessary to adapt the structure of the flow diagram to a particular trial. In some situations, other information may usefully be added. For example, the flow diagram of a parallel group trial of minimal surgery compared with medical management for chronic gastro-oesophageal reflux also included a parallel non-randomised preference group (see fig 3).[196]

The exact form and content of the flow diagram may be varied according to specific features of a trial. For example, many trials of surgery or vaccination do not include the possibility of discontinuation. Although CONSORT strongly recommends using this graphical device to communicate participant flow throughout the study, there is no specific, prescribed format.

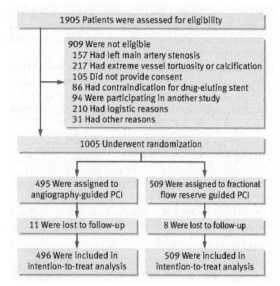

Fig 2 Flow diagram of a multicentre trial of fractional flow reserve versus angiography for guiding percutaneous coronary intervention (PCI) (adapted from Tonino et al[313]). The diagram includes detailed information on the excluded participants.

Table 3 Information required to document the flow of participants through each stage of a randomised trial

Stage	Number of people included	Number of people not included or excluded	Rationale
Enrolment	People evaluated for potential enrolment	People who did not meet the inclusion criteria or met the inclusion criteria but declined to be enrolled	These counts indicate whether trial participants were likely to be representative of all patients seen; they are relevant to assessment of external validity only, and they are often not available.
Randomisation	Participants randomly assigned		Crucial count for defining trial size and assessing whether a trial has been analysed by intention to treat
Treatment allocation	Participants who received treatment as allocated, by study group	Participants who did not receive treatment as allocated, by study group	Important counts for assessment of internal validity and interpretation of results; reasons for not receiving treatment as allocated should be given.
Follow-up	Participants who received treatment as allocated, by study group	Participants who did not complete treatment as allocated, by study group	Important counts for assessment of internal validity and interpretation of results; reasons for not completing treatment or follow-up should be given.
	Participants who completed follow-up as planned, by study group	Participants who did not complete follow-up as planned, by study group	
Analysis	Participants included in main analysis, by study group	Participants excluded from main analysis, by study group	Crucial count for assessing whether a trial has been analysed by intention to treat; reasons for excluding participants should be given.

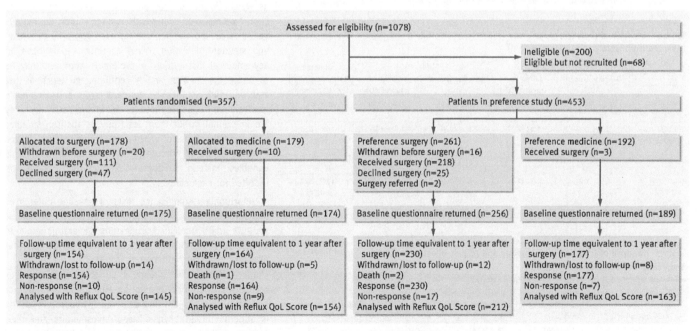

Item 13b. For each group, losses and exclusions after randomisation, together with reasons

Examples—"There was only one protocol deviation, in a woman in the study group. She had an abnormal pelvic measurement and was scheduled for elective caesarean section. However, the attending obstetrician judged a trial of labour acceptable; caesarean section was done when there was no progress in the first stage of labour."[197]

"The monitoring led to withdrawal of nine centres, in which existence of some patients could not be proved, or other serious violations of good clinical practice had occurred."[198]

Explanation—Some protocol deviations may be reported in the flow diagram (see item 13a)—for example, participants who did not receive the intended intervention. If participants were excluded after randomisation (contrary to the intention-to-treat principle) because they were found not to meet eligibility criteria (see item 16), they should be included in the flow diagram. Use of the term "protocol deviation" in published articles is not sufficient to justify exclusion of participants after randomisation. The nature of the protocol deviation and the exact reason for excluding participants after randomisation should always be reported.

Item 14a. Dates defining the periods of recruitment and follow-up

Example—"Age-eligible participants were recruited ... from February 1993 to September 1994 ... Participants attended clinic visits at the time of randomisation (baseline) and at 6-month intervals for 3 years."[199]

Explanation—Knowing when a study took place and over what period participants were recruited places the study in historical context. Medical and surgical therapies, including concurrent therapies, evolve continuously and may affect the routine care given to participants during a trial. Knowing the rate at which participants were recruited may also be useful, especially to other investigators.

The length of follow-up is not always a fixed period after randomisation. In many RCTs in which the outcome is time to an event, follow-up of all participants is ended on a specific date. This date should be given, and it is also useful to report the minimum, maximum, and median duration of follow-up.[200][201]

A review of reports in oncology journals that used survival analysis, most of which were not RCTs,[201] found that nearly 80% (104 of 132 reports) included the starting and ending dates for accrual of patients, but only 24% (32 of 132 reports) also reported the date on which follow-up ended.

Item 14b. Why the trial ended or was stopped

Examples—"At the time of the interim analysis, the total follow-up included an estimated 63% of the total number of patient-years that would have been collected at the end of the study, leading to a threshold value of 0.0095, as determined by the Lan-DeMets alpha-spending function method ... At the interim analysis, the RR was 0.37 in the intervention group, as compared with the control group, with a p value of 0.00073, below the threshold value. The Data and Safety Monitoring Board advised the investigators to interrupt the trial and offer circumcision to the control group, who were then asked to come to the investigation centre, where MC (medical circumcision) was advised and proposed ... Because the study was interrupted, some participants did not have a full follow-up on that date, and their visits that were not yet completed are described as "planned" in this article."[202]

"In January 2000, problems with vaccine supply necessitated the temporary nationwide replacement of the whole cell component of the combined DPT/Hib vaccine with acellular pertussis vaccine. As this vaccine has a different local reactogenicity profile, we decided to stop the trial early."[203]

Explanation—Arguably, trialists who arbitrarily conduct unplanned interim analyses after very few events accrue using no statistical guidelines run a high risk of "catching" the data at a random extreme, which likely represents a large overestimate of treatment benefit.[204]

Readers will likely draw weaker inferences from a trial that was truncated in a data-driven manner versus one that reports its findings after reaching a goal independent of results. Thus, RCTs should indicate why the trial came to an end (see box 5). The report should also disclose

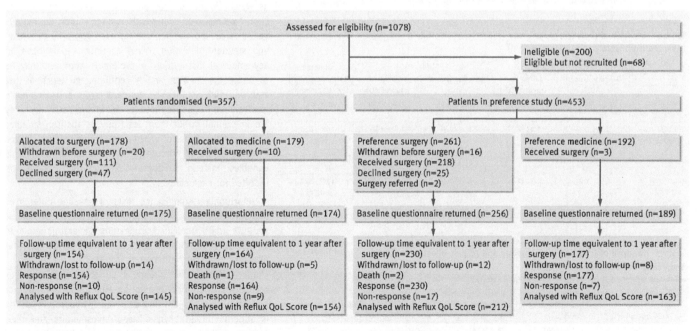

Fig 3 Flow diagram of minimal surgery compared with medical management for chronic gastro-oesophageal reflux disease (adapted from Grant et al[196]). The diagram shows a multicentre trial with a parallel non-randomised preference group.

Table 4 Example of reporting baseline demographic and clinical characteristics.* (Adapted from table 1 of Yusuf et al[209])

	Telmisartan (N=2954)	Placebo (N=2972)
Age (years)	66.9 (7.3)	66.9 (7.4)
Sex (female)	1280 (43.3%)	1267 (42.6%)
Smoking status:		
Current	293 (9.9%)	289 (9.7%)
Past	1273 (43.1%)	1283 (43.2%)
Ethnic origin:		
Asian	637 (21.6%)	624 (21.0%)
Arab	40 (1.3%)	37 (1.3%)
African	51 (1.7%)	55 (1.9%)
European	1801 (61.0%)	1820 (61.2%)
Native or Aboriginal	390 (13.2%)	393 (13.2%)
Other	38 (1.3%)	40 (1.3%)
Blood pressure (mm Hg)	140.7 (16.8/81.8) (10.1)	141.3 (16.4/82.0) (10.2)
Heart rate (beats per min)	68.8 (11.5)	68.8 (12.1)
Cholesterol (mmol/l):		
Total	5.09 (1.18)	5.08 (1.15)
LDL	3.02 (1.01)	3.03 (1.02)
HDL	1.27 (0.37)	1.28 (0.41)
Coronary artery disease	2211 (74.8%)	2207 (74.3%)
Myocardial infarction	1381 (46.8%)	1360 (45.8%)
Angina pectoris	1412 (47.8%)	1412 (47.5%)
Peripheral artery disease	349 (11.8%)	323 (10.9%)
Hypertension	2259 (76.5%)	2269 (76.3%)
Diabetes	1059 (35.8%)	1059 (35.6%)

*Data are means (SD) or numbers (%).

Table 5 Example of reporting of summary results for each study group (binary outcomes).* (Adapted from table 2 of Mease et al[103])

	Number (%)		
Endpoint	Etanercept (n=30)	Placebo (n=30)	Risk difference (95% CI)
Primary endpoint			
Achieved PsARC at 12 weeks	26 (87)	7 (23)	63% (44 to 83)
Secondary endpoint			
Proportion of patients meeting ACR criteria:			
ACR20	22 (73)	4 (13)	60% (40 to 80)
ACR50	15 (50)	1 (3)	47% (28 to 66)
ACR70	4 (13)	0 (0)	13% (1 to 26)

*See also example for item 6a.
PsARC=psoriatic arthritis response criteria. ACR=American College of Rheumatology.

Table 6 Example of reporting of summary results for each study group (continuous outcomes). (Adapted from table 3 of van Linschoten[234])

	Exercise therapy (n=65)		Control (n=66)		Adjusted difference* (95% CI) at 12 months
	Baseline (mean (SD))	12 months (mean (SD))	Baseline (mean (SD))	12 months (mean (SD))	
Function score (0-100)	64.4 (13.9)	83.2 (14.8)	65.9 (15.2)	79.8 (17.5)	4.52 (−0.73 to 9.76)
Pain at rest (0-100)	4.14 (2.3)	1.43 (2.2)	4.03 (2.3)	2.61 (2.9)	−1.29 (−2.16 to −0.42)
Pain on activity (0-100)	6.32 (2.2)	2.57 (2.9)	5.97 (2.3)	3.54 (3.38)	−1.19 (−2.22 to −0.16)

*Function score adjusted for baseline, age, and duration of symptoms.

Table 7 Example of reporting both absolute and relative effect sizes. (Adapted from table 3 of The OSIRIS Collaborative Group[242])

	Percentage (No)			
Primary outcome	Early administration (n=1344)	Delayed selective administration (n=1346)	Risk ratio (95% CI)	Risk difference (95% CI)
Death or oxygen dependence at "expected date of delivery"	31.9 (429)	38.2 (514)	0.84 (0.75 to 0.93)	−6.3 (−9.9 to −2.7)

factors extrinsic to the trial that affected the decision to stop the trial, and who made the decision to stop the trial, including reporting the role the funding agency played in the deliberations and in the decision to stop the trial.[134]

A systematic review of 143 RCTs stopped earlier than planned for benefit found that these trials reported stopping after accruing a median of 66 events, estimated a median relative risk of 0.47 and a strong relation between the number of events accrued and the size of the effect, with smaller trials with fewer events yielding the largest treatment effects (odds ratio 31, 95% confidence interval 12 to 82).[134] While an increasing number of trials published in high impact medical journals report stopping early, only 0.1% of trials reported stopping early for benefit, which contrasts with estimates arising from simulation studies[205] and surveys of data safety and monitoring committees.[206] Thus, many trials accruing few participants and reporting large treatment effects may have been stopped earlier than planned but failed to report this action.

Item 15. A table showing baseline demographic and clinical characteristics for each group

Example—See table 4

Explanation—Although the eligibility criteria (see item 4a) indicate who was eligible for the trial, it is also important to know the characteristics of the participants who were actually included. This information allows readers, especially clinicians, to judge how relevant the results of a trial might be to an individual patient.

Randomised trials aim to compare groups of participants that differ only with respect to the intervention (treatment). Although proper random assignment prevents selection bias, it does not guarantee that the groups are equivalent at baseline. Any differences in baseline characteristics are, however, the result of chance rather than bias.[32] The study groups should be compared at baseline for important demographic and clinical characteristics so that readers can assess how similar they were. Baseline data are especially valuable for outcomes that can also be measured at the start of the trial (such as blood pressure).

Baseline information is most efficiently presented in a table (see table 4). For continuous variables, such as weight or blood pressure, the variability of the data should be reported, along with average values. Continuous variables can be summarised for each group by the mean and standard deviation. When continuous data have an asymmetrical distribution, a preferable approach may be to quote the median and a centile range (such as the 25th and 75th centiles).[177] Standard errors and confidence intervals are not appropriate for describing variability—they are inferential rather than descriptive statistics. Variables with a small number of ordered categories (such as stages of disease I to IV) should not be treated as continuous variables; instead, numbers and proportions should be reported for each category.[48 177]

Unfortunately significance tests of baseline differences are still common[23 32 210]; they were reported in half of 50 RCTs trials published in leading general journals in 1997.[183] Such significance tests assess the probability that observed baseline differences could have occurred by chance; however, we already know that any differences are caused by chance. Tests of baseline differences are not necessarily wrong, just illogical.[211] Such hypothesis testing is superfluous and can mislead investigators and their readers. Rather, comparisons at baseline should be based on consideration of the prognostic strength of the variables measured and the size of any chance imbalances that have occurred.[211]

Item 16. For each group, number of participants (denominator) included in each analysis and whether the analysis was by original assigned groups

Examples—"The primary analysis was intention-to-treat and involved all patients who were randomly assigned."[212]

"One patient in the alendronate group was lost to follow up; thus data from 31 patients were available for the intention-to-treat analysis. Five patients were considered protocol violators ... consequently 26 patients remained for the per-protocol analyses."[213]

Explanation—The number of participants in each group is an essential element of the analyses. Although the flow diagram (see item 13a) may indicate the numbers of participants analysed, these numbers often vary for different outcome measures. The number of participants per group should be given for all analyses. For binary outcomes, (such as risk ratio and risk difference) the denominators or event rates should also be reported. Expressing results as fractions also aids the reader in assessing whether some of the randomly assigned participants were excluded from the analysis. It follows that results should not be presented solely as summary measures, such as relative risks.

Participants may sometimes not receive the full intervention, or some ineligible patients may have been randomly allocated in error. One widely recommended way to handle such issues is to analyse all participants according to their original group assignment, regardless of what subsequently occurred (see box 6). This "intention-to-treat" strategy is not always straightforward to implement. It is common for some patients not to complete a study—they may drop out or be withdrawn from active treatment—and thus are not assessed at the end. If the outcome is mortality, such patients may be included in the analysis based on register information, whereas imputation techniques may need to be used if other outcome data are missing. The term "intention-to-treat analysis" is often inappropriately used—for example, when those who did not receive the first dose of a trial drug are excluded from the analyses.[18]

Conversely, analysis can be restricted to only participants who fulfil the protocol in terms of eligibility, interventions, and outcome assessment. This analysis is known as an "on-treatment" or "per protocol" analysis. Excluding participants from the analysis can lead to erroneous conclusions. For example, in a trial that compared medical with surgical therapy for carotid stenosis, analysis limited to participants who were available for follow-up showed that surgery reduced the risk for transient ischaemic attack, stroke, and death. However, intention-to-treat analysis based on all participants as originally assigned did not show a superior effect of surgery.[214]

Intention-to-treat analysis is generally favoured because it avoids bias associated with non-random loss of participants.[215 216 217] Regardless of whether authors use the term "intention-to-treat," they should make clear which and how many participants are included in each analysis (see item 13). Non-compliance with assigned therapy may mean that the intention-to-treat analysis underestimates the potential benefit of the treatment, and additional analyses, such as a per protocol analysis, may therefore be considered.[218 219] It should be noted, however, that such analyses are often considerably flawed.[220]

In a review of 403 RCTs published in 10 leading medical journals in 2002, 249 (62%) reported the use of intention-to-treat analysis for their primary analysis. This proportion was higher for journals adhering to the CONSORT statement (70% v 48%). Among articles that reported the use of intention-to-treat analysis, only 39% actually analysed all participants as randomised, with more than 60% of articles having missing data in their primary analysis.[221] Other studies show similar findings.[18 222 223] Trials with no reported exclusions are methodologically weaker in other respects than those that report on some excluded participants,[173] strongly indicating that at least some researchers who have excluded participants do not report it. Another study found that reporting an intention-to-treat analysis was associated with other aspects of good study design and reporting, such as describing a sample size calculation.[224]

Item 17a. For each primary and secondary outcome, results for each group, and the estimated effect size and its precision (such as 95% confidence interval)
Examples—See tables 5 and 6.

Explanation—For each outcome, study results should be reported as a summary of the outcome in each group (for example, the number of participants with or without the event and the denominators, or the mean and standard deviation of measurements), together with the contrast between the groups, known as the effect size. For binary outcomes, the effect size could be the risk ratio (relative risk), odds ratio, or risk difference; for survival time data, it could be the hazard ratio or difference in median survival time; and for continuous data, it is usually the difference in means. Confidence intervals should be presented for the contrast between groups. A common error is the presentation of separate confidence intervals for the outcome in each group rather than for the treatment effect.[233] Trial results are often more clearly displayed in a table rather than in the text, as shown in tables 5 and 6.

For all outcomes, authors should provide a confidence interval to indicate the precision (uncertainty) of the estimate.[48 235] A 95% confidence interval is conventional, but occasionally other levels are used. Many journals require or strongly encourage the use of confidence intervals.[236] They are especially valuable in relation to differences that do not meet conventional statistical significance, for which they often indicate that the result does not rule out an important clinical difference. The use of confidence intervals has increased markedly in recent years, although not in all medical specialties.[233] Although P values may be provided in addition to confidence intervals, results should not be reported solely as P values.[237 238] Results should be reported for all planned primary and secondary end points, not just for analyses that were statistically significant or "interesting." Selective reporting within a study is a widespread and serious problem.[55 57] In trials in which interim analyses were performed, interpretation should focus on the final results at the close of the trial, not the interim results.[239]

For both binary and survival time data, expressing the results also as the number needed to treat for benefit or harm can be helpful (see item 21).[240 241]

Item 17b. For binary outcomes, presentation of both absolute and relative effect sizes is recommended

Example—"The risk of oxygen dependence or death was reduced by 16% (95% CI 25% to 7%). The absolute difference was −6.3% (95% CI −9.9% to −2.7%); early administration to an estimated 16 babies would therefore prevent 1 baby dying or being long-term dependent on oxygen" (also see table 7).[242]

Explanation—When the primary outcome is binary, both the relative effect (risk ratio (relative risk) or odds ratio) and the absolute effect (risk difference) should be reported (with confidence intervals), as neither the relative measure nor the absolute measure alone gives a complete picture of the effect and its implications. Different audiences may prefer either relative or absolute risk, but both doctors and lay people tend to overestimate the effect when it is presented in terms of relative risk.[243] [244] [245] The size of the risk difference is less generalisable to other populations than the relative risk since it depends on the baseline risk in the unexposed group, which tends to vary across populations. For diseases where the outcome is common, a relative risk near unity might indicate clinically important differences in public health terms. In contrast, a large relative risk when the outcome is rare may not be so important for public health (although it may be important to an individual in a high risk category).

Item 18. Results of any other analyses performed, including subgroup analyses and adjusted analyses, distinguishing pre-specified from exploratory

Example—"On the basis of a study that suggested perioperative β-blocker efficacy might vary across baseline risk, we prespecified our primary subgroup analysis on the basis of the revised cardiac risk index scoring system. We also did prespecified secondary subgroup analyses based on sex, type of surgery, and use of an epidural or spinal anaesthetic. For all subgroup analyses, we used Cox proportional hazard models that incorporated tests for interactions, designated to be significant at p<0.05 … Figure 3 shows the results of our prespecified subgroup analyses and indicates consistency of effects … Our subgroup analyses were underpowered to detect the modest differences in subgroup effects that one might expect to detect if there was a true subgroup effect."[100]

Explanation—Multiple analyses of the same data create a risk for false positive findings.[246] Authors should resist the temptation to perform many subgroup analyses.[183] [185] [247] Analyses that were prespecified in the trial protocol (see item 24) are much more reliable than those suggested by the data, and therefore authors should report which analyses were prespecified. If subgroup analyses were undertaken, authors should report which subgroups were examined, why, if they were prespecified, and how many were prespecified. Selective reporting of subgroup analyses could lead to bias.[248] When evaluating a subgroup the question is not whether the subgroup shows a statistically significant result but whether the subgroup treatment effects are significantly different from each other. To determine this, a test of interaction is helpful, although the power for such tests is typically low. If formal evaluations of interaction are undertaken (see item 12b) they should be reported as the estimated difference in the intervention effect in each subgroup (with a confidence interval), not just as P values.

In one survey, 35 of 50 trial reports included subgroup analyses, of which only 42% used tests of interaction.[183] It was often difficult to determine whether subgroup analyses had been specified in the protocol. In another survey of surgical trials published in high impact journals, 27 of 72 trials reported 54 subgroup analyses, of which 91% were post hoc and only 6% of subgroup analyses used a test of interaction to assess whether a subgroup effect existed.[249]

Similar recommendations apply to analyses in which adjustment was made for baseline variables. If done, both unadjusted and adjusted analyses should be reported.

Authors should indicate whether adjusted analyses, including the choice of variables to adjust for, were planned. Ideally, the trial protocol should state whether adjustment is made for nominated baseline variables by using analysis of covariance.[187] Adjustment for variables because they differ significantly at baseline is likely to bias the estimated treatment effect.[187] A survey found that unacknowledged discrepancies between protocols and publications were found for all 25 trials reporting subgroup analyses and for 23 of 28 trials reporting adjusted analyses.[92]

Item 19. All important harms or unintended effects in each group

For specific guidance see CONSORT for harms.[42]

Example—"The proportion of patients experiencing any adverse event was similar between the rBPI21 [recombinant bactericidal/permeability-increasing protein] and placebo groups: 168 (88.4%) of 190 and 180 (88.7%) of 203, respectively, and it was lower in patients treated with rBPI21 than in those treated with placebo for 11 of 12 body systems … the proportion of patients experiencing a severe adverse event, as judged by the investigators, was numerically lower in the rBPI21 group than the placebo group: 53 (27.9%) of 190 versus 74 (36.5%) of 203 patients, respectively. There were only three serious adverse events reported as drug-related and they all occurred in the placebo group."[250]

Explanation—Readers need information about the harms as well as the benefits of interventions to make rational and balanced decisions. The existence and nature of adverse effects can have a major impact on whether a particular intervention will be deemed acceptable and useful. Not all reported adverse events observed during a trial are necessarily a consequence of the intervention; some may be a consequence of the condition being treated. Randomised trials offer the best approach for providing safety data as well as efficacy data, although they cannot detect rare harms.

Many reports of RCTs provide inadequate information on adverse events. A survey of 192 drug trials published from 1967 to 1999 showed that only 39% had adequate reporting of clinical adverse events and 29% had adequate reporting of laboratory defined toxicity.[72] More recently, a comparison between the adverse event data submitted to the trials database of the National Cancer Institute, which sponsored the trials, and the information reported in journal articles found that low grade adverse events were underreported in journal articles. High grade events (Common Toxicity Criteria grades 3 to 5) were reported inconsistently in the articles, and the information regarding attribution to investigational drugs was incomplete.[251] Moreover, a review of trials published in six general medical journals in 2006 to 2007 found that, although 89% of 133 reports mentioned adverse events, no information on severe adverse events and withdrawal of patients due to an adverse event was given on 27% and 48% of articles, respectively.[252]

An extension of the CONSORT statement has been developed to provide detailed recommendations on the reporting of harms in randomised trials.[42] Recommendations and examples of appropriate reporting are freely available from the CONSORT website (www.consort-statement.org). They complement the CONSORT 2010 Statement and should be consulted, particularly if the study of harms was a key objective. Briefly, if data on adverse events were collected, events should be listed and defined, with reference to standardised criteria where appropriate. The methods used for data collection and attribution of events should be described. For each study arm the absolute risk of each adverse event, using appropriate metrics for recurrent events, and the number of participants withdrawn due to harms should be presented. Finally, authors should provide a balanced discussion of benefits and harms.[42]

Discussion

Item 20. Trial limitations, addressing sources of potential bias, imprecision, and, if relevant, multiplicity of analyses
Example—"The preponderance of male patients (85%) is a limitation of our study … We used bare-metal stents, since drug-eluting stents were not available until late during accrual. Although the latter factor may be perceived as a limitation, published data indicate no benefit (either short-term or long-term) with respect to death and myocardial infarction in patients with stable coronary artery disease who receive drug-eluting stents, as compared with those who receive bare-metal stents."[253]

Explanation—The discussion sections of scientific reports are often filled with rhetoric supporting the authors' findings[254] and provide little measured argument of the pros and cons of the study and its results. Some journals have attempted to remedy this problem by encouraging more structure to authors' discussion of their results.[255] [256] For example, *Annals of Internal Medicine* recommends that authors structure the discussion section by presenting (1) a brief synopsis of the key findings, (2) consideration of possible mechanisms and explanations, (3) comparison with relevant findings from other published studies (whenever possible including a systematic review combining the results of the current study with the results of all previous relevant studies), (4) limitations of the present study (and methods used to minimise and compensate for those limitations), and (5) a brief section that summarises the clinical and research implications of the work, as appropriate.[255] We recommend that authors follow these sensible suggestions, perhaps also using suitable subheadings in the discussion section.

Although discussion of limitations is frequently omitted from research reports,[257] identification and discussion of the weaknesses of a study have particular importance.[258] For example, a surgical group reported that laparoscopic cholecystectomy, a technically difficult procedure, had significantly lower rates of complications than the more traditional open cholecystectomy for management of acute cholecystitis.[259] However, the authors failed to discuss an obvious bias in their results. The study investigators had completed all the laparoscopic cholecystectomies, whereas 80% of the open cholecystectomies had been completed by trainees.

Authors should also discuss any imprecision of the results. Imprecision may arise in connection with several aspects of a study, including measurement of a primary outcome (see item 6a) or diagnosis (see item 4a). Perhaps the scale used was validated on an adult population but used in a paediatric one, or the assessor was not trained in how to administer the instrument.

The difference between statistical significance and clinical importance should always be borne in mind. Authors should particularly avoid the common error of interpreting a non-significant result as indicating equivalence of interventions. The confidence interval (see item 17a) provides valuable insight into whether the trial result is compatible with a clinically important effect, regardless of the P value.[120]

Authors should exercise special care when evaluating the results of trials with multiple comparisons. Such multiplicity arises from several interventions, outcome measures, time points, subgroup analyses, and other factors. In such circumstances, some statistically significant findings are likely to result from chance alone.

Item 21. Generalisability (external validity, applicability) of the trial findings
Examples—"As the intervention was implemented for both sexes, all ages, all types of sports, and at different levels of sports, the results indicate that the entire range of athletes, from young elite to intermediate and recreational senior athletes, would benefit from using the presented training programme for the prevention of recurrences of ankle sprain. By including non-medically treated and medically treated athletes, we covered a broad spectrum of injury severity. This suggests that the present training programme can be implemented in the treatment of all athletes. Furthermore, as it is reasonable to assume that ankle sprains not related to sports are comparable with those in sports, the programme could benefit the general population."[260]

"This replicates and extends the work of Clarke and colleagues and demonstrates that this CB (cognitive behavioural) prevention program can be reliably and effectively delivered in different settings by clinicians outside of the group who originally developed the intervention. The effect size was consistent with those of previously reported, single-site, indicated depression prevention studies and was robust across sites with respect to both depressive disorders and symptoms … In this generalisability trial, we chose a comparison condition that is relevant to public health—usual care … The sample also was predominantly working class to middle class with access to health insurance. Given evidence that CB therapy can be more efficacious for adolescents from homes with higher incomes, it will be important to test the effects of this prevention program with more economically and ethnically diverse samples."[261]

Explanation—External validity, also called generalisability or applicability, is the extent to which the results of a study can be generalised to other circumstances.[262] Internal validity, the extent to which the design and conduct of the trial eliminate the possibility of bias, is a prerequisite for external validity: the results of a flawed trial are invalid and the question of its external validity becomes irrelevant. There is no absolute external validity; the term is meaningful only with regard to clearly specified conditions that were not directly examined in the trial. Can results be generalised to an individual participant or groups that differ from those enrolled in the trial with regard to age, sex, severity of disease, and comorbid conditions? Are the results applicable to other drugs within a class of similar drugs, to a different dose, timing, and route of administration, and to different concomitant therapies? Can similar results be expected at the primary, secondary, and tertiary levels of care? What about the effect on related outcomes that were not assessed in the trial, and the importance of length of follow-up and duration of treatment, especially with respect to harms?[263]

External validity is a matter of judgment and depends on the characteristics of the participants included in the trial, the trial setting, the treatment regimens tested, and the outcomes assessed.[5] [136] It is therefore crucial that adequate information be described about eligibility criteria and the setting and location (see item 4b), the interventions and how they were administered (see item 5), the definition of outcomes (see item 6), and the period of recruitment and follow-up (see item 14). The proportion of control group participants in whom the outcome develops (control group risk) is also important. The proportion of eligible participants who refuse to enter the trial as indicated on the flowchart (see item 13) is relevant for the generalisability of the trial, as it may indicate preferences for or acceptability of an intervention. Similar considerations may apply to clinician preferences.[264] [265]

Several issues are important when results of a trial are applied to an individual patient.[266] [267] [268] Although some variation in treatment response between an individual patient and the patients in a trial or systematic review is to be expected, the differences tend to be in magnitude rather than direction.

Although there are important exceptions,[268] therapies (especially drugs[269]) found to be beneficial in a narrow range of patients generally have broader application in actual practice. Frameworks for the evaluation of external validity have been proposed, including qualitative studies, such as in integral "process evaluations"[270] and checklists.[271] Measures that incorporate baseline risk when calculating therapeutic effects, such as the number needed to treat to obtain one additional favourable outcome and the number needed to treat to produce one adverse effect, are helpful in assessing the benefit-to-risk balance in an individual patient or group with characteristics that differ from the typical trial participant.[268] [272] [273] Finally, after deriving patient centred estimates for the potential benefit and harm from an intervention, the clinician must integrate them with the patient's values and preferences for therapy. Similar considerations apply when assessing the generalisability of results to different settings and interventions.

Item 22. Interpretation consistent with results, balancing benefits and harms, and considering other relevant evidence
Example—"Studies published before 1990 suggested that prophylactic immunotherapy also reduced nosocomial infections in very-low-birth-weight infants. However, these studies enrolled small numbers of patients; employed varied designs, preparations, and doses; and included diverse study populations. In this large multicenter, randomised controlled trial, the repeated prophylactic administration of intravenous immune globulin failed to reduce the incidence of nosocomial infections significantly in premature infants weighing 501 to 1500 g at birth."[274]

Explanation—Readers will want to know how the present trial's results relate to those of other RCTs. This can best be achieved by including a formal systematic review in the results or discussion section of the report.[83] [275] [276] [277] Such synthesis may be impractical for trial authors, but it is often possible to quote a systematic review of similar trials. A systematic review may help readers assess whether the results of the RCT are similar to those of other trials in the same topic area and whether participants are similar across studies. Reports of RCTs have often not dealt adequately with these points.[277] Bayesian methods can be used to statistically combine the trial data with previous evidence.[278]

We recommend that, at a minimum, the discussion should be as systematic as possible and be based on a comprehensive search, rather than being limited to studies that support the results of the current trial.[279]

Other information
Item 23. Registration number and name of trial registry
Example—"The trial is registered at ClinicalTrials.gov, number NCT00244842. "[280]

Explanation—The consequences of non-publication of entire trials,[281] [282] selective reporting of outcomes within trials, and of per protocol rather than intention-to-treat analysis have been well documented.[55] [56] [283] Covert redundant publication of clinical trials can also cause problems, particularly for authors of systematic reviews when results from the same trial are inadvertently included more than once.[284]

To minimise or avoid these problems there have been repeated calls over the past 25 years to register clinical trials at their inception, to assign unique trial identification numbers, and to record other basic information about the trial so that essential details are made publicly available.[285] [286] [287] [288] Provoked by recent serious problems of withholding data,[289] there has been a renewed effort to register randomised trials. Indeed, the World Health Organisation states that "the registration of all interventional trials is a scientific, ethical and moral responsibility" (www.who.int/ictrp/en). By registering a randomised trial, authors typically report a minimal set of information and obtain a unique trial registration number.

In September 2004 the International Committee of Medical Journal Editors (ICMJE) changed their policy, saying that they would consider trials for publication only if they had been registered before the enrolment of the first participant.[290] This resulted in a dramatic increase in the number of trials being registered.[291] The ICMJE gives guidance on acceptable registries (www.icmje.org/faq.pdf).

In a recent survey of 165 high impact factor medical journals' instructions to authors, 44 journals specifically stated that all recent clinical trials must be registered as a requirement of submission to that journal.[292]

Authors should provide the name of the register and the trial's unique registration number. If authors had not registered their trial they should explicitly state this and give the reason.

Item 24. Where the full trial protocol can be accessed, if available
Example—"Full details of the trial protocol can be found in the Supplementary Appendix, available with the full text of this article at www.nejm.org."[293]

Explanation—A protocol for the complete trial (rather than a protocol of a specific procedure within a trial) is important because it pre-specifies the methods of the randomised trial, such as the primary outcome (see item 6a). Having a protocol can help to restrict the likelihood of undeclared post hoc changes to the trial methods and selective outcome reporting (see item 6b). Elements that may be important for inclusion in the protocol for a randomised trial are described elsewhere.[294]

There are several options for authors to consider ensuring their trial protocol is accessible to interested readers. As described in the example above, journals reporting a trial's primary results can make the trial protocol available on their web site. Accessibility to the trial results and protocol is enhanced when the journal is open access. Some journals (such as *Trials*) publish trial protocols, and such a publication can be referenced when reporting the trial's principal results. Trial registration (see item 23) will also ensure that many trial protocol details are available, as the minimum trial characteristics included in an approved trial registration database includes several protocol items and results (www.who.int/ictrp/en). Trial investigators may also be able to post their trial protocol on a website through their employer. Whatever mechanism is used, we encourage all trial investigators to make their protocol easily accessible to interested readers.

Item 25. Sources of funding and other support (such as supply of drugs), role of funders

Examples—"Grant support was received for the intervention from Plan International and for the research from the Wellcome Trust and Joint United Nations Programme on HIV/AIDS (UNAIDS). The funders had no role in study design, data collection and analysis, decision to publish, or preparation of the manuscript."[295]

"This study was funded by GlaxoSmithKline Pharmaceuticals. GlaxoSmithKline was involved in the design and conduct of the study and provided logistical support during the trial. Employees of the sponsor worked with the investigators to prepare the statistical analysis plan, but the analyses were performed by the University of Utah. The manuscript was prepared by Dr Shaddy and the steering committee members. GlaxoSmithKline was permitted to review the manuscript and suggest changes, but the final decision on content was exclusively retained by the authors."[296]

Explanation—Authors should report the sources of funding for the trial, as this is important information for readers assessing a trial. Studies have showed that research sponsored by the pharmaceutical industry are more likely to produce results favouring the product made by the company sponsoring the research than studies funded by other sources.[297 298 299 300] A systematic review of 30 studies on funding found that research funded by the pharmaceutical industry had four times the odds of having outcomes favouring the sponsor than research funded by other sources (odds ratio 4.05, 95% confidence interval 2.98 to 5.51).[297] A large proportion of trial publications do not currently report sources of funding. The degree of underreporting is difficult to quantify. A survey of 370 drug trials found that 29% failed to report sources of funding.[301] In another survey, of PubMed indexed randomised trials published in December 2000, source of funding was reported for 66% of the 519 trials.[16]

The level of involvement by a funder and their influence on the design, conduct, analysis, and reporting of a trial varies. It is therefore important that authors describe in detail the role of the funders. If the funder had no such involvement, the authors should state so. Similarly, authors should report any other sources of support, such as supply and preparation of drugs or equipment, or in the analysis of data and writing of the manuscript.[302]

Reporting RCTs that did not have a two group parallel design

The primary focus of the CONSORT recommendations is RCTs with a parallel design and two treatment groups. Most RCTs have that design, but a substantial minority do not: 45% (233/519) of RCTs published in December 2000,[16] and 39% (242/616) in December 2006.[17]

Most of the CONSORT statement applies equally to all trial designs, but there are a few additional issues to address for each design. Before the publication of the revised CONSORT statement in 2001, the CONSORT Group decided to develop extensions to the main CONSORT statement relevant to specific trial designs. Extensions have been published relating to reporting of cluster randomised trials[40] and non-inferiority and equivalence trials.[39] Lack of resources has meant that other planned extensions have not been completed; they will cover trials with the following designs: multiarm parallel, factorial, crossover, within-person.

Authors reporting trials with a cluster design or using a non-inferiority or equivalence framework should consult the CONSORT recommendations in addition to those in this document. Here we make a few interim comments about the other designs. In each case, the trial design should be made clear in both the main text and the article's abstract.

Multiarm (>2 group) parallel group trials need the least modification of the standard CONSORT guidance. The flow diagram can be extended easily. The main differences from trials with two groups relate to clarification of how the study hypotheses relate to the multiple groups, and the consequent methods of data analysis and interpretation. For factorial trials, the possibility of interaction between the interventions generally needs to be considered. In addition to overall comparisons of participants who did or did not receive each intervention under study, investigators should consider also reporting results for each treatment combination.[303]

In crossover trials, each participant receives two (or more) treatments in a random order. The main additional issues to address relate to the paired nature of the data, which affect design and analysis.[304] Similar issues affect within-person comparisons, in which participants receive two treatments simultaneously (often to paired organs). Also, because of the risk of temporal or systemic carryover effects, respectively, in both cases the choice of design needs justification.

The CONSORT Group intends to publish extensions to CONSORT to cover all these designs. In addition, we will publish updates to existing guidance for cluster randomised trials and non-inferiority and equivalence trials to take account of this major update of the generic CONSORT guidance.

Discussion

Assessment of healthcare interventions can be misleading unless investigators ensure unbiased comparisons. Random allocation to study groups remains the only method that eliminates selection and confounding biases. Non-randomised trials tend to result in larger estimated treatment effects than randomised trials.[305 306]

Bias jeopardises even RCTs, however, if investigators carry out such trials improperly.[307] A recent systematic review, aggregating the results of several methodological investigations, found that, for subjective outcomes, trials that used inadequate or unclear allocation concealment yielded 31% larger estimates of effect than those that used adequate concealment, and trials that were not blinded yielded 25% larger estimates.[153] As might be expected, there was a strong association between the two.

The design and implementation of an RCT require methodological as well as clinical expertise, meticulous effort,[143 308] and a high level of alertness for unanticipated difficulties. Reports of RCTs should be written with similarly close attention to reducing bias. Readers should not have to speculate; the methods used should be complete and transparent so that readers can readily differentiate trials with unbiased results from those with questionable results.

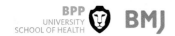

Sound science encompasses adequate reporting, and the conduct of ethical trials rests on the footing of sound science.[309]

We hope this update of the CONSORT explanatory article will assist authors in using the 2010 version of CONSORT and explain in general terms the importance of adequately reporting of trials. The CONSORT statement can help researchers designing trials in future[310] and can guide peer reviewers and editors in their evaluation of manuscripts. Indeed, we encourage peer reviewers and editors to use the CONSORT checklist to assess whether authors have reported on these items. Such assessments will likely improve the clarity and transparency of published trials. Because CONSORT is an evolving document, it requires a dynamic process of continual assessment, refinement, and, if necessary, change, which is why we have this update of the checklist and explanatory article. As new evidence and critical comments accumulate, we will evaluate the need for future updates.

The first version of the CONSORT statement, from 1996, seems to have led to improvement in the quality of reporting of RCTs in the journals that have adopted it.[50][51][52][53][54]. Other groups are using the CONSORT template to improve the reporting of other research designs, such as diagnostic tests[311] and observational studies.[312]

The CONSORT website (www.consort-statement.org) has been established to provide educational material and a repository database of materials relevant to the reporting of RCTs. The site includes many examples from real trials, including all of the examples included in this article. We will continue to add good and bad examples of reporting to the database, and we invite readers to submit further suggestions by contacting us through the website. The CONSORT Group will continue to survey the literature to find relevant articles that address issues relevant to the reporting of RCTs, and we invite authors of any such articles to notify us about them. All of this information will be made accessible through the CONSORT website, which is updated regularly.

More than 400 leading general and specialty journals and biomedical editorial groups, including the ICMJE, World Association of Medical Journal Editors, and the Council of Science Editors, have given their official support to CONSORT. We invite other journals concerned about the quality of reporting of clinical trials to endorse the CONSORT statement and contact us through our website to let us know of their support. The ultimate benefactors of these collective efforts should be people who, for whatever reason, require intervention from the healthcare community.

We are grateful to Frank Davidoff and Tom Lang for their involvement in the 2001 version of CONSORT explanation and elaboration document. A special thanks to Mary Ocampo, the Ottawa CONSORT coordinator, who helped deliver this explanation and elaboration paper and the CONSORT statement.

The CONSORT Group contributors to CONSORT 2010: Douglas G Altman, Centre for Statistics in Medicine, University of Oxford, UK; Virginia Barbour, PLoS Medicine, UK; Jesse A Berlin, Johnson & Johnson Pharmaceutical Research and Development, USA; Isabelle Boutron, University Paris 7 Denis Diderot, Assistance Publique des Hôpitaux de Paris, INSERM, France; PJ Devereaux, McMaster University, Canada; Kay Dickersin, Johns Hopkins Bloomberg School of Public Health, USA; Diana Elbourne, London School of Hygiene & Tropical Medicine, UK; Susan Ellenberg, University of Pennsylvania School of Medicine, USA; Val Gebski, University of Sydney, Australia; Steven Goodman, Journal of the Society for Clinical Trials, USA; Peter C Gøtzsche, Nordic Cochrane Centre, Denmark; Trish Groves, BMJ, UK; Steven Grunberg, American Society of Clinical Oncology, USA; Brian Haynes, McMaster University, Canada; Sally Hopewell, Centre for Statistics in Medicine, University of Oxford, UK; Astrid James, Lancet; Peter Juhn, Johnson & Johnson, USA; Philippa Middleton, University of Adelaide, Australia;

Don Minckler, University of California Irvine, USA; David Moher, Ottawa Methods Centre, Clinical Epidemiology Program, Ottawa Hospital Research Institute, Canada; Victor M Montori, Knowledge and Encounter Research Unit, Mayo Clinic College of Medicine, USA; Cynthia Mulrow, Annals of Internal Medicine, USA; Stuart Pocock, London School of Hygiene & Tropical Medicine, UK; Drummond Rennie, JAMA, USA; David L Schriger, Annals of Emergency Medicine, USA; Kenneth F Schulz, Family Health International, USA; Iveta Simera, EQUATOR Network, UK; Elizabeth Wager, Sideview, UK.

Funding: We gratefully acknowledge financial support from United Kingdom National Institute for Health Research; Canadian Institutes of Health Research; Presidents Fund, Canadian Institutes of Health Research; Johnson & Johnson; BMJ; and the American Society for Clinical Oncology.

In order to encourage dissemination of the CONSORT 2010 Statement, this article is freely accessible on bmj.com and will also be published in the Journal of Clinical Epidemiology. The authors jointly hold the copyright of this article. For details on further use, see the CONSORT website (www.consort-statement.org).

1   Rennie D. CONSORT revised—improving the reporting of randomized trials. JAMA 2001;285:2006-7.
2   Schulz KF, Chalmers I, Hayes RJ, Altman DG. Empirical evidence of bias. Dimensions of methodological quality associated with estimates of treatment effects in controlled trials. JAMA 1995;273:408-12.
3   Moher D. CONSORT: an evolving tool to help improve the quality of reports of randomized controlled trials. Consolidated Standards of Reporting Trials. JAMA 1998;279:1489-91.
4   Kjaergard LL, Villumsen J, Gluud C. Quality of randomised clinical trials affects estimates of intervention efficacy. 7th Cochrane Colloquium, Rome, Italy 1999.
5   Jüni P, Altman DG, Egger M. Systematic reviews in health care: Assessing the quality of controlled clinical trials. BMJ 2001;323:42-6.
6   Veldhuyzen van Zanten SJ, Cleary C, Talley NJ, Peterson TC, Nyren O, Bradley LA, et al. Drug treatment of functional dyspepsia: a systematic analysis of trial methodology with recommendations for design of future trials. Am J Gastroenterol 1996;91:660-73.
7   Talley NJ, Owen BK, Boyce P, Paterson K. Psychological treatments for irritable bowel syndrome: a critique of controlled treatment trials. Am J Gastroenterol 1996;91:277-83.
8   Adetugbo K, Williams H. How well are randomized controlled trials reported in the dermatology literature? Arch Dermatol 2000;136:381-5.
9   Kjaergard LL, Nikolova D, Gluud C. Randomized clinical trials in HEPATOLOGY: predictors of quality. Hepatology 1999;30:1134-8.
10 Schor S, Karten I. Statistical evaluation of medical journal manuscripts. JAMA 1966;195:1123-8.
11 Gore SM, Jones IG, Rytter EC. Misuse of statistical methods: critical assessment of articles in BMJ from January to March 1976. BMJ 1977;1:85-7.
12 Hall JC, Hill D, Watts JM. Misuse of statistical methods in the Australasian surgical literature. Aust N Z J Surg 1982;52:541-3.
13 Altman DG. Statistics in medical journals. Stat Med 1982;1:59-71.
14 Pocock SJ, Hughes MD, Lee RJ. Statistical problems in the reporting of clinical trials. A survey of three medical journals. N Engl J Med 1987;317:426-32.
15 Altman DG. The scandal of poor medical research. BMJ 1994;308:283-4.
16 Chan AW, Altman DG. Epidemiology and reporting of randomised trials published in PubMed journals. Lancet 2005;365:1159-62.
17 Hopewell S, Dutton S, Yu LM, Chan AW, Altman DG. The quality of reports of randomised trials in 2000 and 2006: comparative study of articles indexed in PubMed. BMJ 2010;340:c723
18 Hollis S, Campbell F. What is meant by intention to treat analysis? Survey of published randomised controlled trials. BMJ 1999;319:670-4.
19 Lai TY, Wong VW, Lam RF, Cheng AC, Lam DS, Leung GM. Quality of reporting of key methodological items of randomized controlled trials in clinical ophthalmic journals. Ophthalmic Epidemiol 2007;14:390-8.
20 Moher D, Fortin P, Jadad AR, Jüni P, Klassen T, Le LJ, et al. Completeness of reporting of trials published in languages other than English: implications for conduct and reporting of systematic reviews. Lancet 1996;347:363-6.
21 Junker CA. Adherence to published standards of reporting: a comparison of placebo-controlled trials published in English or German. JAMA 1998;280:247-9.
22 Altman DG. Randomisation. BMJ 1991;302:1481-2.
23 Schulz KF, Chalmers I, Grimes DA, Altman DG. Assessing the quality of randomization from reports of controlled trials published in obstetrics and gynecology journals. JAMA 1994;272:125-8.
24 Streptomycin treatment of pulmonary tuberculosis: a Medical Research Council investigation. BMJ 1948;2:769-82.
25 Schulz KF. Randomized controlled trials. Clin Obstet Gynecol 1998;41:245-56.
26 Greenland S. Randomization, statistics, and causal inference. Epidemiology 1990;1:421-9.
27 Armitage P. The role of randomization in clinical trials. Stat Med 1982;1:345-52.
28 Kleijnen J, Gøtzsche PC, Kunz R, Oxman AD, Chalmers I. So what's so special about randomisation. In: Maynard A, Chalmers I, eds. Non-random reflections on health services research . BMJ Books, 1997:93-106.

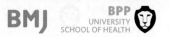

29 Chalmers I. Assembling comparison groups to assess the effects of health care. *J R Soc Med* 1997;90:379-86.

30 Nicolucci A, Grilli R, Alexanian AA, Apolone G, Torri V, Liberati A. Quality, evolution, and clinical implications of randomized, controlled trials on the treatment of lung cancer. A lost opportunity for meta-analysis. *JAMA* 1989;262:2101-7.

31 Ah-See KW, Molony NC. A qualitative assessment of randomized controlled trials in otolaryngology. *J Laryngol Otol* 1998;112:460-3.

32 Altman DG, Doré CJ. Randomisation and baseline comparisons in clinical trials. *Lancet* 1990;335:149-53.

33 Thornley B, Adams C. Content and quality of 2000 controlled trials in schizophrenia over 50 years. *BMJ* 1998;317:1181-4.

34 DerSimonian R, Charette LJ, McPeek B, Mosteller F. Reporting on methods in clinical trials. *N Engl J Med* 1982;306:1332-7.

35 A proposal for structured reporting of randomized controlled trials. The Standards of Reporting Trials Group. *JAMA* 1994;272:1926-31.

36 Call for comments on a proposal to improve reporting of clinical trials in the biomedical literature. Working Group on Recommendations for Reporting of Clinical Trials in the Biomedical Literature. *Ann Intern Med* 1994;121:894-5.

37 Rennie D. Reporting randomized controlled trials. An experiment and a call for responses from readers. *JAMA* 1995;273:1054-5.

38 Begg C, Cho M, Eastwood S, Horton R, Moher D, Olkin I, et al. Improving the quality of reporting of randomized controlled trials: the CONSORT statement. *JAMA* 1996;276:637-9.

39 Piaggio G, Elbourne DR, Altman DG, Pocock SJ, Evans SJ. Reporting of noninferiority and equivalence randomized trials: an extension of the CONSORT statement. *JAMA* 2006;295:1152-60.

40 Campbell MK, Elbourne DR, Altman DG. CONSORT statement: extension to cluster randomised trials. *BMJ* 2004;328:702-8.

41 Zwarenstein M, Treweek S, Gagnier JJ, Altman DG, Tunis S, Haynes B, et al. Improving the reporting of pragmatic trials: an extension of the CONSORT statement. *BMJ* 2008;337:a2390.

42 Ioannidis JP, Evans SJ, Gøtzsche PC, O'Neill RT, Altman DG, Schulz K, et al. Better reporting of harms in randomized trials: an extension of the CONSORT statement. *Ann Intern Med* 2004;141:781-8.

43 Boutron I, Moher D, Altman DG, Schulz KF, Ravaud P. Extending the CONSORT statement to randomized trials of nonpharmacologic treatment: explanation and elaboration. *Ann Intern Med* 2008;148:295-309.

44 Gagnier JJ, Boon H, Rochon P, Moher D, Barnes J, Bombardier C. Reporting randomized, controlled trials of herbal interventions: an elaborated CONSORT statement. *Ann Intern Med* 2006;144:364-7.

45 Hopewell S, Clarke M, Moher D, Wager E, Middleton P, Altman DG, et al. CONSORT for reporting randomized controlled trials in journal and conference abstracts: explanation and elaboration. *PLoS Med* 2008;5:e20.

46 Siegel JE, Weinstein MC, Russell LB, Gold MR. Recommendations for reporting cost-effectiveness analyses. Panel on Cost-Effectiveness in Health and Medicine. *JAMA* 1996;276:1339-41.

47 Drummond MF, Jefferson TO. Guidelines for authors and peer reviewers of economic submissions to the BMJ. The BMJ Economic Evaluation Working Party. *BMJ* 1996;313:275-83.

48 Lang TA, Secic M. *How to report statistics in medicine. Annotated guidelines for authors, editors, and reviewers*. ACP, 1997.

49 Davidoff F. News from the International Committee of Medical Journal Editors. *Ann Intern Med* 2000;133:229-31.

50 Plint AC, Moher D, Morrison A, Schulz K, Altman DG, Hill C, et al. Does the CONSORT checklist improve the quality of reports of randomised controlled trials? A systematic review. *Med J Aust* 2006;185:263-7.

51 Egger M, Jüni P, Bartlett C. Value of flow diagrams in reports of randomized controlled trials. *JAMA* 2001;285:1996-9.

52 Moher D, Schulz KF, Altman DG. The CONSORT statement: revised recommendations for improving the quality of reports of parallel-group randomized trials. *Ann Intern Med* 2001;134:657-62.

53 Moher D, Schulz KF, Altman D. The CONSORT statement: revised recommendations for improving the quality of reports of parallel-group randomized trials. *JAMA* 2001;285:1987-91.

54 Moher D, Schulz KF, Altman DG. The CONSORT statement: revised recommendations for improving the quality of reports of parallel-group randomized trials. *Lancet* 2001;357:1191-4.

55 Chan AW, Hróbjartsson A, Haahr MT, Gøtzsche PC, Altman DG. Empirical evidence for selective reporting of outcomes in randomized trials: comparison of protocols to published articles. *JAMA* 2004;291:2457-65.

56 Al-Marzouki S, Roberts I, Evans S, Marshall T. Selective reporting in clinical trials: analysis of trial protocols accepted by the Lancet. *Lancet* 2008;372:201.

57 Dwan K, Altman DG, Arnaiz JA, Bloom J, Chan AW, Cronin E, et al. Systematic review of the empirical evidence of study publication bias and outcome reporting bias. *PLoS ONE* 2008;3:e3081.

58 Altman DG, Schulz KF, Moher D, Egger M, Davidoff F, Elbourne D, et al. The revised CONSORT statement for reporting randomized trials: explanation and elaboration. *Ann Intern Med* 2001;134:663-94.

59 Schulz KF, Altman DG, Moher D, for the CONSORT Group. CONSORT 2010 Statement: updated guidelines for reporting parallel group randomised trials. *BMJ* 2010;340:c332.

60 Pocock SJ. *Clinical trials: a practical approach*. John Wiley, 1983.

61 Meinert CL. *Clinical trials: design, conduct and analysis*. Oxford University Press, 1986.

62 Friedman LM, Furberg CD, DeMets DL. *Fundamentals of clinical trials*. 3rd ed. Springer, 1998.

63 Bolliger CT, Zellweger JP, Danielsson T, van Biljon X, Robidou A, Westin A, et al. Smoking reduction with oral nicotine inhalers: double blind, randomised clinical trial of efficacy and safety. *BMJ* 2000;321:329-33.

64 Dickersin K, Manheimer E, Wieland S, Robinson KA, Lefebvre C, McDonald S. Development of the Cochrane Collaboration's CENTRAL Register of controlled clinical trials. *Eval Health Prof* 2002;25:38-64.

65 Hopewell S, Clarke M, Moher D, Wager E, Middleton P, Altman DG, et al. CONSORT for reporting randomised trials in journal and conference abstracts. *Lancet* 2008;371:281-3.

66 The impact of open access upon public health. *PLoS Med* 2006;3:e252.

67 Harbourt AM, Knecht LS, Humphreys BL. Structured abstracts in MEDLINE, 1989-1991. *Bull Med Libr Assoc* 1995;83:190-5.

68 Harris AH, Standard S, Brunning JL, Casey SL, Goldberg JH, Oliver L, et al. The accuracy of abstracts in psychology journals. *J Psychol* 2002;136:141-8.

69 Pitkin RM, Branagan MA, Burmeister LF. Accuracy of data in abstracts of published research articles. *JAMA* 1999;281:1110-1.

70 Ward LG, Kendrach MG, Price SO. Accuracy of abstracts for original research articles in pharmacy journals. *Ann Pharmacother* 2004;38:1173-7.

71 Gøtzsche PC. Believability of relative risks and odds ratios in abstracts: cross sectional study. *BMJ* 2006;333:231-4.

72 Ioannidis JP, Lau J. Completeness of safety reporting in randomized trials: an evaluation of 7 medical areas. *JAMA* 2001;285:437-43.

73 Haynes RB, Mulrow CD, Huth EJ, Altman DG, Gardner MJ. More informative abstracts revisited. *Ann Intern Med* 1990;113:69-76.

74 Taddio A, Pain T, Fassos FF, Boon H, Ilersich AL, Einarson TR. Quality of nonstructured and structured abstracts of original research articles in the British Medical Journal, the Canadian Medical Association Journal and the Journal of the American Medical Association. *CMAJ* 1994;150:1611-5.

75 Wager E, Middleton P. Technical editing of research reports in biomedical journals. *Cochrane Database Syst Rev* 2008;MR000002.

76 Hartley J, Sydes M, Blurton A. Obtaining information accurately and quickly: Are structured abstracts more efficient? *J Inform Sci* 1996;22:349-56.

77 Gilligan D, Nicolson M, Smith I, Groen H, Dalesio O, Goldstraw P, et al. Preoperative chemotherapy in patients with resectable non-small cell lung cancer: results of the MRC LU22/NVALT 2/EORTC 08012 multicentre randomised trial and update of systematic review. *Lancet* 2007;369:1929-37.

78 Sandler AD, Sutton KA, DeWeese J, Girardi MA, Sheppard V, Bodfish JW. Lack of benefit of a single dose of synthetic human secretin in the treatment of autism and pervasive developmental disorder. *N Engl J Med* 1999;341:1801-6.

79 World Medical Association. Declaration of Helsinki: ethical principle for medical research involving human subjects. 59th WMA General Assembly, Seoul 2008; www.wma.net/e/policy/b3.htm (accessed 2 June 2009).

80 Lau J, Antman EM, Jimenez-Silva J, Kupelnick B, Mosteller F, Chalmers TC. Cumulative meta-analysis of therapeutic trials for myocardial infarction. *N Engl J Med* 1992;327:248-54.

81 Fergusson D, Glass KC, Hutton B, Shapiro S. Randomized controlled trials of aprotinin in cardiac surgery: could clinical equipoise have stopped the bleeding? *Clin Trials* 2005;2:218-29.

82 Savulescu J, Chalmers I, Blunt J. Are research ethics committees behaving unethically? Some suggestions for improving performance and accountability. *BMJ* 1996;313:1390-3.

83 Sadler LC, Davison T, McCowan LM. A randomised controlled trial and meta-analysis of active management of labour. *BJOG* 2000;107:909-15.

84 Bath FJ, Owen VE, Bath PM. Quality of full and final publications reporting acute stroke trials: a systematic review. *Stroke* 1998;29:2203-10.

85 Blumer JL, Findling RL, Shih WJ, Soubrane C, Reed MD. Controlled clinical trial of zolpidem for the treatment of insomnia associated with attention-deficit/hyperactivity disorder in children 6 to 17 years of age. *Pediatrics* 2009;123:e770-e776.

86 Sabatine MS, Antman EM, Widimsky P, Ebrahim IO, Kiss RG, Saaiman A, et al. Otamixaban for the treatment of patients with non-ST-elevation acute coronary syndromes (SEPIA-ACS1 TIMI 42): a randomised, double-blind, active-controlled, phase 2 trial. *Lancet* 2009;374:787-95.

87 Grant AM, Altman DG, Babiker AB, Campbell MK, Clemens FJ, Darbyshire JH, et al. Issues in data monitoring and interim analysis of trials. *Health Technol Assess* 2005;9:1-iv.

88 Gallo P, Krams M. PhRMA Working Group on adaptive designs, "White Paper." *Drug Information Journal* 2006;40:421-82.

89 Brown CH, Ten Have TR, Jo B, Dagne G, Wyman PA, Muthen B, et al. Adaptive designs for randomized trials in public health. *Annu Rev Public Health* 2009;30:1-25.

90 Kelly PJ, Sooriyarachchi MR, Stallard N, Todd S. A practical comparison of group-sequential and adaptive designs. *J Biopharm Stat* 2005;15:719-38.

91 Pildal J, Chan AW, Hróbjartsson A, Forfang E, Altman DG, Gøtzsche PC. Comparison of descriptions of allocation concealment in trial protocols and the published reports: cohort study. *BMJ* 2005;330:1049.

92 Chan AW, Hróbjartsson A, Jørgensen KJ, Gøtzsche PC, Altman DG. Discrepancies in sample size calculations and data analyses reported in randomised trials: comparison of publications with protocols. *BMJ* 2008;337:a2299.

93 Ndekha MJ, van Oosterhout JJ, Zijlstra EE, Manary M, Saloojee H, Manary MJ. Supplementary feeding with either ready-to-use fortified

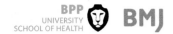

spread or corn-soy blend in wasted adults starting antiretroviral therapy in Malawi: randomised, investigator blinded, controlled trial. *BMJ* 2009;338:1867-75.

94 Rothwell PM. External validity of randomised controlled trials: "to whom do the results of this trial apply?" *Lancet* 2005;365:82-93.

95 Fuks A, Weijer C, Freedman B, Shapiro S, Skrutkowska M, Riaz A. A study in contrasts: eligibility criteria in a twenty-year sample of NSABP and POG clinical trials. National Surgical Adjuvant Breast and Bowel Program. Pediatric Oncology Group. *J Clin Epidemiol* 1998;51:69-79.

96 Shapiro SH, Weijer C, Freedman B. Reporting the study populations of clinical trials. Clear transmission or static on the line? *J Clin Epidemiol* 2000;53:973-9.

97 Gandhi M, Ameli N, Bacchetti P, Sharp GB, French AL, Young M, et al. Eligibility criteria for HIV clinical trials and generalizability of results: the gap between published reports and study protocols. *AIDS* 2005;19:1885-96.

98 Hall JC, Mills B, Nguyen H, Hall JL. Methodologic standards in surgical trials. *Surgery* 1996;119:466-72.

99 Weiss NS, Koepsell TD, Psaty BM. Generalizability of the results of randomized trials. *Arch Intern Med* 2008;168:133-5.

100 Devereaux PJ, Yang H, Yusuf S, Guyatt G, Leslie K, Villar JC, et al. Effects of extended-release metoprolol succinate in patients undergoing non-cardiac surgery (POISE trial): a randomised controlled trial. *Lancet* 2008;371:1839-47.

101 Rannou F, Dimet J, Boutron I, Baron G, Fayad F, Macé Y, et al. Splint for base-of-thumb osteoarthritis: a randomized trial. *Ann Intern Med* 2009;150:661-9.

102 Glasziou P, Meats E, Heneghan C, Shepperd S. What is missing from descriptions of treatment in trials and reviews? *BMJ* 2008;336:1472-4.

103 Mease PJ, Goffe BS, Metz J, VanderStoep A, Finck B, Burge DJ. Etanercept in the treatment of psoriatic arthritis and psoriasis: a randomised trial. *Lancet* 2000;356:385-90.

104 McDowell I, Newell C. Measuring health: a guide to rating scales and questionnaires. 3rd ed. New York: Oxford University Press, 2006.

105 Streiner D, Norman C. Health measurement scales: a practical guide to their development and use. 3rd ed. Oxford: Oxford University Press; 2003.

106 Clarke M. Standardising outcomes for clinical trials and systematic reviews. *Trials* 2007;8:39.

107 Sanders C, Egger M, Donovan J, Tallon D, Frankel S. Reporting on quality of life in randomised controlled trials: bibliographic study. *BMJ* 1998;317:1191-4.

108 Gøtzsche PC. Methodology and overt and hidden bias in reports of 196 double-blind trials of nonsteroidal antiinflammatory drugs in rheumatoid arthritis. *Control Clin Trials* 1989;10:31-56.

109 Marshall M, Lockwood A, Bradley C, Adams C, Joy C, Fenton M. Unpublished rating scales: a major source of bias in randomised controlled trials of treatments for schizophrenia. *Br J Psychiatry* 2000;176:249-52.

110 Jadad AR, Boyle M, Cunnigham C, Kim M, Schachar R. Treatment of Attention-Deficit/Hyperactivity Disorder. Evidence Report/Technology Assessment No. 11. Rockville, MD: U.S. Department of Health and Human Services, Public Health Service, Agency for Healthcare Research and Quality. AHQR publication no. 00-E005; 1999.

111 Schachter HM, Pham B, King J, Langford S, Moher D. The efficacy and safety of methylphenidate in attention deficit disorder: A systematic review and meta-analyis. Prepared for the Therapeutics Initiative, Vancouver, B.C., and the British Columbia Ministry for Children and Families, 2000.

112 Dargie HJ. Effect of carvedilol on outcome after myocardial infarction in patients with left-ventricular dysfunction: the CAPRICORN randomised trial. *Lancet* 2001;357:1385-90.

113 Chan AW, Krleza-Jeric K, Schmid I, Altman DG. Outcome reporting bias in randomized trials funded by the Canadian Institutes of Health Research. *CMAJ* 2004;171:735-40.

114 Vermeulen H, Hofland J, Legemate DA, Ubbink DT. Intravenous fluid restriction after major abdominal surgery: a randomized blinded clinical trial. *Trials* 2009;10:50.

115 Fox K, Ford I, Steg PG, Tendera M, Ferrari R. Ivabradine for patients with stable coronary artery disease and left-ventricular systolic dysfunction (BEAUTIFUL): a randomised, double-blind, placebo-controlled trial. *Lancet* 2008;372:807-16.

116 Campbell MJ, Julious SA, Altman DG. Estimating sample sizes for binary, ordered categorical, and continuous outcomes in two group comparisons. *BMJ* 1995;311:1145-8.

117 Guyatt GH, Mills EJ, Elbourne D. In the era of systematic reviews, does the size of an individual trial still matter. *PLoS Med* 2008;5:e4.

118 Schulz KF, Grimes DA. Sample size calculations in randomised trials: mandatory and mystical. *Lancet* 2005;365:1348-53.

119 Halpern SD, Karlawish JH, Berlin JA. The continuing unethical conduct of underpowered clinical trials. *JAMA* 2002;288:358-62.

120 Altman DG, Bland JM. Absence of evidence is not evidence of absence. *BMJ* 1995;311:485.

121 Moher D, Dulberg CS, Wells GA. Statistical power, sample size, and their reporting in randomized controlled trials. *JAMA* 1994;272:122-4.

122 Freiman JA, Chalmers TC, Smith H Jr, Kuebler RR. The importance of beta, the type II error and sample size in the design and interpretation of the randomized control trial. Survey of 71 "negative" trials. *N Engl J Med* 1978;299:690-4.

123 Charles P, Giraudeau B, Dechartres A, Baron G, Ravaud P. Reporting of sample size calculation in randomised controlled trials: review. *BMJ* 2009;338:b1732.

124 Yusuf S, Collins R, Peto R. Why do we need some large, simple randomized trials? *Stat Med* 1984;3:409-22.

125 Goodman SN, Berlin JA. The use of predicted confidence intervals when planning experiments and the misuse of power when interpreting results. *Ann Intern Med* 1994;121:200-6.

126 Galgiani JN, Catanzaro A, Cloud GA, Johnson RH, Williams PL, Mirels LF, et al. Comparison of oral fluconazole and itraconazole for progressive, nonmeningeal coccidioidomycosis. A randomized, double-blind trial. Mycoses Study Group. *Ann Intern Med* 2000;133:676-86.

127 Connolly SJ, Pogue J, Hart RG, Hohnloser SH, Pfeffer M, Chrolavicius S, et al. Effect of clopidogrel added to aspirin in patients with atrial fibrillation. *N Engl J Med* 2009;360:2066-78.

128 Geller NL, Pocock SJ. Interim analyses in randomized clinical trials: ramifications and guidelines for practitioners. *Biometrics* 1987;43:213-23.

129 Berry DA. Interim analyses in clinical trials: classical vs. Bayesian approaches. *Stat Med* 1985;4:521-6.

130 Pocock SJ. When to stop a clinical trial. *BMJ* 1992;305:235-40.

131 DeMets DL, Pocock SJ, Julian DG. The agonising negative trend in monitoring of clinical trials. *Lancet* 1999;354:1983-8.

132 Buyse M. Interim analyses, stopping rules and data monitoring in clinical trials in Europe. *Stat Med* 1993;12:509-20.

133 Sydes MR, Altman DG, Babiker AB, Parmar MK, Spiegelhalter DJ. Reported use of data monitoring committees in the main published reports of randomized controlled trials: a cross-sectional study. *Clin Trials* 2004;1:48-59.

134 Montori VM, Devereaux PJ, Adhikari NK, Burns KE, Eggert CH, Briel M, et al. Randomized trials stopped early for benefit: a systematic review. *JAMA* 2005;294:2203-9.

135 Coutinho IC, Ramos de Amorim MM, Katz L, Bandeira de Ferraz AA. Uterine exteriorization compared with in situ repair at cesarean delivery: a randomized controlled trial. *Obstet Gynecol* 2008;111:639-47.

136 Jüni P, Altman DG, Egger M. Assessing the quality of controlled clinical trials. In: Egger M, Davey Smith G, Altman DG, eds. *Systematic reviews in health care: meta-analysis in context* . BMJ Books, 2001.

137 Creinin MD, Meyn LA, Borgatta L, Barnhart K, Jensen J, Burke AE, et al. Multicenter comparison of the contraceptive ring and patch: a randomized controlled trial. *Obstet Gynecol* 2008;111:267-77.

138 Tate DF, Jackvony EH, Wing RR. Effects of internet behavioral counseling on weight loss in adults at risk for type 2 diabetes: a randomized trial. *JAMA* 2003;289:1833-6.

139 Lachin JM. Properties of simple randomization in clinical trials. *Control Clin Trials* 1988;9:312-26.

140 Peto R, Pike MC, Armitage P, Breslow NE, Cox DR, Howard SV, et al. Design and analysis of randomized clinical trials requiring prolonged observation of each patient. I. Introduction and design. *Br J Cancer* 1976;34:585-612.

141 Schulz KF, Grimes DA. *The Lancet handbook of essential concepts in clinical research* . Elsevier, 2006.

142 Altman DG, Bland JM. How to randomise. *BMJ* 1999;319:703-4.

143 Schulz KF. Subverting randomization in controlled trials. *JAMA* 1995;274:1456-8.

144 Enas GG, Enas NH, Spradlin CT, Wilson MG, Wiltse CG. Baseline comparability in clinical trials: prevention of poststudy anxiety. *Drug Information Journal* 1990;24:541-8.

145 Treasure T, MacRae KD. Minimisation: the platinum standard for trials? Randomisation doesn't guarantee similarity of groups; minimisation does. *BMJ* 1998;317:362-3.

146 Sinei SK, Schulz KF, Lamptey PR, Grimes DA, Mati JK, Rosenthal SM, et al. Preventing IUCD-related pelvic infection: the efficacy of prophylactic doxycycline at insertion. *Br J Obstet Gynaecol* 1990;97:412-9.

147 Radford JA, Landorf KB, Buchbinder R, Cook C. Effectiveness of low-Dye taping for the short-term treatment of plantar heel pain: a randomised trial. *BMC Musculoskelet Disord* 2006;7:64.

148 Chalmers TC, Levin H, Sacks HS, Reitman D, Berrier J, Nagalingam R. Meta-analysis of clinical trials as a scientific discipline. I: Control of bias and comparison with large co-operative trials. *Stat Med* 1987;6:315-28.

149 Pocock SJ. Statistical aspects of clinical trial design. *Statistician* 1982;31:1-18.

150 Haag U. Technologies for automating randomized treatment assignment in clinical trials. *Drug Information Journal* 1998;32:11.

151 Piaggio G, Elbourne D, Schulz KF, Villar J, Pinol AP, Gülmezoglu AM. The reporting of methods for reducing and detecting bias: an example from the WHO Misoprostol Third Stage of Labour equivalence randomised controlled trial. *BMC Med Res Methodol* 2003;3:19.

152 Pildal J, Hróbjartsson A, Jórgensen KJ, Hilden J, Altman DG, Gøtzsche PC. Impact of allocation concealment on conclusions drawn from meta-analyses of randomized trials. *Int J Epidemiol* 2007;36:847-57.

153 Wood L, Egger M, Gluud LL, Schulz KF, Jüni P, Altman DG, et al. Empirical evidence of bias in treatment effect estimates in controlled trials with different interventions and outcomes: meta-epidemiological study. *BMJ* 2008;336:601-5.

154 McCandlish R, Bowler U, van Asten H, Berridge G, Winter C, Sames L, et al. A randomised controlled trial of care of the perineum during second stage of normal labour. *Br J Obstet Gynaecol* 1998;105:1262-72.

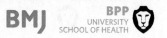

155 Webster J, Clarke S, Paterson D, Hutton A, van Dyk S, Gale C, et al. Routine care of peripheral intravenous catheters versus clinically indicated replacement: randomised controlled trial. *BMJ* 2008;337:a339.

156 Smith SA, Shah ND, Bryant SC, Christianson TJ, Bjornsen SS, Giesler PD, et al. Chronic care model and shared care in diabetes: randomized trial of an electronic decision support system. *Mayo Clin Proc* 2008;83:747-57.

157 Sacks FM, Bray GA, Carey VJ, Smith SR, Ryan DH, Anton SD, et al. Comparison of weight-loss diets with different compositions of fat, protein, and carbohydrates. *N Engl J Med* 2009;360:859-73.

158 Kaptchuk TJ. Intentional ignorance: a history of blind assessment and placebo controls in medicine. *Bull Hist Med* 1998;72:389-433.

159 Guyatt GH, Pugsley SO, Sullivan MJ, Thompson PJ, Berman L, Jones NL, et al. Effect of encouragement on walking test performance. *Thorax* 1984;39:818-22.

160 Gøtzsche PC. Blinding during data analysis and writing of manuscripts. *Control Clin Trials* 1996;17:285-90.

161 Karlowski TR, Chalmers TC, Frenkel LD, Kapikian AZ, Lewis TL, Lynch JM. Ascorbic acid for the common cold. A prophylactic and therapeutic trial. *JAMA* 1975;231:1038-42.

162 Noseworthy JH, Ebers GC, Vandervoort MK, Farquhar RE, Yetisir E, Roberts R. The impact of blinding on the results of a randomized, placebo-controlled multiple sclerosis clinical trial. *Neurology* 1994;44:16-20.

163 Carley SD, Libetta C, Flavin B, Butler J, Tong N, Sammy I. An open prospective randomised trial to reduce the pain of blood glucose testing: ear versus thumb. *BMJ* 2000;321:20.

164 Schulz KF, Chalmers I, Altman DG. The landscape and lexicon of blinding in randomized trials. *Ann Intern Med* 2002;136:254-9.

165 Day SJ, Altman DG. Statistics notes: blinding in clinical trials and other studies. *BMJ* 2000;321:504.

166 Montori VM, Bhandari M, Devereaux PJ, Manns BJ, Ghali WA, Guyatt GH. In the dark: the reporting of blinding status in randomized controlled trials. *J Clin Epidemiol* 2002;55:787-90.

167 Cheng K, Smyth RL, Motley J, O'Hea U, Ashby D. Randomized controlled trials in cystic fibrosis (1966-1997) categorized by time, design, and intervention. *Pediatr Pulmonol* 2000;29:1-7.

168 Lang T. Masking or blinding? An unscientific survey of mostly medical journal editors on the great debate. *Med Gen Med* 2000;2:E25.

169 Devereaux PJ, Manns BJ, Ghali WA, Quan H, Lacchetti C, Montori VM, et al. Physician interpretations and textbook definitions of blinding terminology in randomized controlled trials. *JAMA* 2001;285:2000-3.

170 Haahr MT, Hróbjartsson A. Who is blinded in randomized clinical trials? A study of 200 trials and a survey of authors. *Clin Trials* 2006;3:360-5.

171 Meinert CL. Masked monitoring in clinical trials—blind stupidity? *N Engl J Med* 1998;338:1381-2.

172 Mills E, Prousky J, Raskin G, Gagnier J, Rachlis B, Montori VM, et al. The safety of over-the-counter niacin. A randomized placebo-controlled trial [ISRCTN18054903] . *BMC Clin Pharmacol* 2003;3:4.

173 Schulz KF, Grimes DA, Altman DG, Hayes RJ. Blinding and exclusions after allocation in randomised controlled trials: survey of published parallel group trials in obstetrics and gynaecology. *BMJ* 1996;312:742-4.

174 Fergusson D, Glass KC, Waring D, Shapiro S. Turning a blind eye: the success of blinding reported in a random sample of randomised, placebo controlled trials. *BMJ* 2004;328:432.

175 Sackett DL. Turning a blind eye: why we don't test for blindness at the end of our trials. *BMJ* 2004;328:1136.

176 Astrup A, Rössner S, Van Gaal L, Rissanen A, Niskanen L, Al HM, et al. Effects of liraglutide in the treatment of obesity: a randomised, double-blind, placebo-controlled study. *Lancet* 2009;374:1606-16.

177 Altman DG, Gore SM, Gardner MJ, Pocock SJ. Statistical guidelines for contributors to medical journals. In: Altman DG, Machin D, Bryant TN, Gardner MJ, eds. *Statistics with confidence: confidence intervals and statistical guidelines* . 2nd ed. BMJ Books, 2000:171-90.

178 Altman DG, Bland JM. Statistics notes. Units of analysis. *BMJ* 1997;314:1874.

179 Bolton S. Independence and statistical inference in clinical trial designs: a tutorial review. *J Clin Pharmacol* 1998;38:408-12.

180 Greenland S. Principles of multilevel modelling. *Int J Epidemiol* 2000;29:158-67.

181 Albert CM, Cook NR, Gaziano JM, Zaharris E, MacFadyen J, Danielson E, et al. Effect of folic acid and B vitamins on risk of cardiovascular events and total mortality among women at high risk for cardiovascular disease: a randomized trial. *JAMA* 2008;299:2027-36.

182 Matthews JN, Altman DG. Interaction 3: How to examine heterogeneity. *BMJ* 1996;313:862.

183 Assmann SF, Pocock SJ, Enos LE, Kasten LE. Subgroup analysis and other (mis)uses of baseline data in clinical trials. *Lancet* 2000;355:1064-9.

184 Matthews JN, Altman DG. Statistics notes. Interaction 2: Compare effect sizes not P values. *BMJ* 1996;313:808.

185 Oxman AD, Guyatt GH. A consumer's guide to subgroup analyses. *Ann Intern Med* 1992;116:78-84.

186 Steyerberg EW, Bossuyt PM, Lee KL. Clinical trials in acute myocardial infarction: should we adjust for baseline characteristics? *Am Heart J* 2000;139:745-51.

187 Altman DG. Adjustment for covariate imbalance. In: Armitage P, Colton T, eds. *Encyclopedia of biostatistics* . John Wiley, 1998:1000-5.

188 Mullner M, Matthews H, Altman DG. Reporting on statistical methods to adjust for confounding: a cross-sectional survey. *Ann Intern Med* 2002;136:122-6.

189 Concato J, Feinstein AR, Holford TR. The risk of determining risk with multivariable models. *Ann Intern Med* 1993;118:201-10.

190 Bender R, Grouven U. Logistic regression models used in medical research are poorly presented. *BMJ* 1996;313:628.

191 Khan KS, Chien PF, Dwarakanath LS. Logistic regression models in obstetrics and gynecology literature. *Obstet Gynecol* 1999;93:1014-20.

192 Sackett DL, Gent M. Controversy in counting and attributing events in clinical trials. *N Engl J Med* 1979;301:1410-2.

193 May GS, DeMets DL, Friedman LM, Furberg C, Passamani E. The randomized clinical trial: bias in analysis. *Circulation* 1981;64:669-73.

194 Altman DG, Cuzick J, Peto J. More on zidovudine in asymptomatic HIV infection. *N Engl J Med* 1994;330:1758-9.

195 Meinert CL. Beyond CONSORT: need for improved reporting standards for clinical trials. Consolidated Standards of Reporting Trials. *JAMA* 1998;279:1487-9.

196 Grant AM, Wileman SM, Ramsay CR, Mowat NA, Krukowski ZH, Heading RC, et al. Minimal access surgery compared with medical management for chronic gastro-oesophageal reflux disease: UK collaborative randomised trial. *BMJ* 2008;337:a2664.

197 van Loon AJ, Mantingh A, Serlier EK, Kroon G, Mooyaart EL, Huisjes HJ. Randomised controlled trial of magnetic-resonance pelvimetry in breech presentation at term. *Lancet* 1997;350:1799-804.

198 Brown MJ, Palmer CR, Castaigne A, de Leeuw PW, Mancia G, Rosenthal T, et al. Morbidity and mortality in patients randomised to double-blind treatment with a long-acting calcium-channel blocker or diuretic in the International Nifedipine GITS study: Intervention as a Goal in Hypertension Treatment (INSIGHT). *Lancet* 2000;356:366-72.

199 LaCroix AZ, Ott SM, Ichikawa L, Scholes D, Barlow WE. Low-dose hydrochlorothiazide and preservation of bone mineral density in older adults. A randomized, double-blind, placebo-controlled trial. *Ann Intern Med* 2000;133:516-26.

200 Shuster JJ. Median follow-up in clinical trials. *J Clin Oncol* 1991;9:191-2.

201 Altman DG, de Stavola BL, Love SB, Stepniewska KA. Review of survival analyses published in cancer journals. *Br J Cancer* 1995;72:511-8.

202 Auvert B, Taljaard D, Lagarde E, Sobngwi-Tambekou J, Sitta R, Puren A. Randomized, controlled intervention trial of male circumcision for reduction of HIV infection risk: the ANRS 1265 Trial. *PLoS Med* 2005;2:e298.

203 Diggle L, Deeks J. Effect of needle length on incidence of local reactions to routine immunisation in infants aged 4 months: randomised controlled trial. *BMJ* 2000;321:931-3.

204 Pocock S, White I. Trials stopped early: too good to be true? *Lancet* 1999;353:943-4.

205 Hughes MD, Pocock SJ. Stopping rules and estimation problems in clinical trials. *Stat Med* 1988;7:1231-42.

206 Kiri A, Tonascia S, Meinert CL. Treatment effects monitoring committees and early stopping in large clinical trials. *Clin Trials* 2004;1:40-7.

207 Psaty BM, Rennie D. Stopping medical research to save money: a broken pact with researchers and patients. *JAMA* 2003;289:2128-31.

208 Temple R. FDA perspective on trials with interim efficacy evaluations. *Stat Med* 2006;25:3245-9.

209 Yusuf S, Teo K, Anderson C, Pogue J, Dyal L, Copland I, et al. Effects of the angiotensin-receptor blocker telmisartan on cardiovascular events in high-risk patients intolerant to angiotensin-converting enzyme inhibitors: a randomised controlled trial. *Lancet* 2008;372:1174-83.

210 Senn S. Base logic: tests of baseline balance in randomized clinical trials. *Clin Res Regulatory Affairs* 1995;12:171-82.

211 Altman DG. Comparability of randomised groups. *Statistician* 1985;34:125-36.

212 Heit JA, Elliott CG, Trowbridge AA, Morrey BF, Gent M, Hirsh J. Ardeparin sodium for extended out-of-hospital prophylaxis against venous thromboembolism after total hip or knee replacement. A randomized, double-blind, placebo-controlled trial. *Ann Intern Med* 2000;132:853-61.

213 Haderslev KV, Tjellesen L, Sorensen HA, Staun M. Alendronate increases lumbar spine bone mineral density in patients with Crohn's disease. *Gastroenterology* 2000;119:639-46.

214 Fields WS, Maslenikov V, Meyer JS, Hass WK, Remington RD, Macdonald M. Joint study of extracranial arterial occlusion. V. Progress report of prognosis following surgery or nonsurgical treatment for transient cerebral ischemic attacks and cervical carotid artery lesions. *JAMA* 1970;211:1993-2003.

215 Lee YJ, Ellenberg JH, Hirtz DG, Nelson KB. Analysis of clinical trials by treatment actually received: is it really an option? *Stat Med* 1991;10:1595-605.

216 Lewis JA, Machin D. Intention to treat—who should use ITT? *Br J Cancer* 1993;68:647-50.

217 Lachin JL. Statistical considerations in the intent-to-treat principle. *Control Clin Trials* 2000;21:526.

218 Sheiner LB, Rubin DB. Intention-to-treat analysis and the goals of clinical trials. *Clin Pharmacol Ther* 1995;57:6-15.

219 Nagelkerke N, Fidler V, Bernsen R, Borgdorff M. Estimating treatment effects in randomized clinical trials in the presence of non-compliance. *Stat Med* 2000;19:1849-64.

220 Melander H, Ahlqvist-Rastad J, Meijer G, Beermann B. Evidence b(i)ased medicine--selective reporting from studies sponsored by pharmaceutical industry: review of studies in new drug applications. *BMJ* 2003;326:1171-3.

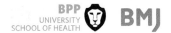

221 Gravel J, Opatrny L, Shapiro S. The intention-to-treat approach in randomized controlled trials: are authors saying what they do and doing what they say? *Clin Trials* 2007;4:350-6.

222 Kruse RL, Alper BS, Reust C, Stevermer JJ, Shannon S, Williams RH. Intention-to-treat analysis: who is in? Who is out? *J Fam Pract* 2002;51:969-71.

223 Herman A, Botser IB, Tenenbaum S, Chechick A. Intention-to-treat analysis and accounting for missing data in orthopaedic randomized clinical trials. *J Bone Joint Surg Am* 2009;91:2137-43.

224 Ruiz-Canela M, Martinez-González MA, de Irala-Estévez J. Intention to treat analysis is related to methodological quality. *BMJ* 2000;320:1007-8.

225 Altman DG. Missing outcomes in randomised trials: addressing the dilemma. *Open Med* 2009;3:e21-3.

226 Wood AM, White IR, Thompson SG. Are missing outcome data adequately handled? A review of published randomized controlled trials in major medical journals. *Clin Trials* 2004;1:368-76.

227 Streiner DL. Missing data and the trouble with LOCF. *Evid Based Ment Health* 2008;11:3-5.

228 Molnar FJ, Hutton B, Fergusson D. Does analysis using "last observation carried forward" introduce bias in dementia research? *CMAJ* 2008;179:751-3.

229 Ware JH. Interpreting incomplete data in studies of diet and weight loss. *N Engl J Med* 2003;348:2136-7.

230 Streiner DL. The case of the missing data: methods of dealing with dropouts and other research vagaries. *Can J Psychiatry* 2002;47:68-75.

231 Lane P. Handling drop-out in longitudinal clinical trials: a comparison of the LOCF and MMRM approaches. *Pharm Stat* 2008;7:93-106.

232 Abraha I, Montedori A, Romagnoli C. Modified intention to treat: frequency, definition and implication for clinical trials [abstract]. Sao Paulo, Brazil: XV Cochrane Colloquium, 2007: 86-7.

233 Altman DG. Confidence intervals in practice. In: Altman DG, Machin D, Bryant TN, Gardner MJ, eds. *Statistics with confidence* . 2nd ed. BMJ Books, 2000:6-14.

234 van Linschoten R, van Middelkoop M, Berger MY, Heintjes EM, Verhaar JA, Willemsen SP, et al. Supervised exercise therapy versus usual care for patellofemoral pain syndrome: an open label randomised controlled trial. *BMJ* 2009;339:b4074.

235 Altman DG. Clinical trials and meta-analyses. In: Altman DG, Machin D, Bryant TN, Gardner MJ, eds. *Statistics with confidence* . 2nd ed. BMJ Books, 2000:120-38.

236 Uniform requirements for manuscripts submitted to biomedical journals. International Committee of Medical Journal Editors. *Ann Intern Med* 1997;126:36-47.

237 Gardner MJ, Altman DG. Confidence intervals rather than P values: estimation rather than hypothesis testing. *BMJ* 1986;292:746-50.

238 Bailar JC, III, Mosteller F. Guidelines for statistical reporting in articles for medical journals. Amplifications and explanations. *Ann Intern Med* 1988;108:266-73.

239 Bland JM. Quoting intermediate analyses can only mislead. *BMJ* 1997;314:1907-8.

240 Cook RJ, Sackett DL. The number needed to treat: a clinically useful measure of treatment effect. *BMJ* 1995;310:452-4.

241 Altman DG, Andersen PK. Calculating the number needed to treat for trials where the outcome is time to an event. *BMJ* 1999;319:1492-5.

242 The OSIRIS Collaborative Group. Early versus delayed neonatal administration of a synthetic surfactant—the judgment of OSIRIS (open study of infants at high risk of or with respiratory insufficiency—the role of surfactant). *Lancet* 1992;340:1363-9.

243 Sorensen L, Gyrd-Hansen D, Kristiansen IS, Nexøe J, Nielsen JB. Laypersons' understanding of relative risk reductions: randomised cross-sectional study. *BMC Med Inform Decis Mak* 2008;8:31.

244 Bobbio M, Demichelis B, Giustetto G. Completeness of reporting trial results: effect on physicians' willingness to prescribe. *Lancet* 1994;343:1209-11.

245 Naylor CD, Chen E, Strauss B. Measured enthusiasm: does the method of reporting trial results alter perceptions of therapeutic effectiveness? *Ann Intern Med* 1992;117:916-21.

246 Tukey JW. Some thoughts on clinical trials, especially problems of multiplicity. *Science* 1977;198:679-84.

247 Yusuf S, Wittes J, Probstfield J, Tyroler HA. Analysis and interpretation of treatment effects in subgroups of patients in randomized clinical trials. *JAMA* 1991;266:93-8.

248 Hahn S, Williamson PR, Hutton JL, Garner P, Flynn EV. Assessing the potential for bias in meta-analysis due to selective reporting of subgroup analyses within studies. *Stat Med* 2000;19:3325-36.

249 Bhandari M, Devereaux PJ, Li P, Mah D, Lim K, Schünemann HJ, et al. Misuse of baseline comparison tests and subgroup analyses in surgical trials. *Clin Orthop Relat Res* 2006;447:247-51.

250 Levin M, Quint PA, Goldstein B, Barton P, Bradley JS, Shemie SD, et al. Recombinant bactericidal/permeability-increasing protein (rBPI21) as adjunctive treatment for children with severe meningococcal sepsis: a randomised trial. rBPI21 Meningococcal Sepsis Study Group. *Lancet* 2000;356:961-7.

251 Scharf O, Colevas AD. Adverse event reporting in publications compared with sponsor database for cancer clinical trials. *J Clin Oncol* 2006;24:3933-8.

252 Pitrou I, Boutron I, Ahmad N, Ravaud P. Reporting of safety results in published reports of randomized controlled trials. *Arch Intern Med* 2009;169:1756-61.

253 Boden WE, O'Rourke RA, Teo KK, Hartigan PM, Maron DJ, Kostuk WJ, et al. Optimal medical therapy with or without PCI for stable coronary disease. *N Engl J Med* 2007;356:1503-16.

254 Horton R. The rhetoric of research. *BMJ* 1995;310:985-7.

255 Annals of Internal Medicine. Information for authors. Available at www.annals.org (accessed 15 Jan 2008).

256 Docherty M, Smith R. The case for structuring the discussion of scientific papers. *BMJ* 1999;318:1224-5.

257 Purcell GP, Donovan SL, Davidoff F. Changes to manuscripts during the editorial process: characterizing the evolution of a clinical paper. *JAMA* 1998;280:227-8.

258 Ioannidis JP. Limitations are not properly acknowledged in the scientific literature. *J Clin Epidemiol* 2007;60:324-9.

259 Kiviluoto T, Sirén J, Luukkonen P, Kivilaakso E. Randomised trial of laparoscopic versus open cholecystectomy for acute and gangrenous cholecystitis. *Lancet* 1998;351:321-5.

260 Hupperets MD, Verhagen EA, van Mechelen W. Effect of unsupervised home based proprioceptive training on recurrences of ankle sprain: randomised controlled trial. *BMJ* 2009;339:b2684.

261 Garber J, Clarke GN, Weersing VR, Beardslee WR, Brent DA, Gladstone TR, et al. Prevention of depression in at-risk adolescents: a randomized controlled trial. *JAMA* 2009;301:2215-24.

262 Campbell D. Factors relevant to the validity of experiments in social settings. *Psychol Bull* 1957;54:297-312.

263 Rothwell PM. Factors that can affect the external validity of randomised controlled trials. *PLoS Clin Trials* 2006;1:e9.

264 King M, Nazareth I, Lampe F, Bower P, Chandler M, Morou M, et al. Conceptual framework and systematic review of the effects of participants' and professionals' preferences in randomised controlled trials. *Health Technol Assess* 2005;9:1-iv.

265 Djulbegovic B, Lacevic M, Cantor A, Fields KK, Bennett CL, Adams JR, et al. The uncertainty principle and industry-sponsored research. *Lancet* 2000;356:635-8.

266 Dans AL, Dans LF, Guyatt GH, Richardson S. Users' guides to the medical literature: XIV. How to decide on the applicability of clinical trial results to your patient. Evidence-Based Medicine Working Group. *JAMA* 1998;279:545-9.

267 Smith GD, Egger M. Who benefits from medical interventions? *BMJ* 1994;308:72-4.

268 McAlister FA. Applying the results of systematic reviews at the bedside. In: Egger M, Davey Smith G, Altman DG, eds. *Systematic reviews in health care: meta-analysis in context* . BMJ Books, 2001.

269 Bartlett C, Doyal L, Ebrahim S, Davey P, Bachmann M, Egger M, et al. The causes and effects of socio-demographic exclusions from clinical trials. *Health Technol Assess* 2005;9:iii-x, 1.

270 Bonell C, Oakley A, Hargreaves J, Strange V, Rees R. Assessment of generalisability in trials of health interventions: suggested framework and systematic review. *BMJ* 2006;333:346-9.

271 Bornhöft G, Maxion-Bergemann S, Wolf U, Kienle GS, Michalsen A, Vollmar HC, et al. Checklist for the qualitative evaluation of clinical studies with particular focus on external validity and model validity. *BMC Med Res Methodol* 2006;6:56.

272 Laupacis A, Sackett DL, Roberts RS. An assessment of clinically useful measures of the consequences of treatment. *N Engl J Med* 1988;318:1728-33.

273 Altman DG. Confidence intervals for the number needed to treat. *BMJ* 1998;317:1309-12.

274 Fanaroff AA, Korones SB, Wright LL, Wright EC, Poland RL, Bauer CB, et al. A controlled trial of intravenous immune globulin to reduce nosocomial infections in very-low-birth-weight infants. National Institute of Child Health and Human Development Neonatal Research Network. *N Engl J Med* 1994;330:1107-13.

275 Randomised trial of intravenous atenolol among 16 027 cases of suspected acute myocardial infarction: ISIS-1. First International Study of Infarct Survival Collaborative Group. *Lancet* 1986;2:57-66.

276 Gøtzsche PC, Gjørup I, Bonnén H, Brahe NE, Becker U, Burcharth F. Somatostatin v placebo in bleeding oesophageal varices: randomised trial and meta-analysis. *BMJ* 1995;310:1495-8.

277 Clarke M, Hopewell S, Chalmers I. Reports of clinical trials should begin and end with up-to-date systematic reviews of other relevant evidence: a status report. *J R Soc Med* 2007;100:187-90.

278 Goodman SN. Toward evidence-based medical statistics. 1: The P value fallacy. *Ann Intern Med* 1999;130:995-1004.

279 Gøtzsche PC. Reference bias in reports of drug trials. *BMJ* 1987;295:654-6.

280 Papp K, Bissonnette R, Rosoph L, Wasel N, Lynde CW, Searles G, et al. Efficacy of ISA247 in plaque psoriasis: a randomised, multicentre, double-blind, placebo-controlled phase III study. *Lancet* 2008;371:1337-42.

281 Dickersin K. How important is publication bias? A synthesis of available data. *AIDS Educ Prev* 1997;9:15-21.

282 Song F, Eastwood AJ, Gilbody S, Duley L, Sutton AJ. Publication and related biases. *Health Technol Assess* 2000;4:1-115.

283 Williamson PR, Gamble C. Identification and impact of outcome selection bias in meta-analysis. *Stat Med* 2005;24:1547-61.

284 Tramèr MR, Reynolds DJ, Moore RA, McQuay HJ. Impact of covert duplicate publication on meta-analysis: a case study. *BMJ* 1997;315:635-40.

285 Simes RJ. Publication bias: the case for an international registry of clinical trials. *J Clin Oncol* 1986;4:1529-41.

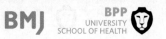

286 Chalmers I. From optimism to disillusion about commitment to transparency in the medico-industrial complex. *J R Soc Med* 2006;99:337-41.

287 Tonks A. A clinical trials register for Europe. *BMJ* 2002;325:1314-5.

288 Dickersin K, Rennie D. Registering clinical trials. *JAMA* 2003;290:516-23.

289 Whittington CJ, Kendall T, Fonagy P, Cottrell D, Cotgrove A, Boddington E. Selective serotonin reuptake inhibitors in childhood depression: systematic review of published versus unpublished data. *Lancet* 2004;363:1341-5.

290 De Angelis CD, Drazen JM, Frizelle FA, Haug C, Hoey J, Horton R, et al. Is this clinical trial fully registered? A statement from the International Committee of Medical Journal Editors. *Lancet* 2005;365:1827-9.

291 Zarin DA, Ide NC, Tse T, Harlan WR, West JC, Lindberg DA. Issues in the registration of clinical trials. *JAMA* 2007;297:2112-20.

292 Hopewell S, Altman DG, Moher D, Schulz KF. Endorsement of the CONSORT Statement by high impact factor medical journals: a survey of journal editors and journal 'instructions to authors'. *Trials* 2008;9:20.

293 Russell JA, Walley KR, Singer J, Gordon AC, Hébert PC, Cooper DJ, et al. Vasopressin versus norepinephrine infusion in patients with septic shock. *N Engl J Med* 2008;358:877-87.

294 Chan AW, Tetzlaff J, Altman D, Gøtzsche PC, Hróbjartsson A, Krleza-Jeric K, et al. The SPIRIT initiative: defining standard protocol items for randomised trials. Oral presentation at the 16th Cochrane Colloquium: Evidence in the era of globalisation; 2008 Oct 3-7; Freiburg, Germany [abstract]. *Zeitschrift fur Evidenz, Fortbildung und Qualitat im Gesundheitswesen* 2008;102:27.

295 Gregson S, Adamson S, Papaya S, Mundondo J, Nyamukapa CA, Mason PR, et al. Impact and process evaluation of integrated community and clinic-based HIV-1 control: a cluster-randomised trial in eastern Zimbabwe. *PLoS Med* 2007;4:e102.

296 Shaddy RE, Boucek MM, Hsu DT, Boucek RJ, Canter CE, Mahony L, et al. Carvedilol for children and adolescents with heart failure: a randomized controlled trial. *JAMA* 2007;298:1171-9.

297 Lexchin J, Bero LA, Djulbegovic B, Clark O. Pharmaceutical industry sponsorship and research outcome and quality: systematic review. *BMJ* 2003;326:1167-70.

298 Kjaergard LL, Als-Nielsen B. Association between competing interests and authors' conclusions: epidemiological study of randomised clinical trials published in the BMJ. *BMJ* 2002;325:249.

299 Bero L, Oostvogel F, Bacchetti P, Lee K. Factors associated with findings of published trials of drug-drug comparisons: why some statins appear more efficacious than others. *PLoS Med* 2007;4:e184.

300 Sismondo S. Pharmaceutical company funding and its consequences: a qualitative systematic review. *Contemp Clin Trials* 2008;29:109-13.

301 Als-Nielsen B, Chen W, Gluud C, Kjaergard LL. Association of funding and conclusions in randomized drug trials: a reflection of treatment effect or adverse events? *JAMA* 2003;290:921-8.

302 Ross JS, Hill KP, Egilman DS, Krumholz HM. Guest authorship and ghostwriting in publications related to rofecoxib: a case study of industry documents from rofecoxib litigation. *JAMA* 2008;299:1800-12.

303 McAlister FA, Straus SE, Sackett DL, Altman DG. Analysis and reporting of factorial trials: a systematic review. *JAMA* 2003;289:2545-53.

304 Senn S. *Crossover trials in clinical research.* 2nd ed. Wiley, 2002.

305 Deeks JJ, Dinnes J, D'Amico R, Sowden AJ, Sakarovitch C, Song F, et al. Evaluating non-randomised intervention studies. *Health Technol Assess* 2003;7:iii-173.

306 Kunz R, Vist G, Oxman AD. Randomisation to protect against selection bias in healthcare trials. *Cochrane Database Syst Rev* 2007;MR000012.

307 Collins R, MacMahon S. Reliable assessment of the effects of treatment on mortality and major morbidity, I: clinical trials. *Lancet* 2001;357:373-80.

308 Schulz KF. Randomised trials, human nature, and reporting guidelines. *Lancet* 1996;348:596-8.

309 Murray GD. Promoting good research practice. *Stat Methods Med Res* 2000;9:17-24.

310 Narahari SR, Ryan TJ, Aggithaya MG, Bose KS, Prasanna KS. Evidence-based approaches for the Ayurvedic traditional herbal formulations: toward an Ayurvedic CONSORT model. *J Altern Complement Med* 2008;14:769-76.

311 Bossuyt PM, Reitsma JB, Bruns DE, Gatsonis CA, Glasziou PP, Irwig LM, et al. Towards complete and accurate reporting of studies of diagnostic accuracy: The STARD Initiative. *Ann Intern Med* 2003;138:40-4.

312 von Elm E, Altman DG, Egger M, Pocock SJ, Gøtzsche PC, Vandenbroucke JP. The Strengthening the Reporting of Observational Studies in Epidemiology (STROBE) statement: guidelines for reporting observational studies. *Ann Intern Med* 2007;147:573-7.

313 Tonino PA, De Bruyne B, Pijls NH, Siebert U, Ikeno F, van't Veer M, et al. Fractional flow reserve versus angiography for guiding percutaneous coronary intervention. *N Engl J Med* 2009;360:213-24.

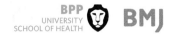

SPIRIT 2013 explanation and elaboration: guidance for protocols of clinical trials

An-Wen Chan, Phelan scientist[1], Jennifer M Tetzlaff, research coordinator[2], Peter C Gøtzsche, professor and director[3], Douglas G Altman, professor and director[4], Howard Mann, programme associate[5], Jesse A Berlin, vice president, epidemiology[6], Kay Dickersin, professor and director[7], Asbjørn Hróbjartsson, senior researcher[3], Kenneth F Schulz, distinguished scientist[8], Wendy R Parulekar, associate professor[9], Karmela Krleža-Jerić, adjunct professor[10], Andreas Laupacis, professor[11], David Moher, senior scientist[2] [10]

[1]Women's College Research Institute at Women's College Hospital, Department of Medicine, University of Toronto, Toronto, Canada, M5G 1N8

[2]Ottawa Methods Centre, Clinical Epidemiology Program, Ottawa Hospital Research Institute, Ottawa, Canada

[3]Nordic Cochrane Centre, Rigshospitalet, Copenhagen, Denmark

[4]Centre for Statistics in Medicine, University of Oxford, Oxford, UK

[5]Division of Medical Ethics and Humanities, University of Utah School of Medicine, Salt Lake City, USA

[6]Janssen Research and Development, Titusville, USA

[7]Center for Clinical Trials, Johns Hopkins Bloomberg School of Public Health, Baltimore, USA

[8]Quantitative Sciences, FHI 360, Research Triangle Park, USA

[9]NCIC Clinical Trials Group, Cancer Research Institute, Queen's University, Kingston, Canada

[10]Department of Epidemiology and Community Medicine, University of Ottawa, Ottawa, Canada

[11]Keenan Research Centre at the Li Ka Shing Knowledge Institute of St Michael's Hospital, Faculty of Medicine, University of Toronto, Toronto, Canada

Correspondence to: A-W Chan
anwen.chan@utoronto.ca

Cite this as: *BMJ* 2013;346:e7586

DOI: 10.1136/bmj.e7586

http://www.bmj.com/content/346/bmj.e7586

ABSTRACT

High quality protocols facilitate proper conduct, reporting, and external review of clinical trials. However, the completeness of trial protocols is often inadequate. To help improve the content and quality of protocols, an international group of stakeholders developed the SPIRIT 2013 Statement (Standard Protocol Items: Recommendations for Interventional Trials). The SPIRIT Statement provides guidance in the form of a checklist of recommended items to include in a clinical trial protocol.

This SPIRIT 2013 Explanation and Elaboration paper provides important information to promote full understanding of the checklist recommendations. For each checklist item, we provide a rationale and detailed description; a model example from an actual protocol; and relevant references supporting its importance. We strongly recommend that this explanatory paper be used in conjunction with the SPIRIT Statement. A website of resources is also available (www.spirit-statement.org).

The SPIRIT 2013 Explanation and Elaboration paper, together with the Statement, should help with the drafting of trial protocols. Complete documentation of key trial elements can facilitate transparency and protocol review for the benefit of all stakeholders.

Every clinical trial should be based on a protocol—a document that details the study rationale, proposed methods, organisation, and ethical considerations.[1] Trial investigators and staff use protocols to document plans for study conduct at all stages from participant recruitment to results dissemination. Funding agencies, research ethics committees/institutional review boards, regulatory agencies, medical journals, systematic reviewers, and other groups rely on protocols to appraise the conduct and reporting of clinical trials.

To meet the needs of these diverse stakeholders, protocols should adequately address key trial elements. However, protocols often lack information on important concepts relating to study design and dissemination plans.[2 3 4 5 6 7 8 9 10 11 12] Guidelines for writing protocols can help improve their completeness, but existing guidelines vary extensively in their content and have limitations, including non-systematic methods of development, limited stakeholder involvement, and lack of citation of empirical evidence to support their recommendations.[13] As a result, there is also variation in the precise definition and scope of a trial protocol, particularly in terms of its relation to other documents such as procedure manuals.[14]

Given the importance of trial protocols, an international group of stakeholders launched the SPIRIT (Standard Protocol Items: Recommendations for Interventional Trials) Initiative in 2007 with the primary aim of improving the content of trial protocols. The main outputs are the SPIRIT 2013 Statement,[14] consisting of a 33 item checklist of minimum recommended protocol items (table 1) plus a diagram (fig1); and this accompanying Explanation and Elaboration (E&E) paper. Additional information and resources are also available on the SPIRIT website (www.spirit-statement.org).The SPIRIT 2013 Statement and E&E paper reflect the collaboration and input of 115 contributors, including trial investigators, healthcare professionals, methodologists, statisticians, trial coordinators, journal editors, as well as representatives from research ethics committees, industry and non-industry funders, and regulatory agencies. Details of the scope and methods have been published elsewhere.[13] [14] [15] Briefly, three complementary methods were specified beforehand, in line with current recommendations for development of reporting guidelines[16]: 1) a Delphi consensus survey[15]; 2) two systematic reviews to identify existing protocol guidelines and empirical evidence supporting the importance of specific checklist items; and 3) two face-to-face consensus meetings to finalise the SPIRIT 2013 checklist. Furthermore, the checklist was pilot tested by graduate course students, and an implementation strategy was developed at a stakeholder meeting.

The SPIRIT recommendations are intended as a guide for those preparing the full protocol for a clinical trial. A clinical trial is a prospective study in which one or more interventions are assigned to human participants in order to assess the effects on health related outcomes. The recommendations are not intended to prescribe how a trial should be designed or conducted. Rather, we call for a transparent and complete description of what is intended, regardless of the characteristics or quality of the plans. The SPIRIT 2013 Statement addresses the minimum content for interventional trials; additional concepts may be important to describe in protocols for trials of specific designs (eg, crossover trials) or in protocols intended for submission to specific groups (eg, funders, research ethics committees/institutional review boards). If information for a recommended item is not yet available when the protocol is being finalised (eg, funding sources), this should be explicitly stated and the protocol updated as new information is obtained. Formatting conventions such as a table of contents, glossary of non-standard or ambiguous terms (eg, randomisation phase or off-protocol), and list of abbreviations and references will facilitate understanding of the protocol.

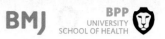

Table 1 SPIRIT 2013 checklist: recommended items to address in a clinical trial protocol and related documents*

Section/item	ItemNo	Description
Administrative information		
Title	1	Descriptive title identifying the study design, population, interventions, and, if applicable, trial acronym
Trial registration	2a	Trial identifier and registry name. If not yet registered, name of intended registry
	2b	All items from the World Health Organization Trial Registration Data Set
Protocol version	3	Date and version identifier
Funding	4	Sources and types of financial, material, and other support
Roles and responsibilities	5a	Names, affiliations, and roles of protocol contributors
	5b	Name and contact information for the trial sponsor
	5c	Role of study sponsor and funders, if any, in study design; collection, management, analysis, and interpretation of data; writing of the report; and the decision to submit the report for publication, including whether they will have ultimate authority over any of these activities
	5d	Composition, roles, and responsibilities of the coordinating centre, steering committee, endpoint adjudication committee, data management team, and other individuals or groups overseeing the trial, if applicable (see Item 21a for data monitoring committee)
Introduction		
Background and rationale	6a	Description of research question and justification for undertaking the trial, including summary of relevant studies (published and unpublished) examining benefits and harms for each intervention
	6b	Explanation for choice of comparators
Objectives	7	Specific objectives or hypotheses
Trial design	8	Description of trial design including type of trial (eg, parallel group, crossover, factorial, single group), allocation ratio, and framework (eg, superiority, equivalence, noninferiority, exploratory)
Methods: Participants, interventions, and outcomes		
Study setting	9	Description of study settings (eg, community clinic, academic hospital) and list of countries where data will be collected. Reference to where list of study sites can be obtained
Eligibility criteria	10	Inclusion and exclusion criteria for participants. If applicable, eligibility criteria for study centres and individuals who will perform the interventions (eg, surgeons, psychotherapists)
Interventions	11a	Interventions for each group with sufficient detail to allow replication, including how and when they will be administered
	11b	Criteria for discontinuing or modifying allocated interventions for a given trial participant (eg, drug dose change in response to harms, participant request, or improving/worsening disease)
	11c	Strategies to improve adherence to intervention protocols, and any procedures for monitoring adherence (eg, drug tablet return, laboratory tests)
	11d	Relevant concomitant care and interventions that are permitted or prohibited during the trial
Outcomes	12	Primary, secondary, and other outcomes, including the specific measurement variable (eg, systolic blood pressure), analysis metric (eg, change from baseline, final value, time to event), method of aggregation (eg, median, proportion), and time point for each outcome. Explanation of the clinical relevance of chosen efficacy and harm outcomes is strongly recommended
Participant timeline	13	Time schedule of enrolment, interventions (including any run-ins and washouts), assessments, and visits for participants. A schematic diagram is highly recommended (see fig 1)
Sample size	14	Estimated number of participants needed to achieve study objectives and how it was determined, including clinical and statistical assumptions supporting any sample size calculations
Recruitment	15	Strategies for achieving adequate participant enrolment to reach target sample size
Methods: Assignment of interventions (for controlled trials)		
Allocation:		
Sequence generation	16a	Method of generating the allocation sequence (eg, computer-generated random numbers) and list of any factors for stratification. To reduce predictability of a random sequence, details of any planned restriction (eg, blocking) should be provided in a separate document that is unavailable to those who enrol participants or assign interventions
Allocation concealment mechanism	16b	Mechanism of implementing the allocation sequence (eg, central telephone; sequentially numbered, opaque, sealed envelopes), describing any steps to conceal the sequence until interventions are assigned
Implementation	16c	Who will generate the allocation sequence, who will enrol participants, and who will assign participants to interventions
Blinding (masking)	17a	Who will be blinded after assignment to interventions (eg, trial participants, care providers, outcome assessors, data analysts) and how
	17b	If blinded, circumstances under which unblinding is permissible and procedure for revealing a participant's allocated intervention during the trial
Methods: Data collection, management, and analysis		
Data collection methods	18a	Plans for assessment and collection of outcome, baseline, and other trial data, including any related processes to promote data quality (eg, duplicate measurements, training of assessors) and a description of study instruments (eg, questionnaires, laboratory tests) along with their reliability and validity, if known. Reference to where data collection forms can be found, if not in the protocol
	18b	Plans to promote participant retention and complete follow-up, including list of any outcome data to be collected for participants who discontinue or deviate from intervention protocols
Data management	19	Plans for data entry, coding, security, and storage, including any related processes to promote data quality (eg, double data entry; range checks for data values). Reference to where details of data management procedures can be found, if not in the protocol
Statistical methods	20a	Statistical methods for analysing primary and secondary outcomes. Reference to where other details of the statistical analysis plan can be found, if not in the protocol
	20b	Methods for any additional analyses (eg, subgroup and adjusted analyses)
	20c	Definition of analysis population relating to protocol non-adherence (eg, as randomised analysis), and any statistical methods to handle missing data (eg, multiple imputation)
Methods: Monitoring		
Data monitoring	21a	Composition of data monitoring committee (DMC); summary of its role and reporting structure; statement of whether it is independent from the sponsor and competing interests; and reference to where further details about its charter can be found, if not in the protocol. Alternatively, an explanation of why a DMC is not needed

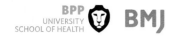

Section/item	ItemNo	Description
	21b	Description of any interim analyses and stopping guidelines, including who will have access to these interim results and make the final decision to terminate the trial
Harms	22	Plans for collecting, assessing, reporting, and managing solicited and spontaneously reported adverse events and other unintended effects of trial interventions or trial conduct
Auditing	23	Frequency and procedures for auditing trial conduct, if any, and whether the process will be independent from investigators and the sponsor
Ethics and dissemination		
Research ethics approval	24	Plans for seeking research ethics committee/institutional review board (REC/IRB) approval
Protocol amendments	25	Plans for communicating important protocol modifications (eg, changes to eligibility criteria, outcomes, analyses) to relevant parties (eg, investigators, REC/IRBs, trial participants, trial registries, journals, regulators)
Consent or assent	26a	Who will obtain informed consent or assent from potential trial participants or authorised surrogates, and how (see Item 32)
	26b	Additional consent provisions for collection and use of participant data and biological specimens in ancillary studies, if applicable
Confidentiality	27	How personal information about potential and enrolled participants will be collected, shared, and maintained in order to protect confidentiality before, during, and after the trial
Declaration of interests	28	Financial and other competing interests for principal investigators for the overall trial and each study site
Access to data	29	Statement of who will have access to the final trial dataset, and disclosure of contractual agreements that limit such access for investigators
Ancillary and post-trial care	30	Provisions, if any, for ancillary and post-trial care and for compensation to those who suffer harm from trial participation
Dissemination policy	31a	Plans for investigators and sponsor to communicate trial results to participants, healthcare professionals, the public, and other relevant groups (eg, via publication, reporting in results databases, or other data sharing arrangements), including any publication restrictions
	31b	Authorship eligibility guidelines and any intended use of professional writers
	31c	Plans, if any, for granting public access to the full protocol, participant-level dataset, and statistical code
Appendices		
Informed consent materials	32	Model consent form and other related documentation given to participants and authorised surrogates
Biological specimens	33	Plans for collection, laboratory evaluation, and storage of biological specimens for genetic or molecular analysis in the current trial and for future use in ancillary studies, if applicable

Amendments to the protocol should be tracked and dated. The SPIRIT checklist is copyrighted by the SPIRIT Group and is reproduced with permission.

	STUDY PERIOD							
	Enrolment	Allocation	Post-allocation					Close-out
TIMEPOINT*	$-t_1$	0	t_1	t_2	t_3	t_4	etc	t_x
ENROLMENT:								
Eligibility screen	X							
Informed consent	X							
(List other procedures)	X							
Allocation		X						
INTERVENTIONS:								
(Intervention A)			●———————●					
(Intervention B)			X		X			
(List other study groups)			●————————————●					
ASSESSMENTS:								
(List baseline variables)	X	X						
(List outcome variables)				X		X	etc	X
(List other data variables)			X	X	X	X	etc	X

* List specific timepoints in this row

Fig 1 Example template for the schedule of enrolment, interventions, and assessments (recommended content can be displayed using other schematic formats)

Purpose and development of explanation and elaboration paper

Modelled after other reporting guidelines,[17] [18] this E&E paper presents each checklist item with at least one model example from an actual protocol, followed by a full explanation of the rationale and main issues to address. This E&E paper provides important information to facilitate full understanding of each checklist item, and is intended to be used in conjunction with the SPIRIT 2013 Statement.[14] These complementary tools serve to inform trial investigators about important issues to consider in the protocol as they relate to trial design, conduct, reporting, and organisation.

To identify examples for each checklist item, we obtained protocols from public websites, journals, trial investigators, and industry sponsors. Model examples were selected to reflect how key elements could be appropriately described in a trial protocol. Some examples illustrate a specific component of a checklist item, while others encompass all key recommendations for an item. Additional examples are also available on the SPIRIT website (www.spirit-statement.org). The availability of examples for all checklist items indicates the feasibility of addressing each recommended item in the main protocol rather than in separate documents.

Examples are quoted verbatim from the trial protocol. Proper names of trial personnel have been abbreviated with italicised initials, and any reference numbers cited in the original quoted text are denoted by [*Reference*] to distinguish them from references cited in this E&E paper.

For each checklist item we also strived to provide references to empirical data supporting its relevance, which we identified through a systematic review conducted to inform the content of the SPIRIT checklist. We searched MEDLINE, the Cochrane Methodology Register, and the Cochrane Database of Systematic Reviews (limited to reviews) up to September 2009, and EMBASE up to August 2007. We searched reference lists, PubMed "related articles," and citation searches using SCOPUS to identify additional relevant studies. We used piloted forms to screen and extract data relevant to specific checklist items.

Studies were included if they provided empirical data to support or refute the importance of a given protocol concept. A summary of the relevant methodological articles was provided to each E&E author for use in preparing the initial draft text for up to six checklist items; each draft was also reviewed and revised by a second author. When citing empirical evidence in the E&E, we aimed to reference a systematic review when available. When no review was identified, we either cited all relevant individual studies, or if too numerous, a representative sample of the literature. Some items had little or no identified empirical evidence (eg, title) but their inclusion in the checklist is supported by a strong pragmatic or ethical rationale. Where relevant, we also provide references to non-empirical publications for further reading.

Two lead authors (AWC, JMT) collated and refined the content and format for all items, and then circulated three iterations of an overall draft to the coauthors for editing and final approval.

SPIRIT 2013 Explanation and Elaboration

Section 1: Administrative information

Item 1: Descriptive title identifying the study design, population, interventions, and, if applicable, trial acronym

> **EXAMPLE**
> "A multi-center, investigator-blinded, randomized, 12-month, parallel-group, non-inferiority study to compare the efficacy of 1.6 to 2.4 g Asacol® Therapy QD [once daily] versus divided dose (BID [twice daily]) in the maintenance of remission of ulcerative colitis."[19]

Explanation
The title provides an important means of trial identification. A succinct description that conveys the topic (study population, interventions), acronym (if any), and basic study design—including the method of intervention allocation (eg, parallel group randomised trial; single-group trial)—will facilitate retrieval from literature or internet searches and rapid judgment of relevance.[20] It can also be helpful to include the trial framework (eg, superiority, non-inferiority), study objective or primary outcome, and if relevant, the study phase (eg, phase II).

Trial registration—registry
Item 2a: Trial identifier and registry name. If not yet registered, name of intended registry

> **EXAMPLE**
> "EudraCT: 2010-019180-10
> ClinicalTrials.gov: NCT01066572
> ISRCTN: 54540667."[21]

Explanation
There are compelling ethical and scientific reasons for trial registration.[22] [23] [24] Documentation of a trial's existence on a publicly accessible registry can help to increase transparency,[24][25] decrease unnecessary duplication of research effort, facilitate identification of ongoing trials for prospective participants, and identify selective reporting of study results.[26] [27] [28] As mandated by the International Committee of Medical Journal Editors (ICMJE) and jurisdictional legislation,[29] [30] [31] registration of clinical trials should occur before recruitment of the first trial participant.

We recommend that registry names and trial identifiers assigned by the registries be prominently placed in the protocol, such as on the cover page. If the trial is not yet registered, the intended registry should be indicated and the protocol updated upon registration. When registration in multiple registries is required (eg, to meet local regulation),

each identifier should be clearly listed in the protocol and each registry.

Trial registration—data set

Item 2b: All items from the World Health Organization Trial Registration Data Set
Explanation

> **EXAMPLE**
> Table 2 Example of trial registration data

In addition to a trial registration number, the World Health Organization (WHO) recommends a minimum standard list of items to be included in a trial registry in order for a trial to be considered fully registered (www.who.int/ictrp/network/trds/en/index.html). These standards are supported by ICMJE, other journal editors, and jurisdictional legislation.[29] [30] [31] We recommend that the WHO Trial Registration Data Set be included in the protocol to serve as a brief structured summary of the trial. Its inclusion in the protocol can also signal updates for the registry when associated protocol sections are amended—thereby promoting consistency between information in the protocol and registry.

Protocol version

Item 3: Date and version identifier

> **EXAMPLE**
> - "Issue date: 25 Jul 2005
> - Protocol amendment number: 05
> - Authors: *MD, JH*
>
> **Revision chronology:**
> - UM . . . 00, 2004-Jan-30 Original
> - UM . . . 01, 2004-Feb-7 Amendment 01.:
> - Primary reason for amendment: changes in Section 7.1 regarding composition of comparator placebo
> - Additional changes (these changes in and of themselves would not justify a protocol amendment): correction of typographical error in Section 3.3 . . .
> - UM . . . 05, 2005-Jul-25 Amendment No.5:
> - At the request of US FDA statements were added to the protocol to better clarify and define the algorithm for determining clinical or microbiological failures prior to the follow-up visit."[33]

Explanation
Sequentially labelling and dating each protocol version helps to mitigate potential confusion over which document is the most recent. Explicitly listing the changes made relative to the previous protocol version is also important (see Item 25). Transparent tracking of versions and amendments facilitates trial conduct, review, and oversight.

Funding

Item 4: Sources and types of financial, material, and other support

> **EXAMPLE**
> "Tranexamic acid will be manufactured by Pharmacia (Pfizer, Sandwich, UK) and placebo by South Devon Healthcare NHS Trust, UK. The treatment packs will be prepared by an independent clinical trial supply company (Brecon Pharmaceuticals Limited, Hereford, UK) . . .

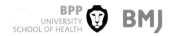

Table 2 Example of trial registration data

Data category	Information[33]
Primary registry and trial identifying number	ClinicalTrials.govNCT01143272
Date of registration in primary registry	11 June, 2010
Secondary identifying numbers	BNI-2009-01, 2009-017374-20, ISRCTN01005546, DRKS00000084
Source(s) of monetary or material support	Bernhard Nocht Institute for Tropical Medicine
Primary sponsor	Bernhard Nocht Institute for Tropical Medicine
Secondary sponsor(s)	German Federal Ministry of Education and Research
Contact for public queries	SE, MD, MPH [email address]
Contact for scientific queries	SE, MD, MPHBernhard Nocht Institute for Tropical Medicine, Hamburg, Germany
Public title	Probiotic*Saccharomyces boulardii* for the prevention of antibiotic associated diarrhoea (SacBo)
Scientific title	*S boulardii* for the prevention of antibiotic associated diarrhoea—randomised, double blind, placebo controlled trial
Countries of recruitment	Germany
Health condition(s) or problem(s) studied	Antibiotic treatment, *Clostridium difficile*,diarrhoea
Intervention(s)	Active comparator: *S boulardii* (500 mg *S boulardii* per day)
	Placebo comparator: microcristallin cellulose (matching capsules containing no active ingredients)
Key inclusion and exclusion criteria	Ages eligible for study: ≥18 years Sexes eligible for study: bothAccepts healthy volunteers: no
	Inclusion criteria: adult patient (≥18 years), patient hospitalised
	Exclusion criteria: allergy against yeast and/or Perenterol forte and/or placebos containing *S cerevisiae* HANSEN CBS 5926, lactose monohydrate, magnesium stearate, gelatine, sodium dodecyl sulfate, titan dioxide, microcrystalline cellulose
Study type	Interventional
	Allocation: randomized intervention model. Parallel assignment masking: double blind (subject, caregiver, investigator, outcomes assessor)
	Primary purpose: prevention
	Phase III
Date of first enrolment	June 2010
Target sample size	1520
Recruitment status	Recruiting
Primary outcome(s)	Cumulative incidence of any antibiotic associated diarrhoea (time frame: 2 years; not designated as safety issue)
Key secondary outcomes	Cumulative incidence of *C difficile* associated diarrhoea (time frame: 2 years; not designated as safety issue)

LSHTM [London School of Hygiene and Tropical Medicine] is funding the run-in costs for the WOMAN trial and up to 2,000 patients' recruitment. The main phase is funded by the UK Department of Health and the Wellcome Trust. Funding for this trial covers meetings and central organisational costs only. Pfizer, the manufacturer of tranexamic acid, have provided the funding for the trial drug and placebo used for this trial. An educational grant, equipment and consumables for ROTEM [thromboelastometry procedure] analysis has been provided by Tem Innovations GmbH, M.-Kollar-Str. 13-15, 81829 Munich, Germany for use in the WOMAN-ETAC study. An application for funding to support local organisational costs has been made to University of Ibadan Senate Research Grant. The design, management, analysis and reporting of the study are entirely independent of the manufacturers of tranexamic acid and Tem Innovations GmbH."[34]

Explanation

A description of the sources of financial and non-financial support provides relevant information to assess study feasibility and potential competing interests (Item 28). Although both industry funded and non-industry funded trials are susceptible to bias,[4] [35] the former are more likely to report trial results and conclusions that favour their own interventions.[27] [36] [37] [38] [39] This tendency could be due to industry trials being more likely to select effective interventions for evaluation (Item 6a), to use less effective control interventions (Item 6b), or to selectively report outcomes (Item 12), analyses (Item 20) or full studies (Item 31).[38] [40] [41] [42] [43] Non-financial support (eg, provision of drugs) from industry has not been shown to be associated with biased results, although few studies have examined this issue.[44] [45]

At a minimum, the protocol should identify the sources of financial and non-financial support; the specific type

(eg, funds, equipment, drugs, services) and time period of support; and any vested interest that the funder may have in the trial. If a trial is not yet funded when the protocol is first written, the proposed sources of support should be listed and updated as funders are confirmed.

No clear consensus exists regarding the level of additional funding details that should be provided in the trial protocol as opposed to trial contracts, although full disclosure of funding information in the protocol can help to better identify financial competing interests. Some jurisdictional guidelines require more detailed disclosure, including monetary amounts granted from each funder, the mechanism of providing financial support (eg, paid in fixed sum or per recruited participant), and the specific fund recipient (eg, trial investigator, department/institute).[46] Detailed disclosure allows research ethics committees/institutional review boards (REC/IRBs) to assess whether the reimbursement amount is reasonable in relation to the time and expenses incurred for trial conduct.

Roles and responsibilities—contributorship

Item 5a: Names, affiliations, and roles of protocol contributors

> **EXAMPLE**
>
> "*RTL* [address], *EJM* [address],*AK* [address] . . .
>
> **Authors' contributions**
>
> *RTL* conceived of the study.*AK, EN,SB, PR, WJ,JH,* and *MC* initiated the study design and *JK* and *LG* helped with implementation. *RTL, JK,LG,* and *FP* are grant holders.*LT* and *EM* provided statistical expertise in clinical trial design and *RN* is conducting the primary statistical analysis. All authors contributed to refinement of the study protocol and approved the final manuscript."[47]

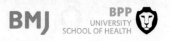

Explanation

Individuals who contribute substantively to protocol development and drafting should have their contributions reported. As with authorship of journal articles,[48] listing the protocol contributors, their affiliations, and their roles in the protocol development process provides due recognition, accountability, and transparency. Naming of contributors can also help to identify competing interests and reduce ghost authorship (Items 28 and 31b).[9] [10] If professional medical writers are employed to draft the protocol, then this should be acknowledged as well.

Naming of authors and statements of contributorship are standard for protocols published in journals such as *Trials*[49] but are uncommon for unpublished protocols. Only five of 44 industry-initiated protocols approved in 1994-95 by a Danish research ethics committee explicitly identified the protocol authors.[9]

Roles and responsibilities—sponsor contact information

Item 5b: Name and contact information for the trial sponsor

> **EXAMPLE**
>
> - "Trial Sponsor: University of Nottingham
> - Sponsor's Reference: RIS 8024 . . .
> - Contact name: Mr *PC*
> - Address: King's Meadow Campus . . .
> - Telephone: . . .
> - Email: . . ."[50]

Explanation

The sponsor can be defined as the individual, company, institution, or organisation assuming overall responsibility for the initiation and management of the trial, and is not necessarily the main funder.[51] [52] In general, the company is the sponsor in industry initiated trials, while the funding agency or institution of the principal investigator is often the sponsor for investigator initiated trials. For some investigator initiated trials, the principal investigator can be considered to be a "sponsor-investigator" who assumes both sponsor and investigator roles.[51] [53]

Identification of the trial sponsor provides transparency and accountability. The protocol should identify the name, contact information, and if applicable, the regulatory agency identifying number of the sponsor.

Roles and responsibilities—sponsor and funder

Item 5c: Role of study sponsor and funders, if any, in study design; collection, management, analysis, and interpretation of data; writing of the report; and the decision to submit the report for publication, including whether they will have ultimate authority over any of these activities

> **EXAMPLE**
>
> "This funding source had no role in the design of this study and will not have any role during its execution, analyses, interpretation of the data, or decision to submit results."[54]

Explanation

There is potential for bias when the trial sponsor or funder (sometimes the same entity) has competing interests (Item 28) and substantial influence on the planning, conduct, or reporting of a trial. Empirical research indicates that specific forms of bias tend to be more prevalent in trials funded by industry compared to those funded by non-commercial sources.[36 37 38 45 55 56 57 58 59 60] The design, analysis, interpretation, and reporting of most industry-initiated

trials are controlled by the sponsor; this authority is often enforced by contractual agreements signed between the sponsor and trial investigators (Item 29).[10 61]

The protocol should explicitly outline the roles and responsibilities of the sponsor and any funders in study design, conduct, data analysis and interpretation, manuscript writing, and dissemination of results. It is also important to state whether the sponsor or funder controls the final decision regarding any of these aspects of the trial.

Despite the importance of declaring the roles of the trial sponsor and funders, few protocols explicitly do so. Among 44 protocols for industry-initiated trials receiving ethics approval in Denmark from 1994-95, none stated explicitly who had contributed to the design of the trial.[9]

Roles and responsibilities—committees

Item 5d: Composition, roles, and responsibilities of the coordinating centre, steering committee, endpoint adjudication committee, data management team, and other individuals or groups overseeing the trial, if applicable (see Item 21a for data monitoring committee)

> **EXAMPLE**
>
> **"Principal investigator and research physician**
> - Design and conduct of RITUXVAS
> - Preparation of protocol and revisions
> - Preparation of investigators brochure (IB) and CRFs [case report forms]
> - Organising steering committee meetings
> - Managing CTO [clinical trials office]
> - Publication of study reports
> - Members of TMC [Trial Management Committee]
>
> **Steering committee (SC)**
> - (see title page for members)
> - Agreement of final protocol
> - All lead investigators will be steering committee members. One lead investigator per country will be nominated as national coordinator.
> - Recruitment of patients and liaising with principle [sic] investigator
> - Reviewing progress of study and if necessary agreeing changes to the protocol and/or investigators brochure to facilitate the smooth running of the study.
>
> **Trial management committee (TMC)**
> - (Principle [sic] investigator, research physician, administrator)
> - Study planning
> - Organisation of steering committee meetings
> - Provide annual risk report MHRA [Medicines and Healthcare Products Regulatory Agency] and ethics committee
> - SUSAR [Serious unexpected suspected adverse events] reporting to MHRA and Roche
> - Responsible for trial master file
> - Budget administration and contractual issues with individual centres
> - Advice for lead investigators
> - Audit of 6 monthly feedback forms and decide when site visit to occur.
> - Assistance with international review, board/independent ethics committee applications
> - Data verification
> - Randomisation
> - Organisation of central serum sample collection

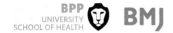

Data manager
- Maintenance of trial IT system and data entry
- Data verification

Lead investigators
In each participating centre a lead investigator (senior nephrologist/rheumatologist/ immunologist) will be identified, to be responsible for identification, recruitment, data collection and completion of CRFs, along with follow up of study patients and adherence to study protocol and investigators brochure. . . . Lead investigators will be steering committee members, with one investigator per country being nominated as national coordinator."[62]

Explanation

The protocol should outline the general membership of the various committees or groups involved in trial coordination and conduct; describe the roles and responsibilities of each; and (when known) identify the chairs and members. This information helps to ensure that roles and responsibilities are clearly understood at the trial onset, and facilitates communication from external parties regarding the trial. It also enables readers to understand the mandate and expertise of those responsible for overseeing participant safety, study design, database integrity, and study conduct. For example, empirical evidence supports the pivotal role of an epidemiologist or biostatistician in designing and conducting higher quality trials.[63] [64]

Section 2: Introduction

Background and rationale

Item 6a: Description of research question and justification for undertaking the trial, including summary of relevant studies (published and unpublished) examining benefits and harms for each intervention

---

EXAMPLE

"Background

Introduction: For people at ages 5 to 45 years, trauma is second only to HIV/AIDS as a cause of death. . . .
Mechanisms: The haemostatic system helps to maintain the integrity of the circulatory system after severe vascular injury, whether traumatic or surgical in origin.[reference] Major surgery and trauma trigger similar haemostatic responses . . . Antifibrinolytic agents have been shown to reduce blood loss in patients with both normal and exaggerated fibrinolytic responses to surgery, and do so without apparently increasing the risk of post-operative complications, . . .
Existing knowledge: Systemic antifibrinolytic agents are widely used in major surgery to prevent fibrinolysis and thus reduce surgical blood loss. A recent systematic review [reference] of randomised controlled trials of antifibrinolytic agents (mainly aprotinin or tranexamic acid) in elective surgical patients identified 89 trials including 8,580 randomised patients (74 trials in cardiac, eight in orthopaedic, four in liver, and three in vascular surgery). The results showed that these treatments reduced the numbers needing transfusion by one third, reduced the volume needed per transfusion by one unit, and halved the need for further surgery to control bleeding. These differences were all highly statistically significant. There was also a statistically non-significant reduction in the risk of death (RR=0.85; 95% CI 0.63 to 1.14) in the antifibrinolytic treated group.

. . .

Need for a trial: A simple and widely practicable treatment that reduces blood loss following trauma might prevent thousands of premature trauma deaths each year and secondly could

---

reduce exposure to the risks of blood transfusion. Blood is a scarce and expensive resource and major concerns remain about the risk of transfusion-transmitted infection. . . . A large randomised trial is therefore needed of the use of a simple, inexpensive, widely practicable antifibrinolytic treatment such as tranexamic acid . . . in a wide range of trauma patients who, when they reach hospital are thought to be at risk of major haemorrhage that could significantly affect their chances of survival.

Dose selection
The systematic review of randomised controlled trials of antifibrinolytic agents in surgery showed that dose regimens of tranexamic acid vary widely.[reference] . . .
In this emergency situation, administration of a fixed dose would be more practicable as determining the weight of a patient would be impossible. Therefore a fixed dose within the dose range which has been shown to inhibit fibrinolysis and provide haemostatic benefit is being used for this trial. . . . The planned duration of administration allows for the full effect of tranexamic acid on the immediate risk of haemorrhage without extending too far into the acute phase response seen after surgery and trauma."[65]

Explanation

The value of a research question, as well as the ethical and scientific justification for a trial, depend to a large degree on the uncertainty of the comparative benefits or harms of the interventions, which depends in turn on the existing body of knowledge on the topic. The background section of a protocol should summarise the importance of the research question, justify the need for the trial in the context of available evidence, and present any available data regarding the potential effects of the interventions (efficacy and harms).[66] [67] This information is particularly important to the trial participants and personnel, as it provides motivation for contributing to the trial.[68] [69] It is also relevant to funders, REC/IRBs, and other stakeholders who evaluate the scientific and ethical basis for trial conduct.

To place the trial in the context of available evidence, it is strongly recommended that an up-to-date systematic review of relevant studies be summarised and cited in the protocol.[70] Several funders request this information in grant applications.[71] [72] Failure to review the cumulated evidence can lead to unnecessary duplication of research or to trial participants being deprived of effective, or exposed to harmful, interventions.[73] [74] [75] [76] A minority of published trial reports cite a systematic review of pre-existing evidence,[77] [78] and in one survey only half of trial investigators were aware of a relevant existing review when they had designed their trial.[79] Given that about half of trials remain unpublished,[80] [81] [82] and that published trials often represent a biased subset of all trials,[80] [83] it is important that systematic reviews include a search of online resources such as trial registries, results databases, and regulatory agency websites.[84]

Background and rationale—choice of comparators
Item 6b: Explanation for choice of comparators

EXAMPLE

"Choice of comparator
In spite of the increasing numbers of resistant strains, chloroquine monotherapy is still recommended as standard blood-stage therapy for patients with P [Plasmodium]vivax malaria in the countries in which this trial will be conducted. Its selection as comparator is therefore justified. The adult dose of chloroquine will be 620 mg for 2 days followed by 310

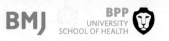

mg on the third day and for children 10 mg/kg for the first two days and 5 mg/kg for the third day. Total dose is in accordance with the current practice in the countries where the study is conducted. The safety profile of chloroquine is well established and known. Although generally well tolerated, the following side-effects of chloroquine treatment have been described:

Gastro-intestinal disturbances, headache, hypotension, convulsions, visual disturbances, depigmentation or loss of hair, skin reactions (rashes, pruritus) and, rarely, bone-marrow suppression and hypersensitivity reactions such as urticaria and angioedema. Their occurrence during the present trial may however be unlikely given the short (3-day) duration of treatment."[85]

Explanation

The choice of control interventions has important implications for trial ethics, recruitment, results, and interpretation. In trials comparing an intervention to an active control or usual care, a clear description of the rationale for the comparator intervention will facilitate understanding of its appropriateness.[86] [87] For example, a trial in which the control group receives an inappropriately low dose of an active drug will overestimate the relative efficacy of the study intervention in clinical practice; conversely, an inappropriately high dose in the control group will lead to an underestimate of the relative harms of the study intervention.[87] [88]

The appropriateness of using placebo-only control groups has been the subject of extensive debate and merits careful consideration of the existence of other effective treatments, the potential risks to trial participants, and the need for assay sensitivity—that is, ability to distinguish an effective intervention from less effective or ineffective interventions.[89] [90] In addition, surveys have demonstrated that a potential barrier to trial participation is the possibility of being allocated a placebo-only or active control intervention that is perceived to be less desirable than the study intervention.[68] [69] [91] [92] Evidence also suggests that enrolled participants perceive the effect of a given intervention differently depending on whether the control group consists of an active comparator or only placebo.[93] [94] [95] [96]

Finally, studies suggest that some "active" comparators in head-to-head randomised trials are presumed by trial investigators to be effective despite having never previously been shown to be superior to placebo.[74] [97] In a systematic review of over 100 head-to-head antibiotic trials for mild to moderate chronic obstructive pulmonary disease,[74] cumulative meta-analysis of preceding placebo controlled trials did not show a significant effect of antibiotics over placebo. Such studies again highlight the importance of providing a thorough background and rationale for a trial and the choice of comparators—including data from an up-to-date systematic review—to enable potential participants, physicians, REC/IRBs, and funders to discern the merit of the trial.

Objectives

Item 7: Specific objectives or hypotheses

EXAMPLE

"1.1 Research hypothesis
Apixaban is noninferior to warfarin for prevention of stroke (hemorrhagic, ischemic or of unspecified type) or systemic

---

embolism in subjects with atrial fibrillation (AF) and additional risk factor(s) for stroke.
. . .

2 STUDY OBJECTIVES

2.1 Primary objective
To determine if apixaban is noninferior to warfarin (INR [international normalized ratio] target range 2.0-3.0) in the combined endpoint of stroke (hemorrhagic, ischemic or of unspecified type) and systemic embolism, in subjects with AF and at least one additional risk factor for stroke.

2.2 Secondary objectives

2.2.1 Key secondary objectives
The key secondary objectives are to determine, in subjects with AF and at least one additional risk factor for stroke, if apixaban is superior to warfarin (INR target range 2.0 - 3.0) for,

- the combined endpoint of stroke (hemorrhagic, ischemic or of unspecified type) and systemic embolism
- major bleeding [International Society of Thrombosis and Hemostasis]
- all-cause death

2.2.2 Other secondary objectives
- To compare, in subjects with AF and at least one additional risk factor for stroke, apixaban and warfarin with respect to:
- The composite endpoint of stroke (ischemic, hemorrhagic, or of unspecified type), systemic embolism and major bleeding, in warfarin naive subjects
- To assess the safety of apixaban in subjects with AF and at least one additional risk factor for stroke."[v]

Explanation

The study objectives reflect the scientific questions to be answered by the trial, and define its purpose and scope. They are closely tied to the trial design (Item 8) and analysis methods (Item 20). For example, the sample size calculation and statistical analyses for superiority trials will differ from those investigating non-inferiority.

The objectives are generally phrased using neutral wording (eg, "to compare the effect of treatment A versus treatment B on outcome X") rather than in terms of a particular direction of effect.[99] A hypothesis states the predicted effect of the interventions on the trial outcomes. For multiarm trials, the objectives should clarify the way in which all the treatment groups will be compared (eg, A versus B; A versus C).

Trial design

Item 8: Description of trial design including type of trial (eg, parallel group, crossover, factorial, single group), allocation ratio, and framework (eg, superiority, equivalence, non-inferiority, exploratory)

EXAMPLE

"The PROUD trial is designed as a randomised, controlled, observer, surgeon and patient blinded multicenter superiority trial with two parallel groups and a primary endpoint of wound infection during 30 days after surgery . . . randomization will be performed as block randomization with a 1:1 allocation."[100]

Explanation

The most common design for published randomised trials is the parallel group, two arm, superiority trial with 1:1 allocation ratio.[101] Other trial types include crossover, cluster, factorial, split body, and n of 1 randomised trials, as well as single group trials and non-randomised comparative trials.

For trials with more than one study group, the allocation ratio reflects the intended relative number of participants in each group (eg, 1:1 or 2:1). Unequal allocation ratios are used for a variety of reasons, including potential cost savings, allowance for learning curves, and ethical considerations when the balance of existing evidence appears to be in favour of one intervention over the other.[102] Evidence also suggests a preference of some participants for enrolling in trials with an allocation ratio that favours allocation to an active treatment.[92]

The framework of a trial refers to its overall objective to test the superiority, non-inferiority, or equivalence of one intervention with another, or in the case of exploratory pilot trials, to gather preliminary information on the intervention (eg, harms, pharmacokinetics) and the feasibility of conducting a full-scale trial.

It is important to specify and explain the choice of study design because of its close relation to the trial objectives (Item 7) and its influence on the study methods, conduct, costs,[103] results,[104] [105] [106] and interpretation. For example, factorial and non-inferiority trials can involve more complex methods, analyses, and interpretations than parallel group superiority trials.[107] [108] In addition, the interpretation of trial results in published reports is not always consistent with the pre-specified trial framework,[6] [109] [110] especially among reports claiming post hoc equivalence based on a failure to demonstrate superiority rather than a specific test of equivalence.[109]

There is increasing interest in adaptive designs for clinical trials, defined as the use of accumulating data to decide how to modify aspects of a study as it continues, without undermining the validity and integrity of the trial.[111] [112] Examples of potential adaptations include stopping the trial early, modifying the allocation ratio, re-estimating the sample size, and changing the eligibility criteria. The most valid adaptive designs are those in which the opportunity to make adaptations is based on prespecified decision rules that are fully documented in the protocol (Item 21b).

Section 3a: Methods—participants, interventions, and outcomes

Study setting

Item 9: Description of study settings (eg, community clinic, academic hospital) and list of countries where data will be collected. Reference to where list of study sites can be obtained

---

EXAMPLE

"Selection of countries
. . . To detect an intervention-related difference in HIV incidences with the desired power, the baseline incidences at the sites must be sufficiently high. We chose the participating sites so that the average baseline annual incidence across all communities in the study is likely to reach at least 3%. The various sites in sub-Saharan Africa met this criterion, but we also wanted sites in Asia to extend the generalizability of the intervention. The only location in Asia with sufficient incidence at the community level is in ethnic minority communities in Northern Thailand, where HIV incidence is currently in excess of 7%;[reference] thus they were invited to participate as well. Our final selection of sites combines rural (Tanzania, Zimbabwe, Thailand, and KwaZulu-Natal) and an urban (Soweto) location. The cultural circumstances between the sub-Saharan African sites vary widely.

. . .

Definition of community
Each of the three southern African sites (Harare, Zimbabwe; and Soweto and Vulindlela, South Africa) selected eight communities, the East African (Tanzanian) site selected 10 communities, and Thailand selected 14 communities . . . They are of a population size of approximately 10,000 . . . which fosters social familiarity and connectedness, and they are geographically distinct. Communities are defined primarily geographically for operational purposes for the study, taking into account these dimensions of social communality. The communities chosen within each country and site are selected to be sufficiently distant from each other so that there would be little cross-contamination or little possibility that individuals from a control community would benefit from the activities in the intervention community."[113]

Explanation

A description of the environment in which a trial will be conducted provides important context in terms of the applicability of the study results; the existence and type of applicable local regulation and ethics oversight; and the type of healthcare and research infrastructure available. These considerations can vary substantially within and between countries.

At a minimum, the countries, type of setting (eg, urban versus rural), and the likely number of study sites should be reported in the protocol. These factors have been associated with recruitment success and degree of attrition for some trials,[68] [91] [92] [114] [115] [116] [117] but not for others.[118] [119] Trial location has also been associated with trial outcome,[120] aspects of trial quality (eg, authenticity of randomisation[121]), and generalisability.[122]

Eligibility criteria

Item 10: Inclusion and exclusion criteria for participants. If applicable, eligibility criteria for study centres and individuals who will perform the interventions (eg, surgeons, psychotherapists)

EXAMPLES

"Patients (or a representative) must provide written, informed consent before any study procedures occur (see Appendix 1 for sample Informed Consent Form) . . .

5.1. Inclusion Criteria
Patients eligible for the trial must comply with all of the following at randomization:
1. Age ≥16 years
2. Current admission under the care of the heart-failure service at the site
. . .

5.2. Exclusion Criteria
1. Acute decompensation thought by the attending heart-failure physician to require or be likely to require PAC [pulmonary-artery catheter] during the next 24 hours. Such patients should be entered into the PAC Registry (see below).
2. Inability to undergo PAC placement within the next 12 hours
. . .

Patients enrolled in other investigational drug studies are potential candidates for ESCAPE. As the ESCAPE protocol does not involve any investigational agents or techniques, patients would be eligible for dual randomization if they are on stable doses of the investigational drugs. . . .

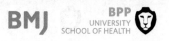

13. Study Network, Training, and Responsibilities

. . . To qualify, physicians responsible for PAC [pulmonary-artery catheter] placements will be required to show proof of insertion of ≥50 PACs in the previous year with a complication rate of <5%. Further, clinicians will need to show competence in the following areas to participate in the study: 1) insertion techniques and cardiovascular anatomy; 2) oxygen dynamics; . . . and 7) common PAC complications.[reference] . . . we will assume basic competence in these areas after satisfactory completion of the PACEP [PAC educational programme] module."[123]

"TRIAL CENTRE REQUIREMENTS

A number of guidelines have stated thrombolysis should only be considered if the patient is admitted to a specialist centre with appropriate experience and expertise.[reference] Hospitals participating in IST-3 [third International Stroke Trial] should have an organized acute stroke service. The components of effective stroke unit care have been identified . . . In brief, the facilities (details of these requirements are specified in the separate operations manual) should include:

- Written protocol for the acute assessment of patients with suspected acute stroke to include interventions to reduce time from onset to treatment.
- Immediate access to CT [computed tomographic] or MR [magnetic resonance] brain scanning (preferably 24 hours a day).

A treatment area where thrombolysis may be administered and the patient monitored according to trial protocol, preferably an acute stroke unit."[124]

EXAMPLE

"Eligible patients will be randomised in equal proportions between IL-1ra [interleukin-1 receptor antagonist] and placebo, receiving either a once daily, subcutaneous (s.c.) injection of IL-1ra (dose 100 mg per 24 h) for 14 days, or a daily s.c. injection of placebo for 14 days . . .

The study drug and placebo will be provided by Amgen Inc in its commercially available recombinant form . . . The study drug and placebo will be relabelled by Amgen, in collaboration with CTEU [Clinical Trials and Evaluation Unit] according to MHRA [Medicines and Healthcare Products Regulatory Agency] guidelines.

The first dose of IL-1ra will be given within 24 h +2 h of the positive Troponin. Injections will be given at a standardised time (24 ± 2 h after the previous dose), immediately after blood sampling. IL-1ra or placebo will [be] administered to the patient by the research nurse while the patient is in hospital. During the hospital stay, the patient will be taught to self-administer the injection by the research nurse and on discharge will continue at home. This has proven possible in other ACS [acute coronary syndrome] trials that required self injection of subcutaneous heparin [reference]. Full written guidance on self injection will also be provided to patients. If self injection is found not to be possible in an individual patient for unexpected reasons, an alternative method will be sought (eg district nurse, or attending the hospital) to try and maintain full compliance with scheduled study drug regimen after discharge. Patients will also be asked to complete a daily injection diary. All personnel will be blinded to the identity of the syringe contents."[145]

Explanation

Eligibility criteria for potential trial participants define the study population. They can relate to demographic information; type or severity of the health condition; comorbidities; previous or current treatment; diagnostic procedures; pregnancy; or other relevant considerations.[125] In trials of operator-dependent interventions such as surgery and psychotherapy, it is usually important to promote consistency of intervention delivery by also defining the eligibility criteria for care providers and centres where the intervention will be administered.[126]

Clear delineation of eligibility criteria serves several purposes. It enables study personnel to apply these criteria consistently throughout the trial.[127] The choice of eligibility criteria can affect recruitment and attrition,[67 114 115 117 118 128 129 130] as well as outcome event rates.[39 131] In addition, the criteria convey key information related to external validity (generalisability or applicability).[132] The importance of transparent documentation is highlighted by evidence that the eligibility criteria listed in publications are often different from those specified in the protocol.[125 133 134]

Certain eligibility criteria warrant explicit justification in the protocol, particularly when they limit the trial sample to a narrow subset of the population.[132 135 136] The appropriateness of restrictive participant selection depends on the trial objectives.[137] When trial participants differ substantially from the overall population to whom the intervention will be applied, the trial results may not reflect the impact in real world practice settings.[134 138 139 140 141 142 143 144]

Interventions

Item 11a: Interventions for each group with sufficient detail to allow replication, including how and when they will be administered

Explanation

Studies of trials and systematic reviews have shown that important elements of the interventions are not described in half of the publications.[146 147] If such elements are also missing from the protocol, or if the protocol simply refers to other documents that are not freely accessible, then it can be impossible for healthcare providers, systematic reviewers, policymakers, and others to fully understand, implement, or evaluate the trial intervention.[148] This principle applies to all types of interventions, but is particularly true for complex interventions (eg, health service delivery; psychotherapy), which consist of interconnected components that can vary between healthcare providers and settings.

For drugs, biological agents, or placebos, the protocol description should include the generic name, manufacturer, constituent components, route of administration, and dosing schedule (including titration and run-in periods, if applicable).[149 150] The description of non-drug interventions—such as devices, procedures, policies, models of care, or counselling—is generally more complex and warrants additional details about the setting (Item 9) and individuals administering the interventions. For example, the level of pre-trial expertise (Item 10) and specific training of individuals administering these complex interventions are often relevant to describe (eg, for surgeons, psychologists, physiotherapists). When intervention delivery is subject to variation, it is important to state whether the same individuals will deliver the trial interventions in all study groups, or whether different individuals will manage each study group—in which case it can be difficult to separate the effect of the intervention from that of the individual delivering it. Interventions that consist of "usual care" or "standard of care" require further elaboration in the protocol, as this care can vary substantially across centres and patients, as well as over the duration of the trial.

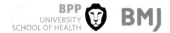

Interventions—modifications
Item 11b: Criteria for discontinuing or modifying allocated interventions for a given trial participant (eg, drug dose change in response to harms, participant request, or improving/worsening disease)

EXAMPLE

"Gastro-Intestinal Upset
The tablets may be taken in two equally divided doses, if necessary, to improve gastro-intestinal tolerance. Should it be necessary the daily dose may be reduced by one tablet at a time to improve gastro-intestinal tolerance.

Renal Function Impairment
Since sodium clodronate is excreted unchanged by the kidney its use is contra-indicated in patients with moderate to severe renal impairment (serum creatinine greater than 2 times upper limit of normal range of the centre). If renal function deteriorates to this extent the trial medication should be withdrawn from the patient.**This should be reported as an adverse event.** In patients with normal renal function or mild renal impairment (serum creatinine less than 2 times upper limit of normal range of the centre) serum creatinine should be monitored during therapy.

Allergic Reactions
Allergic skin reactions have been observed in rare cases. If this is suspected withdraw the trial medication from the patient. **This should be reported as an adverse event.**

Biochemical Disturbances
Asymptomatic hypocalcaemia has been noted rarely. Temporary suspension of the trial medication until the serum calcium returns into the normal range is recommended. The trial medication can be then restarted at half the previous dose. If the situation returns withdraw the trial medication from the patient. **This should be reported as an adverse event.** . . ."[151]

Explanation
For a given trial participant, the assigned study intervention may need to be modified or discontinued by trial investigators for various reasons, including harms, improved health status, lack of efficacy, and withdrawal of participant consent. Comparability across study groups can be improved, and subjectivity in care decisions reduced, by defining standard criteria for intervention modifications and discontinuations in the protocol. Regardless of any decision to modify or discontinue their assigned intervention, study participants should be retained in the trial whenever possible to enable follow-up data collection and prevent missing data (Item 18b).[152]

Interventions—adherence

Item 11c: Strategies to improve adherence to intervention protocols, and any procedures for monitoring adherence (eg, drug tablet return; laboratory tests)

EXAMPLE

"Adherence reminder sessions
Face-to-face adherence reminder sessions will take place at the initial product dispensing and each study visit thereafter. This session will include:

- The importance of following study guidelines for adherence to once daily study product
- Instructions about taking study pills including dose timing, storage, and importance of taking pills whole, and what to

do in the event of a missed dose.

- Instructions about the purpose, use, and care of the MEMS® cap [medication event monitoring system] and bottle
- Notification that there will be a pill count at every study visit
- Reinforcement that study pills may be TDF [tenofovir disproxil fumarate] or placebo
- Importance of calling the clinic if experiencing problems possibly related to study product such as symptoms, lost pills or MEMS® cap.

Subsequent sessions will occur at the follow-up visits. Participants will be asked about any problems they are having taking their study pills or using the MEMS® cap. There will be brief discussion of reasons for missed doses and simple strategies for enhancing adherence, eg, linking pill taking to meals or other daily activities. Participants will have an opportunity to ask questions and key messages from the initial session will be reviewed as needed . . .

Adherence assessments
To enhance validity of data, multiple methods will be used to assess medication adherence including pill count; an electronic medication event monitoring system (MEMS® cap) [reference]; and ACASI [audio-computer administered interview] questionnaire items including a one month visual analogue scale,[reference] reasons for non-compliance, and use of the MEMS® cap. Participants will return the unused tablets and bottle at each follow-up visit. Unused tablets will be counted and recorded on the appropriate CRF [case report form]. Electronic data collected in the MEMS® cap will be downloaded into a designated, secure study computer."[153]

Explanation
Adherence to intervention protocols refers to the degree to which the behaviour of trial participants corresponds to the intervention assigned to them.[154] Distinct but related concepts include trial retention (Item 18b) and adherence to the follow-up protocol of procedures and assessments (Item 13).

On average, adherence to intervention protocols is higher in clinical trials than in non-research settings.[155] Although there is no consensus on the acceptable minimum adherence level in clinical trials, low adherence can have a substantial effect on statistical power and interpretation of trial results.[156] [157] [158] Since fewer participants are receiving the full intervention as intended, non-adherence can reduce the contrast between study groups—leading to decreased study power and increased costs associated with recruiting larger sample sizes for evaluating superiority, or leading to potentially inappropriate conclusions of non-inferiority or equivalence. There is also the possibility of underestimating any efficacy and harms of the study intervention.

Furthermore, if adherence is a marker for general healthy behaviour associated with better prognosis, then different rates of non-adherence between study groups can lead to a biased estimate of an intervention's effect. In support of this "healthy adherer" effect, non-adherers to placebo in clinical studies have been found to have poorer clinical outcomes than adherers.[159]

To help avoid these potential detrimental effects of non-adherence, many trials implement procedures and strategies for monitoring and improving adherence,[67] [156] [157] [158] and any such plans should be described in the protocol.[160] Among applicable drug trials published in 1997-99, 47% reported monitoring the level of adherence.[161] Although each of the many types of monitoring methods has its limitations,[157] [158] adherence data can help to inform the statistical analysis

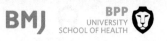

(Item 20c), trial interpretation, and choice of appropriate adherence strategies to implement in the trial as it progresses or in future trials and clinical practice.

A variety of adherence strategies exist,[156] [157] [158] and their use can be tailored to the specific type of trial design, intervention, and participant population. It may be desirable to select strategies that can be easily implemented in clinical practice, so that the level of adherence in the real world setting is comparable to that observed in the trial.[158]

Interventions—concomitant care
Item 11d: Relevant concomitant care and interventions that are permitted or prohibited during the trial

---

EXAMPLE

"**2. Rescue Medication**
For weeks 0-3, topical mometasone furoate 0.1% cream or ointment (30 g/week) will be permitted with participants preferably using ointment. Participants will be instructed to apply the topical mometasone furoate to blisters/lesions as required (not to areas of unaffected skin). If the participant is allergic to mometasone furoate or the hospital pharmacy does not stock it, then an alternative topical steroid may be prescribed but this must be in the potent class. In addition, participants will be advised that they can apply a light moisturiser to blisters/lesions at any time during the study.
For weeks 3-6, use of mometasone furoate (or other topical corticosteroids) is strongly discouraged to prevent potential systemic effects. Accidental use of mometasone furoate or other potent topical steroid during this period will be classified as a protocol deviation.
After week 6, potent topical corticosteroids (up to 30 g/week) may be used to treat symptoms and localised disease if they would have normally been used as part of normal clinical care by the physician in charge of that patient. This must be recorded on the trial treatment log.
However, those patients who are on a dose reducing regime for oral steroids, 30 g/week of a "potent" topical steroid will be allowed.
3. Prohibited Concomitant Medications
The administration of live virus vaccines is not permitted for all participants during weeks 0-6 as the investigator is blinded to treatment allocation, and must therefore warn all participants to refrain for [sic] having a live virus vaccine. However, after week 6, once the investigator knows which medication the participant is on, only those taking prednisolone will not be allowed live virus vaccines.

Participants should continue to take medications for other conditions as normal. However, if it is anticipated that the participant will need a live virus vaccine during the intervention phase, they will be ineligible for entry into the study."[50]

Explanation
In a controlled trial, a key goal is to have comparable study groups that differ only by the intervention being evaluated, so that any difference in outcomes can be attributed to effects of the study intervention. Cointervention bias can arise when the study groups receive different concomitant care or interventions (in addition to the assigned trial interventions) that may affect trial outcomes.[162] To promote comparability of study groups, the protocol should list the relevant concomitant care and interventions that are allowed (including rescue interventions), as well as any that are prohibited.

Outcomes
Item 12: Primary, secondary, and other outcomes, including the specific measurement variable (eg, systolic blood pressure), analysis metric (eg, change from baseline, final value, time to event), method of aggregation (eg, median, proportion), and time point for each outcome. Explanation of the clinical relevance of chosen efficacy and harm outcomes is strongly recommended

---

EXAMPLE

"**1. Primary Outcome Measures**
- Difference between the two treatment arms in the proportion of participants classed as treatment success at 6 weeks. Treatment success is defined as 3 or less significant blisters present on examination at 6 weeks. Significant blisters are defined as intact blisters containing fluid which are at least 5 mm in diameter. However, if the participant has popped a blister, or the blister is at a site that makes it susceptible to bursting such as the sole of the foot, it can be considered part of the blister count, providing there is a flexible (but not dry) roof present over a moist base. Mucosal blisters will be excluded from the count.
- A survey of the UK DCTN [Dermatology Clinical Trials Network] membership showed that a point estimate of 25% inferiority in effectiveness would be acceptable assuming a gain in the safety profile of at least 10%.
- This measure of success was selected as it was considered to be more clinically relevant than a continuous measure of blister count. It would be less clinically relevant to perform an absolute blister count and report a percentage reduction. Instead, to state that treatment is considered a success if remission is achieved (ie the presence of three or less blisters on physical examination at 6 weeks) more closely reflects clinical practice. In addition, it is far less burdensome on investigators than including a full blister count, which would mean counting in the region of 50-60 blisters in many cases. This outcome measure will be performed as a single blind assessment.
- Difference between the two treatment arms in the proportion of participants reporting grade 3, 4 and 5 (mortality) adverse events which are possibly, probably or definitely related to BP [bullous pemphigoid] medication in the 52 weeks following randomisation. A modified version of The Common Terminology Criteria for Adverse Events (CTCAE v3.0) will be used to grade adverse events. At each study visit, participants will be questioned about adverse events they have experienced since the last study visit (using a standard list of known side effects of the two study drugs).

2. Secondary Outcome Measures
For the secondary and tertiary endpoints a participant will be classed as a treatment success if they have 3 or less significant blisters present on examination and have not had their treatment modified (changed or dose increased) on account of a poor response.
- Difference in the proportion of participants who are classed as a treatment success at 6 weeks.
- Difference in the proportion of participants in each treatment arm who are classed as treatment success at 6 weeks and are alive at 52 weeks. This measure will provide a good overall comparison of the two treatment arms. . . ."[50]

Explanation
The trial outcomes are fundamental to study design and interpretation of results. For a given intervention, an outcome can generally reflect efficacy (beneficial effect) or harm (adverse effect). The outcomes of main interest are

designated as primary outcomes, which usually appear in the objectives (Item 7) and sample size calculation (Item 14). The remaining outcomes constitute secondary or other outcomes.

For each outcome, the trial protocol should define four components: the specific measurement variable, which corresponds to the data collected directly from trial participants (eg, Beck Depression Inventory score, all cause mortality); the participant-level analysis metric, which corresponds to the format of the outcome data that will be used from each trial participant for analysis (eg, change from baseline, final value, time to event); the method of aggregation, which refers to the summary measure format for each study group (eg, mean, proportion with score > 2); and the specific measurement time point of interest for analysis.[163]

It is also important to explain the rationale for the choice of trial outcomes. An ideal outcome is valid, reproducible, relevant to the target population (eg, patients), and responsive to changes in the health condition being studied.[67] The use of a continuous versus dichotomous method of aggregation can affect study power and estimates of treatment effect,[164][165] and subjective outcomes are more prone to bias from inadequate blinding (ascertainment bias) and allocation concealment (selection bias) than objective outcomes.[166][167] Although composite outcomes increase event rates and statistical power, their relevance and interpretation can be unclear if the individual component outcomes vary greatly in event rates, importance to patients, or amount of missing data.[168] [169] [170] [171]

The number of primary outcomes should be as small as possible. Although up to 38% of trials define multiple primary outcomes,[435][163] this practice can introduce problems with multiplicity, selective reporting, and interpretation when there are inconsistent results across outcomes. Problems also arise when trial protocols do not designate any primary outcomes, as seen in half (28/59) of protocols for a sample of trials published from 2002-2008,[12] and in 25% of randomised trial protocols that received ethics approval in Denmark in 1994-95.[4] Furthermore, major discrepancies in the primary outcomes designated in protocols/registries/regulatory submissions versus final trial publications are common; favour the reporting of statistically significant primary outcomes over non-significant ones; and are often not acknowledged in final publications.[172] [173] [174] [175] [176] Such bias can only be identified and deterred if trial outcomes are clearly defined beforehand in the protocol and if protocol information is made public.[177]

Where possible, the development and adoption of a common set of key trial outcomes within a specialty can help to deter selective reporting of outcomes and to facilitate comparisons and pooling of results across trials in a meta-analysis.[178] [179] [180] The COMET (Core Outcome Measures in Effectiveness Trials) Initiative aims to facilitate the development and application of such standardised sets of core outcomes for clinical trials of specific conditions (www.comet-initiative.org). Trial investigators are encouraged to ascertain whether there is a core outcome set relevant to their trial and, if so, to include those outcomes in their trial. Existence of a common set of outcomes does not preclude inclusion of additional relevant outcomes for a given trial.

Participant timeline

Item 13: Time schedule of enrolment, interventions (including any run-ins and washouts), assessments, and visits for participants. A schematic diagram is highly recommended (see fig 1)

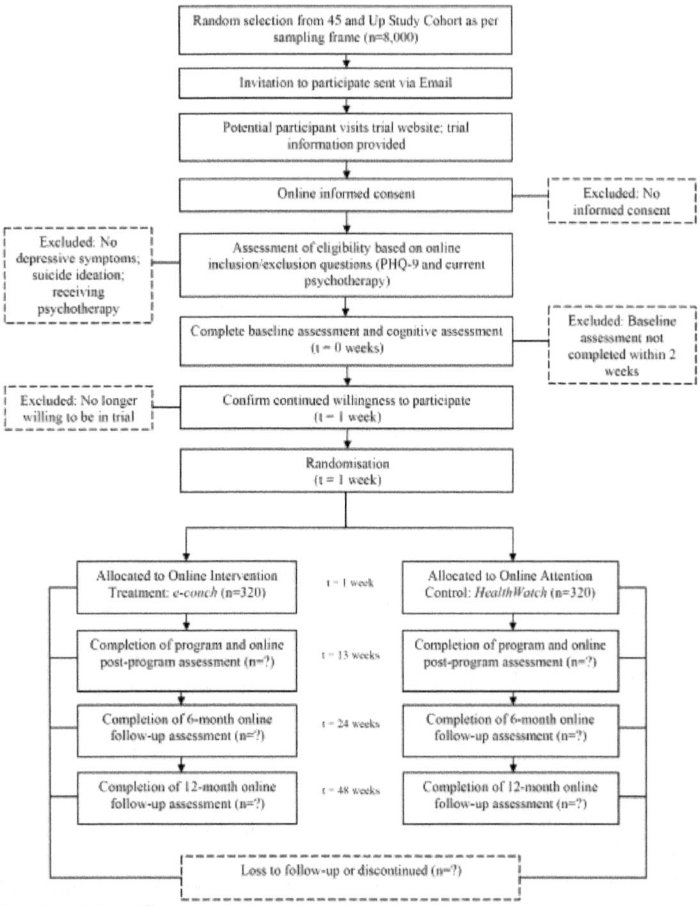

Fig 2 Flow of participants[182]

EXAMPLES

"The main outcomes of interest are the drug and sex-related HIV and HCV [hepatitis C virus] risk behaviors . . . Clients will be assessed using the full battery of instruments from the Common Assessment Battery (CAB), along with the Self-Efficacy and Stages of Change questionnaires and a Urine Drug Screen after consenting . . . questionnaires will take place for all participants 14-30 days after randomization during which they will be given the Stages of Change and Self-Efficacy questionnaires, the Timeline Follow-Back, and a UA [urine analysis]. Follow-up interviews, using the full battery (CAB and questionnaires), will be collected at 2 months (56 days), 4 months (112 days) and 6 months (168 days) after the randomization date. A 14 day window, defined as 7 days before and 7 days after the due date, will be available to complete the 2 and 4 month follow-up interviews and a 28 day window, defined as 7 days before and 21 days after the due date, will be available to complete the 6 month follow up interview . . .

7.1.1 Common Assessment Battery (CAB)
- A Demographic Questionnaire . . .
- The Composite International Diagnostic Interview Version 2.1 . . .
- The Addiction Severity Index-Lite (ASI-Lite) . . .
- The Risk Behavior Survey (RBS), . . .

7.1.2 Additional Interviews/Questionnaires
To assess drug use, urinalysis for morphine, cocaine, amphetamine, and methamphetamine will be performed at the 2-Week Interim Visit, and the 2-, 4-, and 6-month Follow-up visits . . .

Table 3 HIV/HCV risk reduction protocol schedule of forms and procedures (adapted from original table[181])

Activity/ assessment	CRF (Yes/ No)	Staff member	Approximate time to complete (min)	-1 Prestudy screening/ consent	0 Prestudy baseline/ randomisation	T1 Study visit 1	T2 Study/ interim visit 2 and/or 2 week interim	F1 Follow-up 2 months	F2 Follow-up 4-months	F3 Follow-up 6-months
Prescreening consent	No	Study coordinator	5	X						
Screening log	No	Study coordinator	5	X						
Consent form/ quiz	No	Study coordinator	45	X						
Inclusion/ exclusion form	Yes	Study coordinator	N/A	X						
Urine screen	Yes	Study coordinator	10		X		X	X	X	X
Locator form	No	Interviewer	10		X		Update X	Update X	Update X	
Demographics questionnaire	Yes	Interviewer	10		X					
Addiction severity index (ASI) lite	Yes	Interviewer	45		X			X	X	X
Composite international diagnostic interview)	Yes	Interviewer	45		X					
HIV risk behaviour survey	Yes	Interviewer	15		X			X	X	X
Timeline follow back	Yes	Interviewer	5				X	X	X	X
Self efficacy	Yes	Interviewer	5		X		X	X	X	X
Stage of change	Yes	Interviewer	5		X		X	X	X	X
Randomisation	Yes	Study coordinator	15		X					
Voluntary blood sample Counselling and education intervention (treatment group)	Yes	Study phlebotomist	15			X				X
All groups, optional blood sample at study close	Yes	Study phlebotomist	15							X
Termination form	Yes	Study coordinator	N/A							X
Serious adverse event form	Yes	Study coordinator	N/A	As needed throughout protocol						
Progress notes	No	All team members	N/A	X	X	X	X	X	X	X
Communication log	No	All team members	N/A	Every phone or in-person contact outside of a regular visit						

- Stage of change for quitting drug use will be measured using a modification of the Motivation Scales [table 3] . . . " [181]

"The trial consists of a 12-week intervention treatment phase with a 40-week follow-up phase. The total trial period will be 12-months. As shown . . . measurements will be undertaken at four time-points in each group: at baseline, directly after completing the 12-week internet program, and at six and 12-month follow-up" [fig 2].[182]

Explanation

A clear and concise timeline of the study visits, enrolment process, interventions, and assessments performed on participants can help to guide trial conduct and enable external review of participant burden and feasibility. These factors can also affect the decision of potential investigators and participants to join the trial (Item 15).[91]

A schematic diagram is highly recommended to efficiently present the overall schedule and time commitment for trial participants in each study group. Though various presentation formats exist, key information to convey includes the timing of each visit, starting from initial eligibility screening through to study close-out; time periods during which trial interventions will be administered; and the procedures and assessments performed at each visit (with reference to specific data collection forms, if relevant) (fig 1).

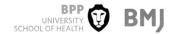

Sample size

Item 14: Estimated number of participants needed to achieve study objectives and how it was determined, including clinical and statistical assumptions supporting any sample size calculations

---

EXAMPLES

"The sample size was calculated on the basis of the primary hypothesis. In the exploratory study,[reference] those referred to PEPS [psychoeducation with problem solving] had a greater improvement in social functioning at 6 month follow-up equivalent to 1.05 points on the SFQ [Social Functioning Questionnaire]. However, a number of people received PEPS who were not included in the trial (eg, the wait-list control) and, for this larger sample (N=93), the mean pre-post-treatment difference was 1.79 (pre-treatment mean=13.85, SD=4.21; post-treatment mean=12.06, SD=4.21). (Note: a lower SFQ score is more desirable). This difference of almost 2 points accords with other evidence that this is a clinically significant and important difference.[reference] A reduction of 2 points or more on the SFQ at 1 year follow-up in an RCT of cognitive behaviour therapy in health anxiety was associated with a halving of secondary care appointments (1.24 vs 0.65), a clinically significant reduction in the Hospital Anxiety and Depression Scale (HADS[reference]) Anxiety score of 2.5 (9.9 vs 7.45) and a reduction in health anxiety (the main outcome) of 5.6 points (17.8 vs 12.2) (11 is a normal population score and 18 is pathological).[reference] These findings suggest that improvements in social functioning may accrue over 1 year, hence we expect to find a greater magnitude of response at the 72 week follow-up than we did in the exploratory trial. Therefore, we have powered this trial to be able to detect a difference in SFQ score of 2 points. SFQ standard deviations vary between treatment, control, and the wait-list samples, ranging from 3.78 to 4.53. We have based our sample size estimate on the most conservative (ie, largest) SD [standard deviation]. To detect a mean difference in SFQ score of 2 point (SD = 4.53) at 72 weeks with a two-sided significance level of 1% and power of 80% with equal allocation to two arms would require 120 patients in each arm of the trial. To allow for 30% drop out, 170 will be recruited per arm, ie, 340 in total."[183]

"Superficial and deep incisional surgical site infection rates for patients in the PDS II® [polydioxanone suture] group are estimated to occur at a rate of 0.12.[reference] The trials by [reference] have shown a reduction of SSI [surgical site infections] of more than 50% (from 10.8% to 4.9% and from 9.2% to 4.3% respectively). Therefore, we estimate a rate of 0.06 for PDS Plus® [triclosan-coated continuous polydioxanone suture].

For a fixed sample size design, the sample size required to achieve a power of 1-β=0.80 for the one-sided chi-square test at level α=0.025 under these assumptions amounts to 2×356=712 (nQuery Advisor®, version 7.0). It can be expected that including covariates of prognostic importance in the logistic regression model as defined for the confirmatory analysis will increase the power as compared to the chi-square test. As the individual results for the primary endpoint are available within 30 days after surgery, the drop-out rate is expected to be small. Nevertheless, a potential dilution of the treatment effect due to drop-outs is taken into account (eg no photographs available, loss to follow up); it is assumed that this can be compensated by additional 5% of patients to be randomized, and therefore the total sample size required for a fixed sample size design amounts to n=712+38=750 patients.

. . .

An adaptive interim analysis [reference] will be performed after availability of the results for the primary endpoint for a total of 375 randomized patients (ie, 50% of the number of patients required in a fixed sample size design). The following type I

---

error rates and decision boundaries for the interim and the final analysis are specified:

- Overall one-sided type I error rate: 0.025
- Boundary for the one-sided p-value of the first stage for accepting the null-hypothesis within the interim analysis: $\alpha_0=0.5$
- One-sided local type I error rate for testing the null-hypothesis within the interim analysis: $\alpha_1=0.0102$
- Boundary for the product of the one-sided p-values of both stages for the rejection of the null-hypothesis in the final analysis: $c\alpha=0.0038$

If the trial will be continued with a second stage after the interim analysis (this is possible if for the one-sided p-value p_1 of the interim analysis $p_1 \in]0.0102,0.5[$ [ie $0.5 \geq P_1 \geq 0.0102$] holds true, the results of the interim analysis can be taken into account for a recalculation of the required sample size. If the sample size recalculation leads to the conclusion that more than 1200 patients are required, the study is stopped, because the related treatment group difference is judged to be of minor clinical importance.

. . .

The actually achieved sample size is then not fixed but random, and a variety of scenarios can be considered. If the sample size is calculated under the same assumptions with respect to the SSI rates for the two groups, applying the same the overall significance level of α=0.025 (one-sided) but employing additionally the defined stopping boundaries and recalculating the sample size for the second stage at a conditional power of 80% on the basis of the SSI rates observed in the interim analysis results in an average total sample size of n=766 patients; the overall power of the study is then 90% (ADDPLAN®, version 5.0)."[100]

Explanation

The planned number of trial participants is a key aspect of study design, budgeting, and feasibility that is usually determined using a formal sample size calculation. If the planned sample size is not derived statistically, then this should be explicitly stated along with a rationale for the intended sample size (eg, exploratory nature of pilot studies; pragmatic considerations for trials in rare diseases).[17][184]

For trials that involve a formal sample size calculation, the guiding principle is that the planned sample size should be large enough to have a high probability (power) of detecting a true effect of a given magnitude, should it exist. Sample size calculations are generally based on one primary outcome; however, it may also be worthwhile to plan for adequate study power or report the power that will be available (given the proposed sample size) for other important outcomes or analyses because trials are often underpowered to detect harms or subgroup effects.[185][186]

Among randomised trial protocols that describe a sample size calculation, 4-40% do not state all components of the calculation.[6][11] The protocol should generally include the following: the outcome (Item 12); the values assumed for the outcome in each study group (eg, proportion with event, or mean and standard deviation) (table 4); the statistical test (Item 20a); alpha (type 1 error) level; power; and the calculated sample size per group—both assuming no loss of data and, if relevant, after any inflation for anticipated missing data (Item 20c). Trial investigators are also encouraged to provide a rationale or reference for the outcome values assumed for each study group.[187] The values

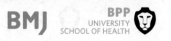

Table 4 Outcome values to report in sample size calculation

Element	Type of summary outcome		
	Binary	**Continuous**	**Time to event**
Assumed result for each study group	Proportion (%) with event	Mean and standard deviation	Proportion (%) with event at a given time point
Effect measure	Relative risk, odds ratio	Difference in means	Hazard ratio

Note: Although the sample size calculation uses the expected outcome value for each group, the corresponding contrast between groups (estimated effect) should also be reported.

of certain prespecified variables tend to be inappropriately inflated (eg, clinically important treatment effect size)[188] [189] or underestimated (eg, standard deviation for continuous outcomes),[190] leading to trials having less power in the end than what was originally calculated. Finally, when uncertainty of a sample size estimate is acknowledged, methods exist for re-estimating sample size.[191] The intended use of such an adaptive design approach should be stated in the protocol.For designs and frameworks other than parallel group superiority trials, additional elements are required in the sample size calculation. For example, an estimate of the standard deviation of within-person changes from baseline should be included for crossover trials[192]; the intracluster correlation coefficient for cluster randomised trials[193]; and the equivalence or non-inferiority margin for equivalence or non-inferiority trials respectively.[108] [194] Such elements are often not described in final trial reports,[110][195] [196] [197] [198] and it is unclear how often they are specified in the protocol.

Complete description of sample size calculations in the protocol enables an assessment of whether the trial will be adequately powered to detect a clinically important difference.[189] [199] [200] [201] [202] [203] [204] [205] [206] It also promotes transparency and discourages inappropriate post hoc revision that is intended to support a favourable interpretation of results or portray consistency between planned and achieved sample sizes.[6] [207]

Recruitment

Item 15: Strategies for achieving adequate participant enrolment to reach target sample size

---

EXAMPLE

"Each center will screen subjects to achieve screening percentages of 50% women and 33% minority; screening will continue until the target population is achieved (12 subjects/site). We recognize that, because of exclusion by genotype and genotypic variation among diverse populations,[reference], the enrolled cohort may not reflect the screened population. The enrollment period will extend over 12 months.

Recruitment strategy
Each clinical center involved in the ACRN [Asthma Clinical Research Network] was chosen based on documentation for patient availability, among other things. It is, however, worthy to note the specific plans of each center.
. . . The Asthma Clinical Research Center at the Brigham & Women's Hospital utilizes three primary resources for identifying and recruiting potential subjects as described below.
1. Research Patient Database
The Asthma Clinical Research Center at the Brigham and Women's Hospital has a database of over 1,500 asthmatics . . .
2. Asthma Patient Lists . . .
3. Advertisements . . .
. . . the Madison ACRN site has utilized some additional approaches to target minority recruitment. We have utilized a marketing expert to coordinate and oversee our overall efforts in recruiting and retaining minorities. . . . As a result of his efforts, we have advertised widely in newspapers and

other publications that target ethnic minorities, established contacts with various ethnic community, university, church, and business groups, and conducted community-based asthma programs . . . For example, student groups such as AHANA (a pre-health careers organization focusing on minority concerns) will be contacted. . . . In addition, we will utilize published examples of successful retention strategies such as frequent payment of subject honoraria as study landmarks are achieved and study participant group social events. Study visits will be carefully planned and scheduled to avoid exam-time and university calendar breaks . . .
The Harlem Hospital Center Emergency Department (ED) sees an average of eight adult patients per day for asthma. Through the REACH (Reducing Emergency Asthma Care in Harlem) project, we have . . . successfully recruited and interviewed 380 patients from the ED . . .
Responses to inquiries about participation in research studies are answered by a dedicated phone line that is manned during business hours and answered by voicemail at all other times. A research assistant responds to each inquiry immediately, using a screening instrument . . .
Patients are recruited for clinical trials at the Jefferson Center through two primary mechanisms: (1) local advertising; and (2) identification in the asthma patient registry (database). Local advertising takes advantage of the printed as well as the audio-visual media. Printed media include . . . All advertising in the printed and audio-visual media has prior approval of the Institutional Review Board.
The Jefferson patient registry (database) has been maintained since 1992 and currently contains 3,100 patients . . . It is estimated that 300-400 new asthmatic patients are seen each year, while a smaller number become inactive due to relocation, change of health care provider, etc. Once identified in the database, patients potentially eligible for a specific study are contacted by the nurse coordinator who explains the study and ascertains the patient's interest. If interested, the patient is seen in the clinical research laboratories where more detailed evaluations are made . . .

Each subject will receive financial compensation within FDA [Food and Drug Administration] guidelines for participation in an amount determined by the local center. For subjects who drop out, payments will be pro-rated for the length of time they stayed in the study, but payment will not be made until the study would have been completed had the subject not dropped out."[208]

Explanation
The main goal of recruitment is to meet the target sample size (Item 14). However, recruitment difficulties are commonly encountered in clinical trials.[209] [210] [211] [212] [213] For example, reviews of government funded trials in the US and UK found that two thirds did not reach their recruitment targets.[214] [215] Low enrolment will reduce statistical power and can lead to early trial stoppage or to extensions with delayed results and greater costs.

Strategies to promote adequate enrolment are thus important to consider during trial planning. Recruitment strategies can vary depending on the trial topic, context, and site. Different recruitment methods can substantially affect the number and type of trial participants recruited[128 209 216 217 218 219 220] and can incur different costs.[221 222 223] Design issues such as the number and stringency of eligibility criteria will also directly affect the number of eligible trial participants.

Protocol descriptions of where participants will be recruited (eg, primary care clinic, community), by whom (eg, surgeon), when (eg, time after diagnosis), and how (eg, advertisements, review of health records) can be helpful for assessing the feasibility of achieving the target sample size and the applicability of the trial results in practice. Other relevant information to explicitly provide in the protocol includes expected recruitment rates, duration of the recruitment period, plans to monitor recruitment during the trial, and any financial or non-financial incentives provided to trial investigators or participants for enrolment (Item 4). If strategies differ by site in multicentre trials, these should be detailed to the extent possible.

Section 3b: Methods—assignment of interventions (for controlled trials)

Allocation—sequence generation

Item 16a: Method of generating the allocation sequence (eg, computer-generated random numbers) and list of any factors for stratification. To reduce predictability of a random sequence, details of any planned restriction (eg, blocking) should be provided in a separate document that is unavailable to those who enrol participants or assign interventions

---

EXAMPLE

"Participants will be randomly assigned to either control or experimental group with a 1:1 allocation as per a computer generated randomisation schedule stratified by site and the baseline score of the Action Arm Research Test (ARAT; <=21 versus >21) using permuted blocks of random sizes. The block sizes will not be disclosed, to ensure concealment."[224]

Explanation

Participants in a randomised trial should be assigned to study groups using a random (chance) process characterised by unpredictability of assignments. Randomisation decreases selection bias in allocation; helps to facilitate blinding/masking after allocation; and enables the use of probability theory to test whether any difference in outcome between intervention groups reflects chance.[17 225 226 227]

Use of terms such as "randomisation" without further elaboration is not sufficient to describe the allocation process, as these terms have been used inappropriately to describe non-random, deterministic allocation methods such as alternation or allocation by date of birth.[121] In general, these non-random allocation methods introduce selection bias and biased estimates of an intervention's effect size,[17 167 228 229] mainly due to the lack of allocation concealment (Item 16b). If non-random allocation is planned, then the specific method and rationale should be stated.

Box 1 outlines the key elements of the random sequence that should be detailed in the protocol. Three quarters of randomised trial protocols approved by a research ethics committee in Denmark (1994-95) or conducted by a US cooperative cancer research group (1968-2006) did not describe the method of sequence generation.[211]

BOX 1 KEY ELEMENTS OF RANDOM SEQUENCE TO SPECIFY IN TRIAL PROTOCOLS

- Method of sequence generation (eg, random number table or computerised random number generator)
- Allocation ratio (Item 8) (eg, whether participants are allocated with equal or unequal probabilities to interventions)
- Type of randomisation (box 2): simple versus restricted; fixed versus adaptive (eg, minimisation); and, where relevant, the reasons for such choices
- If applicable, the factors (eg, recruitment site, sex, disease stage) to be used for stratification (box 2), including categories and relevant cut-off boundaries

---

Box 2 defines the various types of randomisation, including minimisation. When restricted randomisation is used, certain details should not appear in the protocol in order to reduce predictability of the random sequence (box 3). The details should instead be described in a separate document that is unavailable to trial implementers. For blocked randomisation, this information would include details on how the blocks will be generated (eg, permuted blocks by a computer random number generator), the block size(s), and whether the block size will be fixed or randomly varied. Specific block size was provided in 14/102 (14%) randomised trial protocols approved by a Danish research ethics committee in 1994-95, potentially compromising allocation concealment.[2] For trials using minimisation, it is also important to state the details in a separate document, including whether random elements will be used.

Allocation—concealment mechanism

Item 16b: Mechanism of implementing the allocation sequence (eg, central telephone; sequentially numbered, opaque, sealed envelopes), describing any steps to conceal the sequence until interventions are assigned

---

EXAMPLE

"Participants will be randomised using TENALEA, which is an online, central randomisation service . . . Allocation concealment will be ensured, as the service will not release the randomisation code until the patient has been recruited into the trial, which takes place after all baseline measurements have been completed."[240]

Explanation

Successful randomisation in practice depends on two interrelated aspects: 1) generation of an unpredictable allocation sequence (Item 16a) and 2) concealment of that sequence until assignment irreversibly occurs.[233 241] The allocation concealment mechanism aims to prevent participants and recruiters from knowing the study group to which the next participant will be assigned. Allocation concealment helps to ensure that a participant's decision to provide informed consent, or a recruiter's decision to enrol a participant, is not influenced by knowledge of the group to which they will be allocated if they join the trial.[242] Allocation concealment should not be confused with blinding (masking) (Item 17) (table 5).[243]

Without adequate allocation concealment, even random, unpredictable assignment sequences can be subverted.[233 241] For example, a common practice is to enclose assignments in sequentially numbered, sealed envelopes. However, if the envelopes are not opaque and contents are visible when held up to a light source, or if the envelopes can

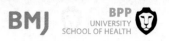

BOX 2 RANDOMISATION AND MINIMISATION (ADAPTED FROM CONSORT 2010 EXPLANATION AND ELABORATION)[17 230 231]

Simple randomisation

Randomisation based solely on a single, constant allocation ratio is known as simple randomisation. Simple randomisation with a 1:1 allocation ratio is analogous to a coin toss, although tossing a coin is not recommended for sequence generation. No other allocation approach, regardless of its real or supposed sophistication, surpasses the bias prevention and unpredictability of simple randomisation.[231]

Restricted randomisation

Any randomised approach that is not simple randomisation is restricted. Blocked randomisation is the most common form. Other forms, used much less frequently, are methods such as replacement randomisation, biased coin, and urn randomisation.[231]

Blocked randomisation

Blocked randomisation (also called permuted block randomisation) assures that study groups of approximately the same size will be generated when an allocation ratio of 1:1 is used. Blocking can also ensure close balance of the numbers in each group at any time during the trial. After every block of eight participants, for example, four would have been allocated to each trial group.[232] Improved balance comes at the cost of reducing the unpredictability of the sequence. Although the order of interventions varies randomly within each block, a person running the trial could deduce some of the next treatment allocations if they discovered the block size.[233] Blinding the interventions, using larger block sizes, and randomly varying the block size will help to avoid this problem.

Biased coin and urn randomisation

Biased coin designs attain the similar objective as blocked designs without forcing strict equality. They therefore preserve much of the unpredictability associated with simple randomisation. Biased-coin designs alter the allocation ratio during the course of the trial to rectify imbalances that might be occurring.[231] Adaptive biased-coin designs, such as the urn design, vary allocation ratios based on the magnitude of the imbalance. However, these approaches are used infrequently.

Stratified randomisation

Stratification is used to ensure good balance of participant characteristics in each group. Without stratification, study groups may not be well matched for baseline characteristics, such as age and stage of disease, especially in small trials. Such imbalances can be avoided without sacrificing the advantages of randomisation. Stratified randomisation is achieved by performing a separate randomisation procedure within each of two or more strata of participants (eg, categories of age or baseline disease severity), ensuring that the numbers of participants receiving each intervention are closely balanced within each stratum. Stratification requires some form of restriction (eg, blocking within strata) in order to be effective. The number of strata should be limited to avoid over-stratification.[234] Stratification by centre is common in multicentre trials.

Minimisation

Minimisation assures similar distribution of selected participant factors between study groups.[230 235] Randomisation lists are not set up in advance. The first participant is truly randomly allocated; for each subsequent participant, the treatment allocation that minimises the imbalance on the selected factors between groups at that time is identified. That allocation may then be used, or a choice may be made at random with a heavy weighting in favour of the intervention that would minimise imbalance (for example, with a probability of 0.8). The use of a random component is generally preferable.[236] Minimisation has the advantage of making small groups closely similar in terms of participant characteristics at all stages of the trial.

Minimisation offers the only acceptable alternative to randomisation, and some have argued that it is superior.[237] On the other hand, minimisation lacks the theoretical basis for eliminating bias on all known and unknown factors. Nevertheless, in general, trials that use minimisation are considered methodologically equivalent to randomised trials, even when a random element is not incorporated. For SPIRIT, minimisation is considered a restricted randomisation approach without any judgment as to whether it is superior or inferior compared to other restricted randomisation approaches.

BOX 3 NEED FOR A SEPARATE DOCUMENT TO DESCRIBE RESTRICTED RANDOMISATION

If some type of restricted randomisation approach is to be used, in particular blocked randomisation or minimisation, then the knowledge of the specific details could lead to bias.[238 239] For example, if the trial protocol for a two arm, parallel group trial with a 1:1 allocation ratio states that blocked randomisation will be used and the block size will be six, then trial implementers know that the intervention assignments will balance every six participants. Thus, if intervention assignments become known after assignment, knowing the block size will allow trial implementers to predict when equality of the sample sizes will arise. A sequence can be discerned from the pattern of past assignments and then some future assignments could be accurately predicted. For example, if part of a sequence contained two "As" and three "Bs," trial implementers would know the last assignment in the sequence would be an "A." If the first three assignments in a sequence contained three "As," trial implementers would know the last three assignments in that sequence would be three "Bs." Selection bias could result, regardless of the effectiveness of allocation concealment (Item 16b).

Of course, this is mainly a problem in open label trials, where everyone becomes aware of the intervention after assignment. It can also be a problem in trials where everyone is supposedly blinded (masked), but the blinding is ineffective or the intervention harms provide clues such that treatments can be guessed.

We recommend that trial investigators do not provide full details of a restricted randomisation scheme (including minimisation) in the trial protocol. Knowledge of these details might undermine randomisation by facilitating deciphering of the allocation sequence. Instead, this specific information should be provided in a separate document with restricted access. However, simple randomisation procedures could be reported in detail in the protocol, because simple randomisation is totally unpredictable.

Table 5 Differences between allocation concealment and blinding (masking) for trials with individual randomisation

	Allocation concealment	Blinding
Definition	Unawareness of the next study group assignment in the allocation sequence	Unawareness of the study group to which trial participants have already been assigned
Purpose	Prevent selection bias by facilitating enrolment of comparable participants in each study group	Prevent ascertainment, performance, and attrition biases by facilitating comparable concomitant care (aside from trial interventions) and evaluation of participants in each study group
Timing of implementation	Before study group assignment	Upon study group assignment and beyond
Who is kept unaware	Trial participants and individuals enrolling them	One or more of the following: trial participants, investigators, care providers, outcome assessors. Other groups: endpoint adjudication committee, data handlers, data analysts
Always possible to implement?	Yes	No

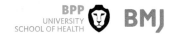

be unsealed and resealed, then this method of allocation concealment can be corrupted.

Protocols should describe the planned allocation concealment mechanism in sufficient detail to enable assessment of its adequacy. In one study of randomised trial protocols in Denmark, over half did not adequately describe allocation concealment methods.[2] In contrast, central randomisation was stated as the allocation concealment method in all phase III trial protocols initiated in 1968-2003 by a cooperative cancer research group that used extensive protocol review processes.[11] Like sequence generation, inadequate reporting of allocation concealment in trial publications is common and has been associated with inflated effect size estimates.[167 244 245]

Allocation—implementation
Item 16c: Who will generate the allocation sequence, who will enrol participants, and who will assign participants to interventions

> **EXAMPLE**
>
> **"Randomization**
> All patients who give consent for participation and who fulfil the inclusion criteria will be randomized. Randomisation will be requested by the staff member responsible for recruitment and clinical interviews from CenTrial [Coordination Centre of Clinical Trials].
> In return, CenTrial will send an answer form to the study therapist who is not involved in assessing outcome of the study. This form will include a randomisation number. In every centre closed envelopes with printed randomisation numbers on it are available. For every randomisation number the corresponding code for the therapy group of the randomisation list will be found inside the envelopes. The therapist will open the envelope and will find the treatment condition to be conducted in this patient. The therapist then gives the information about treatment allocation to the patient. Staff responsible for recruitment and symptom ratings is not allowed to receive information about the group allocation.
> . . .
> The allocation sequence will be generated by the Institute for Medical Biometry (IMB) applying a permuted block design with random blocks stratified by study centre and medication compliance (favourable vs. unfavourable). . . . The block size will be concealed until the primary endpoint will be analysed. Throughout the study, the randomisation will be conducted by CenTrial in order to keep the data management and the statistician blind against the study condition as long as the data bank is open. The randomisation list remains with CenTrial for the whole duration of the study. Thus, randomisation will be conducted without any influence of the principal investigators, raters or therapists."[246]

Explanation
Based on the risk of bias associated with some methods of sequence generation and inadequate allocation concealment, trial investigators should strive for complete separation of the individuals involved in the steps before enrolment (sequence generation process and allocation concealment mechanism) from those involved in the implementation of study group assignments. When this separation is not possible, it is important for the investigators to ensure that the assignment schedule is unpredictable and locked away from even the person who generated it. The protocol should specify who will implement the various stages of the randomisation process, how and where the allocation list

will be stored, and mechanisms employed to minimise the possibility that those enrolling and assigning participants will obtain access to the list.

Blinding (masking)
Item 17a: Who will be blinded after assignment to interventions (eg, trial participants, care providers, outcome assessors, data analysts) and how

> **EXAMPLE**
> "Assessments regarding clinical recovery will be conducted by an assessor blind to treatment allocation. The assessor will go through a profound assessment training program . . . Due to the nature of the intervention neither participants nor staff can be blinded to allocation, but are strongly inculcated not to disclose the allocation status of the participant at the follow up assessments. An employee outside the research team will feed data into the computer in separate datasheets so that the researchers can analyse data without having access to information about the allocation."[247]

Explanation
Blinding or masking (the process of keeping the study group assignment hidden after allocation) is commonly used to reduce the risk of bias in clinical trials with two or more study groups.[166 248] Awareness of the intervention assigned to participants can introduce ascertainment bias in the measurement of outcomes, particularly subjective ones (eg, quality of life)[166 167]; performance bias in the decision to discontinue or modify study interventions (eg, dosing changes) (Item 11b), concomitant interventions, or other aspects of care (Item 11d)[229]; and exclusion/attrition bias in the decision to withdraw from the trial or to exclude a participant from the analysis.[249 250] We have elected to use the term "blinding" but acknowledge that others prefer the term "masking" because "blind" also relates to an ophthalmological condition and health outcome.[251 252]

Many groups can be blinded: trial participants, care providers, data collectors, outcome assessors or committees (Item 5d), data analysts,[253] and manuscript writers. Blinding of data monitoring committees is generally discouraged.[254 255]

When blinding of trial participants and care providers is not possible because of obvious differences between the interventions,[256 257] blinding of the outcome assessors can often still be implemented.[17] It may also be possible to blind participants or trial personnel to the study hypothesis in terms of which intervention is considered active. For example, in a trial evaluating light therapy for depression, participants were informed that the study involved testing two different forms of light therapy, whereas the true hypothesis was that bright blue light was considered potentially effective and that dim red light was considered placebo.[258]

Despite its importance, blinding is often poorly described in trial protocols.[3] The protocol should explicitly state who will be blinded to intervention groups—at a minimum, the blinding status of trial participants, care providers, and outcome assessors. Such a description is much preferred over the use of ambiguous terminology such as "single blind" or "double blind."[259 260] Protocols should also describe the comparability of blinded interventions (Item 11a)[150]—for example, similarities in appearance, use of specific flavours to mask a distinctive taste—and the timing of final unblinding of all trial participants (eg, after the creation of a locked analysis data set).[3]

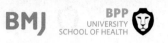

Furthermore, any strategies to reduce the potential for unblinding should be described in the protocol, such as pre-trial testing of blinding procedures.[261] The use of a fixed code (versus a unique code for each participant) to denote each study group assignment (eg, A=Group 1; B=Group 2) can be problematic, as the unblinding of one participant will result in the inadvertent loss of blinding for all trial participants.

Some have suggested that the success of blinding be formally tested by asking key trial persons to guess the study group assignment and comparing these responses to what would be expected by chance.[262] However, it is unclear how best to interpret the results of such tests.[263 264] If done, the planned testing methods should be described in the trial protocol.

Blinding (masking)—emergency unblinding
Item 17b: If blinded, circumstances under which unblinding is permissible and procedure for revealing a participant's allocated intervention during the trial

---

EXAMPLE

"To maintain the overall quality and legitimacy of the clinical trial, code breaks should occur only in exceptional circumstances when knowledge of the actual treatment is absolutely essential for further management of the patient. Investigators are encouraged to discuss with the Medical Advisor or PHRI [Population Health Research Institute] physician if he/she believes that unblinding is necessary.

If unblinding is deemed to be necessary, the investigator should use the system for emergency unblinding through the PHRI toll-free help line as the main system or through the local emergency number as the back-up system.

The Investigator is encouraged to maintain the blind as far as possible. The actual allocation must NOT be disclosed to the patient and/or other study personnel including other site personnel, monitors, corporate sponsors or project office staff; nor should there be any written or verbal disclosure of the code in any of the corresponding patient documents.

The Investigator must report all code breaks (with reason) as they occur on the corresponding CRF [case report form] page. Unblinding should not necessarily be a reason for study drug discontinuation."[265]

Explanation
Among 58 blinded Danish trials approved in 1994-95, three quarters of protocols described emergency unblinding procedures.[3] Such procedures to reveal the assigned intervention in certain circumstances are intended to increase the safety of trial participants by informing the clinical management of harms or other relevant conditions that arise. A clear protocol description of the conditions and procedures for emergency unblinding helps to prevent unnecessary unblinding; facilitates implementation by trial personnel when indicated; and enables evaluation of the appropriateness of the planned procedures. In some cases (eg, minor, reversible harms), stopping and then cautiously reintroducing the assigned intervention in the affected participant can avoid both unblinding and further harm.

Section 3c: Methods—data collection, management, and analysis
Data collection methods

Item 18a: Plans for assessment and collection of outcome, baseline, and other trial data, including any related processes to promote data quality (eg, duplicate measurements, training of assessors) and a description of study instruments (eg, questionnaires, laboratory tests) along with their reliability and validity, if known. Reference to where data collection forms can be found, if not in the protocol

---

EXAMPLES

"Primary outcome
Delirium recognition: In accordance with national guidelines [reference], the study will identify delirium by using the RASS [Richmond Agitation-Sedation Scale] and the CAM-ICU [Confusion Assessment Method for the intensive care unit] on all patients who are admitted directly from the emergency room or transferred from other services to the ICU. Such assessment will be performed after 24 hours of ICU admission and twice daily until discharge from the hospital . . . RASS has excellent inter-rater reliability among adult medical and surgical ICU patients and has excellent validity when compared to a visual analogue scale and other selected sedation scales[reference] . . . The CAM-ICU was chosen because of its practical use in the ICU wards, its acceptable psychometric properties, and based on the recommendation of national guidelines[reference] . . . The CAM-ICU diagnosis of delirium was validated against the DSM-III-R [Diagnostic and Statistical Manual of Mental Disorders, Third Edition—Revised] delirium criteria determined by a psychiatrist and found to have a sensitivity of 97% and a specificity of 92%.[reference] The CAM-ICU has been developed, validated and applied into ICU settings and multiple investigators have used the same method to identify patients with delirium.[reference]
Delirium severity: Since the CAM-ICU does not evaluate delirium severity, we selected the Delirium Rating Scale revised-1998 (DRS-R-98)[reference] . . . The DRS-R-98 was designed to evaluate the breadth of delirium symptoms for phenomenological studies in addition to measuring symptom severity with high sensitivity and specificity . . . The DRS-R-98 is a 16-item clinician-rated scale with anchored items descriptions . . . The DRS-R-98 has excellent inter-rater reliability (intra-class correlation 0.97) and internal consistency (Cronbach's alpha 0.94).[reference]

Secondary outcomes
The study will collect demographic and baseline functional information from the patient's legally authorized representative and/or caregivers. Cognitive function status will be obtained by interviewing the patient's legally authorized representative using the Informant Questionnaire on Cognitive Decline in the Elderly (IQCODE). IQCODE is a questionnaire that can be completed by a relative or other caregiver to determine whether that person has declined in cognitive functioning. The IQCODE lists 26 everyday situations . . . Each situation is rated by the informant for amount of change over the previous 10 years, using a Likert scale ranging from 1-much improved to 5-much worse. The IQCODE has a sensitivity between 69% to 100% and specificity of 80% to 96% for dementia.[reference] Utilizing the electronic medical record system (RMRS), we will collect several data points of interest at baseline and throughout the study period . . . We have previously defined hospital-related consequences to include: the number of patients with documented falls, use of physical restraints . . . These will be assessed using the RMRS, direct daily observation, and retrospective review of the electronic medical record. This definition of delirium related hospital complications has been previously used and published. [reference]"[266]

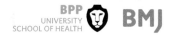

"Training and certification plans

. . . Each center's personnel will be trained centrally in the study requirements, standardized measurement of height, weight, and blood pressure, requirements for laboratory specimen collection including morning urine samples, counseling for adherence and the eliciting of information from study participants in a uniform reproducible manner.

. . . The data to be collected and the procedures to be conducted at each visit will be reviewed in detail. Each of the data collection forms and the nature of the required information will be discussed in detail on an item by item basis. Coordinators will learn how to code medications using the WHODrug software and how to code symptoms using the MedDRA software. Entering data forms, responding to data discrepancy queries and general information about obtaining research quality data will also be covered during the training session.

. . .

13.7. Quality Control of the Core Lab
Data from the Core Lab will be securely transmitted in batches and quality controlled in the same manner as Core Coordinating Center data; ie data will be entered and verified in the database on the Cleveland Clinic Foundation SUN with a subset later selected for additional quality control. Appropriate edit checks will be in place at the key entry (database) level. The Core Lab is to have an internal quality control system established prior to analyzing any FSGS [focal segmental glomerulosclerosis] samples. This system will be outlined in the Manual of Operations for the Core Lab(s) which is prepared and submitted by the Core Lab to the DCC [data coordinating centre] prior to initiating of the study.

At a minimum this system must include:
1) The inclusion of at least two known quality control samples; the reported measurements of the quality control samples must fall within specified ranges in order to be certified as acceptable.
2) Calibration at FDA approved manufacturers' recommended schedules.

13.8. Quality Control of the Biopsy Committee
The chair of the pathology committee will circulate to all of the study pathologists . . . samples [sic] biopsy specimens for evaluation after criteria to establish diagnosis of FSGS has been agreed. This internal review process will serve to ensure common criteria and assessment of biopsy specimens for confirmation of diagnosis of FSGS."[267]

Explanation

The validity and reliability of trial data depend on the quality of the data collection methods. The processes of acquiring and recording data often benefit from attention to training of study personnel and use of standardised, pilot tested methods. These should be identical for all study groups, unless precluded by the nature of the intervention.

The choice of methods for outcome assessment can affect study conduct and results.[268 269 270 271 272 273] Substantially different responses can be obtained for certain outcomes (eg, harms) depending on who answers the questions (eg, the participant or investigator) and how the questions are presented (eg, discrete options or open ended).[269 274 275 276] Also, when compared to paper based data collection, the use of electronic handheld devices and internet websites has the potential to improve protocol adherence, data accuracy, user acceptability, and timeliness of receiving data.[268 270 271 277]

The quality of data also depends on the reliability, validity, and responsiveness of data collection instruments such as questionnaires[278] or laboratory instruments. Instruments with low inter-rater reliability will reduce statistical power,[272] while those with low validity will not accurately measure the intended outcome variable. One study found that only 35% (47/133) of randomised trials in acute stroke used a measure with established reliability or validity.[279] Modified versions of validated measurement tools may no longer be considered validated, and use of unpublished measurement scales can introduce bias and inflate treatment effect sizes.[280]

Standard processes should be implemented by local study personnel to enhance data quality and reduce bias by detecting and reducing the amount of missing or incomplete data, inaccuracies, and excessive variability in measurements.[281 282 283 284 285] Examples include standardised training and testing of outcome assessors to promote consistency; tests of the validity or reliability of study instruments; and duplicate data measurements.

A clear protocol description of the data collection process—including the personnel, methods, instruments, and measures to promote data quality—can facilitate implementation and helps protocol reviewers to assess their appropriateness. Inclusion of data collection forms in the protocol (ie, as appendices) is highly recommended, as the way in which data are obtained can substantially affect the results. If not included in the protocol, then a reference to where the forms can be found should be provided. If performed, pilot testing and assessment of reliability and validity of the forms should also be described.

Data collection methods—retention

Item 18b: Plans to promote participant retention and complete follow-up, including list of any outcome data to be collected for participants who discontinue or deviate from intervention protocols

EXAMPLES

"**5.2.2 Retention**
. . . As with recruitment, retention addresses all levels of participant.

At the parent and student level, study investigators and staff:
• Provide written feedback to all parents of participating students about the results of the "health screenings" . . .
• Maintain interest in the study through materials and mailings . . .
• Send letters to parents and students prior to the final data collection, reminding them of the upcoming data collection and the incentives the students will receive.

At the school level, study investigators and staff:
• Provide periodic communications via newsletters and presentations to inform the school officials/staff, students, and parents about type 2 diabetes, the current status of the study, and plans for the next phase, as well as to acknowledge their support.

• . . .

• Become a presence in the intervention schools to monitor and maintain consistency in implementation, . . . be as flexible as possible with study schedule and proactive in resolving conflicts with schools.

• Provide school administration and faculty with the schedule or grid showing how the intervention fits into the school calendar . . .

• Solicit support from parents, school officials/staff, and teachers . . .

• Provide periodic incentives for school staff and teachers.

• Provide monetary incentives for the schools that increase with each year of the study . . . . [table 6]."[286]

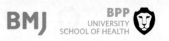

5.4 Infant Evaluations in the Case of Treatment Discontinuation or Study Withdrawal

All randomized infants completing the 18-month evaluation schedule will have fulfilled the infant clinical and laboratory evaluation requirements for the study. . .

All randomized infants who are prematurely discontinued from study drug will be considered *off study drug/on study* and will follow the same schedule of events as those infants who continue study treatment except adherence assessment. All of these infants will be followed through 18 months as scheduled. Randomized infants prematurely discontinued from the study before the 6-month evaluation will have the following clinical and laboratory evaluations performed, if possible: . . .

- Roche Amplicor HIV-1 DNA PCR [polymerase chain reaction] and cell pellet storage
- Plasma for storage (for NVP [nevirapine] resistance, HIV-1 RNA PCR and NVP concentration)
- . . .

Randomized infants prematurely discontinued from the study at any time after the 6-month evaluation will have the following clinical and laboratory evaluations performed, if possible:

. . .

5.5 Participant Retention

Once an infant is enrolled or randomized, the study site will make every reasonable effort to follow the infant for the entire study period . . . It is projected that the rate of loss-to-follow-up on an annual basis will be at most 5% . . . Study site staff are responsible for developing and implementing local standard operating procedures to achieve this level of follow-up.

5.6 Participant Withdrawal

Participants may withdraw from the study for any reason at any time. The investigator also may withdraw participants from the study in order to protect their safety and/or if they are unwilling or unable to comply with required study procedures after consultation with the Protocol Chair, National Institutes of Health (NIH) Medical Officers, Statistical and Data Management Center (SDMC) Protocol Statistician, and Coordinating and Operations Center (CORE) Protocol Specialist.

Participants also may be withdrawn if the study sponsor or government or regulatory authorities terminate the study prior to its planned end date.

Note: Early discontinuation of study product for any reason is not a reason for withdrawal from the study."[287]

Explanation

Trial investigators must often seek a balance between achieving a sufficiently long follow-up for clinically relevant outcome measurement,[122] [288] and a sufficiently short follow-up to decrease attrition and maximise completeness of data collection. Non-retention refers to instances where participants are prematurely "off-study" (ie, consent withdrawn or lost to follow-up) and thus outcome data cannot be obtained from them. The majority of trials will have some degree of non-retention, and the number of these "off-study" participants usually increases with the length of follow-up.[116]

It is desirable to plan ahead for how retention will be promoted in order to prevent missing data and avoid the associated complexities in both the study analysis (Item 20c) and interpretation. Certain methods can improve participant retention,[67] [152] [289] [290] [291] [292] such as financial reimbursement; systematic methods and reminders for contacting patients, scheduling appointments, and monitoring retention; and limiting participant burden related to follow-up visits and procedures (Item 13). A participant who withdraws consent for follow-up assessment of one outcome may be willing to continue with assessments for other outcomes, if given the option.

Non-retention should be distinguished from non-adherence.[293] Non-adherence refers to deviation from intervention protocols (Item 11c) or from the follow-up schedule of assessments (Item 13), but does not mean that the participant is "off-study" and no longer in the trial. Because missing data can be a major threat to trial validity and statistical power, non-adherence should not be an automatic reason for ceasing to collect data from the trial participant prior to study completion. In particular for randomised trials, it is widely recommended that all participants be included in an intention to treat analysis, regardless of adherence (Item 20c).

Protocols should describe any retention strategies and define which outcome data will be recorded from protocol non-adherers.[152] Protocols should also detail any plans to record the reasons for non-adherence (eg, discontinuation of intervention due to harms versus lack of efficacy) and non-retention (ie, consent withdrawn; lost to follow-up), as this information can influence the handling of missing data and interpretation of results.[152] [294] [295]

Data management

Item 19: Plans for data entry, coding, security, and storage, including any related processes to promote data quality (eg, double data entry; range checks for data values). Reference to where details of data management procedures can be found, if not in the protocol

---

Table 6 Excerpts from table showing compensation provided in study[286]

Who	What	Amount
School		
Intervention school	School program enhancement	$2000 in year 1, $3000 in year 3, $4000 in year 3
	Physical education class equipment required to implement intervention	$15 000 over 3 years
	Food service department to defray costs of nutrition intervention	$3000/year
Control school	School program enhancement	$2000 in year 1, $4000 in year 2, $6000 in year 3
Student		
All	Return consent form (signed or not)	Gift item worth ~ $5
	Participation in health screening data collection measures and forms	$50 baseline (6th grade), $10 interim (7th grade), $60 end of study (8th grade)
Family		
Intervention parents	Focus groups to provide input about family outreach events and activities	$35/year per parent, up to two focus groups per field center, 6-10 participants per focus group

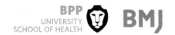

EXAMPLE

"**13.9.2. Data Forms and Data Entry**

In the FSGS-CT [focal segmental glomerulosclerosis—clinical trial], all data will be entered electronically. This may be done at a Core Coordinating Center or at the participating site where the data originated. Original study forms will be entered and kept on file at the participating site. A subset will be requested later for quality control; when a form is selected, the participating site staff will pull that form, copy it, and sent [sic] the copy to the DCC [data coordinating center] for re-entry.

. . . Participant files are to be stored in numerical order and stored in a secure and accessible place and manner. Participant files will be maintained in storage for a period of 3 years after completion of the study.

13.9.3. Data Transmission and Editing

The data entry screens will resemble the paper forms approved by the steering committee. Data integrity will be enforced through a variety of mechanisms. Referential data rules, valid values, range checks, and consistency checks against data already stored in the database (ie, longitudinal checks) will be supported. The option to chose [sic] a value from a list of valid codes and a description of what each code means will be available where applicable. Checks will be applied at the time of data entry into a specific field and/or before the data is written (committed) to the database. Modifications to data written to the database will be documented through either the data change system or an inquiry system. Data entered into the database will be retrievable for viewing through the data entry applications. The type of activity that an individual user may undertake is regulated by the privileges associated with his/her user identification code and password.

13.9.4. Data Discrepancy Inquiries and Reports to Core Coordinating Centers

Additional errors will be detected by programs designed to detect missing data or specific errors in the data. These errors will be summarized along with detailed descriptions for each specific problem in Data Query Reports, which will be sent to the Data Managers at the Core Coordinating Centers . . .

The Data Manager who receives the inquiry will respond by checking the original forms for inconsistency, checking other sources to determine the correction, modifying the original (paper) form entering a response to the query. Note that it will be necessary for Data Managers to respond to each inquiry received in order to obtain closure on the queried item.

The Core Coordinating Center and participating site personnel will be responsible for making appropriate corrections to the original paper forms whenever any data item is changed . . . Written documentation of changes will be available via electronic logs and audit trails.

. . .

Biopsy and biochemistry reports will be sent via e-mail when data are received from the Core Lab.

. . .

13.9.5. Security and Back-Up of Data

. . . All forms, diskettes and tapes related to study data will be kept in locked cabinets. Access to the study data will be restricted. In addition, Core Coordinating Centers will only have access to their own center's data. A password system will be utilized to control access . . . These passwords will be changed on a regular basis. All reports prepared by the DCC will be prepared such that no individual subject can be identified.

A complete back up of the primary DCC database will be performed twice a month. These tapes will be stored off-site in a climate-controlled facility and will be retained indefinitely. Incremental data back-ups will be performed on a daily basis. These tapes will be retained for at least one week on-site. Back-ups of periodic data analysis files will also be kept. These tapes will be retained at the off-site location until the Study is completed and the database is on file with NIH [National Institutes of Health]. In addition to the system back-ups, additional measures will be taken to back-up and export the database on a regular basis at the database management level. . .

13.9.6. Study status reports

The DCC will send weekly email reports with information on missing data, missing forms, and missing visits. Personnel at the Core Coordinating Center and the Participating Sites should review these reports for accuracy and report any discrepancies to the DCC.

. . .

13.9.8. Description of Hardware at DCC

A SUN Workstation environment is maintained in the department with a SUN SPARCstation 10 model 41 as the server . . . Primary access to the departments [sic] computing facilities will be through the Internet . . . For maximum programming efficiency, the Oracle database management system and the SAS and BMDP statistical analysis systems will be employed for this study. . . .

Oracle facilitates sophisticated integrity checks through a variety of mechanisms including stored procedures, stored triggers, and declarative database integrity—for between table verifications. Oracle allows data checks to be programmed once in the database rather than repeating the same checks among many applications . . . Security is enforced through passwords and may be assigned at different levels to groups and individuals."[267]

Explanation

Careful planning of data management with appropriate personnel can help to prevent flaws that compromise data validity. The protocol should provide a full description of the data entry and coding processes, along with measures to promote their quality, or provide key elements and a reference to where full information can be found. These details are particularly important for the primary outcome data. The protocol should also document data security measures to prevent unauthorised access to or loss of participant data, as well as plans for data storage (including timeframe) during and after the trial. This information facilitates an assessment of adherence to applicable standards and regulations.

Differences in data entry methods can affect the trial in terms of data accuracy,[268] cost, and efficiency.[271] For example, when compared with paper case report forms, electronic data capture can reduce the time required for data entry, query resolution, and database release by combining data entry with data collection (Item 18a).[271][277] When data are collected on paper forms, data entry can be performed locally or at a central site. Local data entry can enable fast

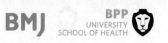

correction of missing or inaccurate data, while central data entry facilitates blinding (masking), standardisation, and training of a core group of data entry personnel.

Raw, non-numeric data are usually coded for ease of data storage, review, tabulation, and analysis. It is important to define standard coding practices to reduce errors and observer variation. When data entry and coding are performed by different individuals, it is particularly important that the personnel use unambiguous, standardised terminology and abbreviations to avoid misinterpretation.

As with data collection (Item 18a), standard processes are often implemented to improve the accuracy of data entry and coding.[281] [284] Common examples include double data entry[296]; verification that the data are in the proper format (eg, integer) or within an expected range of values; and independent source document verification of a random subset of data to identify missing or apparently erroneous values. Though widely performed to detect data entry errors, the time and costs of independent double data entry from paper forms need to be weighed against the magnitude of reduction in error rates compared to single-data entry.[297] [298] [299]

Statistical methods

The planned methods of statistical analysis should be fully described in the protocol. If certain aspects of the analysis plan cannot be prespecified (eg, the method of handling missing data is contingent on examining patterns of "missingness" before study unblinding), then the planned approach to making the final methodological choices should be outlined. Some trials have a separate document—commonly called a statistical analysis plan (SAP)—that fully details the planned analyses. Any SAP should be described in the protocol, including its key elements and where it can be found. As with the protocol, the SAP should be dated, amendments noted and dated, and the SAP authors provided.

Statistical methods—outcomes

Item 20a: Statistical methods for analysing primary and secondary outcomes. Reference to where other details of the statistical analysis plan can be found, if not in the protocol

---

EXAMPLE

"The intervention arm (SMS [short message system (text message)]) will be compared against the control (SOC [standard of care]) for all primary analysis. We will use chi-squared test for binary outcomes, and T-test for continuous outcomes. For subgroup analyses, we will use regression methods with appropriate interaction terms (respective subgroup×treatment group). Multivariable analyses will be based on logistic regression . . . for binary outcomes and linear regression for continuous outcomes. We will examine the residual to assess model assumptions and goodness-of-fit. For timed endpoints such as mortality we will use the Kaplan-Meier survival analysis followed by multivariable Cox proportional hazards model for adjusting for baseline variables. We will calculate Relative Risk (RR) and RR Reductions (RRR) with corresponding 95% confidence intervals to compare dichotomous variables, and difference in means will be used for additional analysis of continuous variables. P-values will be reported to four decimal places with p-values less than 0.001 reported as p < 0.001. Up-to-date versions of SAS (Cary, NC) and SPSS (Chicago, IL) will be used to conduct analyses. For all tests, we will use 2-sided p-values with alpha ≤0.05 level of significance. We will use

---

the Bonferroni method to appropriately adjust the overall level of significance for multiple primary outcomes, and secondary outcomes.
To assess the impact of potential clustering for patients cared by the same clinic, we will use generalized estimating equations [GEE] assuming an exchangeable correlation structure. Table [7] provides a summary of methods of analysis for each variable. Professional academic statisticians (LT, RN) blinded to study groups will conduct all analyses."[47]

Explanation

The protocol should indicate explicitly each intended analysis comparing study groups. An unambiguous, complete, and transparent description of statistical methods facilitates execution, replication, critical appraisal, and the ability to track any changes from the original pre-specified methods.

Results for the primary outcome can be substantially affected by the choice of analysis methods. When investigators apply more than one analysis strategy for a specific primary outcome, there is potential for inappropriate selective reporting of the most interesting result.[6] The protocol should prespecify the main ("primary") analysis of the primary outcome (Item 12), including the analysis methods to be used for statistical comparisons (Items 20a and 20b); precisely which trial participants will be included (Item 20c); and how missing data will be handled (Item 20c). Additionally, it is helpful to indicate the effect measure (eg, relative risk) and significance level that will be used, as well as the intended use of confidence intervals when presenting results.

The same considerations will often apply equally to prespecified secondary and exploratory outcomes. In some instances, descriptive approaches to evaluating rare outcomes such as adverse events—might be preferred over formal analysis given the lack of power.[300] Adequately powered analyses may require preplanned meta-analyses with results from other studies.

Most trials are affected to some extent by multiplicity issues.[301] [302] When multiple statistical comparisons are performed (eg, multiple study groups, outcomes, interim analyses), the risk of false positive (type 1) error is inflated and there is increased potential for selective reporting of favourable comparisons in the final trial report. For trials with more than two study groups, it is important to specify in the protocol which comparisons (of two or more study groups) will be performed and, if relevant, which will be the main comparison of interest. The same principle of specifying the main comparison also applies when there is more than one outcome, including when the same variable is measured at several time points (Item 12). Any statistical approaches to account for multiple comparisons and time points should also be described.

Finally, different trial designs dictate the most appropriate analysis plan and any additional relevant information that should be included in the protocol. For example, cluster, factorial, crossover, and within-person randomised trials require specific statistical considerations, such as how clustering will be handled in a cluster randomised trial.

Statistical methods—additional analyses

Item 20b: Methods for any additional analyses (eg, subgroup and adjusted analyses)

EXAMPLES

"We plan to conduct two subgroup analyses, both with strong biological rationale and possible interaction effects. The first will compare hazard ratios of re-operation based upon the

---

degree of soft tissue injury (Gustilo-Anderson Type I/II open fractures vs. Gustilo-Anderson Type IIIA/B open fractures). The second will compare hazard ratios of re-operation between fractures of the upper and lower extremity. We will test if the treatment effects differ with fracture types and extremities by putting their main effect and interaction terms in the Cox regression. For the comparison of pressure, we anticipate that the low/gravity flow will be more effective in the Type IIIA-B open fracture than in the Type I/II open fracture, and be more effective in the upper extremity than the lower extremity. For the comparison of solution, we anticipate that soap will do better in the Type IIIA-B open fracture than in the Type I/II open fracture, and better in the upper extremity than the lower extremity."[303]

"A secondary analysis of the primary endpoint will adjust for those pre-randomization variables which might reasonably be expected to be predictive of favorable outcomes. Generalized linear models will be used to model the proportion of subjects with neurologically intact (MRS , 3 [Modified Rankin Score]) survival to hospital discharge by ITD [impedance threshold device]/sham device group adjusted for site (dummy variables modeling the 11 ROC [Resuscitation Outcomes Consortium] sites), patient sex, patient age (continuous variable), witness status (dummy variables modeling the three categories of unwitnessed arrest, non-EMS [emergency medical services] witnessed arrest, and EMS witnessed arrest), location of arrest (public versus non-public), time or response (continuous variable modeling minutes between call to 911 and arrival of EMS providers on scene), presenting rhythm (dummy variables modeling asystole, PEA [pulseless electrical activity], VT/VF [ventricular tachycardia/fibrillation], or unknown), and treatment assignment in the Analyze Late vs. Analyze Early intervention. The test statistic used to assess any benefit of the ITD relative to the sham device will be computed as the generalized linear model regression coefficient divided by the estimated "robust" standard error based on the Huber-White sandwich estimator[reference] in order to account for within group variability which might depart from the classical assumptions. Statistical inference will be based on one-sided P values and 95% confidence intervals which adjust for the stopping rule used for the primary analysis."[304]

Explanation

Subgroup analysis

Subgroup analyses explore whether estimated treatment effects vary significantly between subcategories of trial participants. As these data can help tailor healthcare decisions to individual patients, a modest number of prespecified subgroup analyses can be sensible.

However, subgroup analyses are problematic if they are inappropriately conducted or selectively reported. Subgroup analyses described in protocols or grant applications do not match those reported in subsequent publications for more than two thirds of randomised trials, suggesting that subgroup analyses are often selectively reported or not prespecified.[67305] Post hoc (data driven) analyses have a high risk of spurious findings and are discouraged.[306] Conducting a large number of subgroup comparisons leads to issues of multiplicity, even when all of the comparisons have been pre-specified. Furthermore, when subgroups are based on variables measured after randomisation, the analyses are particularly susceptible to bias.[307]

Preplanned subgroup analyses should be clearly specified in the protocol with respect to the precise baseline variables to be examined, the definition of the subgroup categories (including cut-off boundaries for continuous or ordinal variables), the statistical method to be used, and

the hypothesised direction of the subgroup effect based on plausibility.[308309]

Adjusted analysis

Some trials prespecify adjusted analyses to account for imbalances between study groups (eg, chance imbalance across study groups in small trials), improve power, or account for a known prognostic variable. Adjustment is often recommended for any variables used in the allocation process (eg, in stratified randomisation), on the principle that the analysis strategy should match the design.[310] Most trial protocols and publications do not adequately address issues of adjustment, particularly the description of variables.[6310]

It is important that trial investigators indicate in the protocol if there is an intention to perform or consider adjusted analyses, explicitly specifying any variables for adjustment and how continuous variables will be handled. When both unadjusted and adjusted analyses are intended, the main analysis should be identified (Item 20a). It may not always be clear, in advance, which variables will be important for adjustment. In such situations, the objective criteria to be used to select variables should be prespecified. As with subgroup analyses, adjustment variables based on post-randomisation data rather than baseline data can introduce bias.[311312]

Statistical methods—analysis population and missing data

Item 20c: Definition of analysis population relating to protocol non-adherence (eg, as randomised analysis), and any statistical methods to handle missing data (eg, multiple imputation)

EXAMPLE

"Nevertheless, we propose to test non-inferiority using two analysis sets; the intention-to-treat set, considering all patients as randomized regardless of whether they received the randomized treatment, and the "per protocol" analysis set. Criteria for determining the "per protocol" group assignment would be established by the Steering Committee and approved by the PSMB [performance and safety monitoring board] before the trial begins. Given our expectation that very few patients will crossover or be lost to follow-up, these analyses should agree very closely. We propose declaring medical management non-inferior to interventional therapy, only if shown to be non-inferior using both the "intention to treat" and "per protocol" analysis sets.

. . .

10.4.7 Imputation Procedure for Missing Data

While the analysis of the primary endpoint (death or stroke) will be based on a log-rank test and, therefore, not affected by patient withdrawals (as they will be censored) provided that dropping out is unrelated to prognosis; other outcomes, such as the Rankin Score at five years post-randomization, could be missing for patients who withdraw from the trial. We will report reasons for withdrawal for each randomization group and compare the reasons qualitatively . . . The effect that any missing data might have on results will be assessed via sensitivity analysis of augmented data sets. Dropouts (essentially, participants who withdraw consent for continued follow-up) will be included in the analysis by modern imputation methods for missing data.

The main feature of the approach is the creation of a set of clinically reasonable imputations for the respective outcome for each dropout. This will be accomplished using a set of repeated imputations created by predictive models based on the majority of participants with complete data. The imputation models will reflect uncertainty in the modeling process and

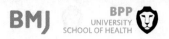

Table 7 Variables, measures, and methods of analysis (reproduced from original table[47])

Variable/outcome	Hypothesis	Outcome measure	Methods of analysis
1) Primary	Intervention improved outcome from baseline to (months		
a) Adherence at 12 months		Percent adherence in previous 30 days >95% [binary]	Chi-squared test
b) Suppression of HIV viral load at 12 months		Viral load ≤400 copies/ml [binary]	Chi-squared test
2) Secondary	improvement occurred	Adherence % (>95%) [binary]	Chi-squared test
Adherence percentage at 12 months			
HIV viral load at 12 months	improvement occurred	Viral load (copies)	T-test
Immune reconstitution (change in CD4 T cell count from baseline)	improvement occurred	CD4 T-cells/mm³ (continuous)	T-test
Time to virological failure	improvement occurred	Virological failure after successful suppression	Kaplan-Meier survival analysis
Weight gain [lbs] and BMI	improvement occurred	Change in weight (lbs) and BMI [continuous]	T-test
Occurrence of opportunistic infections (OIs)	improvement occurred	Presence of AIDS defining opportunistic infection [binary]	Chi-squared test
Time to reporting of adverse drug events (ADEs)	improvement occurred	Presence of drug-related adverse event [time to event]	Kaplan-Meier survival analysis
Deaths (all cause)	improvement occurred	All-cause mortality [binary]	Chi-squared test and Kaplan-Meier survival analysis
SF-12 [short form 12 adapted for regional application in Kiswahili]	improvement occurred	Quality pf [sic] life questionnaire [continuous]	T-test
Satisfaction with care provided	improvement occurred	Questionnaire [continuous]	T-test
Level of disclosure of HIV status	improvement occurred	Disclosed to a family member [binary]	Chi-squared test
Impression of stigma	improvement occurred	Questionnaire [continuous]	T-test
Family dyamics [sic]	improvement occurred	Questionnaire [continuous]	T-test
Employment attendance	improvement occurred	Questionnaire [continuous]	T-test
Household member school attendance	improvement occurred	Questionnaire [continuous]	T-test
Cell phones lost/stolen	improvement occurred	Presence of cellphone [binary]	Poisson regression
Stopped taking HAART [highly active antiretroviral therapy]	improvement occurred	Self-report [binary]	Chi-squared test
Required active tracing for 12 month follow-up	improvement occurred	Field officers [binary]	Chi-squared test
3) Subgroup Analyses:			Regression methods with appropriate interaction term
Urban vs. rural	Distance affects adherence		
Female vs. male	Sex affects adherence		
Phone ownership (owned vs. shared)	Ownership affects adherence		
Level of education	Low education affects adherence		
4) Sensitivity Analyses:	improvement occurred	All outcomes	
a) Per protocol analysis			a) Chi-squared/T-test
b) Adjusting for baseline covariates			b) Multivariable regression
c) clustering among individuals within a clinic			c) GEE

IMPORTANT REMARKS:

- *The GEE [generalised estimating equations] [reference] is a technique that allows to specify the correlation structure between patients within a hospital and this approach produces unbiased estimates under the assumption that missing observations will be missing at random. An amended approach of weighted GEE will be employed if missingness is found not to be at random [reference].*
- *In all analyses results will be expressed as coefficient, standard errors, corresponding 95% and associated p-values.*
- *Goodness-of-fit will be assessed by examining the residuals for model assumptions and chi-squared test of goodness-of-fit.*
- *Bonferroni method will be used to adjust the overall level of significance for multiple secondary outcomes.*

inherent variability in patient outcomes, as reflected in the complete data.

After the imputations are completed, all of the data (complete and imputed) will be combined and the analysis performed for each imputed-and-completed dataset. Rubin's method of multiple (ie, repeated) imputation will be used to estimate treatment effect. We propose to use 15 datasets (an odd number to allow use of one of the datasets to represent the median analytic result).

These methods are preferable to simple mean imputation, or simple "best-worst" or "worst-worst" imputation, because the categorization of patients into clinically meaningful subgroups, and the imputation of their missing data by appropriately different models, accords well with best clinical judgment concerning the likely outcomes of the dropouts, and therefore will enhance the trial's results."[313]

Explanation

In order to preserve the unique benefit of randomisation as a mechanism to avoid selection bias, an "as randomised" analysis retains participants in the group to which they were originally allocated. To prevent attrition bias, outcome data obtained from all participants are included in the data analysis, regardless of protocol adherence (Items 11c and 18b).[249] [250] These two conditions (ie, all participants, as randomised) define an "intention to treat" analysis, which is widely recommended as the preferred analysis strategy.[17]

Some trialists use other types of data analyses (commonly labelled as "modified intention to treat" or "per protocol") that exclude data from certain participants—such as those who are found to be ineligible after randomisation or who deviate from the intervention or follow-up protocols. This exclusion of data from protocol non-adherers can introduce bias, particularly if the frequency of and the reasons for non-adherence vary between the study groups.[314] [315] In some trials, the participants to be included in the analysis will vary by outcome—for example, analysis of harms (adverse events) is sometimes restricted to participants who received the intervention, so that absence or occurrence of harm is not attributed to a treatment that was never received.

Protocols should explicitly describe which participants will be included in the main analyses (eg, all randomised participants, regardless of protocol adherence) and define the study group in which they will be analysed (eg, as randomised). In one cohort of randomised trials approved in 1994-5, this information was missing in half of the protocols.[6] The ambiguous use of labels such as "intention to treat" or "per protocol" should be avoided unless they are fully defined in the protocol.[6 314] Most analyses labelled as "intention to treat" do not actually adhere to its definition because of missing data or exclusion of participants who do not meet certain post-randomisation criteria (eg, specific level of adherence to intervention).[6 316] Other ambiguous labels such as "modified intention to treat" are also variably defined from one trial to another.[314]

In addition to defining the analysis population, it is necessary to address the problem of missing data in the protocol. Most trials have some degree of missing data,[317 318] which can introduce bias depending on the pattern of "missingness" (eg, not missing at random). Strategies to maximise follow-up and prevent missing data, as well as the recording of reasons for missing data, are thus important to develop and document (Item 18b).[152]

The protocol should also state how missing data will be handled in the analysis and detail any planned methods to impute (estimate) missing outcome data, including which variables will be used in the imputation process (if applicable).[152] Different statistical approaches can lead to different results and conclusions,[317 319] but one study found that only 23% of trial protocols specified the planned statistical methods to account for missing data.[6]

Imputation of missing data allows the analysis to conform to intention to treat analysis but requires strong assumptions that are untestable and may be hard to justify.[152 318 320 321] Methods of multiple imputation are more complex but are widely preferred to single imputation methods (eg, last observation carried forward; baseline observation carried forward), as the latter introduce greater bias and produce confidence intervals that are too narrow.[152 320 321 322] Specific issues arise when outcome data are missing for crossover or cluster randomised trials.[323] Finally, sensitivity analyses are highly recommended to assess the robustness of trial results under different methods of handling missing data.[152 324]

Section 3d: Methods—monitoring

Data monitoring—formal committee

Item 21a: Composition of data monitoring committee (DMC); summary of its role and reporting structure; statement of whether it is independent from the sponsor and competing interests; and reference to where further details about its charter can be found, if not in the protocol. Alternatively, an explanation of why a DMC is not needed

---

EXAMPLE

"Appendix 3. Charter and responsibilities of the Data Monitoring Committee

A Data Monitoring Committee (DMC) has been established. The DMC is independent of the study organisers. During the period of recruitment to the study, interim analyses will be supplied, in strict confidence, to the DMC, together with any other analyses that the committee may request. This may include analyses of data from other comparable trials. In the light of these interim analyses, the DMC will advise the TSC [trial steering committee] if, in its view:

---

a) the active intervention has been proved, beyond reasonable doubt*, to be different from the control (standard management) for all or some types of participants, and

b) the evidence on the economic outcomes is sufficient to guide a decision from health care providers regarding recommendation of early lens extraction for PACG [primary angle closure glaucoma].

The TSC can then decide whether or not to modify intake to the trial. Unless this happens, however, the TSC, PMG [project management group], clinical collaborators and study office staff (except those who supply the confidential analyses) will remain ignorant of the interim results.

The frequency of interim analyses will depend on the judgement of the Chair of the DMC, in consultation with the TSC. However, we anticipate that there might be three interim analyses and one final analysis.

The Chair is Mr *D.G.-H.*, with Dr*D.C.*, and Professor *B.D.* Terms of reference for the DMC are available on request from the EAGLE [Effectiveness in Angle Closure Glaucoma of Lens Extraction] study office.

*Appropriate criteria for proof beyond reasonable doubt cannot be specified precisely. A difference of at least three standard deviation [sic] in the interim analysis of a major endpoint may be needed to justify halting, or modifying, such a study prematurely.[reference]"[325]

Explanation

For some trials, there are important reasons for periodic inspection of the accumulating outcome data by study group. In principle, a trial should be modified or discontinued when the accumulated data have sufficiently disturbed the clinical equipoise that justified the initiation of the trial. Data monitoring can also inform aspects of trial conduct, such as recruitment, and identify the need to make adjustments.

The decision to have a data monitoring committee (DMC) will be influenced by local standards. While certain trials warrant some form of data monitoring, many do not need a formal committee,[326] such as trials with a short duration or known minimal risks. A DMC was described in 65% (98/150) of cancer trial protocols with time-to-event outcomes in Italy in 2000-5,[327] and in 17% (12/70) of protocols for Danish randomised trials approved in 1994-5.[6] About 40% of clinical trials registered on ClinicalTrials.gov from 2007-2010 reported having a DMC.[328] The protocol should either state that there will be a DMC and provide further details, as discussed below, or indicate that there will not be a DMC, preferably with reasons.

When formal data monitoring is performed, it is often done by a DMC consisting of members from a variety of disciplines.[254 329] The primary role of a DMC is to periodically review the accumulating data and determine if a trial should be modified or discontinued. The DMC does not usually have executive power; rather, it communicates the outcome of its deliberations to the trial steering committee or sponsor.

Independence, in particular from the sponsor and trial investigators, is a key characteristic of the DMC and can be broadly defined as the committee comprising members who are "completely uninvolved in the running of the trial and who cannot be unfairly influenced (either directly or indirectly) by people, or institutions, involved in the trial."[254] DMC members are usually required to declare any competing interests (Item 28). Among the 12 trial protocols that described a DMC and were approved in Denmark in 1994-5,[6] four explicitly stated that the DMC was independent from

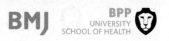

the sponsor and investigators; three had non-independent DMCs; and independence was unclear for the remaining five protocols.

The protocol should name the chair and members of the DMC. If the members are not yet known, the protocol can indicate the intended size and characteristics of the membership until further details are available. The protocol should also indicate the DMC's roles and responsibilities, planned method of functioning, and degree of independence from those conducting, sponsoring, or funding the trial.[254][330][331] A charter is recommended for detailing this information[331]; if this charter is not appended to the protocol, the protocol should indicate whether a charter exists or will be developed, and if so, where it can be accessed.

Data monitoring—interim analysis

Item 21b: Description of any interim analyses and stopping guidelines, including who will have access to these interim results and make the final decision to terminate the trial

---

EXAMPLE

"Premature termination of the study
An interim-analysis is performed on the primary endpoint when 50% of patients have been randomised and have completed the 6 months follow-up. The interim-analysis is performed by an independent statistician, blinded for the treatment allocation. The statistician will report to the independent DSMC [data and safety monitoring committee]. The DSMC will have unblinded access to all data and will discuss the results of the interim-analysis with the steering committee in a joint meeting. The steering committee decides on the continuation of the trial and will report to the central ethics committee. The Peto approach is used: the trial will be ended using symmetric stopping boundaries at P < 0.001 [reference]. The trial will not be stopped in case of futility, unless the DSMC during the course of safety monitoring advices [sic] otherwise. In this case DSMC will discuss potential stopping for futility with the trial steering committee."[332]

Explanation
Interim analyses can be conducted as part of an adaptive trial design to formally monitor the accumulating data in clinical trials. They are generally performed in trials that have a DMC, longer duration of recruitment, and potentially serious outcomes. Interim analyses were described in 71% (106/150) of cancer trial protocols with time-to-event outcomes in Italy in 2000-5,[327] and in 19% (13/70) of protocols for Danish randomised trials approved in 1994-5.[6] The results of these analyses, along with non-statistical criteria, can be part of a stopping guideline that helps inform whether the trial should be continued, modified, or halted earlier than intended for benefit, harm, or futility. Criteria for stopping for harm are often different from those for benefit and might not employ a formal statistical criterion.[333] Stopping for futility occurs in instances where, if the study were to continue, it is unlikely that an important effect would be seen (ie, low chance of rejecting null hypothesis). Multiple analyses of the accumulating data increase the risk of a false positive (type I) error, and various statistical strategies have been developed to compensate for this inflated risk.[254][333][334][335] Aside from informing stopping guidelines, prespecified interim analyses can be used for other trial adaptations such as sample size re-estimation, alteration to the proportion of participants allocated to each study group, and changes to eligibility criteria.[111]

A complete description of any interim analysis plan, even if it is only to be performed at the request of an oversight body (eg, DMC), should be provided in the protocol—including the statistical methods, who will perform the analyses, and when they will be conducted (timing and indications). If applicable, details should also be provided about the decision criteria—statistical or other—that will be adopted to judge the interim results as part of a guideline for early stopping or other adaptations. Among 86 protocols for randomised trials with a time-to-event cancer outcome that proposed efficacy interim analyses, all stated the planned timing of the analyses, 91% specified the overall reason to be used for stopping (eg, superiority, futility), and 94% detailed the statistical approach.[327]

In addition, it is important to state who will see the outcome data while the trial is ongoing, whether these individuals will remain blinded (masked) to study groups, and how the integrity of the trial implementation will be protected (eg, maintaining blinding) when any adaptations to the trial are made. A third of protocols for industry initiated randomised trials receiving Danish ethics approval in 1994-95 stated that the sponsor had access to accumulating trial data, which can introduce potential bias due to competing interests.[10] Finally, the protocol should specify who has the ultimate authority to stop or modify the trial—eg, the principal investigator, trial steering committee, or sponsor.

Harms

Item 22: Plans for collecting, assessing, reporting, and managing solicited and spontaneously reported adverse events and other unintended effects of trial interventions or trial conduct

---

EXAMPLE
"Secondary outcomes
. . . In our study an adverse event will be defined as any untoward medical occurrence in a subject without regard to the possibility of a causal relationship. Adverse events will be collected after the subject has provided consent and enrolled in the study. If a subject experiences an adverse event after the informed consent document is signed (entry) but the subject has not started to receive study intervention, the event will be reported as not related to study drug. All adverse events occurring after entry into the study and until hospital discharge will be recorded. An adverse event that meets the criteria for a serious adverse event (SAE) between study enrollment and hospital discharge will be reported to the local IRB [institutional review board] as an SAE. If haloperidol is discontinued as a result of an adverse event, study personnel will document the circumstances and data leading to discontinuation of treatment. A serious adverse event for this study is any untoward medical occurrence that is believed by the investigators to be causally related to study-drug and results in any of the following: Life-threatening condition (that is, immediate risk of death); severe or permanent disability, prolonged hospitalization, or a significant hazard as determined by the data safety monitoring board. Serious adverse events occurring after a subject is discontinued from the study will NOT be reported unless the investigators feels that the event may have been caused by the study drug or a protocol procedure. Investigators will determine relatedness of an event to study drug based on a temporal relationship to the study drug, as well as whether the event is unexpected or unexplained given the subject's clinical course, previous medical conditions, and concomitant medications.
. . . The study will monitor for the following movement-related adverse effects daily through patient examination and chart

---

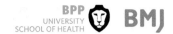

review: dystonia, akathisia, pseudoparkinsonism, akinesia, and neuroleptic malignant syndrome. Study personnel will use the Simpson-Angus [reference] and Barnes Akathisia [reference] scales to monitor movement-related effects.

. . .

For secondary outcomes, binary measures, eg mortality and complications, logistic regression will be used to test the intervention effect, controlling for covariates when appropriate."[266]

. .

Explanation

Evaluation of harms has a key role in monitoring the condition of participants during a trial and in enabling appropriate management of adverse events. Documentation of trial related adverse events also informs clinical practice and the conduct of ongoing and future studies. We use the term "harms" instead of "safety" to better reflect the negative effects of interventions.[300] An adverse event refers to an untoward occurrence during the trial, which may or may not be causally related to the intervention or other aspects of trial participation.[300 336] This definition includes unfavourable changes in symptoms, signs, laboratory values, or health conditions. In the context of clinical trials, it can be difficult to attribute causation for a given adverse event. An adverse effect is a type of adverse event that can be attributed to the intervention.

Harms can be specified as primary or secondary outcomes (Item 12) or can be assessed as part of routine monitoring. To the extent possible, distinctions should be made between adverse events that are anticipated versus unanticipated, and solicited versus unsolicited, because expectation can influence the number and perceived severity of recorded events. For example, providing statements in the informed consent process about the possibility of a particular adverse effect or using structured, as opposed to open ended, questionnaires for data collection, can increase the reporting of specific events ("priming").[269 337 338 339] The timeframe for recording adverse events can also affect the type of data obtained.[340 341]

The protocol should describe the procedures for and frequency of harms data collection, the overall surveillance timeframe, any instruments to be used, and their validity and reliability, if known. Substantial discrepancies have been observed between protocol specified plans for adverse event collection and reporting, and what is described in final publications.[5] Although trials are often not powered to detect important differences in rates of uncommon adverse events, it is also important to describe plans for data analysis, including formal hypothesis testing or descriptive statistics.[300 342]

Finally, the protocol should address the reporting of harms to relevant groups (eg, sponsor, research ethics committee/institutional review board, data monitoring committee, regulatory agency), which is an important process that is subject to local regulation.[343] Key considerations include the severity of the adverse event, determination of potential causality, and whether it represents an unexpected or anticipated event. For multicentre studies, procedures and timing should be outlined for central collection, evaluation, and reporting of pooled harms data.

Auditing

Item 23: Frequency and procedures for auditing trial conduct, if any, and whether the process will be independent from investigators and the sponsor

Explanation

Auditing involves periodic independent review of core trial processes and documents. It is distinct from routine day-to-day measures to promote data quality (Items 18a and 19). Auditing is intended to preserve the integrity of the trial by independently verifying a variety of processes and prompting corrective action if necessary. The processes reviewed can relate to participant enrolment, consent, eligibility, and allocation to study groups; adherence to

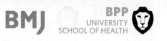

trial interventions and policies to protect participants, including reporting of harms (Item 22); and completeness, accuracy, and timeliness of data collection. In addition, an audit can verify adherence to applicable policies such as the International Conference on Harmonisation*Good Clinical Practice* and regulatory agency guidelines.[160]

In multicentre trials, auditing is usually considered both overall and for each recruiting centre. Audits can be done by exploring the trial dataset or performing site visits. Audits might be initially conducted across all sites, and subsequently conducted using a risk based approach that focuses, for example, on sites that have the highest enrolment rates, large numbers of withdrawals, or atypical (low or high) numbers of reported adverse events.

If auditing is planned, the procedures and anticipated frequency should be outlined in the protocol, including a description of the personnel involved and their degree of independence from the trial investigators and sponsor. If procedures are further detailed elsewhere (eg, audit manual), then the protocol should reference where the full details can be obtained.

Section 4: Ethics and dissemination

Research ethics approval

Item 24: Plans for seeking research ethics committee/ institutional review board (REC/IRB) approval

> **EXAMPLE**
>
> "This protocol and the template informed consent forms contained in Appendix II will be reviewed and approved by the sponsor and the applicable IRBs/ECs [institutional review boards/ethical committees] with respect to scientific content and compliance with applicable research and human subjects regulations. . . .
>
> The protocol, site-specific informed consent forms (local language and English versions), participant education and recruitment materials, and other requested documents—and any subsequent modifications — also will be reviewed and approved by the ethical review bodies. . .
>
> Subsequent to initial review and approval, the responsible local Institutional Review Boards/Ethical Committees (IRBs/ ECs) will review the protocol at least annually. The Investigator will make safety and progress reports to the IRBs/ECs at least annually and within three months of study termination or completion at his/her site. These reports will include the total number of participants enrolled . . . and summaries of each DSMB [data safety and monitoring board] review of safety and/ or efficacy."[287]

Explanation

A universal requirement for the ethical conduct of clinical research is the review and approval of the research protocol by qualified individuals who are not associated with the research team and have no disqualifying competing interests as reviewers.[1] The review is typically conducted by a formal REC/IRB in accordance with jurisdictional policy. Despite the importance of ethics review, approval by a REC/ IRB is not always obtained. Among 767 trials published in leading general medical journals from 1993-95, 37 authors (5%) disclosed that such approval had not been sought for their trials.[344] The protocol should document where approval has been obtained, or outline plans to seek such approval.

Protocol amendments

Item 25: Plans for communicating important protocol modifications (eg, changes to eligibility criteria, outcomes, analyses) to relevant parties (eg, investigators, REC/IRBs, trial participants, trial registries, journals, regulators)

> **EXAMPLE**
>
> **"13.10 Modification of the Protocol**
> Any modifications to the protocol which may impact on the conduct of the study, potential benefit of the patient or may affect patient safety, including changes of study objectives, study design, patient population, sample sizes, study procedures, or significant administrative aspects will require a formal amendment to the protocol. Such amendment will be agreed upon by BCIRG [Breast Cancer International Research Group] and Aventis, and approved by the Ethics Committee/ IRB [institutional review board] prior to implementation and notified to the health authorities in accordance with local regulations.
> Administrative changes of the protocol are minor corrections and/or clarifications that have no effect on the way the study is to be conducted. These administrative changes will be agreed upon by BCIRG and Aventis, and will be documented in a memorandum. The Ethics Committee/IRB may be notified of administrative changes at the discretion of BCIRG."[345]

Explanation

After initial ethics approval, about half of trials have subsequent protocol amendments submitted to the REC/ IRB.[125 346 347] While some amendments may be unavoidable, a study of pharmaceutical industry trials found that according to the sponsors, a third of amendments could have been prevented with greater attention to key issues during protocol development.[346] Substantive amendments can generate challenges to data analysis and interpretation if they occur part way through the trial (eg, changes in eligibility criteria),[348] and can introduce bias if the changes are made based on the trial data.[173 174 175 176] The implementation and communication of amendments are also burdensome and potentially costly.[346]

Numerous studies have revealed substantive changes between prespecified methods (eg, as stated in approved protocols, registries, or regulatory agency submissions) and those described in trial publications, including changes to primary outcomes,[12 172 173 174 175 176] sample size calculations,[6] eligibility criteria,[125 133 134] as well as methods of allocation concealment,[2] blinding,[3] and statistical analysis.[6 7 8 174] These substantive modifications are rarely acknowledged in the final trial reports, providing an inaccurate impression of trial integrity.

It is important that substantive protocol amendments be reviewed by an independent party, such as the REC/IRB, and transparently described in trial reports. The notion of "substantive" is variably defined by authorities, but in general refers to a protocol amendment that can affect the safety of trial participants or the scientific validity, scope, or ethical rigour of the trial.[349 350] To reflect the degree of oversight for the trial and adherence to applicable regulation, the protocol should describe the process for making amendments, including who will be responsible for the decision to amend the protocol and how substantive changes will be communicated to relevant stakeholders (eg, REC/IRBs, trial registries, regulatory agencies). Version control using protocol identifiers and dates (Item 3), as well as a list of amendments, can help to track the history of amendments and identify the most recent protocol version.

Consent or assent

Item 26a: Who will obtain informed consent or assent from potential trial participants or authorised surrogates, and how (see Item 32)

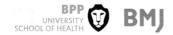

> **EXAMPLE**
>
> " . . . Trained Research Nurses will introduce the trial to patients who will be shown a video regarding the main aspects of the trial. Patients will also receive information sheets. Research Nurses will discuss the trial with patients in light of the information provided in the video and information sheets. Patients will then be able to have an informed discussion with the participating consultant. Research Nurses will obtain written consent from patients willing to participate in the trial. Information sheets and consent forms are provided for all parents involved in the trial however these have been amended accordingly in order to provide separate information sheets and consent form [sic] which are suitable for children and teenagers. All information sheets, consent forms and the video transcript have been translated into Bengali, Punjabi, Gujarati, and Urdu. There are also separate information sheets and consent forms for the cohort group."[351]

Explanation

The notion of acquiring informed consent involves the presentation of comprehensible information about the research to potential participants, confirmation that they understand the research, and assurance that their agreement to participate is voluntary. The process typically involves discussion between the potential participant and an individual knowledgeable about the research; the presentation of written material (eg, information leaflet or consent document); and the opportunity for potential participants to ask questions. Surveys of trial investigators reveal that appropriate informed consent is not always obtained.[344] [352]

The content, quantity, and mode of delivery of consent information can affect trial recruitment, participant comprehension, anxiety, retention rates, and recruitment costs.[68] [114] [218] [292] [353] [354] [355] We recommend that a model consent or assent form be provided as a protocol appendix (Item 32). Assent represents a minor's affirmative agreement to participate in the trial, which typically involves signing a document that provides age appropriate information about the study.

The protocol should include details of the consent process as well as the status, experience, and training (if applicable) of the research team members who will conduct it. In paediatric research, regulations may stipulate obtaining affirmative assent for participation from children above a certain age.[356] The protocol should then describe how pertinent information will be provided to potential participants and how their understanding and assent will be ascertained. When potential participants lack decisional capacity for reasons other than young age (eg, mental status), and proxy consent can be obtained from a legally-authorised representative, the protocol should describe who will determine an individual's decisional capacity, whether a formal capacity instrument will be utilised, and how the individual's informed agreement to continue participation will be secured should they regain decisional capacity. For certain trials, such as cluster randomised trials, it may not be possible to acquire individual informed consent from participants before randomisation, and the consent process may be modified or waived. An explanation should be provided in the protocol in these instances.[357]

Consent or assent—ancillary studies

Item 26b: Additional consent provisions for collection and use of participant data and biological specimens in ancillary studies, if applicable

> **EXAMPLE**
>
> **"6.4.1. Samples for Biorepositories**
> Additional biological samples will be obtained to be stored for use in future studies of the pathobiology of FSGS [focal segmental glomerulosclerosis]. A materials consent will be obtained to specifically address the collection of these . . . urine, serum and plasma specimens . . .
>
> **14.3.4. Instructions for Preparation of Requests for an Ancillary Study**
> . . . A signed consent must be obtained from every participant in the ancillary study, if the data collection/request is not covered in the original informed consent process for the main FSGS Clinical Trial.
> . . .
> A copy of the IRB [institutional review board] letter for the ancillary study should be sent to the DCC [data coordinating centre]. If a separate consent form is required for the ancillary study, a copy of the signed ancillary study consent form for each study participant must be included in the FSGS-CT [clinical trial] record. A data file tracking all signed ancillary consent forms must be maintained by the ancillary study and an electronic copy of that file must be delivered to the FSGS-CT DCC."[267]

Explanation

Ancillary studies involve the collection or derivation of data for purposes that are separate from the main trial. The acquisition and storage of data and biological specimens for ancillary studies is increasingly common in the context of clinical trials (Item 33). Specimens may be used for a specified subset of studies or for submission to biorepositories for future specified or unspecified research.

Ancillary studies have additional processes and considerations relating to consent, which should be detailed in the protocol. Guidance for the creation of a simplified informed consent document for biobanking is available.[358] Participants can be given several options to consider with respect to their participation in ancillary research: consent for the use of their data and specimens in specified protocols; consent for use in future research unrelated to the clinical condition under study; consent for submission to an unrelated biorepository; and consent to be contacted by trial investigators for further informational and consent-related purposes. This is commonly referred to as tiered consent. Participants should also be informed about whether their withdrawal from the ancillary research is possible (eg, the data and specimens are coded and identifiable); what withdrawal means in this context (eg, used specimens and data derived from them cannot be withdrawn); and what information derived from the specimen related research will be provided to them, if any.

Confidentiality

Item 27: How personal information about potential and enrolled participants will be collected, shared, and maintained in order to protect confidentiality before, during, and after the trial

> **EXAMPLE**
>
> **"8.5 Confidentiality**
> All study-related information will be stored securely at the study site. All participant information will be stored in locked file cabinets in areas with limited access. All laboratory specimens, reports, data collection, process, and administrative forms will be identified by a coded ID [identification] number only to maintain participant confidentiality. All records that contain names or other

personal identifiers, such as locator forms and informed consent forms, will be stored separately from study records identified by code number. All local databases will be secured with password-protected access systems. Forms, lists, logbooks, appointment books, and any other listings that link participant ID numbers to other identifying information will be stored in a separate, locked file in an area with limited access. All HIV test results will be kept strictly confidential, all counseling and blood draws will be conducted in private rooms, and study staff will be required to sign agreements to preserve the confidentiality of all participants. Study staff will never inform network members of the serostatus of other members of their group, but counselors will provide general messages about the prevalence of HIV in the study population in the interests of emphasizing harm reduction.

Participants' study information will not be released outside of the study without the written permission of the participant, except as necessary for monitoring by NIAID [National Institute of Allergy and Infectious Diseases] and/or its contractors . . . representatives of the HPTN CORE [HIV Prevention Trials Network Coordinating and Operations Center] . . . and US or in-country government and regulatory authorities."[359]

Explanation

Personal information about participants is acquired during the process of trial recruitment, eligibility screening, and data collection. Much of this information consists of private details over which people customarily wish to maintain control, such as their health status, personal genotype, and social and family history.

The protocol should describe the means whereby personal information is collected, kept secure, and maintained. In general, this involves: 1) the creation of coded, depersonalised data where the participant's identifying information is replaced by an unrelated sequence of characters; 2) secure maintenance of the data and the linking code in separate locations using encrypted digital files within password protected folders and storage media; and 3) limiting access to the minimum number of individuals necessary for quality control, audit, and analysis. The protocol should also describe how the confidentiality of data will be preserved when the data are transmitted to sponsors and coinvestigators (eg, virtual private network internet transmission).

Declaration of interests

Item 28: Financial and other competing interests for principal investigators for the overall trial and each study site

EXAMPLE

"PS:

- 1. Was the Principal Investigator of the second International Stroke Trial (IST-2) to evaluate a neuroprotective compound (619c89). . .
- 2. Has received lecture fees and travel expenses from Bayer and from Boehringer Ingelheim for lectures given at international conferences.
- 3. He serves on the Independent Data Monitoring and Safety Board of the RELY trial, funded by Boehringer Ingelheim and receives attendance fees and travel expenses for attending board meetings.
- 4. He does not have any paid consultancies with pharmaceutical companies, and is not a member of the Speaker's Panel of any company.

KBS:

- Received an honorarium for a lecture from Boehringer Ingelheim and had costs for participating in scientific meetings reimbursed . . . "[124]

Explanation

Competing interests, or conflicts of interest, exist when there is potential for divergence between an individual's or institution's private interests and their responsibilities to scientific and publishing activities.[360] More positive outcomes, larger treatment effect sizes, and more favourable interpretation of results have been found in clinical trials with pharmaceutical industry sponsorship (Item 4)[27 36 37 38 42] and investigators who have declared competing interests,[57 60] compared to those without such interests. Although competing interests are most often associated with drug and device industries, they may exist with support from or affiliation with government agencies, charities, not for profit organisations, and professional and civic organisations.

Competing interests do not in themselves imply wrongdoing. Their disclosure and regular updating enables appropriate management plans to be developed and implemented, and facilitates transparent assessment of the potential for bias.

Many trials and non-industry sponsors have a conflict of interest policy for their investigators, and checklists are available to guide potential interests that should be disclosed and regularly updated by trial investigators.[361 362] Types of financial ties include salary support or grants; ownership of stock or options; honorariums (eg, for advice, authorship, or public speaking); paid consultancy or service on advisory boards and medical education companies; and receipt of patents or patents pending. Non-financial competing interests include academic commitments; personal or professional relationships; and political, religious, or other affiliations with special interests or advocacy positions.

Access to data

Item 29: Statement of who will have access to the final trial dataset, and disclosure of contractual agreements that limit such access for investigators

EXAMPLE

"12.10.1 Intra-Study Data Sharing

The Data Management Coordinating Center will oversee the intra-study data sharing process, with input from the Data Management Subcommittee.

All Principal Investigators (both US and host country) will be given access to the cleaned data sets. Project data sets will be housed on the Project Accept Web site and/or the file transfer protocol site created for the study, and all data sets will be password protected. Project Principal Investigators will have direct access to their own site's data sets, and will have access to other sites data by request. To ensure confidentiality, data dispersed to project team members will be blinded of any identifying participant information."[113]

Explanation

The validity of results from interventional trials can be verified only by individuals who have full access to the complete final dataset. For some multicentre trials, only the steering group has access to the full trial dataset in order to ensure that the overall results are not disclosed by an individual study site prior to the main publication. Many of these trials will allow site investigators to access the full dataset if a formal request describing their plans is approved by the steering group. The World Medical Association supports the principle that trial investigators retain the right to access data.[363] However, among protocols of industry initiated randomised trials published in 2008-9 in the *Lancet* or approved in 2004 by a Danish ethics committee, 30-39% stated that the sponsor owned the data while 0-3% stated that principal investigators had access to all trial data.[10] [364] Similar constraints were found in Danish trial protocols from 1994-5.[10]

The protocol should identify the individuals involved in the trial who will have access to the full dataset. Any restrictions in access for trial investigators should also be explicitly described.

Ancillary and post-trial care
Item 30: Provisions, if any, for ancillary and post-trial care and for compensation to those who suffer harm from trial participation

---

EXAMPLES

"Patients that are enrolled into the study are covered by indemnity for negligent harm through the standard NHS [National Health Service] Indemnity arrangements. The University of Sheffield has insurance to cover for non-negligent harm associated with the protocol . . . This will include cover for additional health care, compensation or damages whether awarded voluntarily by the Sponsor, or by claims pursued through the courts. Incidences judged to arise from negligence (including those due to major protocol violations) will not be covered by study insurance policies. The liability of the manufacturer of IL1RA (Amgen Corporation) is strictly limited to those claims arising from faulty manufacturing of the commercial product and not to any aspects of the conduct of the study."[145]

"13.6 Access to Effective Products
Should this study provide evidence of the effectiveness of TDF [tenofovir disoproxil fumarate], FTC [emtricitabine]/TDF and/or tenofovir 1% gel in preventing HIV infection, it will be critical to provide access to the effective product(s) to study participants, their communities, and the worldwide population at risk for HIV infection in a timely manner. In preparation for this study, discussions have begun with Gilead Sciences, Inc. and CONRAD [Contraceptive Research and Development Organization] to ensure such access. Considerations under discussion include licensing agreements and preferred pricing arrangements for the study communities and other resource-poor settings. While this study is ongoing, the MTN [Microbicide Trials Network] will continue these discussions. In addition, discussions will be initiated with other public and private funding sources such as the WHO, UNAIDS, Gates Foundation, and appropriate site government agencies that may be able to purchase product supplies in bulk and offer them at low or no cost to the study communities and other resource-poor communities most in need of the product(s). Operations and marketing research also may be conducted to determine how best to package and distribute the products, and maximize their acceptability and use, in at-risk populations."[365]

Explanation
The provision of ancillary care refers to the provision of care beyond that immediately required for the proper and safe conduct of the trial, and the treatment of immediate adverse events related to trial procedures. It is generally agreed that trial sponsors and investigators should plan to provide care for participants' healthcare needs that arise as a direct consequence of trial participation (eg, intervention related harms). It is also important to consider whether care should be provided for certain ancillary needs that may otherwise arise during trial participation. Provision of care for ancillary needs reflects the fact that participants implicitly, but unavoidably, entrust certain aspects of their

health to the research team. The scope of entrustment will vary depending on the nature of the trial (eg, setting, health condition under study, investigations performed).[366] Additional factors that influence the strength of the claim to ancillary care include participants' vulnerabilities; uncompensated burdens and harms; the intensity and duration of the participant-researcher relationship; and the degree to which participants are uniquely dependent on the research team for health care.[367]

The Declaration of Helsinki states that "the protocol should describe arrangements for post-study access by study participants to interventions identified as beneficial in the study or access to other appropriate care or benefits."[1] This principle is particularly applicable—and controversial—when research enabling the development and regulatory approval of interventions is performed in countries where subsequent access to the interventions is limited by cost or lack of availability.[368]

The protocol should describe any plans to provide or pay for ancillary care during the trial and identify any interventions, benefits, or other care that the sponsor will continue to provide to participants and host communities after the trial is completed.[369] Any plans to compensate participants for trial related harms should also be outlined.

Dissemination policy—trial results
Item 31a: Plans for investigators and sponsor to communicate trial results to participants, healthcare professionals, the public, and other relevant groups (eg, via publication, reporting in results databases, or other data sharing arrangements), including any publication restrictions

---

EXAMPLE

"XII. Publication Policy
The Publications subcommittee will review all publications following the guidelines given below and report its recommendations to the Steering Committee.

A. Data analysis and release of results
The scientific integrity of the project requires that the data from all BEST [Beta-Blocker Evaluation of Survival Trial] sites be analyzed study-wide and reported as such. Thus, an individual center is not expected to report the data collected from its center alone . . . all presentations and publications are expected to protect the integrity of the major objective(s) of the study; data that break the blind will not be presented prior to the release of mainline results. Recommendations as to the timing of presentation of such endpoint data and the meetings at which they might be presented will be given by the Steering Committee.

B. Review process
Each paper or abstract, as described below, must be submitted to the appropriate Subcommittee for review of its appropriateness and scientific merit prior to submission. The Subcommittee may recommend changes to the authors and will finally submit its recommendations to the Steering Committee for approval.

C. Primary outcome papers
The primary outcome papers of BEST are papers that present outcome data . . . The determination of whether or not a particular analysis represents a primary outcome will be made by the Steering Committee on the recommendation of the Publications Subcommittee . . .

D. Other study papers, abstracts and presentations
All studies other than those designated as "Primary Outcome" fall within this category . . . All papers and abstracts must

---

be approved by the Publications Committee before they are submitted.

It is possible that in certain instances BEST may be asked to contribute papers to workshops, symposia, volumes, etc. The individuals to work on such requests should be appointed by the Executive Committee, but where time permits, a proposal will be circulated soliciting other participants as in the case of other study papers as described in the Application Review Process.

XIII. Close-out Procedures

BEST may terminate at the planned target of 1.5 years after the last participant has been randomized, or at an earlier or later date if the circumstances warrant . . . Regardless of the timing and circumstances of the end of the study, close-out will proceed in two stages:

- Interim period for analysis and documentation of study results.
- Debriefing of participants and dissemination of study results.

A. Interim

Every attempt will be made to reduce to an absolute minimum the interval between the completion of data collection and the release of the study results. We expect to take about 3 to 4 months to compile the final results paper for an appropriate journal.

B. Reporting of study results

The study results will be released to the participating physicians, referring physicians, patients and the general medical community."[370]

Explanation

A fundamental ethical principle in clinical trials is that the potential risks incurred by study participants should be balanced by the benefit of contributing to publicly available knowledge.[371] Unfortunately, about half of clinical trials remain unpublished.[80 83] Trials with statistically non-significant results or industry funding are more prone to non-publication,[36 38 80 81 82 83] although government funded trials are also susceptible.[81] When published, trials with non-significant results often have a longer delay to publication.[80 83] Overall, the medical literature represents a biased subset of existing data, potentially leading to overestimation of benefits, underestimation of harms, and a detrimental impact on patient care and research.[80 372 373 374 375 376 377]

Although peer reviewers can be biased in favour of positive findings,[378] lack of publication appears to be primarily due to trial investigators or sponsors failing to submit negative or null results, rather than journals rejecting them.[80 379] A plan to disseminate trial results to key stakeholders should be outlined in the protocol, including a process and timeframe for approving and submitting reports for dissemination (eg, via journal publication, trial registry, trial website), and an explicit statement that the results will be disseminated regardless of the magnitude or direction of effect.

Furthermore, any conditions relating to the investigators' right to publish or present trial results should be explicitly described. Publication restrictions have been imposed by various groups, including industry sponsors or the trial steering group (eg, to maintain the integrity of the overall dataset).[10 380] These restrictions are sometimes not described in the protocol but rather in separate publication agreements.[10] However, as they can interfere with the ethical responsibility of investigators and sponsors to disseminate trial results in an unbiased and timely manner,[38 381 382 383]

[384] any restrictions should be disclosed in the protocol for review by REC/IRBs, funders, and other stakeholders. A review of industry initiated randomised trial protocols approved in Denmark in 1994-95 revealed that 91% had publication restrictions imposed by sponsors; similar constraints were noted for protocols approved in 2004.[10]

Dissemination policy—authorship

Item 31b: Authorship eligibility guidelines and any intended use of professional writers

---

EXAMPLE

"17.4. Assignment of Writing Committees

Topics suggested for presentation or publication will be circulated to the PIs [principal investigators] of the CCCs [core coordinating centers], the DCC [data coordinating centre], Core Lab and the NIH [National Institutes of Health]. These groups are requested to suggest and justify names for authors to be reviewed by the PC [publications committee]. . . If a topic is suggested by a participant of the FSGS-CT [focal segmental glomerulosclerosis—clinical trial], the writing committee will be formed as just described except that the person making the suggestion may be considered as the lead author. The PI of an ancillary study should be considered for lead author of material derived from this study. Disputes regarding authorship will be settled by the Study Chair after consultation with the Chair of the PC . . .

17.5. Reports of the FSGS-CT: Classes of Reports

There are three classes of reports of the FSGS-CT:

- A. Reports of the major outcomes of the Study.
- B. Reports addressing in detail one aspect of the FSGS-CT, but in which the data are derived from the entire study.
- C. Reports of data derived from a subset of centers by members of the FSGS-CT, (eg, sub-studies or ancillary studies), or reports of investigations initiated outside of the FSGS-CT, but using data or samples collected by the FSGS-CT.
. .

17.6. Authorship Policy

The authors of FSGS publications will be listed as detailed below.

Type A publications:

- abstracts: from the FSGS Clinical Trial Group[x], presented by XXXX.
- papers: from the FSGS Clinical Trial Group[x], prepared by XXXX.

[x]The FSGS participant box, detailed below, must be included in these papers. If a journal's publication policy does not allow authorship by a group, the authors will be listed first as in Type B publications.

Type B publications:

. . .

17.7. Authorship: Professional Participants Listing in the FSGS Participant Box

The FSGS participant box will list all professionals that have participated in the FSGS-CT for a minimum of one year."[267]

Explanation

Substantive contributions to the design, conduct, interpretation, and reporting of a clinical trial are recognised through the granting of authorship on the final trial report. Authorship guidelines in the protocol are intended to help enhance transparency and avoid disputes or misunderstanding after trial completion. These guidelines should define criteria for individually named authors or group authorship.[385]

61

Individuals who fulfil authorship criteria should not remain hidden (ghost authorship) and should have final authority over manuscript content.[9][386][387] Similarly, those who do not fulfil such criteria should not be granted authorship (guest authorship).[386][388] The International Committee of Medical Journal Editors has defined authorship criteria for manuscripts submitted for publication,[389] although these criteria have reportedly been open to abuse.[390] If some protocol authors are not named authors of subsequent publications, their role in protocol design should at least be acknowledged in the published report. Among 44 protocols of industry initiated trials, 75% had evidence of ghost authorship when compared with corresponding journal publications.[9]

Professional medical writers are sometimes hired to improve clarity and structure in a trial report, and guidelines for ethical collaborative writing have been developed.[391] [392] Because the drafting of text can influence how the study results and conclusions are portrayed, plans for the employment of writers and their funding source should be acknowledged in both protocols and trial reports.

Dissemination policy—reproducible research
Item 31c: Plans, if any, for granting public access to the full protocol, participant-level dataset, and statistical code

> **EXAMPLE**
>
> "**Data sharing statement** No later than 3 years after the collection of the 1-year postrandomisation interviews, we will deliver a completely deidentified data set to an appropriate data archive for sharing purposes."[393]

Explanation
Given the central role of protocols in enhancing transparency, reproducibility, and interpretation of trial results, there is a strong ethical and scientific imperative to ensure that full protocols are made publicly available.[24][394][395] High quality protocols contain relevant details on study design and conduct that are generally not available in journal publications or trial registries.[84][396] It is also important to make available the full study report, such as the "clinical study report" submitted to regulatory agencies by industry sponsors.[377][396][397][398][399][400] This detailed report provides the most comprehensive description of trial methods (including the full protocol) and all published and unpublished analyses. In addition, there have increasingly been calls to improve the availability of participant-level datasets and statistical code after journal publication to enable verification and replication of analyses, facilitate pooling with other studies, and accelerate research through open knowledge sharing.[372][401][402][403][404][405][406]

Avenues for providing access to full protocols include journals,[407][408] trial websites, and trial registries.[163] Several journals and funders support the sharing of participant level data,[405][409][410][411] while others routinely publish a statement regarding sharing of protocols, statistical codes, and datasets for all of their published research articles.[412][413]

The protocol should indicate whether the trial protocol, full study report, anonymised participant level dataset, and statistical code for generating the results will be made publicly available; and if so, describe the timeframe and any other conditions for access.

Section 5: Appendices
Informed consent materials
Item 32: Model consent form and other related documentation given to participants and authorised surrogates

> **EXAMPLE**
>
> "APPENDIX 7 SAMPLE PATIENT INFORMED CONSENT
> Note: . . . Each Ethics Committee or Institutional Review Board will revise and adapt according to their own institution's guidelines.
> MULTICENTER PHASE III RANDOMIZED TRIAL COMPARING DOXORUBICIN AND CYCLOPHOSPHAMIDE . . .
> Study number: BCIRG 006 (TAX GMA 302)
> Investigator name:
> Address:
> Consent Form:
> This consent form is part of the informed consent process. It is designed to give you an idea of what this research study is about and what will happen to you if you choose to be in the study . . ."[345]

Explanation
The Declaration of Helsinki states that each potential trial participant must normally, at a minimum, be adequately informed about the purpose of the trial; potential benefits and risks; their right to refuse participation or to withdraw consent at any time; institutional affiliation and potential competing interests of the researcher; and sources of trial funding.[1] There are rare exceptions where deferred consent can be acceptable, such as trials involving unconscious patients in emergency situations.

Special attention is required to ensure that relevant information is provided and appropriate modes of delivery are used during the consent process (Item 26).[414] Consent and participant information forms are often written at a much higher reading level than is acceptable for the general population.[415] Depending on the nature of the trial, several different consent documents may be needed. For example, a paediatric trial may involve both parental permission and participant assent documents. For multicentre trials, a model or sample document is typically drafted for distribution to local investigators, who may then revise the document to comply with local requirements.

Biological specimens
Item 33: Plans for collection, laboratory evaluation, and storage of biological specimens for genetic or molecular analysis in the current trial and for future use in ancillary studies, if applicable

> **EXAMPLE**
>
> "**White Blood Cell and Plasma Collection Procedures**
>
> *1.0 Objectives*
> 1.1 To provide a resource for studies of early markers, etiology, and genetic risk factors for prostate cancer and other diseases.
>
> *2.0 Background*
> The Prostate Cancer Prevention Trial (PCPT) is a randomized double blind chemoprevention trial . . .
> Initial blood collection was specifically for the analysis of PSA [prostate specific antigen] and storage of serum . .
> . an additional blood collection will be carried out using anticoagulant so that plasma and white blood cells can be isolated. Plasma will allow the analysis of additional biomarkers . . . This DNA will be used (among other possible uses) for studies to investigate polymorphisms in genes which may influence prostate cancer risk . . .
> The PCPT WBC [white blood cell] sample will be available to PCPT investigators as well as outside researchers who have important, timely hypotheses to test. Because the sample bank is a limited resource, proposals to use it will be evaluated in terms of scientific relevance, significance, and validity as well

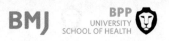

as the potential impact of the proposed study. The amount and type of material needed will also be considered and the efficient use of material will be required. Strict confidentiality will be exercised and the information provided to investigators will not contain personal identifiers.

When specific uses of the WBC samples are approved, the SWOG-9217 protocol will be amended.

Participation in this research is not required for continued participation in the PCPT.

3.0 Methods

3.1 Because the original model consent form did not specifically address genetic studies, participants will be asked to sign an additional consent form to document their consent to the collection and submission of additional blood samples for storage and future testing (including genetic analysis).

3.2 Institutions will be asked to submit additional materials from participants who consent to the additional blood collection. The blood is to be collected, processed and shipped as described in the PCPT Study Manual.

3.3 NCI-Frederick Cancer Research Development Center (FCRDC) in Frederick, Maryland will serve as the processing, aliquotting and storage facility.

3.4 Upon arrival at FCRDC the blood will be pooled and centrifuged. Plasma will be separated into 5 x 1.8 ml aliquots and frozen . . .

3.5 All samples will be logged in and aliquots will be bar coded with a unique storage ID. These data will be electronically transmitted to the Statistical Center for verification.

3.6 The scientists who will carry out analyses on these materials will not have access to personal identifiers and will not be able to link the results of these tests to personal identifier information. No individual results will be presented in publications or other reports. . . .

3.7 Participants will not be informed on an individual basis of any results from these studies . . .

4.0 Sample analysis

4.1 Investigators planning to submit NIH [National Institutes of Health] grant applications must obtain approval for their study and specimen access from the PCPT Serum and Tissue Utilization Committee before submission of a grant proposal. Potential investigators will be required to submit a brief abstract and 1-4 page outline . . . This proposal will be circulated for review to members of the PCPT Serum and Tissue Utilization Committee and two ad hoc members having relevant expertise . . .

4.2 It is anticipated that proposals will be reviewed once a year . . . Approval by this group as well as appropriate Institutional Review Board approval from the investigator's institution will be required before release of samples."[416]

Explanation

Biological specimens (eg, biopsy tissue; blood for DNA extraction) obtained during the conduct of clinical trials can be stored in repositories—often designated as biobanks—for the current trial and future research. This process is usually governed by local regulation and has particular ethical considerations (Item 26b).

If the trial involves genetic or molecular analysis of biological specimens derived from humans, or if any specimens will be stored for future use (specified or unspecified), the protocol should describe details about specimen collection, storage, and evaluation, including the location of repositories. In addition, the protocol should state whether collected samples and associated participant related data will be de-identified or coded to protect participant confidentiality. If a repository is overseen by a named research ethics committee/institutional review board, then this information should also be provided.

Discussion

It is critical that every clinical trial has a complete and transparent protocol, which can then facilitate trial conduct and appraisal by communicating relevant information to key stakeholders. In response to observed deficiencies in protocol content, the SPIRIT Initiative has produced recommendations for minimum relevant protocol items to include in a protocol, published in the form of the SPIRIT 2013 Statement and this Explanation and Elaboration (E&E) paper.[14] The strengths that distinguish SPIRIT from other protocol guidance documents include its systematic and transparent development methods; participation of a wide range of key stakeholders; use of empirical evidence to support its recommendations; and availability of detailed guidance including model examples from protocols.

The overall aim of SPIRIT is to improve the completeness and transparency of trial protocols. The SPIRIT documents can serve as a practical resource for trial investigators and personnel to draft and understand the key elements of a protocol. In doing so, our vision is that the SPIRIT 2013 Statement and E&E paper will also facilitate and expedite the review of protocols by research ethics committees/ institutional review boards, scientific review groups, and funders—for example, by reducing the number of avoidable queries to trial investigators regarding missing or unclear protocol information during the review process. Furthermore, improved protocol content would help facilitate the critical appraisal of final trial reports and results. Finally, several SPIRIT items correspond to items on the CONSORT 2010 checklist (Consolidated Standards of Reporting Trials),[417] which should facilitate the transition from the protocol to the final study report.

The next steps for the SPIRIT Initiative include an implementation strategy to encourage uptake of the SPIRIT 2013 Statement. The SPIRIT website (www.spirit-statement. org) will provide the latest resources and information on the initiative, including a list of supporters. We invite stakeholders to assist in the evaluation of the SPIRIT Statement and E&E paper by using the documents and providing feedback to inform future revisions. Through widespread uptake and support, the potential to improve the completeness and quality of trial protocols, as well as the efficiency of their review, can be fully realised.

We thank Raymond Daniel for his help with reference management and Jessica Kitchen for her work with manuscript formatting and identification of protocol examples. We also acknowledge GlaxoSmithKline for providing a sample of their trial protocols to serve as potential examples.

Contributors: AWC, JT, and DM conceived of the paper. All authors contributed to the drafting and revision of the manuscript, and approve the final version. AWC is the guarantor for the article.

Funding: The SPIRIT meetings were funded by the Canadian Institutes of Health Research (CIHR grant DET - 106068); National Cancer Institute of Canada (now Canadian Cancer Society Research Institute); and Canadian Agency for Drugs and Technologies in Health. CIHR has also funded ongoing dissemination activities (grant MET-117434). KKJ was formerly employed by CIHR (Knowledge Translation Branch), and WRP is affiliated with the NCIC Clinical Trials Group. The funders had no input into the design and conduct of the project; collection, management, analysis, and interpretation of the data; and preparation, review, or approval of the manuscript.

Competing interests: All authors have completed the ICJME unified declaration form at www.icmje.org/coi_disclosure.pdf (available on request from the corresponding author) and declare: JAB is employed by the Janssen Pharmaceutical Companies of Johnson & Johnson; KKJ was formerly employed by CIHR (Knowledge Translation Branch), and WRP is affiliated with the NCIC Clinical Trials Group. Trish Groves is deputy editor of *BMJ* and a member of the SPIRIT group but did not take part in the peer review and decision making process about this publication.

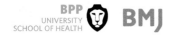

Provenance and peer review: Not commissioned; externally peer reviewed.

1   World Medical Association. WMA Declaration of Helsinki—ethical principles for medical research involving human subjects. 2008.www.wma.net/en/30publications/10policies/b3/index.html.

2   Pildal J, Chan A-W, Hróbjartsson A, Forfang E, Altman DG, Gøtzsche PC. Comparison of descriptions of allocation concealment in trial protocols and the published reports: cohort study.*BMJ* 2005;330:1049.

3   Hróbjartsson A, Pildal J, Chan A-W, Haahr MT, Altman DG, Gøtzsche PC. Reporting on blinding in trial protocols and corresponding publications was often inadequate but rarely contradictory.*J Clin Epidemiol* 2009;62:967-73.

4   Chan A-W, Hróbjartsson A, Haahr MT, Gøtzsche PC, Altman DG. Empirical evidence for selective reporting of outcomes in randomized trials: comparison of protocols to published articles.*JAMA* 2004;291:2457-65.

5   Scharf O, Colevas AD. Adverse event reporting in publications compared with sponsor database for cancer clinical trials.*J Clin Oncol* 2006;24:3933-8.

6   Chan A-W, Hróbjartsson A, Jørgensen KJ, Gøtzsche PC, Altman DG. Discrepancies in sample size calculations and data analyses reported in randomised trials: comparison of publications with protocols.*BMJ* 2008;337:a2299.

7   Al-Marzouki S, Roberts I, Evans S, Marshall T. Selective reporting in clinical trials: analysis of trial protocols accepted by the Lancet.*Lancet* 2008;372:201.

8   Hernández AV, Steyerberg EW, Taylor GS, Marmarou A, Habbema JD, Maas AI. Subgroup analysis and covariate adjustment in randomized clinical trials of traumatic brain injury: a systematic review.*Neurosurgery* 2005;57:1244-53.

9   Gøtzsche PC, Hróbjartsson A, Johansen HK, Haahr MT, Altman DG, Chan A-W. Ghost authorship in industry-initiated randomised trials. *PLoS Med* 2007;4:e19.

10 Gøtzsche PC, Hróbjartsson A, Johansen HK, Haahr MT, Altman DG, Chan A-W. Constraints on publication rights in industry-initiated clinical trials.*JAMA* 2006;295:1645-6.

11 Mhaskar R, Djulbegovic B, Magazin A, Soares HP, Kumar A. Published methodological quality of randomized controlled trials does not reflect the actual quality assessed in protocols. *J Clin Epidemiol* 2012;65:602-9.

12 Smyth RM, Kirkham JJ, Jacoby A, Altman DG, Gamble C, Williamson PR. Frequency and reasons for outcome reporting bias in clinical trials: interviews with trialists.*BMJ* 2011;342:c7153.

13 Tetzlaff JM, Chan A-W, Kitchen J, Sampson M, Tricco AC, Moher D. Guidelines for randomized controlled trial protocol content: a systematic review. *Syst Rev* 2012;1:43.

14 Chan A-W, Tetzlaff JM, Altman DG, Laupacis A, Gøtzsche PC, Krleža-Jerić K, et al. SPIRIT 2013 Statement: Defining standard protocol items for clinical trials. *Ann Intern Med* 2013. www.annals.org/article.aspx?doi=10.7326/0003-4819-158-3-201302050-00583.

15 Tetzlaff JM, Moher D, Chan A-W. Developing a guideline for reporting clinical trial protocols: Delphi consensus survey.*Trials* 2012;13:176.

16 Moher D, Schulz KF, Simera I, Altman DG. Guidance for developers of health research reporting guidelines. *PLoS Med* 2010;7:e1000217.

17 Moher D, Hopewell S, Schulz KF, Montori V, Gøtzsche PC, Devereaux PJ, et al. CONSORT 2010 Explanation and Elaboration: updated guidelines for reporting parallel group randomised trials.*BMJ* 2010;340:c869.

18 Liberati A, Altman DG, Tetzlaff J, Mulrow C, Gøtzsche PC, Ioannidis JP, et al. The PRISMA statement for reporting systematic reviews and meta-analyses of studies that evaluate health care interventions: explanation and elaboration. *J Clin Epidemiol* 2009;62:e1-34.

19 Warner Chilcott. A comparison of once a day dose compared to 2 doses/day. http://clinicaltrials.gov/show/NCT00505778.

20 Dickersin K, Manheimer E, Wieland S, Robinson KA, Lefebvre C, McDonald S. Development of the Cochrane Collaboration's CENTRAL Register of controlled clinical trials. *Eval Health Prof* 2002;25:38-64.

21 Shaw L, Price C, McLure S, Howel D, McColl E, Ford GA. Paramedic Initiated Lisinopril For Acute Stroke Treatment (PIL-FAST): study protocol for a pilot randomised controlled trial [protocol].*Trials* 2011;12:152.

22 Sim I, Chan A-W, Gülmezoglu AM, Evans T, Pang T. Clinical trial registration: transparency is the watchword.*Lancet* 2006;367:1631-3.

23 Dickersin K, Rennie D. Registering clinical trials.*JAMA* 2003;290:516-23.

24 Krleža-Jerić K, Chan A-W, Dickersin K, Sim I, Grimshaw J, Gluud C for the Ottawa Group. Principles for international registration of protocol information and results from human trials of health related interventions: Ottawa statement (part 1).*BMJ* 2005;330:956-8.

25 DeAngelis CD, Drazen JM, Frizelle FA, Haug C, Hoey J, Horton R, et al. Clinical trial registration: a statement from the International Committee of Medical Journal Editors.*JAMA* 2004;292:1363-4.

26 Mathieu S, Boutron I, Moher D, Altman DG, Ravaud P. Comparison of registered and published primary outcomes in randomized controlled trials.*JAMA* 2009;302:977-84.

27 Bourgeois FT, Murthy S, Mandl KD. Outcome reporting among drug trials registered in ClinicalTrials.gov. *Ann Intern Med* 2010;153:158-66.

28 You B, Gan HK, Pond G, Chen EX. Consistency in the analysis and reporting of primary end points in oncology randomized controlled trials from registration to publication: a systematic review. *J Clin Oncol* 2012;30:210-6.

29 United States Congress. Food and Drug Administration Amendments Act of 2007, Title VIII, Section 801. Expanded clinical trial registry data bank. 2007. www.govtrack.us/congress/billtext.xpd?bill=h110-3580.

30 European Commission. Communication from the Commission regarding the guideline on the data fields contained in the clinical trials database provided for in Article 11 of Directive 2001/20/EC to be included in the database on medicinal products provided for in Article 57 of Regulation (EC) No 726/2004 (2008/C 168/02). *Official Journal of the European Union* 2008;51:3-4.

31 Laine C, Horton R, DeAngelis CD, Drazen JM, Frizelle FA, Godlee F, et al. Clinical trial registration.*BMJ* 2007;334:1177-8.

32 Bernhard Nocht Institute for Tropical Medicine. Probiotic Saccharomyces boulardii for the prevention of antibiotic-associated diarrhoea (SacBo). http://clinicaltrials.gov/ct2/show/NCT01143272.

33 Dalessandro M, Hirman J. Protocol SB-275833/030—Studies 030A and 030B: two identical double-blind, double-dummy, multicenter, comparative phase III studies of the safety and efficacy of topical 1% SB-275833, applied twice daily, versus oral Cephalexin, 500 mg in adults, or 12.5 mg/kg (250 mg/5 ml) in children, twice daily, in the treatment of uncomplicated secondarily infected traumatic lesions [protocol]. Version 5 (July 25, 2005). www.spirit-statement.org/wp-content/uploads/2012/12/Protocol-SB-275833.pdf.

34 Effect of tranexamic acid on coagulation in a sample of participants in the WOMAN trial: WOMAN-ETAC study [protocol]. Version 1 (August 3, 2011). www.thewomantrial.lshtm.ac.uk/Images/WOMAN_ETACprotocol.pdf.

35 Chan A-W, Krleža-Jerić K, Schmid I, Altman DG. Outcome reporting bias in randomized trials funded by the Canadian Institutes of Health Research.*CMAJ* 2004;171:735-40.

36 Lexchin J, Bero LA, Djulbegovic B, Clark O. Pharmaceutical industry sponsorship and research outcome and quality: systematic review.*BMJ* 2003;326:1167-70.

37 Als-Nielsen B, Chen W, Gluud C, Kjaergard LL. Association of funding and conclusions in randomized drug trials: a reflection of treatment effect or adverse events?*JAMA* 2003;290:921-8.

38 Bekelman JE, Li Y, Gross CP. Scope and impact of financial conflicts of interest in biomedical research: a systematic review.*JAMA* 2003;289:454-65.

39 Heres S, Davis J, Maino K, Jetzinger E, Kissling W, Leucht S. Why olanzapine beats risperidone, risperidone beats quetiapine, and quetiapine beats olanzapine: an exploratory analysis of head-to-head comparison studies of second-generation antipsychotics. *Am J Psychiatry* 2006;163:185-94.

40 Djulbegovic B, Cantor A, Clarke M. The importance of preservation of the ethical principle of equipoise in the design of clinical trials: relative impact of the methodological quality domains on the treatment effect in randomized controlled trials. *Account Res* 2003;10:301-15.

41 Etter J-F, Burri M, Stapleton J. The impact of pharmaceutical company funding on results of randomized trials of nicotine replacement therapy for smoking cessation: a meta-analysis.*Addiction* 2007;102:815-22.

42 Golder S, Loke YK. Is there evidence for biased reporting of published adverse effects data in pharmaceutical industry-funded studies? *Br J Clin Pharmacol* 2008;66:767-73.

43 Min Y-I, Unalp-Arida A, Scherer R, Dickersin K. Assessment of equipoise using a cohort of randomized controlled trials [abstract]. International congress on peer review and biomedical publication, Chicago, IL, 16-18 September, 2005.

44 Yaphe J, Edman R, Knishkowy B, Herman J. The association between funding by commercial interests and study outcome in randomized controlled drug trials. *Fam Pract* 2001;18:565-8.

45 Ahmer S, Arya P, Anderson D, Faruqui R. Conflict of interest in psychiatry. *Psychiatr Bull* 2005;29:302-4.

46 The Danish National Committee on Biomedical Research Ethics. Guidelines about notification etc. of a biomedical research project to the committee system on biomedical research ethics, No 9154, 5 May 2011. 2011.www.cvk.sum.dk/English/guidelinesaboutnotification.aspx.

47 Lester RT, Mills EJ, Kariri A, Ritvo P, Chung M, Jack W, et al. The HAART cell phone adherence trial (WelTel Kenya1): a randomized controlled trial protocol [protocol].*Trials* 2009;10:87.

48 Rennie D, Yank V, Emanuel L. When authorship fails. A proposal to make contributors accountable.*JAMA* 1997;278:579-85.

49 Trials. Instructions for authors— study protocols. 2012. www.trialsjournal.com/authors/instructions/studyprotocol#formatting-contributions.

50 Williams H. Bullous Pemphigoid Steroids and Tetracyclines (BLISTER) Study. A randomised controlled trial to compare the safety and effectiveness of doxycycline (200 mg/day) with prednisolone (0.5 mg/kg/day) for initial treatment of bullous pemphigoid [protocol]. Version 4.0 (July 20, 2011). www.spirit-statement.org/wp-content/uploads/2012/12/Blister-Protocol-v4-20July2011.pdf.

51 Gertel A, Block P, Gawrylewski H-M, Raymond S, Quinn T, Muhlbradt E. CDISC Clinical research glossary. Version 8.0. 2009. www.cdisc.org/stuff/contentmgr/files/0/be650811feb46f381f0af41ca40ade2e/misc/cdisc_2009_glossary.pdf.

52 World Health Organization. Operational guidelines for ethics committees that review biomedical research. 2000. www.who.int/tdr/publications/documents/ethics.pdf.

53 World Health Organization. Handbook for good clinical research practice (GCP): Guidance for implementation. 2002. http://apps.who.int/prequal/info_general/documents/GCP/gcp1.pdf.

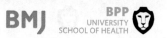

54　Pierce MA, Hess EP, Kline JA, Shah ND, Breslin M, Branda ME, et al. The Chest Pain Choice trial: a pilot randomized trial of a decision aid for patients with chest pain in the emergency department [protocol].*Trials* 2010;11:57.

55　Vlad SC, LaValley MP, McAlindon TE, Felson DT. Glucosamine for pain in osteoarthritis: why do trial results differ?*Arthritis Rheum* 2007;56:2267-77.

56　Kjaergard LL, Als-Nielsen B. Association between competing interests and authors' conclusions: epidemiological study of randomised clinical trials published in the BMJ.*BMJ* 2002;325:249.

57　Liss H. Publication bias in the pulmonary/allergy literature: effect of pharmaceutical company sponsorship. *Isr Med Assoc J* 2006;8:451-4.

58　Montgomery JH, Byerly M, Carmody T, Li B, Miller DR, Varghese F, et al. An analysis of the effect of funding source in randomized clinical trials of second generation antipsychotics for the treatment of schizophrenia. *Control Clin Trials* 2004;25:598-612.

59　Perlis RH, Perlis CS, Wu Y, Hwang C, Joseph M, Nierenberg AA. Industry sponsorship and financial conflict of interest in the reporting of clinical trials in psychiatry. *Am J Psychiatry* 2005;162:1957-60.

60　Jagsi R, Sheets N, Jankovic A, Motomura AR, Amarnath S, Ubel PA, et al. Frequency, nature, effects, and correlates of conflicts of interest in published clinical cancer research.*Cancer* 2009;115:2783-91.

61　Mello MM, Clarridge BR, Studdert DM. Academic medical centers' standards for clinical-trial agreements with industry.*N Engl J Med* 2005;352:2202-10.

62　European Vasculitis Study Group (EUVAS). RITUXVAS Clinical Trial Protocol: An international, randomised, open label trial comparing a rituximab based regimen with a standard cyclophosphamide/ azathioprine regimen in the treatment of active, 'generalised' ANCA associated vasculitis [protocol]. Version 1b (November 15, 2005). www.vasculitis.nl/media/documents/rituxvas.pdf.

63　Delgado-Rodriguez M, Ruiz-Canela M, De Irala-Estevez J, Llorca J, Martinez-Gonzalez MA. Participation of epidemiologists and/or biostatisticians and methodological quality of published controlled clinical trials. *J Epidemiol Community Health* 2001;55:569-72.

64　Llorca J, Martinez-Sanz F, Prieto-Salceda D, Fariñas-Alvarez C, Chinchon MV, Quinones D, et al. Quality of controlled clinical trials on glaucoma and intraocular high pressure. *J Glaucoma* 2005;14:190-5.

65　CRASH2 Clinical Randomisation of an Antifibrinolytic in Significant Haemorrhage. A large randomised placebo controlled trial among trauma patients with or at risk of significant haemorrhage, of the effects of antifibrinolytic treatment on death and transfusion requirement [protocol]. Version 3 (July 2, 2005). www.crash2.lshtm. ac.uk/.

66　Clarke M. Doing new research? Don't forget the old. *PLoS Med* 2004;1:e35.

67　Prescott RJ, Counsell CE, Gillespie WJ, Grant AM, Russell IT, Kiauka S, et al. Factors that limit the quality, number and progress of randomised controlled trials. *Health Technol Assess* 1999;3:1-143.

68　Centre for Reviews and Dissemination. Systematic review of barriers, modifiers and benefits involved in participation in cancer trials. CRD Report 31. York: University of York, 2006.

69　Tournoux C, Katsahian S, Chevret S, Levy V. Factors influencing inclusion of patients with malignancies in clinical trials.*Cancer* 2006;106:258-70.

70　Clarke M, Hopewell S, Chalmers I. Clinical trials should begin and end with systematic reviews of relevant evidence: 12 years and waiting.*Lancet* 2010;376:20-1.

71　Canadian Institutes of Health Research. RCT evaluation criteria and headings. 2010. www.cihr.ca/e/39187.html.

72　National Institute for Health Research. Efficacy and mechanism evaluation program. Important information & guidance notes— preliminary application. 2012. www.eme.ac.uk/funding/Researcher-led.asp.

73　Jüni P, Nartey L, Reichenbach S, Sterchi R, Dieppe PA, Egger M. Risk of cardiovascular events and rofecoxib: cumulative meta-analysis.*Lancet* 2004;364:2021-9.

74　Puhan MA, Vollenweider D, Steurer J, Bossuyt PM, ter Riet G. Where is the supporting evidence for treating mild to moderate chronic obstructive pulmonary disease exacerbations with antibiotics? A systematic review. *BMC Med* 2008;6:28.

75　Fergusson D, Glass KC, Hutton B, Shapiro S. Randomized controlled trials of aprotinin in cardiac surgery: could clinical equipoise have stopped the bleeding? *Clin Trials* 2005;2:218-29.

76　Lau J, Antman EM, Jimenez-Silva J, Kupelnick B, Mosteller F, Chalmers TC. Cumulative meta-analysis of therapeutic trials for myocardial infarction. *N Engl J Med* 1992;327:248-54.

77　Robinson KA, Goodman SN. A systematic examination of the citation of prior research in reports of randomized, controlled trials.*Ann Intern Med* 2011;154:50-5.

78　Goudie AC, Sutton AJ, Jones DR, Donald A. Empirical assessment suggests that existing evidence could be used more fully in designing randomized controlled trials. *J Clin Epidemiol* 2010;63:983-91.

79　Cooper NJ, Jones DR, Sutton AJ. The use of systematic reviews when designing studies. *Clin Trials* 2005;2:260-4.

80　Song F, Parekh S, Hooper L, Loke YK, Ryder J, Sutton AJ, et al. Dissemination and publication of research findings: an updated review of related biases. *Health Technol Assess* 2010;14:iii-193.

81　Ross JS, Tse T, Zarin DA, Xu H, Zhou L, Krumholz HM. Publication of NIH funded trials registered in ClinicalTrials.gov: cross sectional analysis.*BMJ* 2012;344:d7292.

82　Ross JS, Mulvey GK, Hines EM, Nissen SE, Krumholz HM. Trial publication after registration in ClinicalTrials.Gov: a cross-sectional analysis. *PLoS Med* 2009;6:e1000144.

83　Hopewell S, Loudon K, Clarke MJ, Oxman AD, Dickersin K. Publication bias in clinical trials due to statistical significance or direction of trial results. *Cochrane Database Syst Rev* 2009;1:MR000006.

84　Chan A-W. Out of sight but not out of mind: how to search for unpublished clinical trial evidence.*BMJ* 2012;344:d8013.

85　A phase III multi-centre, randomised, double-blind, double-dummy, comparative clinical study to assess the safety and efficacy of a fixed-dose formulation of oral pyronaridine artesunate (180:60 mg tablet) versus chloroquine (155 mg tablet), in children and adult patients with acute Plasmodium vivax malaria [protocol]. Version 2.0 (March 5, 2007). www.plosone.org/article/info%3Adoi%2F10.1371%2Fjournal.pone.0014501#s5

86　Dawson L, Zarin DA, Emanuel EJ, Friedman LM, Chaudhari B, Goodman SN. Considering usual medical care in clinical trial design. *PLoS Med* 2009;6:e1000111.

87　Van Luijn JCF, Van Loenen AC, Gribnau FWJ, Leufkens HGM. Choice of comparator in active control trials of new drugs.*Ann Pharmacother* 2008;42:1605-12.

88　Johansen HK, Gøtzsche PC. Problems in the design and reporting of trials of antifungal agents encountered during meta-analysis.*JAMA* 1999;282:1752-9.

89　Stang A, Hense H-W, Jöckel K-H, Turner EH, Tramèr MR. Is it always unethical to use a placebo in a clinical trial? *PLoS Med* 2005;2:e72.

90　Emanuel EJ, Miller FG. The ethics of placebo-controlled trials—A middle ground. *N Engl J Med* 2001;345:915-9.

91　Ross S, Grant A, Counsell C, Gillespie W, Russell I, Prescott R. Barriers to participation in randomised controlled trials: a systematic review. *J Clin Epidemiol* 1999;52:1143-56.

92　Mills EJ, Seely D, Rachlis B, Griffith L, Wu P, Wilson K, et al. Barriers to participation in clinical trials of cancer: a meta-analysis and systematic review of patient-reported factors. *Lancet Oncol* 2006;7:141-8.

93　Rochon PA, Gurwitz JH, Simms RW. A study of manufacturer supported trials of non-steroidal anti-inflammatory drugs in the treatment of arthritis. *Arch Int Med* 1994;9:157-63.

94　Rutherford BR, Sneed JR, Roose SP. Does study design influence outcome? The effects of placebo control and treatment duration in antidepressant trials. *Psychother Psychosom* 2009;78:172-81.

95　Sneed JR, Rutherford BR, Rindskopf D, Lane DT, Sackeim HA, Roose SP. Design makes a difference: a meta-analysis of antidepressant response rates in placebo-controlled versus comparator trials in late-life depression. *Am J Geriatr Psychiatry* 2008;16:65-73.

96　Sinyor M, Levitt AJ, Cheung AH, Schaffer A, Kiss A, Dowlati Y, et al. Does inclusion of a placebo arm influence response to active antidepressant treatment in randomized controlled trials? Results from pooled and meta-analyses. *J Clin Psychiatry* 2010;71:270-9.

97　Tang J-L, Zhan S-Y, Ernst E. Review of randomised controlled trials of traditional Chinese medicine.*BMJ* 1999;319:160-1.

98　A phase 3, active (Warfarin) controlled, randomized, double-blind, parallel arm study to evaluate efficacy and safety of Apixaban in preventing stroke and systemic embolism in subjects with nonvalvular atrial fibrillation (ARISTOTLE: Apixaban for Reduction In STroke and Other ThromboemboLic Events in Atrial Fibrillation) [protocol]. Version 4 (August 4, 2010). www.nejm.org/doi/full/10.1056/NEJMoa1107039.

99　Fleming TR. Clinical trials: discerning hype from substance. *Ann Intern Med* 2010;153:400-406.

100　Heger U, Voss S, Knebel P, Doerr-Harim C, Neudecker J, Schuhmacher C, et al. Prevention of abdominal wound infection (PROUD trial, DRKS00000390): study protocol for a randomized controlled trial [protocol].*Trials* 2011;12:245.

101　Hopewell S, Dutton S, Yu L-M, Chan A-W, Altman DG. The quality of reports of randomised trials in 2000 and 2006: comparative study of articles indexed in PubMed.*BMJ* 2010;340:c723.

102　Dumville JC, Hahn S, Miles JN, Torgerson DJ. The use of unequal randomisation ratios in clinical trials: a review.*Contemp Clin Trials* 2006;27:1-12.

103　Gilbody S, Bower P, Torgerson D, Richards D. Cluster randomized trials produced similar results to individually randomized trials in a meta-analysis of enhanced care for depression. *J Clin Epidemiol* 2008;61:160-8.

104　Lathyris D, Trikalinos TA, Ioannidis JPA. Evidence from crossover trials: Empirical evaluation and comparison against parallel arm trials. *Int J Epidemiol* 2007;36:422-30.

105　Khan KS, Daya S, Collins JA, Walter SD. Empirical evidence of bias in infertility research: overestimation of treatment effect in crossover trials using pregnancy as the outcome measure. *Fertil Steril* 1996;65:939-45.

106　Katz J, Finnerup NB, Dworkin RH. Clinical trial outcome in neuropathic pain: relationship to study characteristics.*Neurology* 2008;70:263-72.

107　Le Henanff A, Giraudeau B, Baron G, Ravaud P. Quality of reporting of noninferiority and equivalence randomized trials.*JAMA* 2006;295:1147-51.

108　Fleming TR, Odem-Davis K, Rothmann MD, Li SY. Some essential considerations in the design and conduct of non-inferiority trials.*Clin Trials* 2011;8:432-9.

109　Krysan DJ, Kemper AR. Claims of equivalence in randomized controlled trials of the treatment of bacterial meningitis in children. *Pediatr Infect Dis J* 2002;21:753-8.

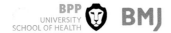

110 Tinmouth JM, Steele LS, Tomlinson G, Glazier GH. Are claims of equivalency in digestive diseases trials supported by the evidence.*Gastroenterol* 2004;126:1700-10.

111 Kairalla JA, Coffey CS, Thomann MA, Muller KE. Adaptive trial designs: a review of barriers and opportunities.*Trials* 2012;13:145.

112 Dragalin V. Adaptive designs: terminology and classification. *Drug Inf J* 2006;40:425-35.

113 Project Accept Study Group. Project Accept (HPTN 043): A phase III randomized controlled trial of community mobilization, mobile testing, same-day results, and post-test support for HIV in Sub-Saharan Africa and Thailand [protocol]. Version 2.4 (April 15, 2011). www.hptn.org/research_studies/hptn043.asp.

114 Ford JG, Howerton MW, Lai GY, Gary TL, Bolen S, Gibbons MC, et al. Barriers to recruiting underrepresented populations to cancer clinical trials: a systematic review.*Cancer* 2008;112:228-42.

115 Elkins JS, Khatabi T, Fung L, Rootenberg J, Johnston SC. Recruiting subjects for acute stroke trials: a meta-analysis.*Stroke* 2006;37:123-8.

116 Heo M, Papademetriou E, Meyers BS. Design characteristics that influence attrition in geriatric antidepressant trials: meta-analysis. *Int J Geriatr Psychiatry* 2009;24:990-1001.

117 Fabricatore AN, Wadden TA, Moore RH, Butryn ML, Gravallese EA, Erondu NE, et al. Attrition from randomized controlled trials of pharmacological weight loss agents: a systematic review and analysis.*Obes Rev* 2009;10:333-41.

118 Lemieux J, Goodwin PJ, Pritchard KI, Gelmon KA, Bordeleau LJ, Duchesne T, et al. Identification of cancer care and protocol characteristics associated with recruitment in breast cancer clinical trials.*J Clin Oncol* 2008;26:4458-65.

119 Jones R, Jones RO, McCowan C, Montgomery AA, Fahey T, Jones R, et al. The external validity of published randomized controlled trials in primary care. *BMC Fam Pract* 2009;10:5.

120 Sood A, Knudsen K, Sood R, Wahner-Roedler DL, Barnes SA, Bardia A, et al. Publication bias for CAM trials in the highest impact factor medicine journals is partly due to geographical bias. *J Clin Epidemiol* 2007;60:1123-6.

121 Wu T, Li Y, Bian Z, Liu G, Moher D. Randomized trials published in some Chinese journals: how many are randomized?*Trials* 2009;10:46.

122 Hotopf M, Lewis G, Normand C. Putting trials on trial--the costs and consequences of small trials in depression: a systematic review of methodology. *J Epidemiol Community Health* 1997;51:354-8.

123 Evaluation study of congestive heart failure and pulmonary artery catheterization effectiveness (ESCAPE) [protocol]. Version 3.0 (November 29, 1999). https://biolincc.nhlbi.nih.gov/studies/escape/?q=escape.

124 Sandercock P, Lindley R, Wardlaw J, Dennis M, Lewis S, Venables G, et al. The third international stroke trial (IST-3) of thrombolysis for acute ischaemic stroke [protocol].*Trials* 2008;9:37.

125 Blümle A, Meerpohl JJ, Rücker G, Antes G, Schumacher M, von Elm E. Reporting of eligibility criteria of randomised trials: cohort study comparing trial protocols with subsequent articles.*BMJ* 2011;342:d1828.

126 Cook JA. The challenges faced in the design, conduct and analysis of surgical randomised controlled trials.*Trials* 2009;10:9.

127 Simpson F, Sweetman EA, Doig GS. Systematic review of techniques and interventions for improving adherence to inclusion and exclusion criteria during enrolment into randomised controlled trials.*Trials* 2010;11:17.

128 Rendell JM, Merritt RK, Geddes JR. Incentives and disincentives to participation by clinicians in randomised controlled trials.*Cochrane Database Syst Rev* 2007;2:MR000021.

129 Weijer C. Characterizing the population in clinical trials: barriers, comparability, and implications for review. *Philosophy Publications.* Paper 250.1995. http://ir.lib.uwo.ca/philosophypub/250.

130 Townsley CA, Selby R, Siu LL. Systematic review of barriers to the recruitment of older patients with cancer onto clinical trials.*J Clin Oncol* 2005;23:3112-24.

131 Uchino K, Billheimer D, Cramer SC. Entry criteria and baseline characteristics predict outcome in acute stroke trials.*Stroke* 2001;32:909-16.

132 Van Spall HGC, Toren A, Kiss A, Fowler RA. Eligibility criteria of randomized controlled trials published in high-impact general medical journals: a systematic sampling review.*JAMA* 2007;297:1233-40.

133 Shapiro SH, Weijer C, Freedman B. Reporting the study populations of clinical trials. Clear transmission or static on the line?*J Clin Epimiol* 2000;53:973-9.

134 Gandhi M, Ameli N, Bacchetti P, Sharp GB, French AL, Young M, et al. Eligibility criteria for HIV clinical trials and generalizability of results: the gap between published reports and study protocols.*AIDS* 2005;19:1885-96.

135 Montori VM, Wang YG, Alonso-Coello P, Bhagra S. Systematic evaluation of the quality of randomized controlled trials in diabetes. *Diabetes Care* 2006;29:1833-8.

136 Mitchell SL, Sullivan EA, Lipsitz LA. Exclusion of elderly subjects from clinical trials for Parkinson disease. *Arch Neurol* 1997;54:1393-8.

137 Thorpe KE, Zwarenstein M, Oxman AD, Treweek S, Furberg CD, Altman DG, et al. A pragmatic-explanatory continuum indicator summary (PRECIS): a tool to help trial designers.*CMAJ* 2009;180:E47-57.

138 Blanco C, Olfson M, Goodwin RD, Ogburn E, Liebowitz MR, Nunes EV, et al. Generalizability of clinical trial results for major depression to community samples: results from the National Epidemiologic Survey on Alcohol and Related Conditions. *J Clin Psychiatry* 2008;69:1276-80.

139 Herland K, Akselsen JP, Skjøonsberg OH, Bjermer L. How representative are clinical study patients with asthma or COPD for a larger "real life" population of patients with obstructive lung disease? *Respir Med* 2005;99:11-9.

140 Bartlett C, Doyal L, Ebrahim S, Davey P, Bachmann M, Egger M, et al. The causes and effects of socio-demographic exclusions from clinical trials. *Health Technol Assess* 2005;9:iii-iiv.

141 Zarin DA, Young JL, West JC. Challenges to evidence-based medicine: a comparison of patients and treatments in randomized controlled trials with patients and treatments in a practice research network.*Soc Psychiatry Psychiatr Epidemiol* 2005;40:27-35.

142 Hordijk-Trion M, Lenzen M, Wijns W, de Jaegere P, Simoons ML, Scholte op Reimer WJ, et al. Patients enrolled in coronary intervention trials are not representative of patients in clinical practice: results from the Euro Heart Survey on Coronary Revascularization. *Eur Heart J* 2006;27:671-8.

143 Kievit W, Fransen J, Oerlemans AJ, Kuper HH, van der Laar MA, de Rooij DJ, et al. The efficacy of anti-TNF in rheumatoid arthritis, a comparison between randomised controlled trials and clinical practice. *Ann Rheum Dis* 2007;66:1473-8.

144 Uijen AA, Bakx JC, Mokkink HG, van Weel C. Hypertension patients participating in trials differ in many aspects from patients treated in general practices. *J Clin Epidemiol* 2007;60:330-5.

145 Crossman DC, Morton AC, Gunn JP, Greenwood JP, Hall AS, Fox KA, et al. Investigation of the effect of Interleukin-1 receptor antagonist (IL-1ra) on markers of inflammation in non-ST elevation acute coronary syndromes (The MRC-ILA-HEART Study) [protocol].*Trials* 2008;9:8.

146 Glasziou P, Meats E, Heneghan C, Shepperd S. What is missing from descriptions of treatment in trials and reviews?*BMJ* 2008;336:1472-4.

147 Duff JM, Leather H, Walden EO, LaPlant KD, George TJ, Jr. Adequacy of published oncology randomized controlled trials to provide therapeutic details needed for clinical application. *J Natl Cancer Inst* 2010;102:702-5.

148 Chalmers I, Glasziou P. Avoidable waste in the production and reporting of research evidence.*Lancet* 2009;374:86-9.

149 Glasziou P, Chalmers I, Altman DG, Bastian H, Boutron I, Brice A, et al. Taking healthcare interventions from trial to practice.*BMJ* 2010;341:c3852.

150 Golomb BA, Erickson LC, Koperski S, Sack D, Enkin M, Howick J. What's in placebos: who knows? Analysis of randomized, controlled trials. *Ann Intern Med* 2010;153:532-5.

151 Medical Research Council Working Party on Prostate Cancer. MRC PR05. A Medical Research Council randomised trial of adjuvant sodium clodronate in patients commencing or responding to hormone therapy for metastatic prostate adenocarcinoma [protocol]. Feb 1995 version. www.ctu.mrc.ac.uk/research_areas/study_details.aspx?s=60.

152 Panel on Handling Missing Data in Clinical Trials, National Research Council. The prevention and treatment of missing data in clinical trials. Washington DC, National Academies Press, 2010.

153 Buchbinder S, Liu A, Thompson M, Mayer K. Phase II extended safety study of tenofovir disoproxil fumarate (TDF) among HIV-1 negative men [protocol]. Version 1.6 (February 16, 2007). www.plosone.org/article/info%3Adoi%2F10.1371%2Fjournal.pone.0023688.

154 World Health Organization. Adherence to long-term therapies: evidence for action. 2012. www.who.int/chp/knowledge/publications/adherence_full_report.pdf.

155 Osterberg L, Blaschke T. Adherence to medication.*N Engl J Med* 2005;353:487-97.

156 Smith D. Patient nonadherence in clinical trials: could there be a link to postmarketing patient safety? *Drug Inf J* 2012;46:27-34.

157 Robiner WN. Enhancing adherence in clinical research. *Contemp Clin Trials* 2005;26:59-77.

158 Matsui D. Strategies to measure and improve patient adherence in clinical trials. *Pharmaceut Med* 2009;23:289-97.

159 Simpson SH, Eurich DT, Majumdar SR, Padwal RS, Tsuyuki RT, Varney J, et al. A meta-analysis of the association between adherence to drug therapy and mortality.*BMJ* 2006;333:15.

160 International Conference on Harmonisation. ICH Harmonised Tripartite Guideline: Good clinical practice, consolidated guideline. International Conference on Harmonisation of Technical Requirements for Registration of Pharmaceuticals for Human Use (June 1996, E6). 1996. http://www.ich.org/fileadmin/Public_Web_Site/ICH_Products/Guidelines/Efficacy/E6_R1/Step4/E6_R1__Guideline.pdf.

161 Jayaraman S, Rieder MJ, Matsui DM. Compliance assessment in drug trials: has there been improvement in two decades?*Can J Clin Pharmacol* 2005;12:e251-3.

162 Sackett DL. Clinician-trialist rounds: 5. Cointervention bias--how to diagnose it in their trial and prevent it in yours.*Clin Trials* 2011;8:440-2.

163 Zarin DA, Tse T, Williams RJ, Califf RM, Ide NC. The ClinicalTrials.gov results database--update and key issues. *N Engl J Med* 2011;364:852-60.

164 Bhandari M, Lochner H, Tornetta P, III. Effect of continuous versus dichotomous outcome variables on study power when sample sizes of orthopaedic randomized trials are small. *Arch Orthop Trauma Surg* 2002;122:96-8.

165 Verhagen AP, de Vet HCW, Willemsen S, Stijnen T. A meta-regression analysis shows no impact of design characteristics on outcome in trials on tension-type headaches. *J Clin Epi* 2008;61:813-8.

166 Hróbjartsson A, Thomsen AS, Emanuelsson F, Tendal B, Hilden J, Boutron I, et al. Observer bias in randomised clinical trials with binary

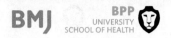

outcomes: systematic review of trials with both blinded and non-blinded outcome assessors.*BMJ* 2012;344:e1119.

167 Savović J, Jones HE, Altman DG, Harris RJ, Jüni P, Pildal J, et al. Influence of reported study design characteristics on intervention effect estimates from randomized, controlled trials. *Ann Intern Med* 2012;157:429-8.

168 Ferreira-González I, Busse JW, Heels-Ansdell D, Montori VM, Akl EA, Bryant DM, et al. Problems with use of composite end points in cardiovascular trials: systematic review of randomised controlled trials.*BMJ* 2007;334:786.

169 Montori VM, Permanyer-Miralda G, Ferreira-González I, Busse JW, Pacheco-Huergo V, Bryant D, et al. Validity of composite end points in clinical trials.*BMJ* 2005;330:596.

170 Freemantle N, Calvert M, Wood J, Eastaugh J, Griffin C. Composite outcomes in randomized trials: greater precision but with greater uncertainty?*JAMA* 2003;289:2554-59.

171 Cordoba G, Schwartz L, Woloshin S, Bae H, Gøtzsche PC. Definition, reporting, and interpretation of composite outcomes in clinical trials: systematic review.*BMJ* 2010;341:c3920.

172 Dwan K, Altman DG, Arnaiz JA, Bloom J, Chan A-W, Cronin E, et al. Systematic review of the empirical evidence of study publication bias and outcome reporting bias. *PLoS One* 2008;3:e3081.

173 Rising K, Bacchetti P, Bero L. Reporting bias in drug trials submitted to the Food and Drug Administration: Review of publication and presentation. *PLoS Med* 2008;5:e217.

174 Turner EH, Matthews AM, Linardatos E, Tell RA, Rosenthal R. Selective publication of antidepressant trials and its influence on apparent efficacy. *N Engl J Med* 2008;358:252-60.

175 Vedula SS, Bero L, Scherer RW, Dickersin K. Outcome reporting in industry-sponsored trials of gabapentin for off-label use.*N Engl J Med* 2009;361:1963-71.

176 Dwan K, Altman DG, Cresswell L, Blundell M, Gamble CL, Williamson PR. Comparison of protocols and registry entries to published reports for randomised controlled trials. *Cochrane Database Syst Rev* 2011;1:MR000031.

177 Chan A-W. Access to clinical trial data.*BMJ* 2011;342:d80.

178 Tugwell P, Boers M, Brooks P, Simon L, Strand V, Idzerda L. OMERACT: an international initiative to improve outcome measurement in rheumatology.*Trials* 2007;8:38.

179 Williamson P, Altman D, Blazeby J, Clarke M, Gargon E. Driving up the quality and relevance of research through the use of agreed core outcomes. *J Health Serv Res Policy* 2012;17:1-2.

180 Clarke M. Standardising outcomes for clinical trials and systematic reviews.*Trials* 2007;8:39.

181 Booth R, Fuller B, Thompson L, McCarty D, Shoptaw S, et al. STUDY #: NIDA-CTN-0017. HIV and HCV risk reduction interventions in drug detoxification and treatment settings [protocol]. Version 4.0 (August 16, 2010).www.dtmi.duke.edu/crflibrary-demo/crf-library-1/crf-library/trials-a-e/ctn-0017.

182 Cockayne NL, Glozier N, Naismith SL, Christensen H, Neal B, Hickie IB. Internet-based treatment for older adults with depression and co-morbid cardiovascular disease: protocol for a randomised, double-blind, placebo controlled trial [protocol]. *BMC Psychiatry* 2011;11:10.

183 McMurran M, Crawford MJ, Reilly JG, McCrone P, Moran P, Williams H, et al. Psycho-education with problem solving (PEPS) therapy for adults with personality disorder: A pragmatic multi-site community-based randomised clinical trial [protocol].*Trials* 2011;12:198.

184 van der Lee JH, Wesseling J, Tanck MW, Offringa M. Efficient ways exist to obtain the optimal sample size in clinical trials in rare diseases. *J Clin Epidemiol* 2008;61:324-30.

185 Yazici Y, Adler NM, Yazici H. Most tumour necrosis factor inhibitor trials in rheumatology are undeservedly called 'efficacy and safety' trials: a survey of power considerations.*Rheumatol* 2008;47:1054-7.

186 Hernández AV, Boersma E, Murray GD, Habbema JD, Steyerberg EW. Subgroup analyses in therapeutic cardiovascular clinical trials: are most of them misleading? *Am Heart J* 2006;151:257-64.

187 Copay AG, Subach BR, Glassman SD, Polly DW Jr, Schuler TC. Understanding the minimum clinically important difference: a review of concepts and methods. *Spine J* 2007;7:541-6.

188 Raju TN, Langenberg P, Sen A, Aldana O. How much 'better' is good enough? The magnitude of treatment effect in clinical trials.*Am J Dis Child* 1992;146:407-11.

189 Charles P, Giraudeau B, Dechartres A, Baron G, Ravaud P. Reporting of sample size calculation in randomised controlled trials: review.*BMJ* 2009;338:b1732.

190 Vickers AJ. Underpowering in randomized trials reporting a sample size calculation. *J Clin Epidemiol* 2003;56:717-20.

191 Proschan MA. Sample size re-estimation in clinical trials. *Biom J* 2009;51:348-57.

192 Julious SA, Campbell MJ, Altman DG. Estimating sample sizes for continuous, binary, and ordinal outcomes in paired comparisons: practical hints. *J Biopharm Stat* 1999;9:241-51.

193 Campbell MK, Elbourne DR, Altman DG, CONSORT group. CONSORT statement: extension to cluster randomised trials.*BMJ* 2004;328:702-8.

194 Piaggio G, Elbourne DR, Altman DG, Pocock SJ, Evans SJW. Reporting of noninferiority and equivalence randomized trials: An extension of the CONSORT statement.*JAMA* 2006;295:1152-60.

195 Pals SL, Murray DM, Alfano CM, Shadish WR, Hannan PJ, Baker WL. Individually randomized group treatment trials: a critical appraisal of frequently used design and analytic approaches. *Am J Pub Health* 2008;98:1418-24.

196 Eldridge S, Ashby D, Bennett C, Wakelin M, Feder G. Internal and external validity of cluster randomised trials: Systematic review of recent trials.*BMJ* 2008;336:876-80.

197 Eldridge SM, Ashby D, Feder GS, Rudnicka AR, Ukoumunne OC. Lessons for cluster randomized trials in the twenty-first century: a systematic review of trials in primary care. *Clin Trials* 2004;1:80-90.

198 Murray DM, Pals SL, Blitstein JL, Alfano CM, Lehman J. Design and analysis of group-randomized trials in cancer: A review of current practices. *J Natl Cancer Inst* 2008;100:483-91.

199 Freiman JA, Chalmers TC, Smith H, Jr., Kuebler RR. The importance of beta, the type II error and sample size in the design and interpretation of the randomized control trial. Survey of 71 "negative" trials.*N Engl J Med* 1978;299:690-4.

200 Bailey CS, Fisher CG, Dvorak MF. Type II error in the spine surgical literature.*Spine* 2004;29:1146-9.

201 Lochner HV, Bhandari M, Tornetta P, III. Type-II error rates (beta errors) of randomized trials in orthopaedic trauma. *J Bone Joint Surg Am* 2001;83-A:1650-5.

202 Enwere G. A review of the quality of randomized clinical trials of adjunctive therapy for the treatment of cerebral malaria.*Trop Med Int Health* 2005;10:1171-5.

203 Breau RH, Carnat TA, Gaboury I. Inadequate statistical power of negative clinical trials in urological literature.*J Urol* 2006;176:263-6.

204 Keen HI, Pile K, Hill CL. The prevalence of underpowered randomized clinical trials in rheumatology. *J Rheumatol* 2005;32:2083-8.

205 Maggard MA, O'Connell JB, Liu JH, Etzioni DA, Ko CY. Sample size calculations in surgery: are they done correctly?*Surgery* 2003;134:275-9.

206 Dimick JB, Diener-West M, Lipsett PA. Negative results of randomized clinical trials published in the surgical literature: equivalency or error? *Arch Surg* 2001;136:796-800.

207 Murray GD. Research governance must focus on research training.*BMJ* 2001;322:1461-2.

208 Asthma Clinical Research Network. Beta Adrenergic Response by Genotype (BARGE) study protocol: a study to compare the effects of regularly scheduled use of inhaled albuterol in patients with mild to moderate asthma who are members of two distinct haplotypes expressed at the β2 -adrenergic receptor [protocol]. Version 5.4 (September 23, 1999). https://biolincc.nhlbi.nih.gov/studies/barge/?q=barge.

209 Campbell MK, Snowdon C, Francis D, Elbourne D, McDonald AM, Knights R, et al. Recruitment to randomised trials: Strategies for trial enrolment and participation study. The STEPS study. *Health Technol Assess* 2007;11:iii-72.

210 Wise P, Drury M. Pharmaceutical trials in general practice: the first 100 protocols. An audit by the clinical research ethics committee of the Royal College of General Practitioners.*BMJ* 1996;313:1245-8.

211 Pich J, Carné X, Arnaiz JA, Gómez B, Trilla A, Rodés J. Role of a research ethics committee in follow-up and publication of results.*Lancet* 2003;361:1015-6.

212 Decullier E, Lhéritier V, Chapuis F. Fate of biomedical research protocols and publication bias in France: retrospective cohort study.*BMJ* 2005;331:19.

213 Dal-Ré R, Ortega R, Espada J. [Efficiency of investigators in recruitment of patients for clinical trials: apropos of a multinational study]. *Med Clin (Barc)* 1998;110:521-3.

214 McDonald AM, Knight RC, Campbell MK, Entwistle VA, Grant AM, Cook JA, et al. What influences recruitment to randomised controlled trials? A review of trials funded by two UK funding agencies.*Trials* 2006;7:9.

215 Charlson ME, Horwitz RI. Applying results of randomised trials to clinical practice: impact of losses before randomisation.*BMJ* 1984;289:1281-4.

216 Caldwell PH, Hamilton S, Tan A, Craig JC. Strategies for increasing recruitment to randomised controlled trials: systematic review. *PLoS Med* 2010;7:e1000368.

217 Treweek S, Pitkethly M, Cook J, Kjeldstrøm M, Taskila T, Johansen M, et al. Strategies to improve recruitment to randomised controlled trials. *Cochrane Database Syst Rev* 2010;4:MR000013.

218 Abraham NS, Young JM, Solomon MJ. A systematic review of reasons for nonentry of eligible patients into surgical randomized controlled trials.*Surgery* 2006;139:469-83.

219 Lai GY, Gary TL, Tilburt J, Bolen S, Baffi C, Wilson RF, et al. Effectiveness of strategies to recruit underrepresented populations into cancer clinical trials. *Clin Trials* 2006;3:133-41.

220 UyBico SJ, Pavel S, Gross CP. Recruiting vulnerable populations into research: a systematic review of recruitment interventions. *J Gen Intern Med* 2007;22:852-63.

221 Miller NL, Markowitz JC, Kocsis JH, Leon AC, Brisco ST, Garno JL. Cost effectiveness of screening for clinical trials by research assistants versus senior investigators. *J Psychiatr Res* 1999;33:81-5.

222 Tworoger SS, Yasui Y, Ulrich CM, Nakamura H, LaCroix K, Johnston R, et al. Mailing strategies and recruitment into an intervention trial of the exercise effect on breast cancer biomarkers.*Cancer Epidemiol Biomarkers Prev* 2002;11:73-7.

223 Schroy P.C. 3rd, Glick JT, Robinson P, Lydotes MA, Heeren TC, Prout M, et al. A cost-effectiveness analysis of subject recruitment strategies in the HIPAA era: results from a colorectal cancer screening adherence trial. *Clin Trials* 2009;6:597-609.

224 Harvey LA, Dunlop SA, Churilov L, Hsueh Y-SA, Galea MP. Early intensive hand rehabilitation after spinal cord injury ("hands on"): a protocol for a randomised controlled trial [protocol].*Trials* 2011;12:14.

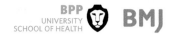

225 Schulz KF, Grimes DA. The Lancet handbook of essential concepts in clinical research. Elsevier, 2006.

226 Greenland S. Randomization, statistics, and causal inference.*Epidemiol* 1990;1:421-9.

227 Armitage P. The role of randomization in clinical trials. *Stat Med* 1982;1:345-52.

228 Odgaard-Jensen J, Vist GE, Timmer A, Kunz R, Akl EA, Schünemann H, et al. Randomisation to protect against selection bias in healthcare trials. *Cochrane Database Syst Rev* 2011;4:MR000012.

229 Jüni P, Altman DG, Egger M. Systematic reviews in health care: assessing the quality of controlled clinical trials.*BMJ* 2001;323:42-6.

230 McEntegart DJ. The pursuit of balance using stratified and dynamic randomization techniques: an overview. *Drug Inf J* 2003;37:293-308.

231 Schulz KF, Grimes DA. Generation of allocation sequences in randomised trials: chance, not choice.*Lancet* 2002;359:515-9.

232 Altman DG, Bland JM. How to randomise.*BMJ* 1999;319:703-4.

233 Schulz KF, Chalmers I, Hayes RJ, Altman DG. Empirical evidence of bias. Dimensions of methodological quality associated with estimates of treatment effects in controlled trials.*JAMA* 1995;273:408-12.

234 Kernan WN, Viscoli CM, Makuch RW, Brass LM, Horwitz RI. Stratified randomization for clinical trials. *J Clin Epidemiol* 1999;52:19-26.

235 Han B, Enas NH, McEntegart D. Randomization by minimization for unbalanced treatment allocation. *Stat Med* 2009;28:3329-46.

236 Altman DG. Practical statistics for medical research. Chapman and Hall/CRC, 1991.

237 Treasure T, MacRae KD. Minimisation: the platinum standard for trials? Randomisation doesn't guarantee similarity of groups; minimisation does.*BMJ* 1998;317:362-3.

238 Berger VW. Varying the block size does not conceal the allocation. *J Crit Care* 2006;21:229-30.

239 Berger VW. Minimization, by its nature, precludes allocation concealment, and invites selection bias. *Contemp Clin Trials* 2010;31:406.

240 Abbott JH, Robertson MC, McKenzie JE, Baxter GD, Theis J-C, Campbell AJ, et al. Exercise therapy, manual therapy, or both, for osteoarthritis of the hip or knee: a factorial randomised controlled trial protocol [protocol].*Trials* 2009;10:11.

241 Schulz KF, Grimes DA. Allocation concealment in randomised trials: defending against deciphering.*Lancet* 2002;359:614-618.

242 Chalmers TC, Levin H, Sacks HS, Reitman D, Berrier J, Nagalingam R. Meta-analysis of clinical trials as a scientific discipline. I: Control of bias and comparison with large co-operative trials. *Stat Med* 1987;6:315-28.

243 Schulz KF, Chalmers I, Grimes DA, Altman DG. Assessing the quality of randomization from reports of controlled trials published in obstetrics and gynecology journals.*JAMA* 1994;272:125-8.

244 Herbison P, Hay-Smith J, Gillespie WJ. Different methods of allocation to groups in randomized trials are associated with different levels of bias. A meta-epidemiological study. *J Clin Epidemiol* 2011;64:1070-5.

245 Kunz R, Vist G, Oxman AD. Randomisation to protect against selection bias in healthcare trials. *Cochrane Database Syst Rev* 2007;2:MR000012.

246 Klingberg S, Wittorf A, Meisner C, Wölwer W, Wiedemann G, Herrlich J, et al. Cognitive behavioural therapy versus supportive therapy for persistent positive symptoms in psychotic disorders: The POSITIVE study, a multicenter, prospective, single-blind, randomised controlled clinical trial [protocol].*Trials* 2010;11:123.

247 Dalum HS, Korsbek L, Mikkelsen JH, Thomsen K, Kistrup K, Olander M, et al. Illness management and recovery (IMR) in Danish community mental health centres [protocol].*Trials* 2011;12:195.

248 Hróbjartsson A, Gøtzsche PC. Placebo interventions for all clinical conditions. *Cochrane Database Syst Rev* 2010;1:CD003974.

249 Tierney JF, Stewart LA. Investigating patient exclusion bias in meta-analysis. *Int J Epidemiol* 2005;34:79-87.

250 Nüesch E, Trelle S, Reichenbach S, Rutjes AW, Bürgi E, Scherer M, et al. The effects of excluding patients from the analysis in randomised controlled trials: meta-epidemiological study.*BMJ* 2009;339:b3244.

251 Schulz KF, Chalmers I, Altman DG. The landscape and lexicon of blinding in randomized trials. *Ann Intern Med* 2002;136:254-59.

252 Ballintine EJ. Randomized controlled clinical trial. National Eye Institute workshop for ophthalmologists. Objective measurements and the double-masked procedure. *Am J Ophthalmol* 1975;79:763-7.

253 Gøtzsche PC. Blinding during data analysis and writing of manuscripts. *Control Clin Trials* 1996;17:285-90.

254 Grant AM, Altman DG, Babiker AB, Campbell MK, Clemens FJ, Darbyshire JH, et al. Issues in data monitoring and interim analysis of trials. *Health Technol Assess* 2005;9:1-238.

255 Meinert CL. Masked monitoring in clinical trials—blind stupidity? *N Engl J Med* 1998;338:1381-2.

256 Boutron I, Estellat C, Guittet L, Dechartres A, Sackett DL, Hróbjartsson A, et al. Methods of blinding in reports of randomized controlled trials assessing pharmacological treatments: a systematic review.*PLoS Med* 2006;3:e425.

257 Boutron I, Guittet L, Estellat C, Moher D, Hróbjartsson A, Ravaud P. Reporting methods of blinding in randomized trials assessing nonpharmacological treatments. *PLoS Med* 2007;4:e61.

258 Lieverse R, Nielen MM, Veltman DJ, Uitdehaag BM, van Someren EJ, Smit JH, et al. Bright light in elderly subjects with nonseasonal major depressive disorder: a double blind randomised clinical trial using early morning bright blue light comparing dim red light treatment.*Trials* 2008;9:48.

259 Devereaux PJ, Manns BJ, Ghali WA, Quan H, Lacchetti C, Montori VM, et al. Physician interpretations and textbook definitions of blinding terminology in randomized controlled trials.*JAMA* 2001;285:2000-3.

260 Haahr MT, Hróbjartsson A. Who is blinded in randomized clinical trials? A study of 200 trials and a survey of authors.*Clin Trials* 2006;3:360-5.

261 Hróbjartsson A, Boutron I. Blinding in randomized clinical trials: imposed impartiality. *Clin Pharmacol Ther* 2011;90:732-6.

262 Fergusson D, Glass KC, Waring D, Shapiro S. Turning a blind eye: the success of blinding reported in a random sample of randomised, placebo controlled trials.*BMJ* 2004;328:432.

263 Sackett DL. Clinician-trialist rounds: 6. Testing for blindness at the end of your trial is a mug's game. *Clin Trials* 2011;8:674-6.

264 Schulz KF, Altman DG, Moher D, Fergusson D. CONSORT 2010 changes and testing blindness in RCTs.*Lancet* 2010;375:1144-6.

265 A randomized, double blind, placebo controlled, parallel group trial for assessing the clinical benefit of Dronedarone 400mg BID on top of standard therapy in patients with permanent atrial fibrillation and additional risk factors. Permanent Atrial fibriLLAtion outcome Study using Dronedarone on top of standard therapy (PALLAS) [protocol]. Version 1 (February 26, 2010). www.nejm.org/doi/full/10.1056/NEJMoa1109867.

266 Campbell NL, Khan BA, Farber M, Campbell T, Perkins AJ, Hui SL, et al. Improving delirium care in the intensive care unit: the design of a pragmatic study [protocol].*Trials* 2011;12:139.

267 FSGS - Clinical trial [protocol]. Version 3c (June 20, 2005). https://clinicalresearch.ccf.org/fsgs/docs/index_docs.html.

268 Lane SJ, Heddle NM, Arnold E, Walker I. A review of randomized controlled trials comparing the effectiveness of hand held computers with paper methods for data collection. *BMC Med Inform Decis Mak* 2006;6:23.

269 Bent S, Padula A, Avins AL. Brief communication: Better ways to question patients about adverse medical events: a randomized, controlled trial. *Ann Intern Med* 2006;144:257-61.

270 Dale O, Hagen KB. Despite technical problems personal digital assistants outperform pen and paper when collecting patient diary data. *J Clin Epidemiol* 2007;60:8-17.

271 Litchfield J, Freeman J, Schou H, Elsley M, Fuller R, Chubb B. Is the future for clinical trials internet-based? A cluster randomised clinical trial. *Clin Trials* 2005;2:72-9.

272 Bedard M, Molloy DW, Standish T, Guyatt GH, D'Souza J, Mondadori C, et al. Clinical trials in cognitively impaired older adults: home versus clinic assessments. *J Am Geriatr Soc* 1995;43:1127-30.

273 Jasperse DM, Ahmed SW. The Mid-Atlantic Oncology Program's comparison of two data collection methods. *Control Clin Trials* 1989;10:282-9.

274 Basch E, Jia X, Heller G, Barz A, Sit L, Fruscione M, et al. Adverse symptom event reporting by patients vs clinicians: relationships with clinical outcomes. *J Natl Cancer Inst* 2009;101:1624-32.

275 Cohen SB, Strand V, Aguilar D, Ofman JJ. Patient- versus physician-reported outcomes in rheumatoid arthritis patients treated with recombinant interleukin-1 receptor antagonist (anakinra) therapy.*Rheumatology (Oxford)* 2004;43:704-11.

276 Fromme EK, Eilers KM, Mori M, Hsieh YC, Beer TM. How accurate is clinician reporting of chemotherapy adverse effects? A comparison with patient-reported symptoms from the Quality-of-Life Questionnaire C30. *J Clin Oncol* 2004;22:3485-90.

277 Walther B, Hossin S, Townend J, Abernethy N, Parker D, Jeffries D. Comparison of electronic data capture (EDC) with the standard data capture method for clinical trial data. *PLoS One* 2011;6:e25348.

278 Kryworuchko J, Stacey D, Bennett C, Graham ID. Appraisal of primary outcome measures used in trials of patient decision support. *Patient Educ Couns* 2008;73:497-503.

279 Roberts L, Counsell C. Assessment of clinical outcomes in acute stroke trials.*Stroke* 1998;29:986-91.

280 Marshall M, Lockwood A, Bradley C, Adams C, Joy C, Fenton M. Unpublished rating scales: a major source of bias in randomised controlled trials of treatments for schizophrenia. *Br J Psychiatry* 2000;176:249-52.

281 Williams GW. The other side of clinical trial monitoring; assuring data quality and procedural adherence. *Clin Trials* 2006;3:530-7.

282 Gassman JJ, Owen WW, Kuntz TE, Martin JP, Amoroso WP. Data quality assurance, monitoring, and reporting. *Control Clin Trials* 1995;16:104S-36S.

283 Meyerson LJ, Wiens BL, LaVange LM, Koutsoukos AD. Quality control of oncology clinical trials. *Hematol Oncol Clin North Am* 2000;14:953-71.

284 Fong DYT. Data management and quality assurance.*Drug Inf J* 2001;35:839-44.

285 Knatterud GL, Rockhold FW, George SL, Barton FB, Davis CE, Fairweather WR, et al. Guidelines for quality assurance in multicenter trials: a position paper. *Control Clin Trials* 1998;19:477-93.

286 Prevention Study Group. HEALTHY primary prevention trial protocol [protocol]. Version 1.4 (July 14, 2008). www.healthystudy.org/.

287 HIV Prevention Trials Network and the International Maternal Pediatric and Adolescent AIDS Clinical Trials Network. HPTN 046: A phase III trial to determine the efficacy and safety of an extended regimen of nevirapine in infants born to HIV-infected women to prevent vertical HIV transmission during breastfeeding [protocol]. Version 3.0 (September 26, 2007).www.hptn.org/research_studies/hptn046.asp.

288 Ioannidis JP, Bassett R, Hughes MD, Volberding PA, Sacks HS, Lau J. Predictors and impact of patients lost to follow-up in a long-

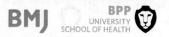

term randomized trial of immediate versus deferred antiretroviral treatment. *J Acquir Immune Defic Syndr Hum Retrovirol* 1997;16:22-30.

289 Ford ME, Havstad S, Vernon SW, Davis SD, Kroll D, Lamerato L, et al. Enhancing adherence among older African American men enrolled in a longitudinal cancer screening trial.*Gerontologist* 2006;46:545-50.

290 Couper MP, Peytchev A, Strecher VJ, Rothert K, Anderson J. Following up nonrespondents to an online weight management intervention: Randomized trial comparing mail versus telephone. *J Med Internet Res* 2007;9:e16.

291 Renfroe EG, Heywood G, Foreman L, Schron E, Powell J, Baessler C, et al. The end-of-study patient survey: methods influencing response rate in the AVID Trial. *Control Clin Trials* 2002;23:521-33.

292 Robinson KA, Dennison CR, Wayman DM, Pronovost PJ, Needham DM. Systematic review identifies number of strategies important for retaining study participants. *J Clin Epi* 2007;60:757-65.

293 Fleming TR. Addressing missing data in clinical trials. *Ann Intern Med* 2011;154:113-7.

294 Liu M, Wei L, Zhang J. Review of guidelines and literature for handling missing data in longitudinal clinical trials with a case study. *Pharm Stat* 2006;5:7-18.

295 Wahlbeck K, Tuunainen A, Ahokas A, Leucht S. Dropout rates in randomised antipsychotic drug trials.*Psychopharmacology (Berl)* 2001;155:230-33.

296 Kawado M, Hinotsu S, Matsuyama Y, Yamaguchi T, Hashimoto S, Ohashi Y. A comparison of error detection rates between the reading aloud method and the double data entry method. *Control Clin Trials* 2003;24:560-9.

297 Day S, Fayers P, Harvey D. Double data entry: what value, what price? *Control Clin Trials* 1998;19:15-24.

298 Reynolds-Haertle RA, McBride R. Single vs. double data entry in CAST. *Control Clin Trials* 1992;13:487-94.

299 Gibson D, Harvey AJ, Everett V, Parmar MK. Is double data entry necessary? The CHART trials. CHART Steering Committee. Continuous, hyperfractionated, accelerated radiotherapy. *Control Clin Trials* 1994;15:482-8.

300 Ioannidis JPA, Evans SJW, Gøtzsche PC, O'Neill RT, Altman DG, Schulz KF, et al. Better reporting of harms in randomized trials: an extension of the CONSORT statement. *Ann Intern Med* 2004;141:781-8.

301 Schulz KF, Grimes DA. Multiplicity in randomised trials I: endpoints and treatments.*Lancet* 2005;365:1591-5.

302 Tendal B, Nüesch E, Higgins JP, Jüni P, Gøtzsche PC. Multiplicity of data in trial reports and the reliability of meta-analyses: empirical study.*BMJ* 2011;343:d4829.

303 Flow Investigators. Fluid lavage of open wounds (FLOW): design and rationale for a large, multicenter collaborative 2 x 3 factorial trial of irrigating pressures and solutions in patients with open fractures [protocol]. *BMC Musculoskelet Disord* 2010;11:85.

304 Resuscitation Outcomes Consortium Prehospital Resuscitation using an IMpedance valve and Early vs Delayed analysis (ROC PRIMED) Trial. A factorial design of an active impedance threshold valve versus sham valve and analyze later versus analyze early [protocol]. Dec 2006 version.www.nejm.org/doi/full/10.1056/NEJMoa1010821.

305 Boonacker CW, Hoes AW, van Liere-Visser K, Schilder AG, Rovers MM. A comparison of subgroup analyses in grant applications and publications. *Am J Epidemiol* 2011;174:219-25.

306 Schulz KF, Grimes DA. Multiplicity in randomised trials II: subgroup and interim analyses.*Lancet* 2005;365:1657-61.

307 Hirji KF, Fagerland MW. Outcome based subgroup analysis: a neglected concern.*Trials* 2009;10:33.

308 Sun X, Briel M, Walter SD, Guyatt GH. Is a subgroup effect believable? Updating criteria to evaluate the credibility of subgroup analyses.*BMJ* 2010;340:c117.

309 Rothwell PM. Treating individuals 2. Subgroup analysis in randomised controlled trials: importance, indications, and interpretation.*Lancet* 2005;365:176-86.

310 Yu L-M, Chan A-W, Hopewell S, Deeks JJ, Altman DG. Reporting on covariate adjustment in randomised controlled trials before and after revision of the 2001 CONSORT statement: a literature review.*Trials* 2010;11:59.

311 Chen X, Liu M, Zhang J. A note on postrandomization adjustment of covariates. *Drug Inf J* 2005;39:373-83.

312 Rochon J. Issues in adjusting for covariates arising postrandomization in clinical trials. *Drug Inf J* 1999;33:1219-28.

313 Mohr JP, Moskowitz A, Ascheim D, Gelijns A, Parides M, et al. A Randomized multicenter clinical trial of unruptured brain AVMs (ARUBA): clinical protocol [protocol]. Version 3.0 (October 16, 2008). http://research.ncl.ac.uk/nctu/ARUBA.html.

314 Abraha I, Montedori A. Modified intention to treat reporting in randomised controlled trials: systematic review.*BMJ* 2010;340:c2697.

315 Fergusson D, Aaron SD, Guyatt G, Hébert P. Post-randomisation exclusions: the intention to treat principle and excluding patients from analysis.*BMJ* 2002;325:652-4.

316 Hollis S, Campbell F. What is meant by intention to treat analysis? Survey of published randomised controlled trials.*BMJ* 1999;319:670-4.

317 Akl EA, Briel M, You JJ, Sun X, Johnston BC, Busse JW, et al. Potential impact on estimated treatment effects of information lost to follow-up in randomised controlled trials (LOST-IT): systematic review.*BMJ* 2012;344:e2809.

318 Wood AM, White IR, Thompson SG. Are missing outcome data adequately handled? A review of published randomized controlled trials in major medical journals. *Clin Trials* 2004;1:368-76.

319 Fielding S, Fayers P, Ramsay CR. Analysing randomised controlled trials with missing data: Choice of approach affects conclusions. *Contemp Clin Trials* 2012;33:461-9.

320 Streiner DL. Missing data and the trouble with LOCF. *Evid Based Ment Health* 2008;11:3-5.

321 Sterne JA, White IR, Carlin JB, Spratt M, Royston P, Kenward MG, et al. Multiple imputation for missing data in epidemiological and clinical research: potential and pitfalls.*BMJ* 2009;338:b2393.

322 Groenwold RH, Donders AR, Roes KC, Harrell FE, Jr., Moons KG. Dealing with missing outcome data in randomized trials and observational studies. *Am J Epidemiol* 2012;175:210-7.

323 Giraudeau B, Ravaud P. Preventing bias in cluster randomised trials. *PLoS Med* 2009;6:e1000065.

324 Berger VW. Conservative handling of missing data.*Contemp Clin Trials* 2012;33:460.

325 Azuara-Blanco A, Burr JM, Cochran C, Ramsay C, Vale L, Foster P, et al. The effectiveness of early lens extraction with intraocular lens implantation for the treatment of primary angle-closure glaucoma (EAGLE): study protocol for a randomized controlled trial [protocol].*Trials* 2011;12:133.

326 Sydes MR, Altman DG, Babiker AB, Parmar MK, Spiegelhalter DJ, DAMOCLES Group. Reported use of data monitoring committees in the main published reports of randomized controlled trials: a cross-sectional study. *Clin Trials* 2004;1:48-59.

327 Floriani I, Rotmensz N, Albertazzi E, Torri V, De Rosa M, Tomino C, et al. Approaches to interim analysis of cancer randomised clinical trials with time to event endpoints: a survey from the Italian National Monitoring Centre for Clinical Trials.*Trials* 2008;9:46.

328 Califf RM, Zarin DA, Kramer JM, Sherman RE, Aberle LH, Tasneem A. Characteristics of clinical trials registered in ClinicalTrials.gov, 2007-2010.*JAMA* 2012;307:1838-47.

329 Ellenberg SS. Independent data monitoring committees: rationale, operations and controversies. *Stat Med* 2001;20:2573-2583.

330 Ellenberg SS, Fleming TR, DeMets DL. Data monitoring committees in clinical trials: a practical perspective. 6th ed. Wiley, 2002.

331 DAMOCLES study group, NHS Health Technology Assessment Programme. A proposed charter for clinical trial data monitoring committees: helping them to do their job well.*Lancet* 2005;365:711-22.

332 Bakker OJ, van Santvoort HC, van Brunschot S, Ali UA, Besselink MG, et al. Pancreatitis, very early compared with normal start of enteral feeding (PYTHON trial): design and rationale of a randomised controlled multicenter trial [protocol].*Trials* 2011;12:73.

333 DeMets DL, Pocock SJ, Julian DG. The agonising negative trend in monitoring of clinical trials.*Lancet* 1999;354:1983-8.

334 Berry DA. Interim analyses in clinical trials: classical vs. Bayesian approaches. *Stat Med* 1985;4:521-6.

335 Pocock SJ. When to stop a clinical trial.*BMJ* 1992;305:235-40.

336 Aronson JK, Ferner RE. Clarification of terminology in drug safety. *Drug Saf* 2005;28:851-70.

337 Myers MG, Cairns JA, Singer J. The consent form as a possible cause of side effects. *Clin Pharmacol Ther* 1987;42:250-3.

338 Wallin J, Sjövall J. Detection of adverse drug reactions in a clinical trial using two types of questioning. *Clin Ther* 1981;3:450-2.

339 Gøtzsche PC. Non-steroidal anti-inflammatory drugs.*BMJ* 2000;320:1058-61.

340 Curfman GD, Morrissey S, Drazen JM. Expression of concern reaffirmed. *N Engl J Med* 2006;354:1193.

341 Wright JM, Perry TL, Bassett KL, Chambers GK. Reporting of 6-month vs 12-month data in a clinical trial of celecoxib.*JAMA* 2001;286:2398-400.

342 Crowe BJ, Xia HA, Berlin JA, Watson DJ, Shi H, Lin SL, et al. Recommendations for safety planning, data collection, evaluation and reporting during drug, biologic and vaccine development: a report of the safety planning, evaluation, and reporting team. *Clin Trials* 2009;6:430-40.

343 Sherman RB, Woodcock J, Norden J, Grandinetti C, Temple RJ. New FDA regulation to improve safety reporting in clinical trials.*N Engl J Med* 2011;365:3-5.

344 Ruiz-Canela M, Martinez-González MA, Gómez-Gracia E, Fernández-Crehuet J. Informed consent and approval by institutional review boards in published reports on clinical trials. *N Engl J Med* 1999;340:1114-5.

345 Breast Cancer International Research Group. BCIRG 006: Multicenter phase III randomized trial comparing doxorubicin and cyclophosphamide followed by docetaxel (AC-->T) with doxorubicin and cyclophosphamide followed by docetaxel and trastuzumab (Herceptin®) (AC-->TH) and with docetaxel, carboplatin and trastuzumab (TCH) in the adjuvant treatment of node positive and high risk node negative patients with operable breast cancer containing the HER2 alteration [protocol]. Version 5www.nejm.org/doi/full/10.1056/NEJMoa0910383.

346 Getz KA, Zuckerman R, Cropp AB, Hindle AL, Krauss R, Kaitin KI. Measuring the incidence, causes, and repercussions of protocol amendments. *Drug Inf J* 2011;45:265-75.

347 Decullier E, Lhéritier V, Chapuis F. The activity of French research ethics committees and characteristics of biomedical research protocols involving humans: a retrospective cohort study. *BMC Med Ethics* 2005;6:e9.

348 Lösch C, Neuhäuser M. The statistical analysis of a clinical trial when a protocol amendment changed the inclusion criteria.*BMC Med Res Methodol* 2008;8:16.

349 US Food and Drug Administration. Code of federal regulations. Title 21, Vol 5. 21CFR312.30. 2011.

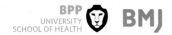

350 European Commission. Communication from the Commission–– Detailed guidance on the request to the competent authorities for authorisation of a clinical trial on a medicinal product for human use, the notification of substantial amendments and the declaration of the end of the trial (CT-1) (2010/C 82/01). *Off J European Union* 2010;53.

351 Bond J, Wilson J, Eccles M, Vanoli A, Steen N, Clarke R, et al. Protocol for north of England and Scotland study of tonsillectomy and adeno-tonsillectomy in children (NESSTAC). A pragmatic randomised controlled trial comparing surgical intervention with conventional medical treatment in children with recurrent sore throats [protocol].*BMC Ear, Nose Throat Disord* 2006;6:13.

352 Williams CJ, Zwitter M. Informed consent in European multicentre randomised clinical trials - Are patients really informed?*Eur J Cancer* 1994;30:907-10.

353 Ryan RE, Prictor MJ, McLaughlin KJ, Hill SJ. Audio-visual presentation of information for informed consent for participation in clinical trials. *Cochrane Database Syst Rev* 2008;1:CD003717.

354 Flory J, Emanuel E. Interventions to improve research participants' understanding in informed consent for research: a systematic review.*JAMA* 2004;292:1593-601.

355 Cohn E, Larson E. Improving participant comprehension in the informed consent process. *J Nurs Scholarsh* 2007;39:273-80.

356 Wendler DS. Assent in paediatric research: theoretical and practical considerations. *J Med Ethic* 2006;32:229.

357 McRae AD, Weijer C, Binik A, Grimshaw JM, Boruch R, Brehaut JC, et al. When is informed consent required in cluster randomized trials in health research?*Trials* 2011;12:202.

358 Beskow LM, Friedman JY, Hardy NC, Lin L, Weinfurt KP. Developing a simplified consent form for biobanking. *PLoS One* 2010;5:e13302.

359 HIV Prevention Trials Network. HPTN 037: A phase III randomized study to evaluate the efficacy of a network-oriented peer educator intervention for the prevention of HIV transmission among injection drug users and their network members [protocol]. Version 2.0 (October 23, 2003). www.hptn.org/research_studies/hptn037.asp.

360 World Association of Medical Editors Editorial Policy and Publication Ethics Committees. Conflict of interest in peer-reviewed medical journals. 2009. www.wame.org/ conflict-of-interest-in-peer-reviewed-medical-journals.

361 Rochon PA, Hoey J, Chan A-W, Ferris LE, Lexchin J, Kalkar SR, et al. Financial conflicts of interest checklist 2010 for clinical research studies. *Open Med* 2010;4:e69-91.

362 Drazen JM, de Leeuw PW, Laine C, Mulrow C, DeAngelis CD, Frizelle FA, et al. Towards more uniform conflict disclosures: the updated ICMJE conflict of interest reporting form.*BMJ* 2010;340:c3239.

363 World Medical Association. WMA statement on conflict of interest. 2012. www.wma.net/en/30publications/10policies/i3/.

364 Lundh A, Krogsbøll LT, Gøtzsche PC. Access to data in industry-sponsored trials.*Lancet* 2011;378:1995-6.

365 Microbicide Trials Network. MTN-003: Phase 2B safety and effectiveness study of tenofovir 1% gel, tenofovir disproxil fumarate tablet and emtricitabine/tenofovir disoproxil fumarate tablet for the prevention of HIV infection in women [protocol]. Version 2.0 (December 31, 2010). www.mtnstopshiv.org/news/studies/mtn003.

366 Richardson HS, Belsky L. The ancillary-care responsibilities of medical researchers. *Hastings Center Report* 2004;34:25-33.

367 Belsky L, Richardson HS. Medical researchers' ancillary clinical care responsibilities.*BMJ* 2004;328:1494-6.

368 Sofaer N, Strech D. Reasons why post-trial access to trial drugs should, or need not be ensured to research participants: A systematic review. *Public Health Ethics* 2011;4:160-84.

369 Participants in the 2006 Georgetown University Workshop on the Ancillary-Care Obligations of Medical Researchers Working in Developing Countries. The ancillary-care obligations of medical researchers working in developing countries. *PLoS Med* 2008;5:e90.

370 Beta-Blocker Evaluation of Survival Trial (BEST) Protocol [protocol]. Version 1 (June 22, 1999). https://biolincc.nhlbi.nih.gov/studies/best/.

371 Mann H. Research ethics committees and public dissemination of clinical trial results.*Lancet* 2002;360:406-8.

372 Gøtzsche PC. Why we need easy access to all data from all clinical trials and how to accomplish it.*Trials* 2011;12:249.

373 Whittington CJ, Kendall T, Fonagy P, Cottrell D, Cotgrove A, Boddington E. Selective serotonin reuptake inhibitors in childhood depression: systematic review of published versus unpublished data.*Lancet* 2004;363:1341-5.

374 Cowley AJ, Skene A, Stainer K, Hampton JR. The effect of lorcainide on arrhythmias and survival in patients with acute myocardial infarction: an example of publication bias. *Int J Cardiol* 1993;40:161-6.

375 McGauran N, Wieseler B, Kreis J, Schüler YB, Kölsch H, Kaiser T. Reporting bias in medical research - a narrative review.*Trials* 2010;11:37.

376 Hart B, Lundh A, Bero L. Effect of reporting bias on meta-analyses of drug trials: reanalysis of meta-analyses.*BMJ* 2012;344:d7202.

377 Doshi P, Jones M, Jefferson T. Rethinking credible evidence synthesis.*BMJ* 2012;344:d7898.

378 Emerson GB, Warme WJ, Wolf FM, Heckman JD, Brand RA, Leopold SS. Testing for the presence of positive-outcome bias in peer review: a randomized controlled trial. *Arch Intern Med* 2010;170:1934-9.

379 Olson CM, Rennie D, Cook D, Dickersin K, Flanagin A, Hogan JW, et al. Publication bias in editorial decision making.*JAMA* 2002;287:2825-8.

380 Rochon PA, Sekeres M, Hoey J, Lexchin J, Ferris LE, Moher D, et al. Investigator experiences with financial conflicts of interest in clinical trials.*Trials* 2011;12:9.

381 Steinbrook R. Gag clauses in clinical-trial agreements. *N Engl J Med* 2005;352:2160-2.

382 McCarthy M. Company sought to block paper's publication.*Lancet* 2000;356:1659.

383 Nathan DG, Weatherall DJ. Academic freedom in clinical research. *N Engl J Med* 2002;347:1368-71.

384 Rennie D. Thyroid storm.*JAMA* 1997;277:1238-43.

385 Flanagin A, Fontanarosa PB, DeAngelis CD. Authorship for research groups.*JAMA* 2002;288:3166-8.

386 Ross JS, Hill KP, Egilman DS, Krumholz HM. Guest authorship and ghostwriting in publications related to rofecoxib: a case study of industry documents from rofecoxib litigation.*JAMA* 2008;299:1800-12.

387 Wislar JS, Flanagin A, Fontanarosa PB, DeAngelis CD. Honorary and ghost authorship in high impact biomedical journals: a cross sectional survey.*BMJ* 2011;343:d6128.

388 Gøtzsche PC, Kassirer JP, Woolley KL, Wager E, Jacobs A, Gertel A, et al. What should be done to tackle ghostwriting in the medical literature? *PLoS Med* 2009;6:e1000023.

389 International Committee of Medical Journal Editors. Uniform requirements for manuscripts submitted to biomedical journals: Writing and editing for biomedical publication. 2010. www.icmje.org/ urm_full.pdf.

390 Matheson A. How industry uses the ICMJE guidelines to manipulate authorship--and how they should be revised. *PLoS Med* 2011;8:e1001072.

391 Graf C, Battisti WP, Bridges D, Bruce-Winkler V, Conaty JM, Ellison JM, et al. Good publication practice for communicating company sponsored medical research: the GPP2 guidelines.*BMJ* 2009;339:b4330.

392 Jacobs A, Wager E. European Medical Writers Association (EMWA) guidelines on the role of medical writers in developing peer-reviewed publications. *Curr Med Res Opin* 2005;21:317-21.

393 Wolinsky FD, Vander Weg MW, Howren MB, Jones MP, Martin R, Luger TM, et al. Protocol for a randomized controlled trial to improve cognitive functioning in older adults: the Iowa Healthy and Active Minds Study [protocol]. *BMJ Open* 2011;1:e000218.

394 Chan A-W. Bias, spin, and misreporting: Time for full access to trial protocols and results. *PLoS Med* 2008;5:e230.

395 Lassere M, Johnson K. The power of the protocol.*Lancet* 2002;360:1620-2.

396 Wieseler B, Kerekes MF, Vervoelgyi V, McGauran N, Kaiser T. Impact of document type on reporting quality of clinical drug trials: a comparison of registry reports, clinical study reports, and journal publications.*BMJ* 2012;344:d8141.

397 Gøtzsche PC, Jørgensen AW. Opening up data at the European Medicines Agency.*BMJ* 2011;342:d2686.

398 European Medicines Agency. European Medicines Agency policy on access to documents (related to medicinal products for human and veterinary use) (EMA/110196/2006). 2010. www.ema.europa.eu/docs/ en_GB/document_library/Other/2010/11/WC500099473.pdf.

399 Doshi P, Jefferson T, Del Mar C. The imperative to share clinical study reports: recommendations from the tamiflu experience.*PLoS Med* 2012;9:e1001201.

400 Eichler H-G, Abadie E, Breckenridge A, Leufkens H, Rasi G. Open clinical trial data for all? A view from regulators. *PLoS Med* 2012;9:e1001202.

401 Committee on Responsibilities of Authorship in the Biological Sciences, National Research Council. Sharing publication-related data and materials: responsibilities of authorship in the life sciences. National Academies Press, 2003.

402 Hrynaszkiewicz I, Norton ML, Vickers AJ, Altman DG. Preparing raw clinical data for publication: guidance for journal editors, authors, and peer reviewers.*Trials* 2010;11:9.

403 Walport M, Brest P. Sharing research data to improve public health.*Lancet* 2011;377:537-9.

404 Ross JS, Lehman R, Gross CP. The importance of clinical trial data sharing: toward more open science. *Circ Cardiovasc Qual Outcomes* 2012;5:238-40.

405 Vickers AJ. Making raw data more widely available.*BMJ* 2011;342:d2323.

406 The Royal Society Science Policy Centre. Science as an open enterprise. 2012. http://royalsociety.org/uploadedFiles/Royal_Society_ Content/policy/projects/sape/2012-06-20-SAOE.pdf

407 Summerskill W, Collingridge D, Frankish H. Protocols, probity, and publication.*Lancet* 2009;373:992.

408 Altman D, Furberg C, Grimshaw J, Rothwell P. Trials—using the opportunities of electronic publishing to improve the reporting of randomised trials.*Trials* 2006;7:6.

409 Sharing of materials, methods, and data. 2011.www.plosone.org/ static/policies.action.

410 Trials. Instructions for authors. Editorial policies. 2012. www. trialsjournal.com/authors/instructions.

411 National Institutes of Health. Final NIH statement on sharing research data. Feb 26, 2003. http://grants.nih.gov/grants/guide/notice-files/ NOT-OD-03-032.html.

412 Laine C, Goodman SN, Griswold ME, Sox HC. Reproducible research: moving toward research the public can really trust.*Ann Intern Med* 2007;146:450-3.

413 BMJ Publishing Group Ltd. Instructions for authors. 2012. http:// bmjopen.bmj.com/site/about/guidelines.xhtml.

414 Sugarman J, McCrory DC, Hubal RC. Getting meaningful informed consent from older adults: a structured literature review of empirical research. *J Am Ger Soc* 1998;46:517-24.

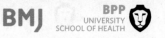

415   Paris A, Cracowski JL, Ravanel N, Cornu C, Gueyffier F, Deygas B, et al. [Readability of informed consent forms for subjects participating in biomedical research: updating is required].*Presse Med* 2005;34:13-8.

416   Southwest Oncology Group. Chemoprevention of prostate cancer with finasteride (Proscar®) Phase III [protocol]. Aug 2001 version. http://swog.org/visitors/pcpt/.

417   Schulz KF, Altman DG, Moher D, the CONSORT Group. CONSORT 2010 Statement: updated guidelines for reporting parallel group randomised trials.*BMJ* 2010;340:c332.

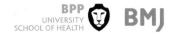

Good publication practice for communicating company sponsored medical research: the GPP2 guidelines

Chris Graf, associate editorial director[1], Wendy P Battisti, associate director, scientific and medical publications[2], Dan Bridges, group programme director[3], Victoria Bruce-Winkler, medical publications consultant[4], Joanne M Conaty, senior director, clinical strategy and planning[5], John M Ellison, senior manager, scientific publications[6], Elizabeth A Field, president[7], James A Gurr, director, publication planning and development[8], Mary-Ellen Marx, senior manager, medical education[9], Mina Patel, senior director, medical communications[10], Carol Sanes-Miller, global publications manager, scientific communications[5], Yvonne E Yarker, senior vice president, medical communications[11], for the International Society for Medical Publication Professionals

[1]John Wiley & Sons, Wiley-Blackwell, Oxford OX4 2DQ

[2]Johnson & Johnson Pharmaceutical Research & Development, Raritan, NJ, USA

[3]Excerpta Medica, Elsevier, London

[4]Dunblane

[5]AstraZeneca Pharmaceuticals, Wilmington, DE, USA

[6]LifeScan, Milpitas, CA, USA

[7]Field Advantage Medical Communications, Chapel Hill, NC, USA

[8]Pfizer Collegeville, PA, USA

[9]PharmaWrite, Princeton, NJ, USA

[10]Cephalon, Frazer, PA, USA

[11]Knowledgepoint 360 Group, Newtown, PA, USA

Correspondence to: C Graf chris.graf@wiley.com

Cite this as: BMJ 2009;339:b4330

http://www.bmj.com/content/339/bmj.b4330

ABSTRACT

In response to changes in the environment in which authors, presenters, and other contributors work together to communicate medical research the **International Society for Medical Publication Professionals** has updated the good publication practice guidelines

Authors and presenters are responsible for how medical research is interpreted and communicated. Often their work is the product of collaborations with other individuals (such as clinical investigators, biostatisticians, and professional medical writers) from around the world. Some or all of the people who contribute to this collaboration may be employees of research sponsors, contract research organisations, or medical communications agencies that may be funded by pharmaceutical, medical device, or biotechnology companies. The authors, collaborators, and organisations share responsibility for developing articles and presentations in a responsible and ethical manner.

The good publication practice (GPP2) guidelines presented here make recommendations that will help

WHAT'S NEW?

GPP2 updates earlier good publication practice guidelines.[6]

New elements include:

- An extensive consultation process was used to write the guidelines
- Authorship guidance recommends assignment of a lead author and guarantor
- Contributorship guidance recommends describing the role of the sponsor
- Recommendations about reimbursement
- Recommendations for specific types of articles and presentations
- Recommendations for publication planning and documentation

Updated elements include:

- Guidance on defining the roles of authors, sponsors, and other contributors
- Guidance on establishing a publication steering committee
- Confirmation of the role of professional medical writers

individuals and organisations maintain ethical practices and comply with current requirements when they contribute to the communication of medical research sponsored by companies. These guidelines apply to peer reviewed journal articles and presentations at scientific congresses.

Evolving standards

The conduct and communication of medical research, including that sponsored by companies, continues to be criticised.[1 2 3 4 5] Since 2003, when the original good publication practice guidelines were published,[6] the environment in which medical research is reported has evolved. The Declaration of Helsinki, updated in 2008, places accuracy and completeness among the primary ethical obligations of individuals communicating medical research, and suggests that "reports of research not in accordance with [its] principles should not be accepted for publication."[7] Information about clinical trials, including results, is being made accessible in new ways driven by regulations and guidelines from around the world.[8 9 10 11 12 13 14 15] Standards for the accurate publication and presentation of research have also evolved,[16] and new or updated codes of practice have been developed (table 1). The International Society for Medical Publication Professionals (www.ismpp.org) has been established and certifies the practice of individuals developing articles and presentations sponsored by companies. These guidelines were written in light of these developments.

Methods

The International Society for Medical Publication Professionals invited members with over 10 years of experience in biomedical publishing to develop these guidelines (figure). The 14 members named as contributors to this article responded to the invitation and formed the steering committee. The steering committee reviewed the original guidelines,[6] discussed items to be included in the revised guidelines (GPP2), and wrote the draft guidelines.

The steering committee recruited an international consultation panel by direct invitation and multiple open requests for volunteers. The draft guidelines were circulated to the 193 people who agreed to be part of the consultation panel for comment. The consultation process was conducted in confidence (table 2). The 116 sets of comments submitted were blinded and collated, and members of the steering committee assessed and ranked them on:

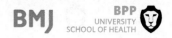

Table 1 New or updated codes of practice since 2003

International Society for Medical Publication Professionals (www.ismpp.org)	Code of ethics
	Position statement: the role of the professional medical writer
Association of American Medical Colleges (www.aamc.org)	Report of task force on industry funding of medical education
American Medical Writers Association (www.amwa.org)	Code of ethics
	Position statement: the contribution of medical writers to scientific publications
Committee on Publication Ethics (http://publicationethics.org)	Multiple resources for editors
Council of Science Editors (www.councilscienceeditors.org)	White paper on promoting integrity in scientific journal publications
Elsevier (www.elsevier.com/wps/find/editorshome.editors/Introduction)	Publishing ethics resource kit
European Medical Writers Association (www.emwa.org)	Guidelines on the role of medical writers in developing peer reviewed publications
EQUATOR Network (www.equator-network.org)	Reporting guidelines—for example, CONSORT, STROBE, QUOROM/PRISMA, STARD, MOOSE
Federation of American Societies for Experimental Biology (www.faseb.org)	Conflicts of interest in biomedical research—the FASEB guidelines
International Committee of Medical Journal Editors (www.icmje.org)	Uniform requirements for manuscripts submitted to biomedical journals: writing and editing for biomedical publication
Institute of Medicine (www.iom.edu/CMS/3740/47464/65721.aspx)	Conflict of interest in medical research, education, and practice
International Federation of Pharmaceutical Manufacturers and Associations (www.ifpma.org/fileadmin/pdfs/webnews/Revised_Joint_Industry_Position_26Nov08.pdf)	Joint position on the disclosure of clinical trial information via clinical trial registries and databases
International Society for Pharmacoeconomics and Outcomes Research (www.ispor.org/PEguidelines/index.asp)	Pharmacoeconomic guidelines around the world
Pharmaceutical Research and Manufacturers of America (www.phrma.org)	Principles on conduct of clinical trials and communication of clinical trial results
World Association of Medical Editors (www.wame.org/resources /policies)	WAME policy statements prepared by the editorial policy committee, including conflict of interest in peer reviewed medical journals
Wiley-Blackwell (www.wiley.com/bw/publicationethics)	Best practice guidelines on publication ethics: a publisher's perspective

Step 1 - ISMPP
International Society for Medical Publication Professionals (ISMPP)
Recruited steering committee from ISMPP membership

Step 2 - Steering committee
Reviewed original good practice guidelines
Considered new literature
Wrote first draft for new guidelines
Recruited the consultation panel by direct invitation and open request

Step 3 - Consultation panel
Reviewed first draft
Submitted comments to steering committee
Gave each comment critical or beneficial rating and line number

Step 4 - Steering committee
Ranked comments from consultation panel by frequency (using line numbers), critical or beneficial rating, and individual judgment
Finalised guidelines

Fig Methods used to write GPP2

- The frequency of comments received on a particular line number
- The critical or beneficial rating given by members of the consultation panel
- The steering committee member's interpretation of the importance of the comments.

Ranked comments submitted by steering committee members were combined into a composite rank, which was used to create the final guidelines.

Guidelines and recommendations

Roles and responsibilities

Written agreement

We recommend that companies describe obligations for good publication practice in written publication agreements with authors of articles or presentations and with members of writing groups or publication steering committees. We recommend that the written agreement confirms the sponsors' responsibilities to:

- Grant authors full access to study data
- Confirm the authors' freedom to make public or publish the study results
- Provide authors with copies of the sponsor's publication policy.

We recommend that the written agreement confirms the authors' responsibilities to:

- Plan and produce articles or presentations that are accurate and complete in a timely manner
- Avoid premature publication or release of study information
- Avoid duplicate publication
- Make decisions about practical issues concerning presentation and publication (for example, choice of congress or journal)
- Disclose potential conflicts of interest in all articles and presentations
- Identify funding sources in all articles and presentations
- Ensure authorship is attributed appropriately
- Acknowledge in all articles and presentations all significant contributions made by individuals and organisations
- Provide the sponsor with copies of publication policies from the authors' institutions

We recommend that the written agreement confirms the shared responsibilities of all contributors, including authors and sponsors, and that it:

- Confirms that sponsors will work with investigators, authors, and contributors to report and publish studies in a timely and responsible manner
- Defines the criteria that will be used to determine authorship for articles and presentations
- Confirms that the sponsor and the investigators will be informed about the publication process
- Provides protection to parties with intellectual property rights, and establishes a reasonable period before study results are made public for intellectual property rights to be protected
- Establishes the right of the sponsor to review, in a timely manner, articles and abstracts before they are submitted, and to share scientific comments with the authors
- Describes what, if any, support for the development of the article or presentation will be provided
- Establishes a process founded on honest scientific debate as the means to resolve scientific differences in interpretation of findings or study presentation

- Establishes that all articles and presentations will conform to good publication practice and other recognised standards (table 1)

We recommend that written agreements for articles and presentations from research studies are made at the earliest opportunity—for example, when the protocol is finalised. Written agreements for other articles and presentations (for example, meta-analyses, sub-analyses, review articles) should be made before the authors begin work.

Written agreements must respect the institutional policies of authors, investigators, and other contributors, as well as those of the sponsor. Individuals must not be asked to violate the policies of their institutions.

Access to data

Sponsors have a responsibility to share the data and the analyses with the investigators who participated in the study. Sponsors must provide authors and other contributors (for example, members of a publication steering committee or professional medical writers) with full access to study data and should do so before the manuscript writing process begins or before the first external presentation of the data. Information provided to the authors should include study protocols, statistical analysis plans, statistical reports, data tables, clinical study reports, and results intended for posting on clinical trial results websites. Sufficient time should be allowed for authors and contributors to review and interpret the data provided and to seek further information if they wish (for example, access to raw data tables or the study database).

Reimbursement

It may be appropriate for companies to reimburse reasonable out of pocket expenses (for example, travel expenses) incurred by contributors or pay for specialised services such as statistical analysis. Details of this reimbursement must be disclosed. We recommend that no honorariums are paid for authorship of peer reviewed articles or presentations.

Publication steering committee

It may be useful to form a publication steering committee of authors and contributors to oversee and produce articles and presentations from a research study. This committee should be a small working group of individuals; its composition may change over time, and it may include:

- Members of the study steering committee and the protocol development team
- Investigators and other individuals who have expertise in the area and who are willing to interpret the data and write or review articles and presentations
- Employees of, or contributors contracted by, the sponsor company who are involved in the study (for example, clinicians, statisticians, or professional medical writers)

Members of the publication steering committee may become authors, but membership of the committee does not automatically confer authorship. For any given study, we recommend that:

- The publication steering committee is formed early (for example, when the protocol is finalised or at the end of enrolment)
- All study investigators are informed of the committee's membership and responsibilities
- Authors and contributors agree to their roles in the development of an article or presentation before writing begins.

Authors

Recognised criteria should be used to determine which of the contributors to an article or presentation should be identified as authors.

We recommend using the criteria for authorship described in the International Committee of Medical Journal Editors (ICMJE) uniform requirements (box 1).[8] Guidance regarding authorship is also available from the World Association of Medical Editors[17] and the Council of Science Editors.[18] Criteria used to define authorship may vary among journals and congresses, and we recommend following individual journal and congress requirements when these differ from ICMJE criteria. ICMJE criteria allow assignment of authorship to individuals who have contributed to the analysis and interpretation of a study but who may not have contributed to its conception and design. In these instances, or if authors differ from initial plans, particular care should be taken to attribute authorship and to acknowledge contributions appropriately.

We recommend that authorship criteria are applied consistently to all contributors to an article or presentation, including investigators, sponsor employees, and individuals contracted by the sponsor. All authors listed on an article or presentation must fulfil authorship criteria, and all those who fulfil the criteria must be listed as authors. All authors should agree on the order in which they appear in an article or presentation (if possible before writing begins) and should agree on any changes in authorship (for example, to ensure authorship reflects actual contributions made) before submission. Before writing begins one author (a lead author, who may also be guarantor) should take the lead for writing and managing each publication or presentation. One author (identified as guarantor) should take overall responsibility for the integrity of a study and its report.

Contributorship and acknowledgments

Contributorship and contributors

Interpretation of authorship criteria varies, and using a contributorship model to describe who did what helps to remove ambiguity.[8][19][20][21] We support this approach and recommend that clear, concise descriptions of the role of each contributor during preparation of the article or presentation (including but not limited to the authors)

BOX 1 INTERNATIONAL COMMITTEE OF MEDICAL JOURNAL EDITORS CRITERIA FOR AUTHORSHIP[8]

Authors "should have participated sufficiently in the work to take public responsibility for relevant portions of the content" and should meet all three conditions below:

- Substantial contributions to conception and design, acquisition of data, or analysis and interpretation of data; and
- Drafting the article or revising it critically for important intellectual content; and
- Final approval of the version to be published

Table 2   Consultation on first draft of GPP2

Place of work	No invited or volunteered	No agreed to comment	No who commented
Academic centre or university	10	4	4
Journal editor	11	8	7
Journal publisher	18	5	2
Medical communication agency, freelance medical writer	119*	83	52
Drug, medical device, or biotechnology company	109†	76‡	43
Professional organisation	21	17	8

*One email invitation was sent but not delivered.
†Two email invitations were sent but not delivered.
‡One person was lost between invitation and opening of the consultation period.

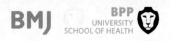

are made in an acknowledgment within the article or presentation.

Individual contributions to an article or presentation that should be acknowledged include study conception and design, conceiving the idea for an article, conducting or managing a study, collecting data, performing statistical analysis, interpreting data, analysing published literature, drafting a manuscript, critically reviewing a manuscript, and approving a manuscript. Permission should be obtained from each individual acknowledged.

Acknowledgments

We recommend that all articles and presentations include an acknowledgment, even if not requested by the journal or congress, to describe:

- Author contributions—for example: "A and B designed the study. C was the study statistician. A and C analysed and interpreted the study data. A reviewed the literature. A, B, and C critically reviewed the manuscript and approved the final version for submission. A accepts overall responsibility for the accuracy of the data, its analysis, and this report"
- Contributions to the article or presentation from people who are not listed as authors, including name and affiliation or employer—for example: "The authors would like to thank D, YZ Pharmaceuticals, for overall management of the trial and E, WX Medical Writing, for drafting the manuscript"
- The role of the sponsor in the study and its reporting, including how the sponsor was involved in the "study design; collection, analysis, and interpretation of data; writing the report; and the decision to submit the report for publication."[8] For example: "In collaboration with A and B, YZ Pharmaceuticals, designed the study, analysed, and interpreted the data, and edited the report. Data were recorded at participating clinical centres and maintained by YZ Pharmaceuticals. All authors had full access to the data. The authors had final responsibility for the decision to submit for publication"
- Funding sources, if any, for the research and for the article or presentation, such as for the work of a professional medical writer. For example: "The study was funded by YZ Pharmaceuticals, the manufacturer of drug F. Medical writing services from WX Medical Writing were funded by YZ Pharmaceuticals."

When journal or congress submission requirements do not allow inclusion of this information within the article or presentation, we recommend that it is included in a letter that accompanies the submission.

Professional medical writers

Professional medical writers work with authors to prepare abstracts, posters, slides, and manuscripts. They should ensure that authors control and direct writing and that disclosures of funding, potential conflicts of interest, and acknowledgment of contributions are made. They are required to have a good understanding of publication ethics and conventions, and ensure, in part through their collaborations with authors, that their work is scientifically appropriate.[21] [22] [23] Professional medical writers are not ghostwriters. The Association of American Medical Colleges states "transparent writing collaboration with attribution between academic and industry investigators, medical writers and/or technical experts is not ghostwriting."[24] This

is echoed by the US Institute of Medicine.[25] We recommend that authors and professional medical writers working with authors use a published checklist to discourage ghostwriting.[26]

We recommend that particular care is taken to ensure appropriate acknowledgment of the contributions made by medical writers and to describe their funding. Companies funding the work of medical writers should ensure that writers follow good publication practice. We refer readers to guidelines from the European Medical Writers Association.[23]

Working with authors

Professional medical writers must be directed by the lead author from the earliest possible stage (for example, when the outline is written), and all authors must be aware of the medical writer's involvement. The medical writer should remain in frequent contact with the authors throughout development of the article or presentation. The authors must critically review and comment on the outline and drafts, approve the final version of the article or presentation before it is submitted to the journal or congress, approve changes made during the peer review process, and approve the final version before it is published or accepted for presentation. Authors may delegate to the medical writer (or to an assistant) the administrative tasks associated with submitting the article or presentation to a journal or congress.

As authors

Professional medical writers, depending on the contributions they make, may qualify for authorship. For example, if a medical writer contributed extensive literature searches and summarised the literature discovered, and by doing so helped define the scope of a review article, and if he or she is willing to "take public responsibility for relevant portions of the content"[8] then he or she may be in a position to meet the remaining ICMJE criteria for authorship.

Conflicts of interest

We recommend that authors disclose financial relationships (for example, any financial relationships or obligation to the research sponsor or other companies, including contractual relations or consultancy fees for scientific, government, or legal services, or equity in the company) and non-financial relationships (for example, personal relationships, including those of immediate family members, and participation in litigation) that could inappropriately influence or seem to influence professional judgment. We recommend that these disclosures are made in all articles submitted for publication in peer reviewed journals, as well as in abstracts and posters submitted to congresses at the time of submission, if space requirements allow, and that they are included in oral presentations and posters at the time of presentation, regardless of whether disclosure is requested by the journal or congress.

For example: "A is a member of a speakers' bureau, has been a consultant for, and has received research grants from YZ Pharmaceuticals. C is an employee of YZ Pharmaceuticals. B has stated that she has no conflicts of interest."

There is no universal standard applied by journals and congresses for disclosure of potential conflicts of interest. Until discussions about how to address conflicts of interest are resolved,[25] [27] [28] [29] we recommend authors favour greater, rather than lesser, disclosure.

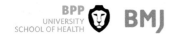

Recommendations for specific types of articles and presentations

Primary and secondary publications

A primary article is the first full report of a study. We recommend that all articles and presentations include statements to indicate whether they are the primary article or first presentation from a study, including for randomised clinical trials; epidemiological, observational, and descriptive studies; non-clinical outcomes research studies; and health economics studies.

Authors preparing secondary articles and presentations (including those that describe exploratory secondary analyses, national or single centre data taken from international or multicentre studies, and alternative analyses or pooled analyses of already published data) must avoid duplicate publication. All post-hoc and exploratory analyses must be clearly identified as such.

Authorship of secondary articles and presentations may differ from that of primary articles and presentations from the same study, depending on, for example, the topic of the article or presentation. We recommend that one or more authors of the primary article from a study contribute to the secondary articles and presentations from the same study.

Duplicate publication

We recommend that the same study results are not published in more than one peer reviewed journal article unless:

- The results are substantially re-analysed, re-interpreted for a different audience, or translated into a different language; and
- The primary publication is clearly acknowledged and cited; and
- The article is clearly presented as an analysis derived from the previously published primary results or is a translation, is not presented as reporting the primary results, and respects copyright law.

Presentations

Congress guidelines should be followed for presentations that describe study results that have been presented at an earlier congress. We recommend that, at the time of submission, authors disclose whether the same results will have already been presented at the time of the congress. With approval from the authors of the primary article,

research submitted for presentation at national or local meetings may include authors who do not appear on the primary article (for example, to enable accurate presentation in the appropriate language).

Review articles

We recommend that review articles are comprehensive and that the methods for searching, selecting, and summarising information are clearly stated. We recommend that discussions in review articles founded principally on opinion are clearly identified as such. We also recommend that care is taken to ensure appropriate description of contributions from professional medical writers and other contributors, particularly when they may have contributed to the design of a review article or when they may have suggested the idea for the article. We refer readers to the *BMJ*'s "Who prompted this submission?" guidance (box 2).[20]

Reporting standards

We recommend that authors follow established reporting standards such as CONSORT, CONSORT for Abstracts, STROBE, PRISMA, MOOSE, and STARD.[16] We offer the following brief recommendations:

- Articles and presentations should be complete, balanced, and clear
- Reference to the unique trial identifier should be included in all articles and presentations that report research from applicable clinical trials
- Interpretation of results should be unbiased, based on findings, and relevant to the audience
- Discussion of results should be unbiased, placed in the context of other relevant literature, and the evidence cited should be balanced
- Limitations of the study design and methodology should be described
- Studies with related findings should be cited, especially when previous results conflict with the results being reported.

Planning, registering, posting, and documenting

Publication planning

Publication plans can help study sponsors ensure that clinical trial results are communicated by presentation or publication to the scientific and medical community in an effective and timely manner. They can also enable sponsors to identify the timelines and resources necessary to meet their obligations for reporting and publishing clinical trial results. Authors retain responsibility for decisions about articles and presentations from individual studies, which may be described in a publication plan.

A publication plan should support authors and publication steering committees (if they exist) in their efforts to ensure appropriate, efficient, and complete communication of results by:

- Identifying submission deadlines for relevant congresses and determining which studies are appropriate to present and might have data available in time
- Identifying areas for new publications (for example, subgroup analyses, topics for pooled data analyses, post-hoc analyses, systematic reviews) and the resources required for them, such as statistical analyses
- Avoiding premature release of results
- Avoiding duplicate publication.

BOX 2 *BMJ*'S "WHO PROMPTED THIS SUBMISSION?" QUESTIONS[20]

We may ask authors submitting or offering unsolicited articles, particularly reviews and editorials covering topics with related commercial interests, several questions before proceeding. Even if the answers to all of these questions were "yes," we wouldn't necessarily reject the proposal or article. We appreciate that companies can commission some excellent evidence based work and that professional writers can present that evidence in a particularly readable and clear way that benefits readers and learners. We would, however, expect such companies' and writers' contributions to be mentioned in the article. And we would want to know that the *BMJ* article did not overlap by more than 15% with any similar publications or submissions written by the same authors elsewhere. Here are the questions:

- Has anyone (particularly a company or public relations agency) prompted or paid you to write this article?
- Would/did a professional writer contribute to the article, and to what extent?
- Would the *BMJ* article be original, or would it be similar to articles submitted or published elsewhere?

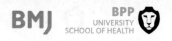

Before publication

Research sponsors must register and post all applicable clinical trials according to the definitions and timelines required of them by relevant legislation and guidelines.[8] [9] [10] [11] [12] [13] [14] [15] Posting clinical trial results according to the US Food and Drug Administration Amendment Act of 2007[10] and the *Joint Position on the Disclosure of Clinical Trial Information*,[11] whether before or after submission to a peer reviewed journal, should not preclude consideration for publication.[8]

Authors may present clinical study results at congresses before publication in a peer reviewed journal. Authors and other parties with access to study results should avoid further and more detailed public reporting before publication in a peer reviewed journal, unless the circumstances are exceptional.

Authors should not submit their work for consideration by more than one peer reviewed journal at any one time. All parties should respect embargoes set by journals, congresses, and other media. For example, authors should follow journal instructions when articles are "in press" or published online ahead of print.

Documentation

We recommend that companies, and the organisations or individuals working for them, document how publications are initiated and developed. We recommend that companies implement policies detailing the types of documentation to be retained, including:

- Agreements to participate in the writing process (for example, signed and dated letter, email)
- Details of intellectual input, direction, and contributions, including comments on drafts (emails, notes from teleconferences) or drafts that contain revisions
- Main versions of the draft, to document how comments on previous versions were incorporated
- Workflow and timelines that were used to develop the document, including time taken to review and revise the document
- Approval from authors of the final version to be submitted
- Lists of participants other than authors who were allowed to review or comment on the document.

We recommend that this documentation is maintained for a period defined by the sponsor company's retention policy.

Checklists

Articles and presentations following good publication practice will show the characteristics described in table 3. Written agreements using good publication practice will cover, at a minimum, the items described in table 4.

The International Society for Medical Publication Professionals initiated the development of these guidelines. The opinions expressed here do not necessarily represent those of the authors' employers. We thank the consultation panel for their comments. We thank Elizabeth Wager, Sideview, for her work on the original guidelines[6] that GPP2 updates (some of the earlier guidance remains in these new guidelines) and for her willingness for ISMPP to sponsor the authors to write GPP2. We thank Sheema Sheikh at Excerpta Medica, Elsevier for compiling comments from the consultation.

Contributors: Jane Moore, Medtronic, and John Draper, Peloton Advantage, were members of the steering committee and contributed to discussions about the recommendations made in this document (JD in particular on managed care, pharmacoeconomic, and health outcomes). CG wrote the first and final draft; WPB wrote the draft sections on publication planning, documentation, and conflict of interest; DB, EAF, CSM, and MP contributed to outline, intermediate drafts, and revisions; VBW wrote the draft sections on authors, contributorship, acknowledgments, and medical writers; JMC the draft duplicate publication section, JME the draft review articles section, JAG the draft publication steering committee section, and YEY the draft access to data section. MEM compiled steering committee comments after the consultation, and contributed to outline, intermediate drafts, and revisions. All the authors contributed to the literature analysis and review before writing these guidelines. All the authors contributed to the outline and to the first and subsequent drafts, to interpretation of the comments gathered during the consultation phase, and reviewed the final draft. All the authors approve this document and CG is the guarantor.

Funding: The International Society for Medical Publication Professionals provided the contributors with meeting and teleconferencing facilities and web conferencing technology.

Competing interests: All authors are members of the International Society for Medical Publication Professionals a not for profit organisation with membership comprising pharmaceutical, biotechnology, and device industries; medical communications agencies; publishers; and independent medical writers. The society is funded by its membership. WPB and JME have stock in Johnson & Johnson; VBW has stock in Novo Nordisk and Parexel; JMC has stock in AstraZeneca; JAG has stock in Wyeth; and MP has stock in Cephalon. CG is a council member of the Committee on Publication Ethics. JAG was an employee of Wyeth, which was acquired by Pfizer in October 2009. VBW was previously employed by Novo Nordisk to work with publications.

Provenance and peer review: Not commissioned; externally peer reviewed.

Table 3 GPP2 checklist for articles and presentations

Characteristic	Check
Integrity	
Accurate, objective, balanced writing	
Full access to data for authors and contributors	
Absence of duplicative publications	
Honest attribution of authorship	
Completeness	
Clear description of research hypotheses	
Reporting the detail required to ensure unbiased presentation	
Complete and honest reference to related work	
Use of unique trial identifiers	
Discussion of limitations of study design and findings	
Making public or publishing results regardless of outcome	
Transparency	
Making clear sources of funding	
Disclosure of potential conflicts of interest	
Acknowledging individuals who have made significant contributions, including but not limited to those made by authors, and by description of these contributions	
Recognising the contributions of research sponsors	
Accountability	
Being accountable for the work and, in the case of authors and presenters, taking public responsibility for the work	
Assigning a guarantor	
Responsibility	
Making public or publishing results in a timely manner	
Respecting intellectual property	
Respecting the responsibilities of contributing individuals and organisations for good publication practice	

Table 4 GPP2 checklist of basic requirements for written publication agreements

	Check
Does the agreement describe the roles and responsibilities of the sponsor, authors, and contributors?	
Confirmation of full access to data for authors and contributors	
Confirmation of authors' freedom to make public or publish the study results	
Confirmation of the intent to report or publish studies in a timely and responsible manner	
Definition of criteria that will be used to determine authorship	
Requirement that premature and duplicate publication are avoided	
Establishment of right of sponsor to review articles and presentations and responsibility to do so in a timely manner	
Establishment of process founded on honest scientific debate to resolve differences in study interpretation or presentation	
Requirement that intellectual property rights are respected	
Does the agreement confirm that all articles and presentations will conform to good publication practice and other recognised standards?	
Was the agreement established at the earliest opportunity (for example, when protocol was finalised)?	

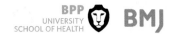

1   Angell M. Industry-sponsored clinical research: a broken system. *JAMA* 2008;300:1069-71.

2   Ross JS, Hill KP, Egilman DS, Krumholz HM. Guest authorship and ghostwriting in publications related to rofecoxib: a case study of industry documents from rofecoxib litigation. *JAMA* 2008;299:1800-12.

3   Hill KP, Ross JS, Egilman DS, Krumholz HM. The ADVANTAGE seeding trial: a review of internal documents. *Ann Intern Med* 2008;149:251-8.

4   Titus SL, Wells JA, Rhoades LJ. Repairing research integrity. *Nature* 2008;453:980-2.

5   Woloshin S, Schwartz LM, Casella SL, Kennedy AT, Larson RJ. Press releases by academic medical centers: not so academic? *Ann Intern Med* 2009;150:613-8.

6   Wager E, Field EA, Grossman L. Good publication practice for pharmaceutical companies. *Curr Med Res Opin* 2003;19:149-54.

7   World Medical Association. *Declaration of Helsinki: ethical principles for medical research involving human subjects, 22 October 2008* . www.wma.net/en/30publications/10policies/b3/index.html.

8   International Committee of Medical Journal Editors. *Uniform requirements for manuscripts submitted to biomedical journals* . www.icmje.org.

9   World Health Organization. *International clinical trials registry platform (ICTRP)*. www.who.int/ictrp/en/.

10 *Food and Drug Administration Amendments Act of 2007*. www.fda.gov/RegulatoryInformation/Legislation/FederalFoodDrugandCosmeticActFDCAct/SignificantAmendmentstotheFDCAct/FoodandDrugAdministrationAmendmentsActof2007/default.htm.

11 International Federation of Pharmaceutical Manufacturers and Associations, European Federation of Pharmaceutical Industries and Associations, Japan Pharmaceutical Manufacturers Association, Pharmaceutical Research and Manufacturers of America. *Joint position on the disclosure of clinical trial information via clinical trial registries and databases*. http://clinicaltrials.ifpma.org/fileadmin/files/pdfs/EN/Revised_Joint_Industry_Position_Nov_2008.pdf.

12 Legisalud Argentina. *Créase el registro de ensayos clínicos en seres humanos*. http://test.e-legis-ar.msal.gov.ar/leisref/public/showAct.php?id=12916.

13 Sociedade Brasileira de Profissionais em Pesquisa Clínica. *Legislação Brasileira Secretaria De Vigilância Sanitária E Anvisa* . www.sbppc.org.br.

14 South African National Clinical Trial Register. www.sanctr.gov.za/InvestigatorbrnbspInformation/Registrationandregulation/tabid/194/Default.aspx.

15 European Commission. *List of fields contained in the 'EudraCT' clinical trials database to be made public, in accordance with article 57(2) of regulation (EC) No 726/2004 and its implementing guideline 2008/C168/02*. 2009. http://ec.europa.eu/enterprise/pharmaceuticals/eudralex/vol-10/2009_02_04_guideline.pdf.

16 EQUATOR Network. *Library for health research reporting* . www.equator-network.org/resource-centre/library-of-health-research-reporting.

17 World Association of Medical Editors. *Policy statements* . www.wame.org/resources/policies#authorship.

18 Council of Science Editors. *CSE task force on authorship. Draft white paper: solutions*. 1999. www.councilscienceeditors.org/services/atf_whitepaper.cfm#5.

19 Rennie D, Flanagin A, Yank V. The contributions of authors. *JAMA* 2000;284:89-91.

20 BMJ. *Submitting an article to the BMJ*. http://resources.bmj.com/bmj/authors/article-submission.

21 Norris R, Bowman A, Fagan JM, Gallagher ER, Geraci AB, Gertel A, et al. International Society for Medical Publication Professionals (ISMPP) position statement: the role of the professional medical writer. *Curr Med Res Opin* 2007;23:1837-40.

22 Hamilton CW, Royer MG; AMWA 2002 task force on the contributions of medical writers to scientific publications. AMWA position statement on the contributions of medical writers to scientific publications. *AMWA Journal* 2003;18:13-6.

23 Jacobs A, Wager E. EMWA guidelines on the role of medical writers in developing peer-reviewed publications. *Curr Med Res Opin* 2005;21:317-21.

24 Association of American Medical Colleges. *Industry funding of medical education. Report of an AAMC task force*. 2008. http://services.aamc.org/publications/showfile.cfm?file=version114.pdf&prd_id=232.

25 Lo B, Field MJ, Institute of Medicine. *Conflict of interest in medical research, education, and practice*. Washington, DC: National Academies Press, 2009.

26 Gøtzsche PC, Kassirer JP, Woolley KL, Wager E, Jacobs A, Gertel A, et al. What should be done to tackle ghostwriting in the medical literature? *PLoS Med* 2009;6(2):e1000023.

27 Stossel TP. Has the hunt for conflicts of interest gone too far? Yes. *BMJ* 2008;336:476.

28 Lee K. Has the hunt for conflicts of interest gone too far? No. *BMJ* 2008;336:477.

29 Drazen JM, van der Weyden MB, Sahni P, Rosenberg J, Marusic A, Laine C, et al. Uniform format for disclosure of competing interests in ICMJE journals. *N Engl J Med* 2009 Oct 13 [Epub ahead of print].

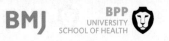

CONSORT 2010 Statement: updated guidelines for reporting parallel group randomised trials

Kenneth F Schulz, distinguished scientist and vice president[1], Douglas G Altman, professor[2], David Moher, senior scientist[3], for the CONSORT Group

[1]Family Health International, Research Triangle Park, NC 27709, USA

[2]Centre for Statistics in Medicine, University of Oxford, Wolfson College, Oxford

[3]Ottawa Methods Centre, Clinical Epidemiology Program, Ottawa Hospital Research Institute, Department of Epidemiology and Community Medicine, University of Ottawa, Ottawa, Canada

Cite this as: *BMJ* 2010;340:c332

DOI: 10.1136/bmj.c332

http://www.bmj.com/content/340/bmj.c332

ABSTRACT

The CONSORT statement is used worldwide to improve the reporting of randomised controlled trials. **Kenneth Schulz and colleagues** describe the latest version, CONSORT 2010, which updates the reporting guideline based on new methodological evidence and accumulating experience

Introduction

Randomised controlled trials, when appropriately designed, conducted, and reported, represent the gold standard in evaluating healthcare interventions. However, randomised trials can yield biased results if they lack methodological rigour.[1] To assess a trial accurately, readers of a published report need complete, clear, and transparent information on its methodology and findings. Unfortunately, attempted assessments frequently fail because authors of many trial reports neglect to provide lucid and complete descriptions of that critical information.[2 3 4]

That lack of adequate reporting fuelled the development of the original CONSORT (Consolidated Standards of Reporting Trials) statement in 1996[5] and its revision five years later.[6 7 8] While those statements improved the reporting quality for some randomised controlled trials,[9 10] many trial reports still remain inadequate.[2] Furthermore, new methodological evidence and additional experience has accumulated since the last revision in 2001. Consequently, we organised a CONSORT Group meeting to update the 2001 statement.[6 7 8] We introduce here the result of that process, CONSORT 2010.

Intent of CONSORT 2010

The CONSORT 2010 Statement is this paper including the 25 item checklist in the table and the flow diagram. It provides guidance for reporting all randomised controlled trials, but focuses on the most common design type—individually randomised, two group, parallel trials. Other trial designs, such as cluster randomised trials and non-inferiority trials, require varying amounts of additional information. CONSORT extensions for these designs,[11 12] and other CONSORT products, can be found through the CONSORT website (www.consort-statement.org). Along with the CONSORT statement, we have updated the explanation and elaboration article,[13] which explains the inclusion of each checklist item, provides methodological background, and gives published examples of transparent reporting.Diligent adherence by authors to the checklist items facilitates clarity, completeness, and transparency of reporting. Explicit descriptions, not ambiguity or omission, best serve the interests of all readers. Note that the CONSORT 2010 Statement does not include recommendations for designing, conducting, and analysing trials. It solely addresses the reporting of what was done and what was found.

Nevertheless, CONSORT does indirectly affect design and conduct. Transparent reporting reveals deficiencies in research if they exist. Thus, investigators who conduct inadequate trials, but who must transparently report, should not be able to pass through the publication process without revelation of their trial's inadequacies. That emerging reality should provide impetus to improved trial design and conduct in the future, a secondary indirect goal of our work. Moreover, CONSORT can help researchers in designing their trial.

Background to CONSORT

Efforts to improve the reporting of randomised controlled trials accelerated in the mid-1990s, spurred partly by methodological research. Researchers had shown for many years that authors reported such trials poorly, and empirical evidence began to accumulate that some poorly conducted or poorly reported aspects of trials were associated with bias.[14] Two initiatives aimed at developing reporting guidelines culminated in one of us (DM) and Drummond Rennie organising the first CONSORT statement in 1996.[5] Further methodological research on similar topics reinforced earlier findings[15] and fed into the revision of 2001.[6 7 8] Subsequently, the expanding body of methodological research informed the refinement of CONSORT 2010. More than 700 studies comprise the CONSORT database (located on the CONSORT website), which provides the empirical evidence to underpin the CONSORT initiative.

Indeed, CONSORT Group members continually monitor the literature. Information gleaned from these efforts provides an evidence base on which to update the CONSORT statement. We add, drop, or modify items based on that evidence and the recommendations of the CONSORT Group, an international and eclectic group of clinical trialists, statisticians, epidemiologists, and biomedical editors. The CONSORT Executive (KFS, DGA, DM) strives for a balance of established and emerging researchers. The membership of the group is dynamic. As our work expands in response to emerging projects and needed expertise, we invite new members to contribute. As such, CONSORT continually assimilates new ideas and perspectives. That process informs the continually evolving CONSORT statement.

Over time, CONSORT has garnered much support. More than 400 journals, published around the world and in many languages, have explicitly supported the CONSORT statement. Many other healthcare journals support it without our knowledge. Moreover, thousands more have implicitly supported it with the endorsement of the CONSORT statement by the International Committee of Medical Journal Editors (www.icmje.org). Other prominent editorial groups, the Council of Science Editors and the World Association of Medical Editors, officially support CONSORT. That support seems warranted: when used by authors and journals, CONSORT seems to improve reporting.[9]

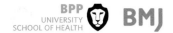

Development of CONSORT 2010

Thirty one members of the CONSORT 2010 Group met in Montebello, Canada, in January 2007 to update the 2001 CONSORT statement. In addition to the accumulating evidence relating to existing checklist items, several new issues had come to prominence since 2001. Some participants were given primary responsibility for aggregating and synthesising the relevant evidence on a particular checklist item of interest. Based on that evidence, the group deliberated the value of each item. As in prior CONSORT versions, we kept only those items deemed absolutely fundamental to reporting a randomised controlled trial. Moreover, an item may be fundamental to a trial but not included, such as approval by an institutional ethical review board, because funding bodies strictly enforce ethical review and medical journals usually address reporting ethical review in their instructions for authors. Other items may seem desirable, such as reporting on whether on-site monitoring was done, but a lack of empirical evidence or any consensus on their value cautions against inclusion at this point. The CONSORT 2010 Statement thus addresses the minimum criteria, although that should not deter authors from including other information if they consider it important.

After the meeting, the CONSORT Executive convened teleconferences and meetings to revise the checklist. After seven major iterations, a revised checklist was distributed to the larger group for feedback. With that feedback, the executive met twice in person to consider all the comments and to produce a penultimate version. That served as the basis for writing the first draft of this paper, which was then distributed to the group for feedback. After consideration of their comments, the executive finalised the statement.

The CONSORT Executive then drafted an updated explanation and elaboration manuscript, with assistance from other members of the larger group. The substance of the 2007 CONSORT meeting provided the material for the update. The updated explanation and elaboration manuscript was distributed to the entire group for additions, deletions, and changes. That final iterative process converged to the CONSORT 2010 Explanation and Elaboration.[13]

Changes in CONSORT 2010

The revision process resulted in evolutionary, not revolutionary, changes to the checklist (table), and the flow diagram was not modified except for one word (figure). Moreover, because other reporting guidelines augmenting the checklist refer to item numbers, we kept the existing items under their previous item numbers except for some renumbering of items 2 to 5. We added additional items either as a sub-item under an existing item, an entirely new item number at the end of the checklist, or (with item 3) an interjected item into a renumbered segment. We have summarised the noteworthy general changes in box 1 and specific changes in box 2. The CONSORT website contains a side by side comparison of the 2001 and 2010 versions.

Implications and limitations

We developed CONSORT 2010 to assist authors in writing reports of randomised controlled trials, editors and peer reviewers in reviewing manuscripts for publication, and readers in critically appraising published articles. The CONSORT 2010 Explanation and Elaboration provides elucidation and context to the checklist items. We strongly recommend using the explanation and elaboration in conjunction with the checklist to foster complete, clear, and transparent reporting and aid appraisal of published trial reports.

CONSORT 2010 focuses predominantly on the two group, parallel randomised controlled trial, which accounts for over half of trials in the literature.[2] Most of the items from the CONSORT 2010 Statement, however, pertain to all types of randomised trials. Nevertheless, some types of trials or trial situations dictate the need for additional information in the trial report. When in doubt, authors, editors, and readers should consult the CONSORT website for any CONSORT extensions, expansions (amplifications), implementations, or other guidance that may be relevant.

The evidence based approach we have used for CONSORT also served as a model for development of other reporting guidelines, such as for reporting systematic reviews and meta-analyses of studies evaluating interventions,[16] diagnostic studies,[17] and observational studies.[18] The explicit goal of all these initiatives is to improve reporting. The Enhancing the Quality and Transparency of Health Research (EQUATOR) Network will facilitate development of reporting guidelines and help disseminate the guidelines: www.equator-network.org provides information on all reporting guidelines in health research.

With CONSORT 2010, we again intentionally declined to produce a rigid structure for the reporting of randomised trials. Indeed, SORT[19] tried a rigid format, and it failed in a pilot run with an editor and authors.[20] Consequently, the format of articles should abide by journal style, editorial directions, the traditions of the research field addressed, and, where possible, author preferences. We do not wish to standardise the structure of reporting. Authors should simply address checklist items somewhere in the article,

---

BOX 1 NOTEWORTHY GENERAL CHANGES IN CONSORT 2010 STATEMENT

- We simplified and clarified the wording, such as in items 1, 8, 10, 13, 15, 16, 18, 19, and 21
- We improved consistency of style across the items by removing the imperative verbs that were in the 2001 version
- We enhanced specificity of appraisal by breaking some items into sub-items. Many journals expect authors to complete a CONSORT checklist indicating where in the manuscript the items have been addressed. Experience with the checklist noted pragmatic difficulties when an item comprised multiple elements. For example, item 4 addresses eligibility of participants and the settings and locations of data collection. With the 2001 version, an author could provide a page number for that item on the checklist, but might have reported only eligibility in the paper, for example, and not reported the settings and locations. CONSORT 2010 relieves obfuscations and forces authors to provide page numbers in the checklist for both eligibility and settings

---

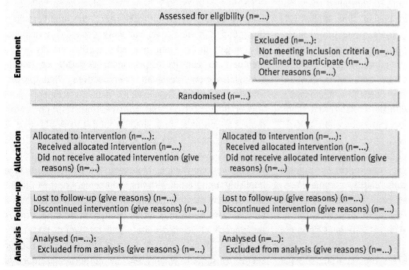

Fig Flow diagram of the progress through the phases of a parallel randomised trial of two groups (that is, enrolment, intervention allocation, follow-up, and data analysis)

with ample detail and lucidity. That stated, we think that manuscripts benefit from frequent subheadings within the major sections, especially the methods and results sections.

CONSORT urges completeness, clarity, and transparency of reporting, which simply reflects the actual trial design and conduct. However, as a potential drawback, a reporting guideline might encourage some authors to report fictitiously the information suggested by the guidance rather than what was actually done. Authors, peer reviewers, and editors should vigilantly guard against that potential drawback and refer, for example, to trial protocols, to information on trial registers, and to regulatory agency websites. Moreover, the CONSORT 2010 Statement does not include recommendations for designing and conducting randomised trials. The items should elicit clear pronouncements of how and what the authors did, but do not contain any judgments on how and what the authors should have done. Thus, CONSORT 2010 is not intended as an instrument to evaluate the quality of a trial. Nor is it appropriate to use the checklist to construct a "quality score."

Nevertheless, we suggest that researchers begin trials with their end publication in mind. Poor reporting allows authors, intentionally or inadvertently, to escape scrutiny of any weak aspects of their trials. However, with wide adoption of CONSORT by journals and editorial groups, most authors should have to report transparently all important aspects of their trial. The ensuing scrutiny rewards well conducted trials and penalises poorly conducted trials. Thus, investigators should understand the CONSORT 2010 reporting guidelines before starting a trial as a further incentive to design and conduct their trials according to rigorous standards.

CONSORT 2010 supplants the prior version published in 2001. Any support for the earlier version accumulated from journals or editorial groups will automatically extend to this newer version, unless specifically requested otherwise. Journals that do not currently support CONSORT may do so by registering on the CONSORT website. If a journal supports or endorses CONSORT 2010, it should cite one of the original versions of CONSORT 2010, the CONSORT 2010 Explanation and Elaboration, and the CONSORT website in their "Instructions to authors." We suggest that authors who wish to cite CONSORT should cite this or another of the original journal versions of CONSORT 2010 Statement, and, if appropriate, the CONSORT 2010 Explanation and Elaboration.[13]. All CONSORT material can be accessed through the original publishing journals or the CONSORT website. Groups or individuals who desire to translate the CONSORT 2010 Statement into other languages should first consult the CONSORT policy statement on the website.

We emphasise that CONSORT 2010 represents an evolving guideline. It requires perpetual reappraisal and, if necessary, modifications. In the future we will further revise the CONSORT material considering comments, criticisms, experiences, and accumulating new evidence. We invite readers to submit recommendations via the CONSORT website.

BOX 2 NOTEWORTHY SPECIFIC CHANGES IN CONSORT 2010 STATEMENT

- *Item 1b (title and abstract)*—We added a sub-item on providing a structured summary of trial design, methods, results, and conclusions and referenced the CONSORT for abstracts article[21]
- *Item 2b (introduction)*—We added a new sub-item (formerly item 5 in CONSORT 2001) on "Specific objectives or hypotheses"
- *Item 3a (trial design)*—We added a new item including this sub-item to clarify the basic trial design (such as parallel group, crossover, cluster) and the allocation ratio
- *Item 3b (trial design)*—We added a new sub-item that addresses any important changes to methods after trial commencement, with a discussion of reasons
- *Item 4 (participants)*—Formerly item 3 in CONSORT 2001
- *Item 5 (interventions)*—Formerly item 4 in CONSORT 2001. We encouraged greater specificity by stating that descriptions of interventions should include "sufficient details to allow replication"[3]
- *Item 6 (outcomes)*—We added a sub-item on identifying any changes to the primary and secondary outcome (endpoint) measures after the trial started. This followed from empirical evidence that authors frequently provide analyses of outcomes in their published papers that were not the prespecified primary and secondary outcomes in their protocols, while ignoring their prespecified outcomes (that is, selective outcome reporting).[4][22] We eliminated text on any methods used to enhance the quality of measurements
- *Item 9 (allocation concealment mechanism)*—We reworded this to include mechanism in both the report topic and the descriptor to reinforce that authors should report the actual steps taken to ensure allocation concealment rather than simply report imprecise, perhaps banal, assurances of concealment
- *Item 11 (blinding)*—We added the specification of how blinding was done and, if relevant, a description of the similarity of interventions and procedures. We also eliminated text on "how the success of blinding (masking) was assessed" because of a lack of empirical evidence supporting the practice as well as theoretical concerns about the validity of any such assessment[23][24]
- *Item 12a (statistical methods)*—We added that statistical methods should also be provided for analysis of secondary outcomes
- *Sub-item 14b (recruitment)*—Based on empirical research, we added a sub-item on "Why the trial ended or was stopped"[25]
- *Item 15 (baseline data)*—We specified "A table" to clarify that baseline and clinical characteristics of each group are most clearly expressed in a table
- *Item 16 (numbers analysed)*—We replaced mention of "intention to treat" analysis, a widely misused term, by a more explicit request for information about retaining participants in their original assigned groups[26]
- *Sub-item 17b (outcomes and estimation)*—For appropriate clinical interpretability, prevailing experience suggested the addition of "For binary outcomes, presentation of both relative and absolute effect sizes is recommended"[27]
- *Item 19 (harms)*—We included a reference to the CONSORT paper on harms[28]
- *Item 20 (limitations)*—We changed the topic from "Interpretation" and supplanted the prior text with a sentence focusing on the reporting of sources of potential bias and imprecision
- *Item 22 (interpretation)*—We changed the topic from "Overall evidence." Indeed, we understand that authors should be allowed leeway for interpretation under this nebulous heading. However, the CONSORT Group expressed concerns that conclusions in papers frequently misrepresented the actual analytical results and that harms were ignored or marginalised. Therefore, we changed the checklist item to include the concepts of results matching interpretations and of benefits being balanced with harms
- *Item 23 (registration)*—We added a new item on trial registration. Empirical evidence supports the need for trial registration, and recent requirements by journal editors have fostered compliance[29]
- *Item 24 (protocol)*—We added a new item on availability of the trial protocol. Empirical evidence suggests that authors often ignore, in the conduct and reporting of their trial, what they stated in the protocol.[4][22] Hence, availability of the protocol can instigate adherence to the protocol before publication and facilitate assessment of adherence after publication
- *Item 25 (funding)*—We added a new item on funding. Empirical evidence points toward funding source sometimes being associated with estimated treatment effects[30]

Author contributions: KFS, DM, and DGA participated in meetings and regular conference calls, planned the CONSORT 2007 meeting at Montebello, developed the agenda, prepared background research, identified and invited participants, contributed to the CONSORT meeting, drafted the manuscript, and, after critical review by the CONSORT Group, finalised the text of the manuscript. Members of the CONSORT Group attended the meeting, except for those noted below, and provided input on and review of the revised checklist and text of this article. Some members also prepared background material.

The CONSORT Group contributors to CONSORT 2010: DG Altman, Centre for Statistics in Medicine, University of Oxford; Virginia Barbour, *PLoS Medicine*; Jesse A Berlin, Johnson & Johnson Pharmaceutical Research and Development, USA; Isabelle Boutron, University Paris 7 Denis Diderot, Assistance Publique des Hôpitaux de Paris, INSERM, France; PJ Devereaux, McMaster University, Canada; Kay Dickersin, Johns Hopkins Bloomberg School of Public Health, USA; Diana Elbourne, London School of Hygiene & Tropical Medicine; Susan Ellenberg, University of Pennsylvania School of Medicine, USA; Val Gebski, University of Sydney, Australia; Steven Goodman, *Journal of the Society for Clinical Trials*, USA; Peter C Gøtzsche, Nordic Cochrane

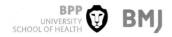

Table CONSORT 2010 checklist of information to include when reporting a randomised trial*

Section/Topic	Item No	Checklist item	Reported on page No
Title and abstract			
	1a	Identification as a randomised trial in the title	
	1b	Structured summary of trial design, methods, results, and conclusions (for specific guidance see CONSORT for abstracts[21 31])	
Introduction			
Background and objectives	2a	Scientific background and explanation of rationale	
	2b	Specific objectives or hypotheses	
Methods			
Trial design	3a	Description of trial design (such as parallel, factorial) including allocation ratio	
	3b	Important changes to methods after trial commencement (such as eligibility criteria), with reasons	
Participants	4a	Eligibility criteria for participants	
	4b	Settings and locations where the data were collected	
Interventions	5	The interventions for each group with sufficient details to allow replication, including how and when they were actually administered	
Outcomes	6a	Completely defined pre-specified primary and secondary outcome measures, including how and when they were assessed	
	6b	Any changes to trial outcomes after the trial commenced, with reasons	
Sample size	7a	How sample size was determined	
	7b	When applicable, explanation of any interim analyses and stopping guidelines	
Randomisation:			
Sequence generation	8a	Method used to generate the random allocation sequence	
	8b	Type of randomisation; details of any restriction (such as blocking and block size)	
Allocation concealment mechanism	9	Mechanism used to implement the random allocation sequence (such as sequentially numbered containers), describing any steps taken to conceal the sequence until interventions were assigned	
Implementation	10	Who generated the random allocation sequence, who enrolled participants, and who assigned participants to interventions	
Blinding	11a	If done, who was blinded after assignment to interventions (for example, participants, care providers, those assessing outcomes) and how	
	11b	If relevant, description of the similarity of interventions	
Statistical methods	12a	Statistical methods used to compare groups for primary and secondary outcomes	
	12b	Methods for additional analyses, such as subgroup analyses and adjusted analyses	
Results			
Participant flow (a diagram is strongly recommended)	13a	For each group, the numbers of participants who were randomly assigned, received intended treatment, and were analysed for the primary outcome	
	13b	For each group, losses and exclusions after randomisation, together with reasons	
Recruitment	14a	Dates defining the periods of recruitment and follow-up	
	14b	Why the trial ended or was stopped	
Baseline data	15	A table showing baseline demographic and clinical characteristics for each group	
Numbers analysed	16	For each group, number of participants (denominator) included in each analysis and whether the analysis was by original assigned groups	
Outcomes and estimation	17a	For each primary and secondary outcome, results for each group, and the estimated effect size and its precision (such as 95% confidence interval)	
	17b	For binary outcomes, presentation of both absolute and relative effect sizes is recommended	
Ancillary analyses	18	Results of any other analyses performed, including subgroup analyses and adjusted analyses, distinguishing pre-specified from exploratory	
Harms	19	All important harms or unintended effects in each group (for specific guidance see CONSORT for harms[28])	
Discussion			
Limitations	20	Trial limitations, addressing sources of potential bias, imprecision, and, if relevant, multiplicity of analyses	
Generalisability	21	Generalisability (external validity, applicability) of the trial findings	
Interpretation	22	Interpretation consistent with results, balancing benefits and harms, and considering other relevant evidence	
Other information			
Registration	23	Registration number and name of trial registry	
Protocol	24	Where the full trial protocol can be accessed, if available	
Funding	25	Sources of funding and other support (such as supply of drugs), role of funders	

We strongly recommend reading this statement in conjunction with the CONSORT 2010 Explanation and Elaboration[13] for important clarifications on all the items. If relevant, we also recommend reading CONSORT extensions for cluster randomised trials,[11] non-inferiority and equivalence trials,[12] non-phar-macological treatments,[32] herbal interventions,[33] and pragmatic trials.[34] Additional extensions are forthcoming: for those and for up to date references relevant to this checklist, see www.consort-statement.org.

Centre, Denmark; Trish Groves, *BMJ*; Steven Grunberg, American Society of Clinical Oncology, USA; Brian Haynes, McMaster University, Canada; Sally Hopewell, Centre for Statistics in Medicine, University of Oxford; Astrid James, *Lancet*; Peter Juhn, Johnson & Johnson, USA; Philippa Middleton, University of Adelaide, Australia; Don Minckler, University of California Irvine, USA; D Moher, Ottawa Methods Centre, Clinical Epidemiology Program, Ottawa Hospital Research Institute, Canada; Victor M Montori, Knowledge and Encounter Research Unit, Mayo Clinic College of Medicine, USA; Cynthia Mulrow, *Annals of Internal Medicine*, USA; Stuart Pocock, London School of Hygiene & Tropical Medicine; Drummond Rennie, *JAMA*, USA; David L Schriger, *Annals of Emergency Medicine*, USA; KF Schulz, Family Health International, USA; Iveta Simera, EQUATOR Network; Elizabeth Wager, Sideview.

Contributors to CONSORT 2010 who did not attend the Montebello meeting: Mike Clarke, UK Cochrane Centre; Gordon Guyatt, McMaster University, Canada.

Funding: We received financial support from United Kingdom National Institute for Health Research and the Medical Research Council; Canadian Institutes of Health Research; Presidents Fund, Canadian Institutes of Health Research; Johnson & Johnson; *BMJ*; and the American Society for Clinical Oncology. DGA is supported by Cancer Research UK, DM by a University of Ottawa Research Chair, and KFS by Family Health International. None of the sponsors had any involvement in the planning, execution, or writing of the CONSORT documents. Additionally, no funder played a role in drafting the manuscript.

Competing interests: Uniform disclosure of potential conflicts of interest: all authors have completed the ICMJE unified competing interest form at www.icmje.org/coi_disclosure.pdf (available from the corresponding author) and declare (1) DM received grants for this work from Johnson & Johnson, BMJ, and American Society for Clinical Oncology; KFS and DGA received support for travel to meetings for this work from Johnson & Johnson, BMJ, and American Society for Clinical Oncology; (2) KFS and DA had travel expenses reimbursed by the EQUATOR Network; KFS has received honoraria for delivering educational presentations for the American Board of Obstetrics and Gynecology Foundation for Excellence in Women's Health Care, Ortho-McNeil Janssen Scientific Affairs, and the American College of Obstetrics and Gynecology; and has done consultancy for Wyeth. All authors also declare (3) no spouses, partners, or children with relationships with commercial entities that might have an interest in the submitted work; (4) no non-financial interests that may be relevant to the submitted work.

In order to encourage dissemination of the CONSORT 2010 Statement, this article is freely accessible on bmj.com and will also be published in the *Lancet, Obstetrics and Gynecology, PLoS Medicine, Annals of Internal Medicine, Open Medicine, Journal of Clinical Epidemiology, BMC Medicine,* and *Trials.* The authors jointly hold the copyright of this article. For details on further use, see the CONSORT website (www.consort-statement.org).

1 Jüni P, Altman DG, Egger M. Systematic reviews in health care: assessing the quality of controlled clinical trials. *BMJ* 2001;323:42-6.
2 Chan AW, Altman DG. Epidemiology and reporting of randomised trials published in PubMed journals. *Lancet* 2005;365:1159-62.
3 Glasziou P, Meats E, Heneghan C, Shepperd S. What is missing from descriptions of treatment in trials and reviews? *BMJ* 2008;336:1472-4.
4 Dwan K, Altman DG, Arnaiz JA, Bloom J, Chan AW, Cronin E, et al. Systematic review of the empirical evidence of study publication bias and outcome reporting bias. *PLoS ONE* 2008;3:e3081.
5 Begg C, Cho M, Eastwood S, Horton R, Moher D, Olkin I, et al. Improving the quality of reporting of randomized controlled trials. The CONSORT statement. *JAMA* 1996;276:637-9.
6 Moher D, Schulz KF, Altman DG. The CONSORT statement: revised recommendations for improving the quality of reports of parallel-group randomised trials. *Lancet* 2001;357:1191-4.
7 Moher D, Schulz KF, Altman DG. The CONSORT statement: revised recommendations for improving the quality of reports of parallel-group randomized trials. *Ann Intern Med* 2001;134:657-62.
8 Moher D, Schulz KF, Altman D. The CONSORT statement: revised recommendations for improving the quality of reports of parallel-group randomized trials. *JAMA* 2001;285:1987-91.
9 Plint AC, Moher D, Morrison A, Schulz K, Altman DG, Hill C, et al. Does the CONSORT checklist improve the quality of reports of randomised controlled trials? A systematic review. *Med J Aust* 2006;185:263-7.
10 Hopewell S, Dutton S, Yu L-M, Chan A-W, Altman DG. The quality of reports of randomised trials in 2000 and 2006: a comparative study of articles indexed by PubMed. *BMJ* 2010;340:c723.
11 Campbell MK, Elbourne DR, Altman DG. CONSORT statement: extension to cluster randomised trials. *BMJ* 2004;328:702-8.
12 Piaggio G, Elbourne DR, Altman DG, Pocock SJ, Evans SJ. Reporting of noninferiority and equivalence randomized trials: an extension of the CONSORT statement. *JAMA* 2006;295:1152-60.
13 Moher D, Hopewell S, Schulz KF, Montori V, Gøtzsche PC, Devereaux PJ, et al. CONSORT 2010 Explanation and Elaboration: updated guidelines for reporting parallel group randomised trials. *BMJ* 2010;340:c869.
14 Schulz KF, Chalmers I, Hayes RJ, Altman DG. Empirical evidence of bias. Dimensions of methodological quality associated with estimates of treatment effects in controlled trials. *JAMA* 1995;273:408-12.
15 Moher D, Pham B, Jones A, Cook DJ, Jadad AR, Moher M, et al. Does quality of reports of randomised trials affect estimates of intervention efficacy reported in meta-analyses? *Lancet* 1998;352:609-13.
16 Moher D, Liberati A, Tetzlaff J, Altman DG, for the PRISMA Group. Preferred reporting items for systematic reviews and meta-analyses: the PRISMA statement. *BMJ* 2009;339:b2535.
17 Bossuyt PM, Reitsma JB, Bruns DE, Gatsonis CA, Glasziou PP, Irwig LM, et al. Towards complete and accurate reporting of studies of diagnostic accuracy: the STARD initiative. *BMJ* 2003;326:41-4.
18 von Elm E, Altman DG, Egger M, Pocock SJ, Gøtzsche PC, Vandenbroucke JP, for the STROBE Initiative. Strengthening the reporting of observational studies in epidemiology (STROBE) statement: guidelines for reporting observational studies. *BMJ* 2007;335:806-8.
19 Standards of Reporting Trials Group. A proposal for structured reporting of randomized controlled trials. *JAMA* 1994;272:1926-31.
20 Rennie D. Reporting randomized controlled trials. An experiment and a call for responses from readers. *JAMA* 1995;273:1054-5.
21 Hopewell S, Clarke M, Moher D, Wager E, Middleton P, Altman DG, et al. CONSORT for reporting randomised trials in journal and conference abstracts. *Lancet* 2008;371:281-3.
22 Chan AW, Hróbjartsson A, Haahr MT, Gøtzsche PC, Altman DG. Empirical evidence for selective reporting of outcomes in randomized trials: comparison of protocols to published articles. *JAMA* 2004;291:2457-65.
23 Sackett DL. Commentary: Measuring the success of blinding in RCTs: don't, must, can't or needn't? *Int J Epidemiol* 2007;36:664-5.
24 Schulz KF, Grimes DA. Blinding in randomised trials: hiding who got what. *Lancet* 2002;359:696-700.
25 Montori VM, Devereaux PJ, Adhikari NK, Burns KE, Eggert CH, Briel M, et al. Randomized trials stopped early for benefit: a systematic review. *JAMA* 2005;294:2203-9.
26 Hollis S, Campbell F. What is meant by intention to treat analysis? Survey of published randomised controlled trials. *BMJ* 1999;319:670-4.
27 Nuovo J, Melnikow J, Chang D. Reporting number needed to treat and absolute risk reduction in randomized controlled trials. *JAMA* 2002;287:2813-4.
28 Ioannidis JP, Evans SJ, Gøtzsche PC, O'Neill RT, Altman DG, Schulz K, et al. Better reporting of harms in randomized trials: an extension of the CONSORT statement. *Ann Intern Med* 2004;141:781-8.
29 De Angelis C, Drazen JM, Frizelle FA, Haug C, Hoey J, Horton R, et al. Clinical trial registration: a statement from the International Committee of Medical Journal Editors. *Lancet* 2004;364:911-2.
30 Lexchin J, Bero LA, Djulbegovic B, Clark O. Pharmaceutical industry sponsorship and research outcome and quality: systematic review. *BMJ* 2003;326:1167-70.
31 Hopewell S, Clarke M, Moher D, Wager E, Middleton P, Altman DG, et al. CONSORT for reporting randomized controlled trials in journal and conference abstracts: explanation and elaboration. *PLoS Med* 2008;5:e20.
32 Boutron I, Moher D, Altman DG, Schulz KF, Ravaud P. Extending the CONSORT statement to randomized trials of nonpharmacologic treatment: explanation and elaboration. *Ann Intern Med* 2008;148:295-309.
33 Gagnier JJ, Boon H, Rochon P, Moher D, Barnes J, Bombardier C. Reporting randomized, controlled trials of herbal interventions: an elaborated CONSORT statement. *Ann Intern Med* 2006;144:364-7.
34 Zwarenstein M, Treweek S, Gagnier JJ, Altman DG, Tunis S, Haynes B, et al. Improving the reporting of pragmatic trials: an extension of the CONSORT statement. *BMJ* 2008;337:a2390.

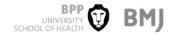

Improving the reporting of pragmatic trials: an extension of the CONSORT statement

Merrick Zwarenstein, director[1] [2] [3], Shaun Treweek, senior research fellow[4] [5],
Joel J Gagnier, post-graduate fellow[5] [6], Douglas G Altman, director[7],
Sean Tunis, director[8] [9] [10], Brian Haynes, Michael Gent professor and chair[11],
Andrew D Oxman, senior researcher[5], David Moher,
senior scientist[12] [13], for the CONSORT and Pragmatic Trials in Healthcare (Practihc) groups

[1]Health Services Sciences, Sunnybrook Hospital, Toronto, Ontario, Canada

[2]Institute for Clinical Evaluative Sciences, Toronto Department of Health Policy, Management and Evaluation, University of Toronto, Toronto

[3]Division of International Health (IHCAR), Karolinska Institute, Stockholm, Sweden

[4]Clinical and Population Sciences and Education, University of Dundee, Dundee

[5]Norwegian Knowledge Centre for the Health Services, Oslo, Norway

[6]Faculty of Medicine, University of Toronto

[7]Centre for Statistics in Medicine, University of Oxford, Oxford

[8]Center for Medical Technology Policy, Baltimore, MD, USA

[9]Division of General Internal Medicine, Johns Hopkins School of Medicine, Baltimore, MD

[10]Center for Healthcare Policy, Stanford University School of Medicine, Palo Alto, CA, USA

[11]Department of Clinical Epidemiology and Biostatistics and Department of Medicine, McMaster University Faculty of Health Sciences, Hamilton, ON, Canada

[12]Clinical Epidemiology Program, Ottawa Health Research Institute, Ottawa, Canada

[13]Department of Epidemiology and Community Medicine, Faculty of Medicine, University of Ottawa, Ottawa

Cite this as: BMJ 2008;337:a2390

DOI: 10.1136/bmj.a2390

http://www.bmj.com/content/337/bmj.a2390

ABSTRACT

Background The CONSORT statement is intended to improve reporting of randomised controlled trials and focuses on minimising the risk of bias (internal validity). The applicability of a trial's results (generalisability or external validity) is also important, particularly for pragmatic trials. A pragmatic trial (a term first used in 1967 by Schwartz and Lellouch) can be broadly defined as a randomised controlled trial whose purpose is to inform decisions about practice. This extension of the CONSORT statement is intended to improve the reporting of such trials and focuses on applicability.

Methods At two, two-day meetings held in Toronto in 2005 and 2008, we reviewed the CONSORT statement and its extensions, the literature on pragmatic trials and applicability, and our experiences in conducting pragmatic trials.

Recommendations We recommend extending eight CONSORT checklist items for reporting of pragmatic trials: the background, participants, interventions, outcomes, sample size, blinding, participant flow, and generalisability of the findings. These extensions are presented, along with illustrative examples of reporting, and an explanation of each extension. Adherence to these reporting criteria will make it easier for decision makers to judge how applicable the results of randomised controlled trials are to their own conditions. Empirical studies are needed to ascertain the usefulness and comprehensiveness of these CONSORT checklist item extensions. In the meantime we recommend that those who support, conduct, and report pragmatic trials should use this extension of the CONSORT statement to facilitate the use of trial results in decisions about health care.

Pragmatic trials are designed to inform decisions about practice, but poor reporting can reduce their usefulness. The **CONSORT and Practihc groups** describe modifications to the CONSORT guidelines to help readers assess the applicability of the results.

Randomised controlled trials are used to assess the benefits and harms of interventions in health care. If conducted properly, they minimise the risk of bias (threats to internal validity), particularly selection bias.[1] [2] There is, however, considerable evidence that trials are not always well reported,[3] [4] and this can be associated with bias, such as selective reporting of outcomes.[5]

The usefulness of a trial report also depends on the clarity with which it details the relevance of its interventions, participants, outcomes, and design to the clinical, health service, or policy question it examines. Furthermore, a trial may be valid and useful in the healthcare setting in which it was conducted but have limited applicability (also known as generalisability or external validity) beyond this because of differences between the trial setting and other settings to which its results are to be extrapolated.

Schwartz and Lellouch[6] coined the terms "pragmatic" to describe trials designed to help choose between options for care, and "explanatory" to describe trials designed to test causal research hypotheses—for example, that an intervention causes a particular biological change. Table 1 shows some key differences between explanatory and pragmatic trials. Table 2 compares a trial that was highly explanatory in attitude[7] with one that was highly pragmatic.[8] There is a continuum rather than a dichotomy between explanatory and pragmatic trials. In fact, Schwartz and Lellouch characterised pragmatism as an attitude to trial design rather than a characteristic of the trial itself. The pragmatic attitude favours design choices that maximise applicability of the trial's results to usual care settings, rely on unarguably important outcomes such as mortality and severe morbidity, and are tested in a wide range of participants.[9] [10] [11] As Schwartz and Lellouch wrote: "Most trials done hitherto have adopted the explanatory approach without question; the pragmatic approach would often have been more justifiable."[6]

Calls have been made for more pragmatic trials in general,[6] [12] [13] and in relation to specific clinical problems.[14] [15] [16] Articles have been published discussing the characteristics and value of pragmatic trials[17] [18] [19] [20] [21] [22] [23] [24] [25] [26] [27] [28] [29] [30] [31] [32] [33] [34] [35] or proposing improvements in the design and conduct of these trials.[36] [37] [38] Patients, advocacy groups, clinicians, systematic reviewers, funders, and policymakers want to use the results of randomised controlled trials. As such, a clear description of the design and execution of the trial, the intervention and comparator, and the setting in which health care is provided may simplify their decision on the likely benefits, harms, and costs to be expected when implementing the intervention in their own situation. There is, however, no accepted standard to guide reporting on the aspects of design and conduct of trials that affect their usefulness for decision making, particularly considerations that would affect the applicability of the results.

We propose here guidance for reporting pragmatic trials, as a specific extension of the CONSORT statement. Our aim is to identify information which, if included in reports of pragmatic trials, will help users determine whether the results are applicable to their own situation and whether the intervention might be feasible and acceptable. Reporting this information is crucial for any trial that is intended to inform decisions about practice.

CONSORT initiative

The original CONSORT statement (www.consort-statement.org), last revised in 2001, was developed by clinical trialists, methodologists, and medical journal editors to help improve the reporting of parallel (two) group randomised trials.[39] The

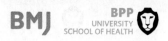

Table 1 Key differences between trials with explanatory and pragmatic attitudes, adapted from a table presented at the 2008 Society for Clinical Trials meeting by Marion Campbell, University of Aberdeen

Question	Efficacy—can the intervention work?	Effectiveness—does the intervention work when used in normal practice?
Setting	Well resourced, "ideal" setting	Normal practice
Participants	Highly selected. Poorly adherent participants and those with conditions which might dilute the effect are often excluded	Little or no selection beyond the clinical indication of interest
Intervention	Strictly enforced and adherence is monitored closely	Applied flexibly as it would be in normal practice
Outcomes	Often short term surrogates or process measures	Directly relevant to participants, funders, communities, and healthcare practitioners
Relevance to practice	Indirect—little effort made to match design of trial to decision making needs of those in usual setting in which intervention will be implemented	Direct—trial is designed to meet needs of those making decisions about treatment options in setting in which intervention will be implemented

Table 2 Comparison of trial that was highly explanatory in attitude with trial that was highly pragmatic

	Highly explanatory attitude (NASCET[7])	Highly pragmatic attitude (Thomas et al[8])
Question	Among patients with symptomatic 70-99% stenosis of carotid artery can carotid endarterectomy plus best medical therapy reduce outcomes of major stroke or death over next two years compared with best medical therapy alone?	Does a short course of acupuncture delivered by a qualified acupuncturist reduce pain in patients with persistent non-specific low-back pain?
Setting	Volunteer academic and specialist hospitals with multidisciplinary neurological-neurosurgical teams and high procedure volumes with low mortality in US and Canada	General practice and private acupuncture clinics in UK
Participants	Symptomatic patients stratified for carotid stenosis severity, with primary interest in severe carotid stenosis (high risk) group, who were thought to be most likely to respond to endarterectomy. Exclusions included mental incompetence and another illness likely to cause death within 5 years. Patients also were temporarily ineligible if they had any of seven transient medical conditions (eg, uncontrolled hypertension or diabetes)	Anyone aged 18-65 with non-specific low back pain of 4-52 weeks' duration who were judged to be suitable by their general practitioner. There were some exclusion criteria, eg those with spinal disease
Intervention	Endarterectomy had to be carried out (rather than stenting or some other operation), but the surgeon was given leeway in how it was performed. Surgeons had to be approved by an expert panel, and were restricted to those who had performed at least 50 carotid endarterectomies in the past 24 months with a postoperative complication rate (stroke or death within 30 days) of less than 6%. Centre compliance with the study protocol was monitored, with the chief investigator visiting in the case of deficiencies	Acupuncturists determined the content and number of treatments according to patients' needs
Outcomes	The primary outcome was time to ipsilateral stroke, the outcome most likely to be affected by carotid endarterectomy. Secondary outcomes: all strokes, major strokes, and mortality	Primary outcome was bodily pain as measured by SF-36. Secondary outcomes included use of pain killers and patient satisfaction
Relevance to practice	Indirect—patients and clinicians are highly selected and it isn't clear how widely applicable the results are	Direct—general practitioners and patients can immediately use the trial results in their decision making

objective of the statement is to enable readers to critically appraise and interpret trials by providing authors with guidance about how to improve the clarity, accuracy, and transparency of their trial reports. It consists of a 22-item checklist and a diagram, detailing the flow of participants through the trial. It is a living document that is updated as needed, incorporating new evidence.[40] The guidelines have been endorsed by more than 300 journals,[41] and by several editorial groups, including the International Committee of Medical Journal Editors.[42] The CONSORT statement has been translated into several languages.[43] Since its original publication in 1996 the quality of reports of controlled trials has improved.[44]

The CONSORT recommendations are intentionally generic, and necessarily do not consider in detail all types of trials. Extensions of the CONSORT statement have been developed for non-inferiority and equivalence,[45] cluster randomised designs,[46] reporting of abstracts,[47] data on harms,[48] trials of herbal interventions,[49] and of non-pharmacological interventions,[50] [51] but not yet for the reporting of pragmatic trials, although some issues pertaining to pragmatic trials were discussed in the CONSORT explanation and elaboration paper.[4]

Methods

In January 2005 and in March 2008, we held two-day meetings in Toronto, Canada, to discuss ways to increase the contribution of randomised controlled trials to healthcare decision making, focusing on pragmatic trials. Participants included people with experience in clinical care, commissioning research, healthcare financing, developing clinical practice guidelines, and trial methodology and reporting. Twenty four people participated in 2005 and 42

in 2008, including members of the CONSORT and Pragmatic Trials in Healthcare (Practihc) groups.[52]

After the 2005 meeting a draft revised checklist for the extension was circulated to a writing group, including some of those invited to the meeting but unable to attend. After several revisions the writing group produced a draft summary paper. At the 2008 meeting the draft was discussed and modified. It was circulated to the CONSORT group for feedback, modified, and submitted for publication.

Recommendations for reporting pragmatic trials

Meeting participants agreed that no items needed to be added to the CONSORT checklist and that the flow diagram did not need modification. However, participants felt that eight items (2-4, 6, 7, 11, 13, and 21) needed additional text specific to the reporting of pragmatic trials (see table 3). Although participants discussed additional text for item 1 of the checklist (title/abstract), principally adding the word pragmatic to the title or abstract, we decided against making this recommendation because it may reinforce the misconception that there is a dichotomy between pragmatic and explanatory trials rather than a continuum. We elected not to extend item 5 (objectives), although we would encourage trialists to report the purpose of the trial in relation to the decisions that it is intended to inform and in which settings; we have included this recommendation in connection with the extension of item 2 (background).

For each of the eight items we present the standard CONSORT text and additional guidance, an example of good reporting for the item, and an explanation of the issues. The selection of examples is illustrative for a specific item and should not be interpreted as a marker of quality for other

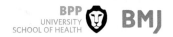

Table 3 Checklist of items for reporting pragmatic trials

Section	Item	Standard CONSORT description	Extension for pragmatic trials
Title and abstract	1	How participants were allocated to interventions (eg, "random allocation," "randomised," or "randomly assigned")	
Introduction			
Background	2	Scientific background and explanation of rationale	Describe the health or health service problem that the intervention is intended to address and other interventions that may commonly be aimed at this problem
Methods			
Participants	3	Eligibility criteria for participants; settings and locations where the data were collected	Eligibility criteria should be explicitly framed to show the degree to which they include typical participants and/or, where applicable, typical providers (eg, nurses), institutions (eg, hospitals), communities (or localities eg, towns) and settings of care (eg, different healthcare financing systems)
Interventions	4	Precise details of the interventions intended for each group and how and when they were actually administered	Describe extra resources added to (or resources removed from) usual settings in order to implement intervention. Indicate if efforts were made to standardise the intervention or if the intervention and its delivery were allowed to vary between participants, practitioners, or study sites
			Describe the comparator in similar detail to the intervention
Objectives	5	Specific objectives and hypotheses	
Outcomes	6	Clearly defined primary and secondary outcome measures and, when applicable, any methods used to enhance the quality of measurements (eg, multiple observations, training of assessors)	Explain why the chosen outcomes and, when relevant, the length of follow-up are considered important to those who will use the results of the trial
Sample size	7	How sample size was determined; explanation of any interim analyses and stopping rules when applicable	If calculated using the smallest difference considered important by the target decision maker audience (the minimally important difference) then report where this difference was obtained
Randomisation—sequence generation	8	Method used to generate the random allocation sequence, including details of any restriction (eg, blocking, stratification)	
Randomisation—allocation concealment	9	Method used to implement the random allocation sequence (eg, numbered containers or central telephone), clarifying whether the sequence was concealed until interventions were assigned	
Randomisation—implementation	10	Who generated the allocation sequence, who enrolled participants, and who assigned participants to their groups	
Blinding (masking)	11	Whether participants, those administering the interventions, and those assessing the outcomes were blinded to group assignment	If blinding was not done, or was not possible, explain why
Statistical methods	12	Statistical methods used to compare groups for primary outcomes; methods for additional analyses, such as subgroup analyses and adjusted analyses	
Results			
Participant flow	13	Flow of participants through each stage (a diagram is strongly recommended)—specifically, for each group, report the numbers of participants randomly assigned, receiving intended treatment, completing the study protocol, and analysed for the primary outcome; describe deviations from planned study protocol, together with reasons	The number of participants or units approached to take part in the trial, the number which were eligible, and reasons for non-participation should be reported
Recruitment	14	Dates defining the periods of recruitment and follow-up	
Baseline data	15	Baseline demographic and clinical characteristics of each group	
Numbers analysed	16	Number of participants (denominator) in each group included in each analysis and whether analysis was by "intention-to-treat"; state the results in absolute numbers when feasible (eg, 10/20, not 50%)	
Outcomes and estimation	17	For each primary and secondary outcome, a summary of results for each group and the estimated effect size and its precision (eg, 95% CI)	
Ancillary analyses	18	Address multiplicity by reporting any other analyses performed, including subgroup analyses and adjusted analyses, indicating which are prespecified and which are exploratory	
Adverse events	19	All important adverse events or side effects in each intervention group	
Discussion			
Interpretation	20	Interpretation of the results, taking into account study hypotheses, sources of potential bias or imprecision, and the dangers associated with multiplicity of analyses and outcomes	
Generalisability	21	Generalisability (external validity) of the trial findings	Describe key aspects of the setting which determined the trial results. Discuss possible differences in other settings where clinical traditions, health service organisation, staffing, or resources may vary from those of the trial
Overall evidence	22	General interpretation of the results in the context of current evidence	

aspects of those trial reports. The suggestions in this paper should be seen as additional to the general guidance in the main CONSORT explanatory paper and where relevant, other CONSORT guidance.

Item 2: introduction; background

Scientific background and explanation of rationale
Extension for pragmatic trials: Describe the health or health service problem that the intervention is intended to

address, and other interventions that may commonly be aimed at this problem.

Example (a): Describe the health or health service problem which the intervention is intended to address—"Although interventions such as telephone or postal reminders from pharmacists improve compliance their effect on clinical outcome is not known. We investigated whether periodic telephone counselling by a pharmacist . . . reduced mortality in patients" receiving polypharmacy.[53]

Explanation—Users of pragmatic trial reports seek to solve a health or health service problem in a particular setting. The problem at which the intervention is targeted should thus be described. This enables readers to understand whether the problem confronting them is similar to the one described in the trial report, and thus whether the study is relevant to them. Ideally, the report should state that the trial is pragmatic in attitude (and why) and explain the purpose of the trial in relationship to the decisions that it is intended to inform and in which settings.

Example (b): Describe other interventions that may commonly be aimed at this problem—"Sublingual buprenorphine is increasingly being prescribed by General Practitioners for opiate detoxification, despite limited clinical and research evidence. Comparing methadone, dihydrocodeine and buprenorphine it is important to note several factors which may impact upon prescribing and use of these agents".[54]

Explanation—The background of the trial report should mention the intervention under investigation and the usual alternative(s) in relevant settings. To help place the trial in the context of other settings authors should explain key features that make the intervention feasible in their trial setting and elsewhere (such as, the widespread availability of the trial drug, the availability of trained staff to deliver the intervention, electronic databases that can identify eligible patients).

Item 3: methods; participants

Eligibility criteria for participants and the settings and the locations where the data were collected
Extension for pragmatic trials: Eligibility criteria should be explicitly framed to show the degree to which they include typical participants and, where applicable, typical providers (eg, nurses), institutions (eg, hospitals), communities (or localities eg, towns) and settings of care (eg, different healthcare financing systems).

Examples—"The study population included all National Health System physicians in the Northern Region of Portugal except for those not involved in any clinical activity (eg, administrators, laboratory analysis); those working in substance abuse and rehabilitation centers or specialty hospitals (because they cover multiple geographical areas); and those working at the regional pharmacosurveillance center or any department having a specific voluntary ADR reporting program."[55]

"Our study took place in the three public hospitals (totalling 850 beds) in southern Adelaide, Australia, with a regional population of about 350 000. In Australia, entry to long term care (nursing home) can occur only after an independent clinical assessment by the aged care assessment team (ACAT), who determine level of dependency."[56]

Explanation—Treatments may perform better when evaluated among selected, highly adherent patients with severe but not intractable disease and few comorbidities. Reports of these restricted trials may be of limited applicability. Excessively stringent inclusion and exclusion

criteria reduce the applicability of the results and may result in safety concerns,[57] so the method of recruitment should be completely described. This stringency seems to be reducing over time but remains a problem.[58]

In some trials the unit of randomisation and intervention might be healthcare practitioners, communities, or healthcare institutions such as clinics (that is, cluster randomised pragmatic trials). In these trials volunteer institutions may be atypically well resourced or experienced, successful innovators. Since the feasibility and success of an intervention may depend on attributes of the healthcare system and setting, reporting this information enables readers to assess the relevance and applicability of the results in their own, possibly different, settings.

Item 4: methods; interventions

Precise details of the interventions intended for each group and how and when they were actually administered.
Extension for pragmatic trials: Describe extra resources added to (or resources removed from) usual settings in order to implement the intervention. Indicate if efforts were made to standardise the intervention or if the intervention and its delivery were allowed to vary between participants, practitioners or study sites. Describe the comparator in similar detail to the intervention.

Example: (a) Describe extra resources added to (or resources removed from) usual settings in order to implement the intervention—"The hospitals and a private long term care provider developed and ran the off-site transitional care facility, which was 5-25 km from the study hospitals. The private provider supplied accommodation, catering, cleaning, nursing (5.0 full time equivalents in 24 hours), and career staff (10.0 full time equivalents in 24 hours) while the hospitals provided the allied health staff (4.4 full time equivalents), medical staff, and a transitional care nurse coordinator (1.0 full time equivalent). The whole team assessed all patients on admission to the transitional care unit and had weekly case conferences. Specialist medical staff visited the site for the case conferences and reviewed all admissions. On-call medical care was available 24 hours a day."[56]

Explanation—If the extra resources to deliver the intervention are not described, readers cannot judge the feasibility of the intervention in their own setting. When relevant, authors should report details (experience, training etc) of those who delivered the intervention[51] and its frequency and intensity. If multicomponent interventions are being evaluated, details of the different components should be described.

Example: (b) Indicate if efforts were made to standardise the intervention or if the intervention and its delivery were allowed to vary between participants, practitioners or study sites—"Two trained leaders introduced a structured sequence of topics using a collaborative approach. All leaders had run at least one previous group. Throughout the 12 week programme leaders received three hours of supervision each week from a certified trainer.[59]

Explanation—In explanatory trials the intervention is standardised, and thus the results may not apply under usual conditions of care where no such standardisation is enforced. Pragmatic trials are conducted in typical care settings, and so care may vary between similar participants, by chance, by practitioner preference, and according to institutional policies.[60] For pragmatic trials, efforts that may reduce this natural variation in the intervention and its delivery should be described. However, if reducing variation in a care process or shifting practice patterns is itself the main purpose of the intervention, this should be explicit in the title, abstract, and introduction.

Regardless of the extent to which the intervention was standardised, pragmatic trials should describe the intervention in sufficient detail that it would be possible for someone to replicate it, or include a reference or link to a detailed description of the intervention. Unfortunately, this information is often lacking in reports of trials.[61]

Examples: (c) Describe the comparator in similar detail to the intervention—"Standard advice was given as for the naproxen group. Participants were provided with cocodamol for additional pain relief and an information leaflet about "tennis elbow" based on the Arthritis Research Campaign publication but omitting specific treatment recommendations."[62]

"Women assigned to the control group received usual care from the healthcare team and completed all outcome measures on the same time frame as the intervention group. After randomisation, this group received a two page leaflet entitled "Exercise after cancer diagnosis," which provided safe guidelines. After the six month follow-up, these women were helped to construct their own personalised exercise plan and invited to join a local general practice exercise referral scheme."[63]

Explanation—In a randomised controlled trial the effects of the intervention are always related to a comparator. To increase applicability, and feasibility, pragmatic trials often compare new interventions to usual care. The chosen comparator should be described in sufficient detail for readers to assess whether the incremental benefits or harms reported are likely to apply in their own setting, where usual care may be more, or less, effective.

Item 6: methods; outcomes

Clearly defined primary and secondary outcome measures, and, when applicable, any methods used to enhance the quality of measurements (eg, multiple observations, training of assessors)
Extension for pragmatic trials: Explain why the chosen outcomes and, when relevant, the length of follow-up are considered important to those who will use the results of the trial.

Example—"The patient-based outcomes used in the evaluation were selected on the basis of empirical evidence from consumers about the most important outcomes from SDM [shared decision making] and risk communication."[64]

The total number of days off work in the year after inclusion was calculated for each patient. Days off were defined as days 100% compensated by the NIA [National Insurance Administration]. Thus, days on ASL [Active Sick Leave] were considered as days absent. After a full year of sick leave, administrative proceedings are initiated to transfer the beneficiary to other measures of rehabilitation or disability pension within the NIA system. One year of absence was therefore a proxy measure for long-term disability."[65]

Explanation—The primary outcome(s)[66] in pragmatic trials are chosen to be relevant to the participants and key decision makers at whom the trial is aimed. The length of follow-up should be appropriate to the decision the trial is designed to inform. If the target decision makers are patients and their clinicians, the primary outcome is likely to be a health outcome, while trials aimed at policymakers and institutional leaders may focus on a process or system efficiency or equity outcome. Explicitly indicating that the chosen outcome is important to decision makers, and specifying the decision makers to whom it was important

will assist other readers to decide whether the results are relevant to them.

Item 7: methods; sample size

How sample size was determined; when applicable, explanation of any interim analyses and stopping rules
Extension for pragmatic trials: If calculated using the smallest difference considered important by the target decision maker audience (the minimally important difference) then report where this difference was obtained.

Example—"There were no previous data using the main outcome measure on which to base the sample size calculation, and therefore the sample size was calculated on the number of days with URTI [upper respiratory tract infection]. It was decided, in line with other rigorous pragmatic studies that the smallest difference worth detecting was a 20% reduction in number of days with URTI."[67]

Explanation—The minimally important difference (MID) is the size of a change in the primary outcome which would be important to the key decision making audience. The MID may differ between settings, consequently readers need to know what MID was considered important in the trial setting, and by whom, to contrast with their own expectations.

Item 11: methods; blinding (masking)

Whether participants, those administering the interventions, and those assessing the outcomes were blinded to group assignment
Extension for pragmatic trials: If blinding was not done, or was not possible, explain why.

Example—"Randomisation was done by telephone to an interactive voice response system. We entered and managed all data in an anonymised format; we held data on patient contacts and other administrative data in a separate database. The study was a pragmatic, randomised, prospective, open trial. In exercise studies, blinding the participants to allocation is not possible. We took steps to blind the evaluation of outcomes by having questionnaire responses in sealed envelopes and ensuring that outcome measures were taken by researchers who were not involved in exercise classes."[63]

Explanation—In explanatory trials blinding[68] prevents belief in the effectiveness of the intervention (by participant, clinician and/or assessor) from confounding the causal link between the intervention and the primary outcome. In pragmatic trials, as in the real world delivery of care, blinding of participants and clinicians may be impossible. Belief (or disbelief) in the intervention, extra enthusiasm and effort (or less), and optimism (or pessimism) in the self-assessment of outcomes may thus add to (or detract from) the effects of an intervention. Pragmatic trials may incorporate these factors into the estimate of effectiveness, rendering the findings more applicable to usual care settings. Authors should speculate on the effect of any suspected modifying factors, such as belief in the intervention, in the discussion (item 20). Moreover, in pragmatic trials, it is still desirable and often possible to blind the assessor or obtain an objective source of data for evaluation of outcomes.

Item 13: results; participant flow

Flow of participants through each stage (a diagram is strongly recommended). Specifically, for each group report the numbers of participants randomly assigned, receiving intended treatment, completing the study protocol, and analyzed for the primary outcome. Describe protocol

deviations from study as planned, together with reasons
Extension for pragmatic trials: The number of participants or units approached to take part in the trial, the number which were eligible and reasons for non-participation should be reported.

Example—"These practices ascertained 3392 registered patients with Parkinson's disease; 3124 were eligible for study of whom 1859 (59.5%) agreed to participate (fig 3). Twenty-three patients died during recruitment, leaving 1836 patients when the intervention began. Seventeen of the 1836 patients were not traced at the NHS central registry and are therefore not included in mortality analyses".[69]

Explanation—The more similar the participants, practitioners, or other units of intervention or randomisation are to those in usual care, the more likely that the results of the trial will be applicable to usual care. Consequently the text and/or the trial flow diagram should mention, if known, the number of participants or units approached to take part in the trial, the number whom were eligible, and reasons for non-participation. Although this information is requested in the CONSORT statement, the need for it is greater when reporting a pragmatic trial.

Item 21: generalisability (applicability, external validity)
Generalisability of the trial findings
Extension for pragmatic trials: Describe key aspects of the setting which determined the trial results. Discuss possible differences in other settings where clinical traditions, health service organisation, staffing, or resources may vary from those of the trial.

Examples—"The intervention was tailored to the specific study population and may not be as effective in a different group. The positive results may reflect in part unique aspects of the Portuguese health care system or the regional physician culture. Willingness to report adverse drug reactions may be less in countries in which there is greater concern about malpractice liability."[55]

"The incentive for implementing the clinical pathway will be different for a single-payer third-party system, as exists in Canada, in which costs of the pathway and offsetting hospital costs are realized by the same payer, than for a multiple payer system as exists in the United States, in which hospital cost offsets will be realized by the hospital and not the nursing home payer."[70]

Explanation—The usefulness of the trial report is critically dependent on how applicable the trial and its results are and how feasible the intervention would be. The authors are well placed to suggest how feasible the intervention might be, which aspects of their setting were essential to achieve the trial result, and how that result might differ in other settings. The applicability of the study result could be encapsulated here by reference to the setting (is it a usual care setting), the participants and providers (how selected were they), intensity of intervention and follow up (how much like usual care was this), adherence to the intervention and whether efforts were made to standardise its delivery, the use of intention to treat analysis, and the amount of loss to follow up. Feasibility can be encapsulated by reference to economic, political, and logistic barriers to implementation and by the range of settings and societies in which these barriers would be low.

Discussion
As demand rises for more pragmatic trials to inform real world choices,[13] so too does the need to ensure that the results are clearly reported. Readers need to be able to evaluate the validity of the results, the extent to which they are applicable to their settings, and the feasibility of the tested interventions. The existing CONSORT statement applies fully and directly to pragmatic trials. Here we have proposed extensions for eight items in the statement to make more explicit the important attributes of pragmatic trials and thus to ease the task of users in assessing feasibility, relevance, and likely effects of the intervention in their own setting.

We reached consensus that the trial results are likely to be more widely applicable if the participants, communities, practitioners, or institutions were not narrowly selected; if the intervention was implemented without intense efforts to standardise it; if the comparator group received care or other interventions already widely used; and if the outcomes studied were of importance to the relevant decision makers. The intervention needs to be precisely described if readers are to be able to assess its feasibility.

The multiplicity and independence of the elements constituting the design of pragmatic trials guarantee that pragmatism is not an all or none attribute; rather, it might be best conceived as a continuum along several dimensions. For example, a randomised trial could have broad inclusion criteria for participants but rely primarily on a short term, physiological outcome rather than one that is more meaningful to the participants. Alternatively, a trial might include a wide range of participants, meaningfully assess the effect, but evaluate an intervention that is enforced or tightly monitored and thus not widely feasible. Other permutations probably exist. It is not the case that more pragmatic is always better; a trial's design should be such that the results will meet the needs of the intended users. A trial intended to inform a research decision about the biological effect of a new drug is likely to be more explanatory in design. At a later date, a trial of that same drug aimed at helping patients, practitioners, or policymakers to decide whether it should be prescribed is likely to be more pragmatic in design. To help display this multidimensionality, we have developed of a tool, primarily intended to be used in designing a trial, for characterising where it will stand along the pragmatic-explanatory continuum in relation to each design decision.[71]

We hope that these reporting guidelines will help editors, reviewers, trialists, and policy makers in reporting, reviewing, and using pragmatic trials. Journals that have endorsed the CONSORT statement could also support CONSORT for pragmatic trials, by including reference to this extension paper in the journal's instructions to authors. We also invite editorial groups to consider endorsing the CONSORT extension for pragmatic trials and encourage authors to adhere to it. Up to date versions of all CONSORT guidelines can be found on the CONSORT website (www.consort-statement.org).

We thank Eduardo Bergel, Curt Furberg, Jeremy Grimshaw, Jan Hux, Andreas Laupacis, John Lavis, Simon Lewin, Carl Lombard, Malcolm Maclure, Dale Needham, Dave Sackett, Kevin Thorpe, and the Practihc and CONSORT groups for their contributions.

Funding: The Practihc group was supported by the European Commission's 5th Framework INCO programme, contract ICA4-CT-2001-10019. The 2005 Toronto meeting was supported by the Canadian Institutes for Health Research grant number FRN 63095. The 2008 Toronto meeting was supported by the UK Medical Research Council, the Centre for Health Services Sciences at Sunnybrook Hospital, Toronto, Canada, the Centre for Medical Technology Policy, Balitimore, Maryland, USA and the National Institute for Health and Clinical Excellence, UK. DM is supported by a University of Ottawa research chair; much of his contribution to this paper was while he was with the Children's Hospital of Eastern Ontario Research Institute. DA is supported by Cancer Research UK.

Competing interests: None declared.

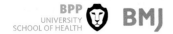

Provenance and peer review: Not commissioned; externally peer reviewed.

1 Altman DG, Bland JM. Statistics notes. Treatment allocation in controlled trials: why randomise? *BMJ* 1999;318:1209.

2 Guyatt GH, Haynes RB, Jaeschke RZ, Cook DJ, Green L, Naylor CD, et al. Users' guides to the medical literature: XXV. Evidence-based medicine: principles for applying the users' guides to patient care. *JAMA* 2000;284:1290-6.

3 Chan AW, Altman DG. Epidemiology and reporting of randomised trials published in PubMed journals. *Lancet* 2005;365:1159-62.

4 Altman DG, Schulz KF, Moher D, Egger M, Davidoff F, Elbourne DG, et al. The revised CONSORT statement for reporting randomized trials: explanation and elaboration. *Ann Intern Med* 2001;134:663-94.

5 Gluud LL. Bias in clinical intervention research. *Am J Epidemiol* 2006;163:493-501.

6 Schwartz D, Lellouch J. Explanatory and pragmatic attitudes in therapeutical trials. *J Chronic Dis* 1967;20:637-48.

7 North American Symptomatic Carotid Endarterectomy Trial Collaborators. Beneficial effect of carotid endarterectomy in symptomatic patients with high-grade carotid stenosis. *N Engl J Med* 1991;325:445-53.

8 Thomas KJ, MacPherson H, Thorpe L, Brazier J, Fitter M, Campbell MJ, et al. Randomised controlled trial of a short course of traditional acupuncture compared with usual care for persistent non-specific low back pain. *BMJ* 2006;333:623-8.

9 Coca SG, Krumholz HM, Garg AX, Parikh CR. Underrepresentation of renal disease in randomized controlled trials of cardiovascular disease. *JAMA* 2006;296:1377-84.

10 Lee PY, Alexander KP, Hammill BG, Pasquali SK, Peterson ED. Representation of elderly persons and women in published randomized trials of acute coronary syndromes. *JAMA* 2001;286:708-13.

11 Zarin DA, Young JL, West JC. Challenges to evidence-based medicine: a comparison of patients and treatments in randomized controlled trials with patients and treatments in a practice research network. *Soc Psychiatry Psychiatr Epidemiol* 2005;40:27-35.

12 Liberati A. The relationship between clinical trials and clinical practice: the risks of underestimating its complexity. *Stat Med* 1994;13:1485-91.

13 Tunis SR, Stryer DB, Clancy CM. Practical clinical trials: increasing the value of clinical research for decision making in clinical and health policy. *JAMA* 2003;290:1624-32.

14 Marson A, Kadir Z, Chadwick D. Large pragmatic randomised studies of new antiepileptic drugs are needed. *BMJ* 1997;314:1764.

15 Williams H. Fungal infections of skin and nails of feet. Pragmatic clinical trial is now needed. *BMJ* 1999;319:1070-1.

16 Lieberman JA, Stroup TS. Guest editors' introduction: what can large pragmatic clinical trials do for public mental health care? *Schizophr Bull* 2003;29:1-6.

17 Roland M, Torgerson DJ. What are pragmatic trials? *BMJ* 1998;316:285.

18 Rothwell PM. External validity of randomised controlled trials: "to whom do the results of this trial apply?" *Lancet* 2005;365:82-93.

19 Macpherson H. Pragmatic clinical trials. *Complement Ther Med* 2004;12:136-40.

20 Godwin M, Ruhland L, Casson I, MacDonald S, Delva D, Birtwhistle R, et al. Pragmatic controlled clinical trials in primary care: the struggle between external and internal validity. *BMC Med Res Methodol* 2003;3:28.

21 Hotopf M, Churchill R, Lewis G. Pragmatic randomised controlled trials in psychiatry. *Br J Psychiatry* 1999;175:217-23.

22 Engel CC. Explanatory and pragmatic perspectives regarding idiopathic physical symptoms and related syndromes. *CNS Spectr* 2006;11:225-32.

23 Whittaker K, Sutton C, Burton C. Pragmatic randomised controlled trials in parenting research: the issue of intention to treat. *J Epidemiol Community Health* 2006;60:858-64.

24 Coutinho ES, Huf G, Bloch KV. [Pragmatic clinical trials: an option in the construction of health-related evidence]. *Cad Saude Publica* 2003;19:1189-93.

25 Ernst E, Canter PH. Limitations of "pragmatic" trials. *Postgrad Med J* 2005;81:203.

26 Vallve C. [A critical review of the pragmatic clinical trial]. *Med Clin (Barc)* 2003;121:384-8.

27 Thompson SG, Barber JA. How should cost data in pragmatic randomised trials be analysed? *BMJ* 2000;320:1197-200.

28 Silverman WA. Sample size, representativeness, and credibility in pragmatic neonatal trials. *Am J Perinatol* 1987;4:129-30.

29 Andersen B. [Principles of medical statistics. XII. Causal or pragmatic clinical research?]. *Nord Med* 1971;86:1434-6.

30 Flamant R. [From the explanatory to the pragmatic]. *Bull Cancer* 1987;74:169-76.

31 Eschwege E, Bouvenot G. [Explanatory or pragmatic trials, the dualism]. *Rev Med Interne* 1994;15:357-61.

32 Califf RM, Woodlief LH. Pragmatic and mechanistic trials. *Eur Heart J* 1997;18:367-70.

33 Resch K. Pragmatic randomised controlled trials for complex therapies. *Forsch Komplementarmed* 1998;5(suppl S1):136-9.

34 Charlton BG. Understanding randomized controlled trials: explanatory or pragmatic? *Fam Pract* 1994;11:243-4.

35 Algra A, van der Graff Y. [Roaming through methodology. XII. Pragmatic and pathophysiologic trials: a question of goal formulation]. *Ned Tijdschr Geneeskd* 1999 6;143:514-7.

36 Green LW, Glasgow RE. Evaluating the relevance, generalization, and applicability of research: issues in external validation and translation methodology. *Eval Health Prof* 2006;29:126-53.

37 Glasgow RE, Magid DJ, Beck A, Ritzwoller D, Estabrooks PA. Practical clinical trials for translating research to practice: design and measurement recommendations. *Med Care* 2005;43:551-7.

38 Tansella M, Thornicroft G, Barbui C, Cipriani A, Saraceno B. Seven criteria for improving effectiveness trials in psychiatry. *Psychol Med* 2006;36:711-20.

39 CONSORT Group. *CONSORT statement 2007* . www.consort-statement. org/?o=1004.

40 Moher D, Schulz KF, Altman DG. The CONSORT statement: revised recommendations for improving the quality of reports of parallel-group randomised trials. *Lancet* 2001;357:1191-4.

41 CONSORT Group. *CONSORT endorsers—journals* . 2007. www.consort-statement.org/index.aspx?o=1096.

42 Davidoff F. News from the International Committee of Medical Journal Editors. *Ann Intern Med* 2000;133:229-31.

43 CONSORT Group. *CONSORT translations*. 2007. www.consort-statement. org/?o=1216.

44 Plint AC, Moher D, Morrison A, Schulz K, Altman DG, Hill C, et al. Does the CONSORT checklist improve the quality of reports of randomised controlled trials? A systematic review. *Med J Aust* 2006;185:263-7.

45 Piaggio G, Elbourne DR, Altman DG, Pocock SJ, Evans SJ. Reporting of noninferiority and equivalence randomized trials: an extension of the CONSORT statement. *JAMA* 2006;295:1152-60.

46 Campbell MK, Elbourne DR, Altman DG. CONSORT statement: extension to cluster randomised trials. *BMJ* 2004;328:702-8.

47 Hopewell S, Clarke M, Moher D, Wager E, Middleton P, Altman DG, et al. CONSORT for reporting randomised trials in journal and conferences abstracts. *Lancet* 2008;371:281-3.

48 Ioannidis JP, Evans SJ, Gotzsche PC, O'Neill RT, Altman DG, Schulz K, et al. Better reporting of harms in randomized trials: an extension of the CONSORT statement. *Ann Intern Med* 2004;141:781-8.

49 Gagnier JJ, Boon H, Rochon P, Moher D, Barnes J, Bombardier C. Reporting randomized, controlled trials of herbal interventions: an elaborated CONSORT statement. *Ann Intern Med* 2006;144:364-7.

50 Boutron I, Moher D, Altman DG, Schulz KF, Ravaud P, the CONSORT Group. Reporting of nonpharmacological treatment interventions: an extension of the CONSORT statement. *Ann Intern Med* 2008;w60-66.

51 Boutron I, Moher D, Altman DG, Schulz KF, Ravaud P, the CONSORT Group. Extending the CONSORT statement to trials reporting nonpharmacological treatments: extension and elaboration. *Ann Intern Med* 2008;148:295-309.

52 Pragmatic Randomized Controlled Trials in HealthCare. www.practihc. org.

53 Wu JY, Leung WY, Chang S, Lee B, Zee B, Tong PC, et al. Effectiveness of telephone counselling by a pharmacist in reducing mortality in patients receiving polypharmacy: randomised controlled trial. *BMJ* 2006;333:522.

54 Wright NM, Sheard L, Tompkins CN, Adams CE, Allgar VL, Oldham NS. Buprenorphine versus dihydrocodeine for opiate detoxification in primary care: a randomised controlled trial. *BMC Fam Pract* 2007;8:3.

55 Figueiras A, Herdeiro MT, Polonia J, Gestal-Otero JJ. An educational intervention to improve physician reporting of adverse drug reactions: a cluster-randomized controlled trial. *JAMA* 2006;296:1086-93.

56 Crotty M, Whitehead CH, Wundke R, Giles LC, Ben-Tovim D, Phillips PA. Transitional care facility for elderly people in hospital awaiting a long term care bed: randomised controlled trial. *BMJ* 2005;331:1110.

57 Juurlink DN, Mamdani MM, Lee DS, Kopp A, Austin PC, Laupacis A, et al. Rates of hyperkalemia after publication of the randomized aldactone evaluation study. *N Engl J Med* 2004;351:543-51.

58 Van Spall HG, Toren A, Kiss A, Fowler RA. Eligibility criteria of randomized controlled trials published in high-impact general medical journals: a systematic sampling review. *JAMA* 2007;297:1233-40.

59 Hutchings J, Gardner F, Bywater T, Daley D, Whitaker C, Jones K, et al. Parenting intervention in Sure Start services for children at risk of developing conduct disorder: pragmatic randomised controlled trial. *BMJ* 2007;334:678.

60 Hawe P, Shiell A, Riley T. Complex interventions: how "out of control" can a randomised controlled trial be? *BMJ* 2004;328:1561-3.

61 Schroter S, Glasziou PP, Heneghan CJ. Quality of descriptions of treatments: a review of published randomised controlled trials. *BMJ* (in press).

62 Hay EM, Paterson SM, Lewis M, Hosie G, Croft P. Pragmatic randomised controlled trial of local corticosteroid injection and naproxen for treatment of lateral epicondylitis of elbow in primary care. *BMJ* 1999;319:964-8.

63 Mutrie N, Campbell AM, Whyte F, McConnachie A, Emslie C, Lee L, et al. Benefits of supervised group exercise programme for women being treated for early stage breast cancer: pragmatic randomised controlled trial. *BMJ* 2007;334:517.

64 Edwards A, Elwyn G, Hood K, Atwell C, Robling M, Houston H, et al. Patient-based outcome results from a cluster randomized trial of shared decision making skill development and use of risk communication aids in general practice. *Fam Pract* 2004;21:347-54.

65 Scheel IB, Hagen KB, Herrin J, Carling C, Oxman AD. Blind faith? The effects of promoting active sick leave for back pain patients. A cluster-randomised trial. *Spine* 2002;27:2734-40.

66 Roland M, Torgerson D. Understanding controlled trials: what outcomes should be measured? *BMJ* 1998;317:1075.

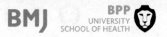

67 Steinsbekk A, Fonnebo V, Lewith G, Bentzen N. Homeopathic care for the prevention of upper respiratory tract infections in children: a pragmatic, randomised, controlled trial comparing individualised homeopathic care and waiting-list controls. *Complement Ther Med* 2005;13:231-8.

68 Schulz KF, Altman DG, Moher D. Blinding is better than masking. *BMJ* 2007;334:918.

69 Jarman B, Hurwitz B, Cook A, Bajekal M, Lee A. Effects of community based nurses specialising in Parkinson's disease on health outcome and costs: randomised controlled trial. *BMJ* 2002;324:1072-5.

70 Loeb M, Carusone SC, Goeree R, Walter SD, Brazil K, Krueger P, et al. Effect of a clinical pathway to reduce hospitalizations in nursing home residents with pneumonia: a randomized controlled trial. *JAMA* 2006;295:2503-10.

71 Thorpe KE, Zwarenstein M, Oxman A, Treweek S, Furberg CD, Altman DG, et al. A proposal for graphing randomized controlled trials within the pragmatic-explanatory continuum: PRECIS. *J Clin Epidemiol* (in press).

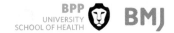

Preparing raw clinical data for publication: guidance for journal editors, authors, and peer reviewers

Iain Hrynaszkiewicz, managing editor[1], Melissa L Norton, editorial director (medicine)[1], Andrew J Vickers, associate attending research methodologist[2], Douglas G Altman, professor of statistics in medicine[3]

[1]BioMed Central, 236 Gray's Inn Road, London WC1X 8HL

[2]Department of Epidemiology and Biostatistics, Memorial Sloan Kettering Cancer Center, 1275 York Avenue, NY, NY 10021, USA

[3]Centre for Statistics in Medicine, University of Oxford, Wolfson College Annexe, Oxford OX2 6UD

Cite this as: BMJ 2010;340:c181

DOI: 10.1136/bmj.c181

http://www.bmj.com/content/340/bmj.c181

ABSTRACT

Many peer reviewed journals now require authors to be prepared to share their raw, unprocessed data with other scientists or state the availability of raw data in published articles, but little information on how such data should be prepared for sharing has emerged. **Iain Hrynaszkiewicz and colleagues** propose a minimum standard for de-identifying datasets to ensure patient privacy when sharing clinical research data

Background

Many peer-reviewed journals' instructions for authors require that authors should be prepared to share their raw (that is, unprocessed) data with other scientists on request. Although data sharing is commonplace in some scientific disciplines and is a requirement of a number of major research funding agencies' policies, this culture has not yet been widely adopted by the clinical research community. Some journals have appealed to their authors to increase the availability of medical research data,[1][2][3] recognising the benefits of such transparency. These benefits are well documented and include replication of previous findings, comparisons with independent datasets, testing of additional hypotheses, teaching, and patient safety.[3][4][5][6] Moreover, patients themselves are increasingly seeing the benefits of openly sharing their experiences with others (www.patientslikeme.com/).

Online journals with unlimited space now provide the platform for publishing large, raw datasets as supplementary material,[5][7] but a common concern is confidentiality. If there is any doubt over anonymity, publishing data that have arisen from the doctor-patient or researcher-participant relationship will raise issues of privacy unless explicit and properly informed consent to all of the intended uses of that data has been obtained. The International Committee of Medical Journal Editors' *Uniform Requirements for Manuscripts Submitted to Biomedical Journals* require that patient privacy be protected, and maintaining confidentiality

and privacy is ingrained in various legal statutes such as the UK Data Protection Act and the Health Insurance Portability and Accountability Act (HIPAA) in the US.[8]

In Europe, the Data Protection Directive (Directive 95/46/EC) provides some harmony in data protection legislation, but in the US there is no overarching data protection law. Therefore, in an increasingly global research and publishing industry, universally agreed definitions as to what constitutes anonymised patient information would benefit clinical researchers. The HIPAA provides a list of 18 items that need to be removed from patient information in order for it to be considered anonymous for the purposes of sharing information between the "covered entities" specified in the act, but the list was not designed with publication in biomedical journals in mind. A number of publications from UK bodies provide some form of guidance on identifying information,[9][10][11][12] but none is as explicit as the HIPAA.

This article aims to provide practical guidance for those involved in the publication process by proposing a minimum standard for anonymising (or de-identifying) data for the purposes of publication in a peer reviewed biomedical journal or sharing with other researchers, either directly, where appropriate, or via a third party. Basic advice on file preparation is also provided, along with procedural guidance on prospective and retrospective publication of raw clinical data. Although the focus of this discussion is on data from randomised trials, the same issues of confidentiality apply to data from any research study involving human subjects, including cohort, case-control, and case series designs.

Data preparation guidance

What is the dataset?

For the purposes of this guidance, the dataset is the aggregated collection of patient observations (including sociodemographic and clinical information) used for the purposes of producing the summary statistical findings presented in the main report of the research project, whether previously published or not.

Data are almost always collected at a greater level of detail than are reported in a journal article. For example, each participant in a pain study may complete a pain diary twice a day for 30 days, with the authors reporting "mean post-treatment pain" for one or more groups of participants. Similarly, a quality of life questionnaire may include a large number of questions divided into domains such as physical, mental, emotional, and social wellbeing.

Here we define a dataset as that containing the minimum level of detail necessary to reproduce all numbers reported in the paper. The dataset for the pain trial, for example, might therefore consist of one value per individual for mean post-treatment pain rather than 30 values for pain

SUMMARY POINTS

- Despite journal and funder policies requiring data sharing, there has been little practical guidance on how data should be shared
- Confidentiality and anonymity are key considerations when publishing or sharing data relating to individuals, and this article provides practical advice on data sharing while minimising risks to patient privacy
- Consent for publication of appropriately anonymised raw data should ideally be sought from participants in clinical research
- Direct identifiers such as patients' names should be removed from datasets; datasets that contain three or more indirect identifiers, such as age or sex, should be reviewed by an independent researcher or ethics committee before being submitted for publication

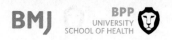

levels on each day. However, if more detailed, underlying data are available and can be shared then that should also be encouraged, provided the data conform to the same standards—as proposed in this article—as the main dataset. If possible, authors should present all outcomes and variables, regardless of significance.

Anonymisation

A list of 28 patient identifiers has been formulated, based on information aggregated from policy documents and research guidance from major UK and US funding agencies, governmental health departments and statutes, and three internationally recognised publication ethics resources for editors of biomedical journals.[8][9][10][11][12][13][14][15] This list is provided in the table.

Types of identifying information have been classified as either direct or indirect. Publication of any direct identifiers places individuals in the dataset at risk of being identified. Although none of the indirect identifiers on its own would point to an individual, a dataset with several indirect identifiers, especially those relating to attributes, might do. The consensus of the authors, and working group members acknowledged in the current manuscript, is that a dataset including three or more indirect identifiers should be assessed by an independent researcher or ethics committee to evaluate the risk that individuals might be identifiable. If the risk of identification is considered non-negligible, before publication can proceed approval should be sought from a relevant advisory body (see below). An explicit justification for publication of a dataset with three or more indirect identifiers should be given by the researcher—as an annotation to the dataset and in any accompanying articles. This should include the name of any oversight bodies consulted.

Use of dates relevant to individuals

In circumstances where it is essential for the scientific validity of the study to include dates, such as dates of treatment (a direct identifier), data must be presented in such a way that is unlikely to affect statistical analyses but preserves anonymity. For example, one could add or subtract a small, randomly chosen number of days to all dates, so that the true dates are not published. In cases where it is necessary to include dates, this fact and any supporting information should be disclosed on submission to the journal.

File preparation

Authors should provide a clean, well annotated dataset in a suitable format so that statistical analyses could be conducted. By "clean," we mean reviewed systematically for duplicates, errors, and missing data; by "well annotated," we mean that sufficient information is given about each variable to allow replication of the originally published results. For example, the dataset included as supplementary material by Vickers[5] includes a brief description of the study and data and a detailed explanation of each variable on the dataset. It is recommended that file formats be as general as possible. Microsoft Excel is widely used and delimited text format is universally convertible, so these formats are preferable to files saved in formats specific to statistical software such as SAS or STATA. If a dataset may be updated in the future—for example, in cancer studies where follow-up is continued over many years—it could be given a version number or date.

Copyright

Where datasets are being published as supplementary material in a journal that requires transfer of copyright to the publisher, it is recommended the supporting data be separated from the article itself and that transfer of copyright for the data is not required as a condition of publication. Of note, there is no protection by intellectual property law on data that are gathered for research purposes[16]—facts themselves are not copyrightable, only the way in which they are expressed.

Prospective data publication

With the increasing prevalence of data sharing policies from research funding agencies, researchers should be encouraged to make allowances for data sharing or publication when preparing study protocols. Although consent is not required in law to process anonymised data, ideally informed consent should be obtained from research participants for the publication of suitably anonymised raw data, as part of the recruitment process, for all new studies. Researchers should inform participants of all possibilities for the use of their information and allow them to choose. Participants who do not agree to publication of potentially identifying information may need to be removed from the dataset.[15] Approval or consent should include use of the data in subsequent meta-analyses. Research ethics committees should also encourage researchers to include details of the intention to publish data in the study information sheets that are provided to study participants, and to ensure that safeguards are in place to protect patient privacy. In the absence of mandates for data sharing or publication,

Table   List of potential patient identifiers in datasets

Identifier (information sources)	Comments
Direct	
Name ([8-15])	
Initials ([13])	
Address, including full or partial postal code ([8-15])	
Telephone or fax numbers or contact information ([8][10][12][15])	
Electronic mail addresses ([8])	
Unique identifying numbers ([8-15])	Generalised HIPAA items 7-10, 18
Vehicle identifiers ([8])	
Medical device identifiers ([8])	
Web or internet protocol addresses ([8])	
Biometric data ([8])	
Facial photograph or comparable image ([8][10][11][13])	
Audiotapes ([11])	
Names of relatives ([10])	
Dates related to an individual (including date of birth) ([8][9][11][15])	
Indirect—may present a risk if present in combination with others in the list	
Place of treatment or health professional responsible for care ([10][15])	Could be inferred from investigator affiliations
Sex ([9])	
Rare disease or treatment ([10])	
Sensitive data, such as illicit drug use or "risky behaviour" ([15])	
Place of birth ([10][15])	
Socioeconomic data, such as occupation or place of work, income, or education ([9][10][12][15])	MRC requirement is for "rare" occupations only
Household and family composition ([15])	
Anthropometry measures ([15])	
Multiple pregnancies ([15])	
Ethnicity ([9])	
Small denominators—population size of <100 ([14])	
Very small numerators—event counts of <3 ([14])	
Year of birth or age (this article)	Age is potentially identifying if the recruitment period is short and is fully described
Verbatim responses or transcripts ([15])	

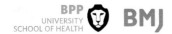

research funding agencies should give greater scrutiny to data sharing plans referred to in their policy documents and check their enforcement.

Retrospective data publication

There will be instances when researchers wish to publish a dataset retrospectively. This might be from current clinical research that was conducted without explicit consent for data sharing or publication from the participants (due to a lack of specific requirements of funders or regulators) or use of data from a historic piece of research conducted before data sharing policies were established.

In such cases, researchers may publish raw data if it is clear and demonstrable that there is no threat to anonymity—for example, if the dataset includes no direct identifiers and fewer than three indirect identifiers. If it is not certain that data are completely anonymous, and where consent of all participants is not possible, a careful case-by-case assessment must be made—taking into account public interest and scientific imperative for publication—before publishing the data. Where there is a risk of identification, we recommend authors consult local ethics committees about their wish to publish their raw data in a freely accessible manner before submitting it for publication. When the relevant committee no longer exists, the authors are encouraged to consult an appropriate national advisory body. In the UK, for example, the National Information Governance Board for Health and Social Care (NIGB), formerly the Patient Information Advisory Group, provides advice on issues of national significance involving the use of patient information. The NIGB includes the Ethics and Confidentiality Committee. Such bodies may not be in a position to approve the decision to publish raw data, but they could provide a valuable opinion. Advice may also be sought from the Caldicott Guardian (a person responsible for protecting patient confidentiality) or equivalent person within the author's institution. In the US, a research ethics consultation could be considered in addition to institutional review board approval.

A case-by-case judgment, whether this is by an advisory body or the journal editor, will need to take into account the sample size, the ways in which results will be published and used, and all other circumstances of the study. For example, the fact that research findings are increasingly being published in open access journals, so that a published dataset would be visible to anyone with an internet connection, arguably makes any issues of confidentiality and anonymity even more important.

Preparing for journal submission—statement in submitted manuscript

Authors should be asked to state in their manuscript if informed consent for data publication has been obtained. If consent was not obtained, authors should be asked to state the reasons for this and the name of the body that gave approval or any guidance adhered to in preparing their data for publication. In practice, authors could make one of three statements:

• Consent for publication of raw data obtained from study participants
• Consent for publication of raw data not obtained but dataset is fully anonymous in a manner that can easily be verified by any user of the dataset. Publication of the dataset clearly and obviously presents minimal risk to confidentiality of study participants
• Consent for publication of raw data not obtained and dataset could in theory pose a threat to confidentiality.

For statements 2 and 3, authors should also provide:
• Reasons why it was not possible to obtain consent
• Reasons why publication of data constituted a negligible risk to confidentiality or reasons why benefit of publishing data outweighs a non-negligible risk to confidentiality, plus the name of an oversight body consulted for approval of publication or guidance.

Alternatives to journal publication

There will be circumstances where raw data cannot be published in journals, because of policy or space restrictions, but alternatives do exist. These include online repositories and databases such as the Dataverse Network Project (http://thedata.org/). Specialist data centres or archives are also emerging, such as the UK Data Archive (www.data-archive.ac.uk/). But in all cases, whether data are published or deposited, restrictions on access to certain aspects of data may be warranted, such as when removal of information that could identify the data would negate its scientific value. In circumstances where data must be behind a barrier to universal access, the data could be made accessible only to those who agree to certain conditions of use, and to individuals who meet certain professional criteria. Embargoes on access to data could also be applied.[3]

Limitations of this guidance

This guidance is directed at quantitative research data and should be applicable to most observational studies and randomised controlled trials. Qualitative or mixed methods researchers should seek alternative advice. The UK Data Archive, for example, has produced guidance on anonymisation techniques for qualitative data.[17] An important limitation of the search strategy used in preparing the table is that it is restricted to US HIPAA guidance and known UK bodies with an interest in maintaining confidentiality in human subjects research. Investigation of requirements of non-English speaking nations would be beneficial. This guidance is aimed at those producing data: guidelines for use of published data have been reported separately.[5]

Some advocates of clinical data sharing are also keen for data to be shared in agreed, standardised formats to facilitate its automated re-use for statistical analysis.[18] Although basic principles of data preparation have been provided, how this relates to initiatives aimed at standardising raw data are beyond the scope of this document.

In order to encourage its wide dissemination, this article is freely accessible on bmj.com and will also be published in the journal Trials (www.trialsjournal.com).

We thank the following individuals for their review of earlier drafts of the manuscript: Trish Groves and Jane Smith of the BMJ, Sabine Kleinert and Jessica Clark of the Lancet, David Neal of the National Research Ethics Service, and Sara Tobin of Stanford Center for Biomedical Ethics.

Contributors: The idea for the manuscript was conceived at a meeting (described by Groves[2] and Hrynaszkiewicz et al[3]) in September 2008 chaired by IH, and was attended by MLN, AJV, and DGA. IH wrote the first draft of the manuscript. MLN, AJV, and DGA all reviewed the manuscript and were involved in its critical revision before submission. All authors read and approved the final manuscript. IH is guarantor for the manuscript.

Competing interests: All authors have completed the Unified Competing Interest form at www.icmje.org/coi_disclosure.pdf (available on request from the corresponding author) and declare that all authors had: (1) No financial support for the submitted work from anyone other than their employer; (2) IH and MN are employees of BioMed Central, the open access publisher, and receive fixed salaries, but work on this manuscript has not been at the urging of BioMed Central; (3) No spouses, partners, or children with relationships with commercial entities that might have an interest in the submitted work; (4) AJV is an associate editor for the BioMed

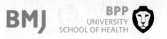

Central journal *Trials*, which hopes to encourage greater prevalence of raw clinical data sharing and publication; DGA is coeditor-in-chief of *Trials*. All authors are supporters of data sharing and release from all types of research.

Provenance and peer review: Not commissioned; externally peer reviewed.

1 Laine C, Goodman SN, Griswold ME, Sox HC. Reproducible research: moving toward research the public can really trust. *Ann Intern Med* 2007;146:450-3.

2 Groves T. Managing UK research data for future use. *BMJ* 2009;338:b1252.

3 Hrynaszkiewicz I, Altman DG. Towards agreement on best practice for publishing raw clinical trial data. *Trials* 2009;10:17.

4 Kirwan JR. Making original data from clinical studies available for alternative analyses. *J Rheumatol* 1997;24:822-5.

5 Vickers AJ. Whose data set is it anyway? Sharing raw data from randomized trials. *Trials* 2006;7:15.

6 Smith R, Roberts I. Patient safety requires a new way to publish clinical trials. *PLoS Clin Trials* 2006;1:e6.

7 Hutchon DJ. Publishing raw data and real time statistical analysis on e-journals. *BMJ* 2001;322:530.

8 Partners Human Research Committee. HIPAA frequently asked questions: 5) What is identifiable information? How can information be deidentified? What is a "limited data set?" http://healthcare.partners.org/phsirb/hipaafaq.htm#b5.

9 National Information Governance Board. Information about patients. www.advisorybodies.doh.gov.uk/piag/InformationAboutPatients.pdf.

10 Medical Research Council. Personal information in medical research. www.mrc.ac.uk/consumption/idcplg?IdcService=GET_FILE&dID=6233&dDocName=MRC002452&allowInterrupt=1.

11 Department of Health. Confidentiality: NHS code of practice. 2003. www.dh.gov.uk/en/Publicationsandstatistics/Publications/PublicationsPolicyAndGuidance/DH_4069253?IdcService=GET_FILE&dID=9722&Rendition=Web.

12 UK Data Archive. Training module II: Dealing with confidential research information. Data Management and Sharing Workshop, Edinburgh, 17 June 2008. www.data-archive.ac.uk/news/eventsdocs/anon17jun08.doc.

13 International Committee of Medical Journal Editors: Uniform requirements for manuscripts submitted to biomedical journals. Ethical considerations in the conduct and reporting of research: privacy and confidentiality. 2009. www.icmje.org/ethical_5privacy.html.

14 Washington State Department of Health. Health data guidelines: guidelines for working with small numbers. 2009. www.doh.wa.gov/Data/guidelines/SmallNumbers.htm.

15 National Hearth Lung and Blood Institute. Policy for dataset preparation. https://biolincc.nhlbi.nih.gov/static/Policy_for_Dataset_Preparation.pdf.

16 Association of Learned and Professional Society Publishers (ALPSP) and International Association of Scientific, Technical, & Medical Publishers (STM). ALPSP and STM issue joint statement clarifying publishers' views on access to raw data, data sets, and databases. 2006. www.alpsp.org/ForceDownload.asp?id=128.

17 UK Data Archive. Managing and sharing data: a best practice guide for researchers. 2009. www.data-archive.ac.uk/news/publications/managingsharing.pdf.

18 Tu SW, Carini S, Rector A, Maccallum P, Toujilov I, Harris S, et al. OCRe: an ontology of clinical research. 2009. http://protege.stanford.edu/conference/2009/abstracts/S8P2Tu.pdf.

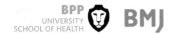

Comparative effectiveness research in cancer screening programmes

Michael Bretthauer, professor and endoscopist[1] [2], Geir Hoff, professor and head of screening programme[2] [3] [4]

[1]University of Oslo, Oslo, Norway

[2]Oslo University Hospital, Oslo

[3]Cancer Registry of Norway, Oslo

[4]Department of Research, Telemark Hospital, Skien, Norway

Cite this as: BMJ 2012;344:e2864

DOI: 10.1136/bmj.e2864

http://www.bmj.com/content/344/bmj.e2864

ABSTRACT

Large scale cancer screening programmes are not amenable to generating or responding to new evidence about their effectiveness. The authors outline a new approach in Norway intended to overcome these drawbacks by means of comparative effectiveness research

In recent decades, cancer screening programmes (screening that is publicly organised and includes invitation procedures for eligible people of the average risk population in the screening area) have been established in many countries. While cancer screening in the context of clinical trials is innovative and investigative, cancer screening programmes themselves are largely static and not designed to generate new, evidence based knowledge. However, screening programmes themselves affect health and healthcare, which may in turn substantially affect the effectiveness of the programmes. Many screening programmes today can be regarded as supertankers; once under way, they are difficult to halt or alter in direction or content. In mammography, increasing concern about the benefits and harms of screening programmes has led to the announcement of an independent review of mammography screening in the United Kingdom.[1] Here, we outline new approaches that aim to overcome this obstacle, using the principles of comparative effectiveness research.

Screening programmes change medicine

Breast cancer mortality in Norway has declined since the introduction of the Norwegian breast cancer screening programme in the 1990s. According to new evidence, however, most of the observed decline in mortality is not due to the screening itself but is because of the improved patient care that resulted from the introduction of the screening programme (which was accompanied by reorganisation of breast cancer care, improving quality and awareness).[2] This surprising finding indicates that screening tests themselves may be of minor importance for the reduced morbidity and mortality achieved by implementing a screening programme.

SUMMARY POINTS

- Cancer screening programmes are generally static and are not designed to include research studies
- Cancer screening programmes change the environment they are operating in, and this may change the effectiveness of the programme
- Comparative effectiveness research may be used to continuously optimise effectiveness of screening services within running programmes
- In Norway, the entire population of two areas is being randomised within a new bowel cancer screening programme from 2012, to generate new evidence for effectiveness and harms of screening

In the case of the Norwegian breast cancer screening programme, it was possible to tease out the effect of the reorganised care from that of the screening itself only because the programme was introduced in stages, and control groups that were parallel in time with the intervention groups could be established. Such control groups (so called concurrent groups) are important for the evaluation of screening programmes because of changes in risk factors and improvements in diagnostics and treatment over time and socioeconomic imbalance between screening areas and non-screening areas. Most screening programmes, however, do not include concurrent control groups, which makes it difficult to obtain valid comparisons between individuals who are invited to screening and those who are not. This precludes a scientific evaluation of the effects of the programmes.

Comparative effectiveness research

Comparative effectiveness research is "the generation and synthesis of evidence that compares the benefits and harms of alternative methods to prevent, diagnose, treat, and monitor a clinical condition, or to improve the delivery of care ... The purpose of [comparative effectiveness research] is to assist consumers, clinicians, purchasers, and policy makers to make informed decisions that will improve health care at both the individual and population levels."[3] This approach has been used most often in the context of clinical trials comparing different therapies such as drugs or devices. However, it may also be applicable for other types of interventions, such as disease prevention and screening. Comparative effectiveness research can also be used to improve the quality and effectiveness of applied concepts of healthcare services, such as screening programmes for cancer.

Lack of evidence

Cancer screening trials are costly and difficult to perform compared with most clinical trials. There is a long lag time—often exceeding 10 years—between a screening intervention and the time when the most important effect of screening, disease specific mortality, can be observed. Because relatively few people die from cancer, screening trials have to include a large number of participants; and high compliance rates are difficult to obtain because screening trials approach presumptively healthy people who will have no immediate gain from participation (unlike trials among symptomatic patients). These challenges may account for the lack of scientific evidence for many of the large cancer screening programmes currently in place. Cervical smear screening for cervical cancer, introduced in the 1960s, has never been investigated in a randomised trial. Prostate specific antigen (PSA) screening for prostate cancer became endemic before any randomised trials were even started, with the consequence of contamination bias and controversy about the validity of the obtained results.[4]

However, the scientific evidence which screening programmes are based on should arise from randomised trials. To disentangle the different options of screening methods, intervals, thresholds for follow-up and surveillance, head to head randomised comparisons of the different screening options and tests available are needed, as recently emphasised by Baum in the *BMJ*.[5] Screening programmes, rather than independent randomised trials, may be the natural platforms for these studies.

Colorectal cancer is one of the major causes of death from cancer worldwide.[6] A range of screening tests exists—such as faecal occult blood testing, flexible sigmoidoscopy, and colonoscopy—but evidence on the performance of one test compared with the others is limited. Furthermore, the different tests may have different cost effectiveness profiles in different settings, populations, and cultures. Head to head comparisons are needed to evaluate the efficacy, effectiveness, and cost effectiveness of the tests. Best clinical practice changes with time. A good health service programme should integrate development and testing of new modalities as part of the programme itself. The introduction of organised screening programmes for colorectal cancer is an ideal opportunity to establish comparative effectiveness research. Randomised comparisons of different screening strategies are the best means of obtaining valid, high quality data.

The Norwegian approach

Norway has one of the highest incidences of colorectal cancer worldwide. In 2009 the Norwegian Directorate of Health established a national board of experts to advise the government about colorectal cancer screening. The board recognised an imminent need to control the burden of colorectal cancer and the part screening might play in achieving this. However, in light of the ongoing harsh debate about other cancer screening programmes (particularly mammography) in Norway and other countries, a strong recommendation was given to evaluate the possibility of integrating high quality research into the colorectal cancer screening programme. The Norwegian Centre of Knowledge in Health Care, an independent publicly owned research institute, was asked to produce a report on the current evidence for the different colorectal cancer screening tests. As a prerequisite, the Norwegian government requested that only screening modalities that had been shown to be effective compared with no screening in randomised trials should be considered for inclusion in a future screening programme. The report, available in 2010, concluded that two screening tests have been proved to reduce colorectal cancer mortality in randomised trials (faecal occult blood test and flexible sigmoidoscopy), but that there was insufficient evidence to show which was the better of the two.[7] Further, there were substantial differences between the studies with regard to effect sizes for mortality and incidence, and with regard to population and test performance settings.

The board therefore concluded that a future national colorectal cancer screening programme would need to establish its own evidence on a continuous basis to be able to monitor the effectiveness and adverse effects of the screening programme. The board recommended the use of clinical trial methodology, through randomised comparisons within comparative effectiveness research projects whenever possible, combined with rigorous data gathering and evaluation. On the advice of the board, the Norwegian government established a national comparative effectiveness screening programme for colorectal cancer. This programme's aim is to generate evidence on the comparative effectiveness of the screening tests and strategies available.[8]

The entire population aged 50–74 years in two geographical areas of Norway will be randomised to one of two screening options: half to biennial screening by immunochemical faecal occult blood test, and half to once only screening by flexible sigmoidoscopy (figure). The primary evaluation end point is the comparison of the two tests with regard to mortality from colorectal cancer after 10 years. Within the two primary comparison groups, additional randomised trials will be performed to evaluate other important measures such as anxiety and lifestyle changes due to screening, invitation procedures, appointment assignments, and bowel cleansing regimens. The entire screening programme will essentially be set up as a series of adaptive randomised trials, ensuring continuous evaluation of the effectiveness of the different measures compared by establishing concurrent comparison groups through randomisation.

This will result in a continuously updated programme that can rapidly take into account new, self generated evidence and integrate it into the programme. Also, when future screening tests show promising results in clinical trials (such as molecular markers), these new methods can be enrolled into the programme in a randomised fashion as additional arms along the two established ones, and thus rigorously tested within the setting of a real life screening programme.

Although the randomised trial is the optimal method in clinical research, not all unanswered questions can be resolved by applying this method. Observational studies with

Fig Design of the comparative effectiveness research screening programme for colorectal cancer currently implemented in Norway. Screening by immunochemical faecal occult blood testing is offered biennially, whereas flexible sigmoidoscopy screening is once only. The time from start of screening until evaluation of the primary end point is 10 years

iFOBT = immunochemical faecal occult blood test

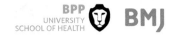

case-control or cohort design or registry based observations are useful to evaluate health services and will be applied in the planned screening programme. For example, a system for continuous monitoring of all endoscopies in the programme will be set up. These observational data will be used to improve the quality of the service, and may also be used in research projects.

Comparative research in public health programmes

Cancer screening addresses large numbers of presumptively healthy individuals, who are subjected to medical interventions that are not risk-free, often cumbersome, and frequently result in false positive or false negative results. The vast majority of people invited to screening will never get the disease. For example, the lifetime risk for colorectal cancer in Western countries is around 5%. This means that 95% of the population will not get the disease irrespective of attending screening, and that screening only affects the course of the disease for the 5% who would get the disease if screening had not been an option. The others will not have any personal gain by participating in screening, but are prone to the adverse effects and the complications. The integration of randomised, head to head comparison trials within new or established screening programmes provides healthcare providers, funding bodies, and the public with population specific, updated, and reliable evidence on the effectiveness and risks of different options and strategies in cancer screening. There is no opposing interest between proponents of cancer screening programmes and those advocating randomised trials.

Some may argue that it is too late for many screening programmes to incorporate comparative research strategies. However, even in established programmes, such as for mammography or cervical cancer screening, many new concepts and innovations can be tested by means of comparative effectiveness research. Examples for comparison trials within the programmes would include evaluation of "watch and wait" versus radiotherapy for screen detected ductal carcinoma in situ (www.clinicaltrials. gov; NCT 00077168), or comparisons of different human papillomavirus tests in cervical cancer screening.

The establishment of comparative effectiveness screening programmes does not require significantly more resources compared with conventional programmes. Comparing two or more screening tools, different modes for invitation, or strategies for reminders and follow-up (such as telephone versus letters versus emails) are easily handled with most available information technology and database management systems. Many new methods to be tested are less resource demanding or improve compliance and thereby effectiveness. Therefore, incorporation of comparative effectiveness research will help to save costs and increase cost effectiveness, and is attractive also for developing countries with limited resources and a high level of uncertainty about the effect of public health programmes (due to the lack of own data).

The overarching aim of the new comparative effectiveness screening programme for colorectal cancer in Norway is to achieve continuous optimisation of the screening service. This includes comparisons of different screening tests to find the best test for the Norwegian population. The programme will produce comparative data on effectiveness, adverse events, side effects such as overdiagnosis, and costs. The programme, however, is not designed to evaluate the effectiveness of screening versus no screening because everyone is offered screening. Thus, we will not be able to find out if screening is effective, only help find the most effective of different screening options.

Contributors: MB and GH had the idea for the paper. MB drafted the first version of the manuscript. MB is a member of the Norwegian Directorate of Health national advisory board for colorectal cancer screening. GH is head of the Norwegian colorectal cancer screening programme.

Provenance and peer review: Not commissioned; peer reviewed.

Competing interests: All authors have completed the ICMJE uniform disclosure form at www.icmje.org/coi_disclosure.pdf (available on request from the corresponding author) and declare: no support from any organisation for the submitted work; no financial relationships with any organisations that might have an interest in the submitted work in the previous three years; no other relationships or activities that could appear to have influenced the submitted work.

1   Richards M. An independent review is under way. *BMJ* 2011;343:d6843.
2   Kalager M, Zelen M, Langmark F, Adami HO. Effect of screening mammography on breast-cancer mortality in Norway. *N Engl J Med* 2010;363:1203-10.
3   Sox H. Better evidence about screening for lung cancer. *N Engl J Med* 2011;365:455-7.
4   Djulbegovic M, Beyth RJ, Neuberger MM, Stoffs TL, Vieweg J, Djulbegovic B, et al. Screening for prostate cancer: systematic review and meta-analysis of randomised controlled trials. *BMJ* 2010;341:c4543.
5   Baum M. Screening for breast cancer: an appeal to Mike Richards. *BMJ* 2011;343:d7535.
6   Cancer Mondial. Globocan 2002 database. www-dep.iarc.fr (accessed 22 Aug 2011).
7   Fretheim A, Bretthauer M. *Expected impact of introducing screening for colorectal cancer in Norway: rapid review* . National Centre of Knowledge in Health Care, 2010.
8   Ministry of Health and Care Services. Press release: Kraftig satsing på helse og omsorg [in Norwegian]. www.regjeringen.no/nb/dep/ hod/pressesenter/pressemeldinger/2010/kraftig-satsing-pa-helse-og-omsorg.html?id=620271 .

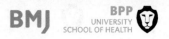

Economic evaluation using decision analytical modelling: design, conduct, analysis, and reporting

Stavros Petrou, professor of health economics[1], Alastair Gray, professor of health economics[2]

[1]Clinical Trials Unit, Warwick Medical School, University of Warwick, Coventry CV4 7AL, UK

[2]Health Economics Research Centre, Department of Public Health, University of Oxford, Oxford, UK

Correspondence to: S Petrou S.Petrou@warwick.ac.uk

Cite this as:
BMJ 2011;342:d1766

DOI: 10.1136/bmj.d1766

http://www.bmj.com/content/342/bmj.d1766

ABSTRACT

Evidence relating to healthcare decisions often comes from more than one study. Decision analytical modelling can be used as a basis for economic evaluations in these situations.

Economic evaluations are increasingly conducted alongside randomised controlled trials, providing researchers with individual patient data to estimate cost effectiveness.[1] However, randomised trials do not always provide a sufficient basis for economic evaluations used to inform regulatory and reimbursement decisions. For example, a single trial might not compare all the available options, provide evidence on all relevant inputs, or be conducted over a long enough time to capture differences in economic outcomes (or even measure those outcomes).[2] In addition, reliance on a single trial may mean ignoring evidence from other trials, meta-analyses, and observational studies. Under these circumstances, decision analytical modelling provides an alternative framework for economic evaluation.

Decision analytical modelling compares the expected costs and consequences of decision options by synthesising information from multiple sources and applying mathematical techniques, usually with computer software. The aim is to provide decision makers with the best available evidence to reach a decision—for example, should a new drug be adopted? Following on from our article on trial based economic evaluations,[1] we outline issues relating to the design, conduct, analysis, and reporting of economic evaluations using decision analytical modelling.

Defining the question

The first stage in the development of any model is to specify the question or decision problem. It is important to define all relevant options available for evaluation, the recipient population, and the geographical location and setting in which the options are being delivered.[3] The requirements of the decision makers should have a crucial role in identifying the appropriate perspective of the analysis, the time horizon, the relevant outcome measures, and, more broadly, the scope or boundaries of the model.[4] If these factors are unclear, or different decision makers have conflicting requirements, the perspective and scope should be broad enough to allow the results to be disaggregated in different ways.[5]

Decision trees

The simplest form of decision analytical modelling in economic evaluation is the decision tree. Alternative options are represented by a series of pathways or branches as in figure 1, which examines whether it is cost effective to screen for breast cancer every two years compared with not screening. The first point in the tree, the decision node (drawn as a square) represents this decision question. In this instance only two options are represented, but additional options could easily be added. The pathways that follow each option represent a series of logically ordered alternative events, denoted by branches emanating from chance nodes (circular symbols). The alternatives at each chance node must be mutually exclusive and their probabilities should sum exactly to one. The end points of each pathway are denoted by terminal nodes (triangular symbols) to which values or pay-offs, such as costs, life years, or quality adjusted life years (QALYs), are assigned. Once the probabilities and pay-offs have been entered, the decision tree is "averaged out" and "folded back" (or rolled back), allowing the expected values of each option to be calculated.[4]

Decision trees are valued for their simplicity and transparency, and they can be an excellent way of clarifying the options of interest. However, they are limited by the lack of any explicit time variable, making it difficult to deal with time dependent elements of an economic evaluation.[6] Recursion or looping within the decision tree is also not allowed, so that trees representing chronic diseases with recurring events can be complex with numerous lengthy pathways.

Markov models

An alternative form of modelling is the Markov model. Unlike decision trees, which represent sequences of events as a large number of potentially complex pathways, Markov models permit a more straightforward and flexible sequencing of outcomes, including recurring outcomes, through time. Patients are assumed to reside in one of a finite number of health states at any point in time and make transitions between those health states over a series of discrete time intervals or cycles.[3][6] The probability of staying in a state or moving to another one in each cycle is determined by a set of defined transition probabilities. The definition and number of health states and the duration

SUMMARY POINTS

- Decision analytical modelling for economic evaluation uses mathematical techniques to determine the expected costs and consequences of alternative options
- Methods of modelling include decision trees, Markov models, patient level simulation models, discrete event simulations, and system dynamic models
- The process of identifying and synthesising evidence for a model should be transparent and appropriate to decision makers' objectives
- The results of decision analytical models are subject to the influences of variability, uncertainty, and heterogeneity, and these must be handled appropriately
- Validation of model based economic evaluations strengthens the credibility of their results

of the cycles will be governed by the decision problem: one study of treatment for gastro-oesophageal reflux disease used one month cycles to capture treatment switches and side effects,[7] whereas an analysis of cervical cancer screening used six monthly cycles to model lifetime outcomes.[8]

Figure 2 presents a state transition diagram and matrix of transition probabilities for a Markov model of a hypothetical breast cancer intervention. There are three health states: well, recurrence of breast cancer, and dead. In this example, the probability of moving from the well state at time t to the recurrence state at time $t+1$ is 0.3, while the probability of moving from well to dead is 0.1. At each cycle the sum of the transition probabilities out of a health state (the row probabilities) must equal 1. In order for the Markov process to end, some termination condition must be set. This could be a specified number of cycles, a proportion passing through or accumulating in a particular state, or the entire population reaching a state that cannot be left (in our example, dead); this is called an absorbing state.

An important limitation of Markov models is the assumption that the transition probabilities depend only on the current health state, independent of historical experience (the Markovian assumption). In our example, the probability of a person dying from breast cancer is independent of the number of past recurrences and also independent of how long the person spent in the well state before moving to the recurrent state. This limitation can be overcome by introducing temporary states that patients can only enter for one cycle or by a series of temporary states that must be visited in a fixed sequence.[4]

GLOSSARY OF TERMS

- *Cost effectiveness acceptability curve*—Graphical depiction of the probability that a health intervention is cost effective across a range of willingness to pay thresholds held by decision makers for the health outcome of interest
- *Cost effectiveness plane*—Graphical depiction of difference in effectiveness between the new treatment and the comparator against the difference in cost
- *Discounting*—The practice of reducing future costs and health outcomes to present values
- *Health utilities*—Preference based outcomes normally represented on a scale where 0 represents death and 1 represents perfect health
- *Incremental cost effectiveness ratio*—A measure of cost effectiveness of a health intervention compared with an alternative, defined as the difference in costs divided by the difference in effects
- *Multiparameter evidence synthesis*—A generalisation of meta-analysis in which multiple variables are estimated jointly
- *Quality adjusted life year* (QALY)—Preference-based measure of health outcome that combines length of life and health related quality of life (utility scores) in a single metric
- *Time horizon*—The start and end points (in time) over which the costs and consequences of a health intervention will be measured and valued
- *Value of information analysis*—An approach for estimating the monetary value associated with collecting additional information within economic evaluation

---

The final stage is to assign values to each health state, typically costs and health utilities.[6][9] Most commonly, such models simulate the transition of a hypothetical cohort of individuals through the Markov model over time, allowing the analyst to estimate expected costs and outcomes. This simply involves, for each cycle, summing costs and outcomes across health states, weighted by the proportion of the cohort expected to be in each state, and then summing across cycles.[3] If the time horizon of the model is over one year, discounting is usually applied to generate the present values of expected costs and outcomes.[1]

Alternative modelling approaches

Although Markov models alone or in combination with decision trees are the most common models used in economic evaluations, other approaches are available.

Patient level simulation (or microsimulation) models the progression of individuals rather than hypothetical cohorts. The models track the progression of potentially heterogeneous individuals with the accumulating history of each individual determining transitions, costs, and health outcomes.[3][10] Unlike Markov models, they can simulate the time to next event rather than requiring equal length cycles and can also simulate multiple events occurring in parallel.[10]

Discrete event simulations describe the progress of individuals through healthcare processes or systems, affecting their characteristics and outcomes over unrestricted time periods.[10] Discrete event simulations are not restricted to the use of equal time periods or the Markovian assumption and, unlike patient level simulation models, also allow individuals to interact with each other[11]— for example, in a transplant programme where organs are scarce and transplant decisions and outcomes for any individual affect everyone else in the queue.

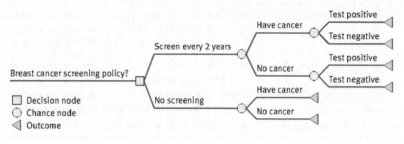

Fig 1 Decision tree for breast cancer screening options[4]

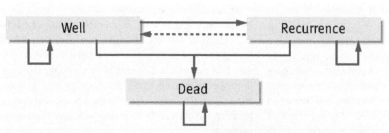

State at time t	State at t + 1		
	Well	**Recurrence**	**Dead**
Well	1-(0.3 + 0.1)	0.3	0.1
Recurrence	0.1	1-(0.1 + 0.2)	0.2
Dead	0	0	1

Fig 2 Markov state diagram and transition probability matrix for hypothetical breast cancer intervention. The arrows represent possible transitions between the three health states (well, recurrence, and dead), loops indicate the possibility of remaining in a health state in successive cycles, and the dashed line indicates the possibility of backwards transition from recurrence of breast cancer to the well state after successful treatment. The cycle length is set at one year

Dynamic models allow internal feedback loops and time delays that affect the behaviour of the entire health system or population being studied. They are particularly valuable in studies of infectious diseases, where analysts may need to account for the evolving effects of factors such as herd immunity on the likelihood of infection over time, and their results can differ substantially from those obtained from static models.[12]

The choice of modelling approach will depend on various factors, including the decision maker's requirements.[10 11 13]

Identifying, synthe sising, and transforming data inputs

The process of identifying and synthesising evidence to populate a decision analytical model should be consistent with the general principles of evidence based medicine.[3] [14] These principles are broadly established for clinical evidence.[15] Less clear is the strategy that should be adopted to identify and synthesise evidence on other variables, such as costs and health utilities, other than it should be transparent and appropriate given the objectives of the model.[16] Indeed, many health economists recognise that the time and resource constraints imposed by many funders of health technology assessments will tend to preclude systematic reviews of the evidence for all variables.[17]

If evidence is not available from randomised trials, it has to be drawn from other sources, such as epidemiological or observational studies, medical records, or, more controversially, expert opinion. And sometimes the evidence from randomised trials may not be appropriate for use in the model—for example, cost data drawn from a trial might reflect protocol driven resource use rather than usual practice[18] or might not be generalisable to the jurisdiction of interest.[5] These methodological considerations have increased interest in multiparameter evidence synthesis (box)[19] in decision analytical modelling. These techniques acknowledge the importance of trying to incorporate correlations between variables in models, which may have an important influence on the resulting estimates of cost effectiveness.[2] However, accurately assessing the correlation between different clinical events, or between events and costs or health utilities, may be difficult without patient level data from a single source. Another complication is that evidence may have to be transformed in complex ways to meet the requirements of the model—for example, interval probabilities reported in the literature may have to be transformed into instantaneous rates and then into transition probabilities corresponding to the cycle length used in a Markov model.[3 4 14]

Quantifying and reporting cost effectiveness

Once data on all variables required by the model have been assembled, the model is run for each intervention being evaluated in order to estimate its expected costs and expected outcomes (or effects). The results are typically compared in terms of incremental cost effectiveness ratios and depicted on the cost effectiveness plane (box).[1]

Handling variability, uncertainty, and heterogeneity

The results of a decision analytical model are subject to the influences of variability, uncertainty, and heterogeneity, and these must be handled appropriately if decision makers are to be confident about the estimates of cost effectiveness.[3 13]

Variability reflects the randomness arising from the modelling process itself—that is, the fact that models typically use random numbers when determining whether an event with a given probability of occurring happens or not in any given cycle or model run, so that an identical patient will experience different outcomes each time they proceed through the model. This variability, sometimes referred to as Monte Carlo uncertainty, is not informative and needs to be eliminated by running the model repeatedly until a stable estimate of the central tendency has been obtained.[20] There is little evidence or agreement on how many model runs are needed to eliminate such variability, but it may be many thousands.

Parameter uncertainty reflects the uncertainty and imprecision surrounding the value of model variables such as transition probabilities, costs, and health utilities. Standard sensitivity analysis, in which each variable is varied separately and independently, does not give a complete picture of the effects of joint uncertainty and correlation between variables.[6] Probabilistic sensitivity analysis, in which all variables are varied simultaneously using probability distributions informed by estimates of the sample mean and sampling error from the best available evidence, is therefore the preferred way of assessing parameter uncertainty.[13] Probabilistic sensitivity analysis is usually executed by running the model several thousand times, each time varying the parameter values across the specified distributions and recording the outputs—for example, costs and effects—until a distribution has been built up and confidence intervals can be estimated. Probabilistic sensitivity analysis also allows the analyst to present cost effectiveness acceptability curves, which show the probability that each intervention is cost effective at an assumed maximum willingness to pay for health gains.[21] If a model has been derived from a single dataset, bootstrapping can be used to model uncertainty—that is, repeatedly re-estimating the model using random subsamples drawn with replacement from the full sample.[22]

Structural or model uncertainty reflects the uncertainty surrounding the structure of the model and the assumptions underpinning it—for example, the way a disease pathway is modelled. Such model uncertainty is usually examined with a sensitivity analysis, re-running the model with alternative structural assumptions.[6] Alternatively, several research groups could model the same decision problem in different ways and then compare their results in an agreed way. This approach has been used extensively in fields such as climate change but less commonly in health economics. However, one example is provided by the Mount Hood Challenge, which invited eight diabetes modelling groups to independently predict clinical trial outcomes on the basis of changes in risk factors and then compare their predictions.[23] How the results from different models can be reconciled in the absence of a gold standard is unclear; however, Bojke and colleagues have recommended some form of model averaging, whereby each model's results could be weighted by a measure of model adequacy.[24]

Finally, heterogeneity should be clearly differentiated from variability because it reflects differences in outcomes or in cost effectiveness that can in principle be explained by variations between subgroups of patients, either in terms of baseline characteristics such as age, risk level, or disease severity or in terms of both baseline characteristics and relative treatment effects. As in the analysis of clinical trials, subgroups should be predefined and carefully justified in terms of their clinical and economic relevance.[25] A model can then be re-run for different subgroups of patients.

Alternatively, heterogeneity can be addressed by making model variables functions of other variables—for example, transition probabilities between events or health states might be transformed into functions of age or disease severity. As with subgroup analysis in clinical trials, care must be taken to avoid generating apparently large differences in cost effectiveness that are not based on genuine evidence of heterogeneity. For example, Mihaylova et al, recognising the absence of evidence of heterogeneity in treatment effect across subgroups in the Heart Protection Study, applied the same relative risk reduction to different subgroups defined in terms of absolute risk levels at baseline, resulting in large but reliable differences in cost effectiveness.[26] [27]

Model evaluation

Evaluation is an important, and often overlooked, step in the development of a decision analytical model. Well evaluated models are more likely to be believed by decision makers. Three steps in model validation of escalating difficulty are face validation, internal validation, and external validation:

Face or descriptive validation entails checking whether the assumptions and structure of a model are reliable, sensible, and can be explained intuitively.[14] This may also require experiments to assess whether setting some variables at null or extreme values generates predictable effects on model outputs.

Internal validation requires thorough internal testing of the model—for example by getting an independent researcher or using different software to construct a replicate of the model and assess whether the results are consistent.[14] [28] Internal validation of a model derived from a single data source, for example a Markov model being used to simulate long term outcomes beyond the end of a clinical trial, may involve proving that the model's predicted results also fit the observed data used in the estimation.[22] In these circumstances some analysts also favour splitting the initial data in two and using one set to "train" or estimate the model and the other to test or validate the model. Some analysts also calibrate the model, adjusting variables to ensure that the results accord with aggregate and observable outcomes, such as overall survival.[29] This approach has been criticised as an ad hoc search for values that makes it impossible to characterise the uncertainty in the model correctly.[30]

External validation assesses whether the model's predictions match the observed results in a population or over a time period that was not used to construct the model. This might entail assessing whether the model can accurately predict future events. For example, the Mount Hood Challenge compared the predictions of the diabetes models with each other and the reported trial outcomes.[23] External validation might also be appropriate for calibrated models.

Value of additional research

Decision analytical models are increasingly used as a framework for indicating the need for and value of additional research. We have established that the analyst will never be certain that the value placed on each variable is correct. As a result, there are distributions surrounding the outputs of decision analytical models that can be estimated using probabilistic sensitivity analysis and synthesised using cost effectiveness acceptability curves.[6] These techniques indicate the probability that the decision to adopt an intervention on grounds of cost effectiveness is correct. The techniques also allow a quantification of the cost of making an incorrect decision, which when combined with the probability of making an incorrect decision generates the

expected cost of uncertainty. This has become synonymous with the expected value of perfect information (EVPI)—that is, the monetary value associated with eliminating the possibility of making an incorrect decision by eliminating parameter uncertainty in the model.[31] A population-wide EVPI can be estimated by multiplying the EVPI estimate produced by a decision analytical model by the number of decisions expected to be made on the basis of the additional information.[32] This can then be compared with the potential costs of further research to determine whether further studies are economically worthwhile.[33] [34] The approach has been extended in the form of expected value of partial perfect information (EVPPI), which estimates the value of obtaining perfect information on a subset of parameters in the model, and the expected value of sample information (EVSI), which focuses on optimal study design issues such as the optimal sample size of further studies.[3]

Conclusions

Further detail on the design, conduct, analysis, and reporting of economic evaluations using decision analytical modelling is available elsewhere.[4] [6] This article and our accompanying article[1] show that there is considerable overlap between modelling based and trial based economic evaluations, not only in their objectives but, for example, in dealing with heterogeneity and presenting results, and in both cases we have argued the benefits of using individual patient data. These two broad approaches should be viewed as complements rather than as competing alternatives.

Contributors: SP conceived the idea for this article. Both authors contributed to the review of the published material in this area, as well as the writing and revising of the article. SP is the guarantor.

Competing interests: All authors have completed the unified competing interest form at www.icmje.org/coi_disclosure.pdf (available on request from the corresponding author) and declare no support from any organisation for the submitted work; The Warwick Clinical Trials Unit benefited from facilities funded through the Birmingham Science City Translational Medicine Clinical Research and Infrastructure Trials Platform, with support from Advantage West Midlands. The Health Economics Research Centre receives funding from the National Institute of Health Research. SP started working on this article while employed by the National Perinatal Epidemiology Unit, University of Oxford, and the Health Economics Research Centre, University of Oxford, and funded by a UK Medical Research Council senior non-clinical research fellowship. AG is an NIHR senior investigator. They have no other relationships or activities that could appear to have influenced the submitted work.

Provenance and peer review: Commissioned; externally peer reviewed.

1   Petrou S, Gray A. Economic evaluation alongside randomised clinical trials: design, conduct, analysis and reporting. *BMJ* 2011;342:d1548.
2   Sculpher MJ, Claxton K, Drummond M, McCabe C. Whither trial-based economic evaluation for health care decision making? *Health Econ* 2006;15:677-87.
3   Briggs A, Claxton C, Sculpher M. *Decision modelling for health economic evaluation* . Oxford University Press, 2006.
4   Gray A, Clarke P, Wolstenholme J, Wordsworth S. *Applied methods of cost-effectiveness analysis in health care* . Oxford University Press, 2010.
5   Drummond M, Manca A, Sculpher M. Increasing the generalizability of economic evaluations: recommendations for the design, analysis, and reporting of studies. *Int J Technol Assess* 2005;21:165-71.
6   Drummond MF, Sculpher MJ, Torrance GW, O'Brien BJ, Stoddart G. *Methods for the economic evaluation of health care programmes* . 3rd ed. Oxford University Press, 2005.
7   Bojke L, Hornby E, Sculpher M. A comparison of the cost-effectiveness of pharmacotherapy or surgery (laparoscopic fundoplication) in the treatment of GORD. *Pharmacoeconomics* 2007;25:829-41.
8   Legood R, Gray A, Wolstenholme J, Moss S, LBC/HPV Cervical Screening Pilot Studies Group. The lifetime effects, costs and cost-effectiveness of using HPV testing to manage low-grade cytological abnormalities: results of the NHS pilot studies. *BMJ* 2006;332:79-83.
9   Torrance GW, Feeny D. Utilities and quality-adjusted life years. *Int J Technol Assess Health Care* 1989;5:559-75.

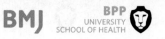

10 Brennan A, Chick SE, Davies R. A taxonomy of model structures for economic evaluation of health technologies. *Health Econ* 2006;15:1295-310.

11 Cooper K, Brailsford SC, Davies R. Choice of modelling technique for evaluating health care interventions. *J Oper Res Soc* 2007;58:168-76.

12 Brisson M, Edmunds WJ. Economic evaluation of vaccination programs: the impact of herd-immunity. *Med Decis Making* 2003;23:76-82.

13 Barton P, Bryan S, Robinson S. Modelling in the economic evaluation of health care: selecting the appropriate approach. *J Health Serv Res Policy* 2004;9:110-8.

14 Weinstein MC, O'Brien B, Hornberger J, Jackson J, Johannesson M, McCabe C, et al. Principles of good practice for decision analytic modeling in health-care evaluation: report of the ISPOR Task Force on Good Research Practices—modeling studies. *Value Health* 2003;6:9-17.

15 NHS Centre for Reviews and Dissemination. *Undertaking systematic reviews of research on effectiveness: CRD's guidance for those carrying out or commissioning reviews* . NHS CRD, University of York, 2001.

16 Philips Z, Ginnelly L, Sculpher M, Claxton K, Golder S, Riemsma R, et al. Review of guidelines for good practice in decision-analytic modelling in health technology assessment. *Health Technol Assess* 2004;8:iii-xi,1.

17 Golder S, Glanville J, Ginnelly L. Populating decision-analytic models: the feasibility and efficiency of database searching for individual parameters. *Int J Technol Assess Health Care* 2005;21:305-11.

18 Coyle D, Lee LM. The problem of protocol driven costs in pharmacoeconomic analysis. *Pharmacoeconomics* 1998;14:357-63.

19 Ades AE, Sutton A. Multiparameter evidence synthesis in epidemiology and medical decision-making: current approaches. *J R Stat Soc* 2006;169:5-35.

20 Weinstein MC. Recent developments in decision-analytic modelling for economic evaluation. *Pharmacoeconomics* 2006;24:1043-53.

21 Fenwick E, O'Brien BJ, Briggs A. Cost-effectiveness acceptability curves: facts, fallacies and frequently asked questions. *Health Econ* 2004;13:405-15.

22 Clarke PM, Gray AM, Briggs A, Farmer A, Fenn P, Stevens R, et al. A model to estimate the lifetime health outcomes of patients with type 2 diabetes: the United Kingdom Prospective Diabetes Study (UKPDS) outcomes model. *Diabetologia* 2004;47:1747-59.

23 Mount Hood. Computer modeling of diabetes and its complications: a report on the fourth Mount Hood challenge meeting. *Diabetes Care* 2007;30:1638-46.

24 Bojke L, Claxton K, Sculpher M, Palmer S. Characterizing structural uncertainty in decision analytic models: a review and application of methods. *Value Health* 2009;12:739-49.

25 Rothwell PM. Treating individuals 2. Subgroup analysis in randomised controlled trials: importance, indications, and interpretation. *Lancet* 2005;365:176-86.

26 Mihaylova B, Briggs A, Armitage J, Parish S, Gray A, Collins R, et al. Cost-effectiveness of simvastatin in people at different levels of vascular disease risk: a randomised trial in 20 536 individuals. *Lancet* 2005;365:1779-85.

27 Mihaylova B, Briggs A, Armitage J, Parish S, Gray, A, Collins R. Lifetime cost effectiveness of simvastatin in a range of risk groups and age groups derived from a randomised trial of 20 536 people. *BMJ* 2006;333:1145-8.

28 Philips Z, Bojke L, Sculpher M, Claxton K, Golder S. Good practice guidelines for decision-analytic modelling in health technology assessment: a review and consolidation of quality assessment. *Pharmacoeconomics* 2006;24:355-71.

29 Stout NK, Knudsen AB, Kong CK, McMahon PM, Gazelle GS. Calibration methods used in cancer simulation models and suggested reporting guidelines. *Pharmacoeconomics* 2009;27:533-45.

30 Ades AE, Cliffe S. Markov chain Monte Carlo estimation of a multi-parameter decision model: consistency of evidence and the accurate assessment of uncertainty. *Med Decis Making* 2002;22:359-71.

31 Claxton K, Ginnelly L, Sculpher M, Philips Z, Palmer S. A pilot study on the use of decision theory and value of information analysis as part of the NHS health technology assessment programme. *Health Technol Assess* 2004;8:1-103,iii.

32 Philips Z, Claxton K, Palmer S. The half-life of truth: appropriate time horizons for research decisions? *Med Decis Making* 2008;28:287-99.

33 Speight PM, Palmer S, Moles DR, Downer MC, Smith DH, Henriksson M, et al. The cost-effectiveness of screening for oral cancer in primary care. *Health Technol Assess* 2006;10:1-144,iii-iv.

34 Castelnuovo E, Thompson-Coon J, Pitt M, Cramp M, Siebert U, Price A, et al. The cost-effectiveness of testing for hepatitis C in former injecting drug users. *Health Technol Assess* 2006;10:iii-iv,ix-xii,1-93.

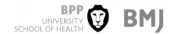

Consort 2010 statement: extension to cluster randomised trials

Marion K Campbell, director[1], Gilda Piaggio, honorary professor[2], Diana R Elbourne, professor of healthcare evaluation[2], Douglas G Altman, director[3], for the CONSORT Group

[1]Health Services Research Unit, University of Aberdeen, Aberdeen AB25 2ZD, UK

[2]Department of Medical Statistics, London School of Hygiene and Tropical Medicine, London, UK

[3]Centre for Statistics in Medicine, University of Oxford, Oxford, UK

Correspondence to: M K Campbell m.k.campbell@abdn.ac.uk

Cite this as:
BMJ 2012;345:e5661

DOI: 10.1136/bmj.e5661

http://www.bmj.com/content/345/bmj.e5661

ABSTRACT

The Consolidated Standards of Reporting Trials (CONSORT) statement was developed to improve the reporting of randomised controlled trials. It was initially published in 1996 and focused on the reporting of parallel group randomised controlled trials. The statement was revised in 2001, with a further update in 2010. A separate CONSORT statement for the reporting of abstracts was published in 2008. In earlier papers we considered the implications of the 2001 version of the CONSORT statement for the reporting of cluster randomised trial. In this paper we provide updated and extended guidance, based on the 2010 version of the CONSORT statement and the 2008 CONSORT statement for the reporting of abstracts.

Many journals now require that reports of trials conform to the guidelines in the Consolidated Standards of Reporting Trials (CONSORT) statement, first published in 1996,[1] revised in 2001,[2] and revised most recently in 2010.[3] The statement includes a checklist of items that should be included in the trial report. These items are evidence based whenever possible and are regularly reviewed.[4] The statement also recommends including a flow diagram to show the progression of participants from group assignment through to the final analysis. An explanation and elaboration of the rationale for the checklist items is provided in an accompanying article.[4]

The standard CONSORT statement focuses on reporting parallel group randomised controlled trials in which individual participants are randomly assigned to study groups. However, in some situations it is preferable to randomly assign groups of people (such as communities, families, or medical practices) rather than individuals. Reasons include the threat of "contamination" (the unintentional spill-over of intervention effects from one treatment group to another) of some interventions if individual randomisation is used.[5][6] Also, in certain settings, randomisation by group may be the only feasible method of conducting a trial.[7] Trials with this design are variously

SUMMARY POINTS

- Reports of randomised trials should include key information on their methods and findings
- Custer randomised trials have additional reporting considerations; we previously provided guidance on these in 2004
- This paper provides updated guidance on the reporting of cluster randomised trials based on the 2010 revision of the CONSORT statement
- New guidance is provided on the reporting of abstracts of cluster randomised trials
- Routine use of this guidance should lead to improved quality of reporting

known as field trials, community based trials, group randomised trials, place based trials, or (as in this paper) cluster randomised trials.[8] Although we would recommend the standard use of the term "cluster randomised trial" we recognise that those searching electronically for cluster trials may need to expand their search strategy to ensure that cluster trials using the terms "community" or "group" randomised trials are included.

In earlier papers we considered the implications of the CONSORT statement for the reporting of cluster randomised trials.[9][10] Here we present updated guidance, based on the 2010 revision of the CONSORT statement,[3] and the 2008 CONSORT extension for the reporting of abstracts.[11][12]

Scope of this paper

Cluster randomised trials are characterised by their multilevel nature; most often cluster trials involve two levels—the cluster and their individual members, such as general practice and patient—although trials of more than two levels, such as hospital-ward-patient, do exist. In this paper we focus on two level cluster trials for simplicity and refer to the groups that are randomised as "clusters" (these could be families, wards, etc) and we refer to the individual members of the clusters as "participants" (as they are usually individual people) unless there is ambiguity in a particular context. On occasion, however, a single person may be a cluster, with their teeth or eyes or limbs or multiple lesions as the members of the cluster. Measurements of these teeth, eyes, etc, within one individual will be correlated and so should not be treated as independent observations. A particular context for such trials is split mouth trials in dentistry.[13] However, those studies have additional considerations relating to the randomisation and the comparisons being within individuals. We do not consider them in detail in this paper.

In some situations another form of clustering can be observed in individually randomised trials—for example, several patients receiving care from the same therapist or surgeon.[14] This type of clustering is also not the focus of this paper—it is discussed in the CONSORT extension for non-pharmacological treatments.[15] Nor are we interested in trials with one cluster per intervention. Trials with one cluster per arm should be avoided as they cannot give a valid analysis, as the intervention effect is completely confounded with the cluster effect.[16] It has been recommended that the minimum number of clusters per arm to ensure a valid analysis should be at least four.[17] Sometimes trials are inappropriately referred to as using cluster randomisation—for example, "To avoid patient interference a cluster randomisation was performed to alternate months."[18] This study was in fact not truly randomised nor was it a cluster trial. However, there is a particular design within the scope of cluster randomised trials, the cluster randomised crossover trial, where each participating cluster receives both intervention and control treatments consecutively, in separate periods, but the

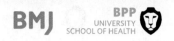

order of treatment is randomised.[19] Similarly, many stepped wedge designs, which randomise in terms of the period for receipt of the intervention, may be seen as a type of cluster crossover trial if the unit of randomisation is a cluster.[20] [21]

We note that cluster randomised trials have no connection to cluster analysis; an exploratory multivariate statistical technique used to define clusters of similar people. We also note that the statistical issues raised by cluster randomised trials are different to those raised by cluster sampling, in which natural clusters such as geographical areas are identified and some clusters are chosen to be studied (for example, as in Mucklebecker 2006),[22] preferably at random.

In summary, our focus is on trials that are cluster randomised by design and have two or more clusters per intervention arm.

Updating the CONSORT statement for cluster randomised trials

The updated CONSORT 2010 statement includes a 25 item checklist. The wording was simplified and clarified and the specificity of certain elements of the statement made more explicit, for example by breaking some items into sub-items. Methodological advances reported in the literature since the 2001 statement were also reviewed and taken into account where appropriate.

To ensure that the extension for cluster trials reflected the wording of the updated CONSORT statement, and to integrate any important advances in the methodology for cluster trials since 2004, we decided to update the cluster extension in the summer of 2010.

BOX 1 NOTEWORTHY CHANGES FROM CONSORT 2004 EXTENSION FOR CLUSTER RANDOMISED TRIALS

- Separate presentation of the standard CONSORT checklist items and extension specific to cluster trials (table 1)
- Provision of updated examples of good reporting practice
- Provision of an augmented checklist for abstracts of cluster randomised controlled trials
- Expansion of item 7a (sample size) to include the possibility of unequal cluster sizes
- Discussion of CONSORT 2010 item 7b (interim analysis guidelines) included in the context of cluster randomised controlled trials
- Item 10 (generation of random allocation sequence for participants) replaced by items 10a, 10b, and 10c

---

BOX 2 METHODOLOGICAL CONSIDERATIONS IN CLUSTER RANDOMISED TRIALS

Design

- Observations on participants in the same cluster tend to be correlated (non-independent), so the effective sample size is less than that suggested by the actual number of individual participants. The reduction in effective sample size depends on average cluster size and the degree of correlation within clusters, ρ, also known as the intracluster (or intraclass) correlation coefficient (ICC).
- The intracluster correlation coefficient is the proportion of the total variance of the outcome that can be explained by the variation between clusters. A related coefficient of variation, k, between clusters has also been described.[90] Although no simple relation exists between k and ρ for continuous outcomes, another study described the relation for binary outcomes.[91] For both types of variable, when $k=0$, ρ also=0. Unlike k, the intracluster correlation coefficient cannot be defined for time to event data.
- Adjusting for the intracluster correlation is necessary for a valid analysis, but it reduces statistical power. For the same statistical power the overall sample size needs to be larger in a cluster randomised trial than in an individually randomised trial.
- If m is the cluster size (assumed to be the same for all clusters), then the inflation factor, or "design effect," associated with cluster randomisation is $1+(m-1)\rho$. Although typically ρ is small (often <0.05) and it is often not known when a trial is planned (and only estimated with error after a trial is completed), its impact on the inflation factor can be considerable if the clusters are large. In general, the power is increased more easily by increasing the number of clusters rather than the cluster size.
- Cluster randomised trials may use a simple, completely randomised design, a matched cluster design, or a stratified design. If an appropriate matching factor is used, the matched design gains power relative to the completely randomised design. However, such matching variables may be difficult to identify, especially if the number of clusters to be matched is large. In addition, calculating the intracluster correlation coefficient from a matched design is generally problematic because the variation between clusters cannot be disentangled from the effects of the intervention or interventions and the matching factors.[8] The use of stratified designs is therefore generally preferable.[92]

Conduct

- The conduct of cluster randomised controlled trials differs in some ways from that of trials that randomise individuals. In particular, random allocation is done at the cluster level. Clusters are usually randomised all at once (or in batches) rather than one at a time, as in most individually randomised trials. This feature of the cluster randomised trial facilitates the use of a matched design.
- Sometimes consent can be sought both at cluster level and at individual participant level before randomisation. Commonly, however, prior consent to randomisation by individual cluster participants is not feasible.[93] In such circumstances, once clusters have been randomly assigned, participants in the clusters can no longer be asked for their consent to be randomised to receive either of the interventions, only for consent to receive the intervention to which their group has been assigned, and for consent to follow-up. This introduces the possibility of post-randomisation selection bias[5] [94] as well as ethical concerns,[95] [96] [97] which have been explored in qualitative studies.[98] These concerns are analogous to those arising from randomised consent designs[99] [100] [101] for individually randomised trials.
- The concept of what blinding means in the context of a cluster randomised controlled trial is also complex—some patients may know which intervention they are allocated to but not that they are in a trial.

Analysis

- Cluster randomised controlled trials also present special requirements for analysis.[102] If the inference is intended at the participant level, they should not be analysed as if the trial was individually randomised as, if ρ is greater than zero, this gives spurious precision.
- The data could be analysed as if each cluster was a single individual, but this approach ignores the information collected on participants within a cluster and hence may not use the full richness of the dataset. Advances in software for the analysis of cluster randomised controlled trials have been reviewed.[24]
- Bayesian approaches to the analysis of cluster randomised trials have also been developed.[103] [104] [105]
- For in depth discussion of survival analysis that links to k, see Hayes and Moulton.[17]

Interpretation

- The interpretation of the results from cluster randomised trials may be more complicated than individually randomised trials as the conclusions may relate to the clusters, to the participants in those clusters, or to both.

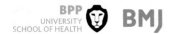

The updating process

To identify papers relevant to the methodology for cluster randomised trials published between 2004 and 2010, we undertook an electronic search of Medline, Embase, and the Cochrane Methodology Register and a full text search of *Statistics in Medicine*, *Clinical Trials*, *Contemporary Clinical Trials*, and *BMC Medical Research Methodology*. The search yielded 1198 abstracts. One researcher (MKC) initially assessed the abstracts for relevance and classified 155 as potentially relevant to the update of the CONSORT extension. Each author took primary responsibility for aggregating and synthesising evidence most relevant to the reporting of a trial in particular areas—for example, analysis, intracluster correlation coefficients. We also reviewed all correspondence that had been received after the publication of the 2004 extension for cluster trials. We decided to reformat the checklist for cluster trials in line with the style currently promoted by the CONSORT Group, as used, for example, in the extensions for non-pharmacological interventions[15] and pragmatic trials.[23] In this updated style, additions to the main CONSORT checklist items are presented in a separate column rather than being integrated directly into the text of the checklist.

The researchers met face to face and by teleconference on several occasions to discuss updating the checklist and revision of the text, with additional discussion in conference calls and by email. A draft revised paper was distributed to the larger CONSORT Group for feedback. After consideration of their comments a final version of the extension was prepared and approved by the CONSORT executive.

Box 1 presents the noteworthy changes from the 2004 cluster extension paper. As for previous CONSORT checklists, we have included only those items deemed fundamental to the reporting of a cluster randomised controlled trial— that is, providing a minimum standard for the reporting of cluster trials. Moreover, a few items may be crucial to a trial but not included, such as approval by an institutional ethical review board, because funding bodies strictly enforce ethical review and medical journals usually address reporting ethical review in their instructions for authors. It is also not the purpose of this paper to provide a best practice guide on the design, conduct, and analysis of cluster randomised trials—these issues have been outlined by several other authors.

Advances in methodology since 2004

The 2004 extension paper[10] outlined the principal implications of adopting a cluster randomised trial (summarised in box 2). These included the need to account for the non-independence of participants within clusters and the need to be explicit about the level of inference at which the trial interventions and trial outcomes are targeted. Since 2004 there have been several methodological advances in the specialty. Detailed overviews of these methodological developments are presented elsewhere.[17 24 25 26 27]

Advances in reporting requirements since 2004

In 2008 the CONSORT Group also produced a separate reporting checklist for abstracts of reports of randomised controlled trials,[11 12] which presented a minimum list of essential items that should be reported within a trial abstract. The motivation for the extension for the reporting of abstracts was multi-fold but it was clear that readers of journals often base their assessment of a trial on the information presented in the abstract and as such quality reporting was particularly important within this aspect of the trial report. Therefore as part of the update process for the reporting of cluster trials we also reviewed the CONSORT extension for abstracts and highlighted the key areas where cluster trial specific reporting requirements would apply.

Quality of reporting of cluster trials

Early surveys of published cluster trials found that the conduct and reporting of the trials were often poor.[5 27 28 29 30 31 32 33] One study, however, found clear signs of improvement in the methods and reporting of cluster trials published in the *BMJ* from 1983 to 2003.[34]

Recent reviews have shown that deficiencies in reports of cluster trials remain common.[35 36 37 38 39 40 41 42] For example, the unit of analysis error (where results were analysed without accounting for the clustering) was seen in 19/40 (48%) of medical care trials,[35] and among 75 reports of cluster trials in cancer prevention and control a third (34%) "failed to report any analyses that were judged to be appropriate."[37] Among 50 reports of cluster trials of screening interventions, 32 (64%) reported using a method of analysis that took account of clustering, but in several the method used was not stated explicitly.[40] Those authors found that reporting was much better in high influence journals.

Three recent reviews have considered reporting in relation to the CONSORT extension for cluster trials. The first of these reviews examined the reports of 106 cluster randomised trials in children, published from 2004 to 2010.[41] Issues specific to cluster trials were poorly reported. The rationale for using a cluster design was given in 32% of the articles; how clustering was accounted for in sample size calculation and in analysis were reported in 59% and 65% of trials; and 55% of flow diagrams (which were included in 80% of the articles) omitted some information on the numbers of participants or clusters. Overall, 37% of the articles reported an intracluster correlation coefficient. The second review examined 300 randomly sampled cluster randomised trials published during 2000-08.[42] Of those presenting sample size calculations, 60% accounted for clustering in the design, whereas 70% accounted for clustering in analysis. Only 18% of the articles reported an intracluster correlation coefficient. Both of these studies saw only a slight improvement in reporting over time, but the third review suggested the opposite.[40]

In summary, there is some evidence for improved reporting of cluster randomised trials but the quality of reporting remains well below an acceptable level.

Extension of CONSORT 2010 to cluster trials

Table 1 presents the revised checklist for the reporting of a cluster randomised controlled trial (updated in line with CONSORT 2010). Some items are extended to cover the reporting requirements relating to the cluster design, and item 10 is replaced by items 10a, 10b, and 10c, acknowledging the added complexity imposed on the randomisation and recruitment by the cluster design. Items requiring an extension from the CONSORT 2010 statement, and those items particularly relevant to the reporting of cluster randomised trials, are explained, with illustrative examples. As all our examples have been taken from previously published papers, it is inevitable that several do not display all the desirable elements of good reporting. Where this is the case, or where there might be ambiguity,

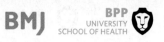

Table 1 CONSORT 2010 checklist of information to include when reporting a cluster randomised trial

Section/topic and item No	Standard checklist item	Extension for cluster designs	Page No*
Title and abstract			
1a	Identification as a randomised trial in the title	Identification as a cluster randomised trial in the title	
1b	Structured summary of trial design, methods, results, and conclusions (for specific guidance see CONSORT for abstracts)[11 12]	See table 2	
Introduction			
Background and objectives:			
2a	Scientific background and explanation of rationale	Rationale for using a cluster design	
2b	Specific objectives or hypotheses	Whether objectives pertain to the cluster level, the individual participant level, or both	
Methods			
Trial design:			
3a	Description of trial design (such as parallel, factorial) including allocation ratio	Definition of cluster and description of how the design features apply to the clusters	
3b	Important changes to methods after trial commencement (such as eligibility criteria), with reasons		
Participants:			
4a	Eligibility criteria for participants	Eligibility criteria for clusters	
4b	Settings and locations where the data were collected		
Interventions:			
5	The interventions for each group with sufficient details to allow replication, including how and when they were actually administered	Whether interventions pertain to the cluster level, the individual participant level, or both	
Outcomes:			
6a	Completely defined prespecified primary and secondary outcome measures, including how and when they were assessed	Whether outcome measures pertain to the cluster level, the individual participant level, or both	
6b	Any changes to trial outcomes after the trial commenced, with reasons		
Sample size:			
7a	How sample size was determined	Method of calculation, number of clusters(s) (and whether equal or unequal cluster sizes are assumed), cluster size, a coefficient of intracluster correlation (ICC or k), and an indication of its uncertainty	
7b	When applicable, explanation of any interim analyses and stopping guidelines		
Randomisation			
Sequence generation:			
8a	Method used to generate the random allocation sequence		
8b	Type of randomisation; details of any restriction (such as blocking and block size)	Details of stratification or matching if used	
Allocation concealment mechanism:			
9	Mechanism used to implement the random allocation sequence (such as sequentially numbered containers), describing any steps taken to conceal the sequence until interventions were assigned	Specification that allocation was based on clusters rather than individuals and whether allocation concealment (if any) was at the cluster level, the individual participant level, or both	
Implementation:			
10	Who generated the random allocation sequence, who enrolled participants, and who assigned participants to interventions	Replaced by 10a, 10b, and 10c	
10a		Who generated the random allocation sequence, who enrolled clusters, and who assigned clusters to interventions	
10b		Mechanism by which individual participants were included in clusters for the purposes of the trial (such as complete enumeration, random sampling)	
10c		From whom consent was sought (representatives of the cluster, or individual cluster members, or both) and whether consent was sought before or after randomisation	
Blinding:			
11a	If done, who was blinded after assignment to interventions (for example, participants, care providers, those assessing outcomes) and how		
11b	If relevant, description of the similarity of interventions		
Statistical methods:			
12a	Statistical methods used to compare groups for primary and secondary outcomes	How clustering was taken into account	
12b	Methods for additional analyses, such as subgroup analyses and adjusted analyses		
Results			
Participant flow (a diagram is strongly recommended):			
13a	For each group, the numbers of participants who were randomly assigned, received intended treatment, and were analysed for the primary outcome	For each group, the numbers of clusters that were randomly assigned, received intended treatment, and were analysed for the primary outcome	
13b	For each group, losses and exclusions after randomisation, together with reasons	For each group, losses and exclusions for both clusters and individual cluster members	
Recruitment:			

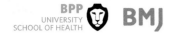

Section/topic and item No	Standard checklist item	Extension for cluster designs	Page No*
14a	Dates defining the periods of recruitment and follow-up		
14b	Why the trial ended or was stopped		
Baseline data:			
15	A table showing baseline demographic and clinical characteristics for each group	Baseline characteristics for the individual and cluster levels as applicable for each group	
Numbers analysed:			
16	For each group, number of participants (denominator) included in each analysis and whether the analysis was by original assigned groups	For each group, number of clusters included in each analysis	
Outcomes and estimation:			
17a	For each primary and secondary outcome, results for each group, and the estimated effect size and its precision (such as 95% confidence interval)	Results at the individual or cluster level as applicable and a coefficient of intracluster correlation (ICC or k) for each primary outcome	
17b	For binary outcomes, presentation of both absolute and relative effect sizes is recommended		
Ancillary analyses:			
18	Results of any other analyses performed, including subgroup analyses and adjusted analyses, distinguishing prespecified from exploratory		
Harms:			
19	All important harms or unintended effects in each group (for specific guidance see CONSORT for harms106)		
Discussion			
Limitations:			
20	Trial limitations, addressing sources of potential bias, imprecision, and, if relevant, multiplicity of analyses		
Generalisability:			
21	Generalisability to clusters and/or individual participants (as relevant)	Generalisability (external validity, applicability) of the trial findings	
Interpretation:			
22	Interpretation consistent with results, balancing benefits and harms, and considering other relevant evidence		
Other information			
Registration:			
23	Registration number and name of trial registry		
Protocol:			
24	Where the full trial protocol can be accessed, if available		
Funding:			
25	Sources of funding and other support (such as supply of drugs), role of funders		

Page numbers optional depending on journal requirements.

Original abstract (Acolet et al)[52]

ABSTRACT (original)

Background Research findings are not rapidly or fully implemented into policies and practice in care.

Objectives To assess whether an "active" strategy was more likely to lead to changes in policy and practice in preterm baby care than traditional information dissemination.

Design Cluster randomised trial.

Participants 180 neonatal units (87 active, 93 control) in England; clinicians from active arm units; babies born <27 weeks' gestation.

Control arm Dissemination of research report; slides; information about newborn care position statement.

Active arm As above plus offer to become "regional champion" (attend two workshops, support clinicians to implement research evidence regionally), or attend one workshop, promote implementation of research evidence locally.

Main outcome measures Timing of surfactant administration; admission temperature; staffing of resuscitation team present at birth.

Results 48/87 lead clinicians in the active arm attended one or both workshops. There was no evidence of difference in post-intervention policies between trial arms. Practice outcomes based on babies in the active (169) and control arms (186), in 45 and 49 neonatal units respectively, showed active arm babies were more likely to have been given surfactant on labour ward (RR=1.30; 95% CI 0.99 to1.70); P=0.06); to have a higher temperature on admission to neonatal intensive care unit (mean difference=0.29°C; 95% CI 0.22 to 0.55; P=0.03); and to have had the baby's trunk delivered into a plastic bag (RR=1.27; 95% CI 1.01 to 1.60; P=0.04) than the control group. The effect on having an "ideal" resuscitation team at birth was in the same direction of benefit for the active arm (RR=1.18; 95% CI 0.97 to 1.43; P=0.09). The costs of the intervention were modest.

Conclusions This is the first trial to evaluate methods for transferring information from neonatal research into local policies and practice in England. An active approach to research dissemination is both feasible and cost-effective.

Trial registration Current controlled trials ISRCTN89683698

Enhanced abstract (with changes outlined in red)

Background Research findings are not rapidly or fully implemented into policies and practice in care.

Objectives To assess whether an "active" strategy was more likely to lead to changes in unit-level policies, and in practice for preterm babies than traditional information dissemination.

Design Cluster randomised trial.

Participants 180 neonatal units (87 active, 93 control) in England; clinicians from active arm units; babies born <27 weeks' gestation.

Control arm Dissemination of research report; slides; information about newborn care position statement.

Active arm As above plus offer to become "regional champion" (attend two workshops, support clinicians to implement research evidence regionally), or attend one workshop, promote implementation of research evidence locally.

Randomisation Neonatal units were stratified by level of care and randomly allocated to control or active intervention within blocks of varying size; all eligible babies within these units were assessed for practice outcomes.

Main outcome measures Timing of surfactant administration at cluster (policy) level; admission temperature; staffing of resuscitation team present at birth (at policy and individual practice level). Clinicians in active arm not blind to allocation but blind in control arm; outcomes assessed by assessors independent of the trial.

Results 48/87 lead clinicians in the active arm attended one or both workshops. There was no evidence of difference in post-intervention policies between trial arms based on 62 and 69 clusters (RR for policy specifying which paediatric staff should be present 0.92 (0.84 to 0.99); for delivery in plastic bag or wrapping 0.98 (95% CI 0.90 to 1.07; P=0.71)). Practice outcomes based on babies in the active (169) and control arms (186), in 45 and 49 neonatal units respectively, showed active arm babies were more likely to have been given surfactant on labour ward (RR=1.30; 95% CI 0.99 to1.70); P=0.06); to have a higher temperature on admission to neonatal intensive care unit (mean difference=0.29°C; 95% CI 0.22 to 0.55; P=0.03); and to have had the baby's trunk delivered into a plastic bag (RR=1.27; 95% CI 1.01 to 1.60; P=0.04) than the control group. The effect on having an 'ideal' resuscitation team at birth was in the same direction of benefit for the active arm (RR=1.18; 95% CI 0.97 to 1.43; P=0.09). There were no important adverse events. The costs of the intervention were modest.

Conclusions This is the first trial to evaluate methods for transferring information from neonatal research into local policies and practice in England. An active approach to research dissemination by neonatal units is both feasible and cost effective.

Trial registration Current controlled trials ISRCTN89683698

Funding Bliss Innovation in Care Programme, and CEMACH

Fig 1 Example of abstract for report of cluster randomised trial

we have attempted to identify which specific aspects of reporting are addressed.

We reviewed the checklist for abstracts and provide an augmented checklist for reporting of abstracts within cluster randomised controlled trials in table 2.

Title and abstract

Item 1a

Standard CONSORT item: identification as a randomised trial in the title

Extension for cluster trials: identification as a cluster randomised trial in the title

Example

Cluster randomised trial of a targeted multifactorial intervention to prevent falls among older people in hospital[43]

Explanation

The primary reason for identifying the design in the title is to ensure appropriate indexing of the study as a cluster randomised trial in Medline. This indexing ensures ease of identification of these studies for inclusion in systematic reviews. "Community" randomised and "group" randomised are also widely used descriptions for such trials (for example, the trial report by Cavalcante et al)[44], especially when entire communities are randomised. A recent review of cluster randomised trials showed that identification of cluster randomised trials remains problematic, with only 48% of cluster randomised controlled trials published in 78 journals between 2000 and 2007 being clearly identified as cluster randomised in titles or abstracts.[45] Identification of the trial as a cluster randomised trial also ensures that readers will not be misled by apparently large sample sizes.

Item 1b

Standard CONSORT item: structured summary of trial design, methods, results, and conclusions (for specific guidance see CONSORT for abstracts)[11] [12]

Extension for cluster trials: outlined in table 2

Example: presented in figure 1

Explanation

In 2008 a CONSORT extension on reporting abstracts was published.[11] [12] We have provided an augmented checklist for this aspect of trial reporting in this update (table 2). As the extension on reporting abstracts was published only recently, and the 2004 extension to cluster trials did not specifically deal with abstracts, we were not able to find examples of good reporting tackling all the items required. We have therefore developed an abstract based on enhancing a published abstract (fig 1). Although this increases the word count by over a third, many journals now follow PubMed in no longer setting a limit.

In addition to the items recommended for all trials it is important that abstracts for cluster randomised controlled trials give the number of clusters per arm (and numbers of participants) and the level of inference (that is, the level at which hypotheses and conclusions are to be made) for the primary outcome, to allow appropriate interpretation.

Introduction

Background and objectives

Item 2a

Standard CONSORT item: scientific background and explanation of rationale

Extension for cluster trials: rationale for using cluster design

Example 1

Our intention was to enhance the application of evidence by the whole labour ward team so, to minimise contamination, the unit of randomisation and analysis was the obstetric unit[46]

Example 2

A cluster randomization was chosen for practical reasons and to prevent contamination by preference of patient or physician (selection bias)[47]

Explanation

Under the principles of the Helsinki declaration it is unethical to expose people unnecessarily to the risks of

Table 2 Extension of CONSORT for abstracts[11] [12] to reports of cluster randomised trials*Relevant to conference abstracts.*

Item	Standard checklist item	Extension for cluster trials
Title	Identification of study as randomised	Identification of study as cluster randomised
Trial design	Description of the trial design (for example, parallel, cluster, non-inferiority)	
Methods:		
Participants	Eligibility criteria for participants and the settings where the data were collected	Eligibility criteria for clusters
Interventions	Interventions intended for each group	
Objective	Specific objective or hypothesis	Whether objective or hypothesis pertains to the cluster level, the individual participant level, or both
Outcome	Clearly defined primary outcome for this report	Whether the primary outcome pertains to the cluster level, the individual participant level or both
Randomisation	How participants were allocated to interventions	How clusters were allocated to interventions
Blinding (masking)	Whether or not participants, care givers, and those assessing the outcomes were blinded to group assignment	
Results:		
Numbers randomised	Number of participants randomised to each group	Number of clusters randomised to each group
Recruitment	Trial status*	
Numbers analysed	Number of participants analysed in each group	Number of clusters analysed in each group
Outcome	For the primary outcome, a result for each group and the estimated effect size and its precision	Results at the cluster or individual level as applicable for each primary outcome
Harms	Important adverse events or side effects	
Conclusions	General interpretation of the results	
Trial registration	Registration number and name of trial register	
Funding	Source of funding	

Relevant to conference abstracts.

research.[48] Because a cluster randomised design increases the complexity of the research and usually requires more participants than an individually randomised design (to ensure equivalent statistical power), it is particularly important that the rationale for adopting a cluster design is outlined in the introduction.[49] In a recent review of cluster randomised trials, the reviewers[50] found that a third of published cluster trials could have used individual randomisation instead. As such, it is important that all alternatives are considered and that if a cluster trial is adopted it is clear why it was judged to be the most appropriate and robust design to adopt.[51]

Item 2b

Standard CONSORT item: specific objectives or hypotheses

Extension for cluster trials: whether objectives pertain to cluster level, individual participant level, or both

Example

The main aim of the present study is to use the rigour of a RCT [randomised controlled trial] in an evaluation comparing the effects of different approaches to knowledge transfer on policy and practice in the care of preterm babies in another setting . . . The main outcomes were at the level of unit policy and practice [neonatal units were the clusters][52]

Explanation

Descriptions of specific objectives and hypotheses need to make it clear whether they pertain to the individual participant level, the cluster level, or both. When objectives and hypotheses are targeted at the cluster level, analysis and interpretation of results at the cluster level might be appropriate. When the objectives and hypotheses are targeted at the individual participant level, statistical techniques at the individual level are usually required.

Methods

The main difference when reporting a cluster trial, as opposed to an individually randomised trial, is that there are two levels of inference rather than one: the cluster level and the individual participant level.[53] Thus, to allow readers to interpret the results appropriately, it is important to indicate explicitly the level at which the interventions were targeted, hypotheses generated, randomisation done, and outcomes measured.

Trial design

Item 3a

Standard CONSORT item: description of trial design (such as parallel, factorial) including allocation ratio

Extension for cluster trials: definition of cluster and description of how design features apply to clusters

Example 1 (definition of clusters)

Clusters were health centers with more than 400 residents aged 65.0-67.9 y in low-middle socioeconomic status municipalities (average population 127,000 individuals) in the Santiago Metropolitan area[54]

Example 2 (description of how the design applied to clusters)

This study was a pragmatic, cluster randomised, factorial, controlled trial. A 2×2 factorial design was used to assess the effect of each intervention and to explore the effect of the interventions combined . . . The four allocated groups were general practitioners' [the cluster] use of C reactive protein testing (1), training in enhanced communication skills (2), the interventions combined (3), and usual care (4)[55]

Example 3 (definition of how the design applied to clusters)

Hospitals [the clusters] were matched by country, type of hospital (public, private or social security), and baseline caesarean section rate (15-20%, 21-35%, or >35%), and the paired units were randomly assigned to intervention or control[56]

Explanation

The cluster is the unit of randomisation and it should be appropriately defined so that it can be adequately taken into account in the analysis. Whether the cluster randomised design is parallel, matched pair, or other, and whether the treatments have a factorial structure, has implications for the appropriate analysis of the outcome data and thus should be reported. Random assignment generally ensures that any baseline differences in group characteristics are the result of chance rather than of some systematic bias.[57] In individually randomised trials the sample size can be sufficiently large to ensure balanced baseline characteristics across groups. In cluster randomised designs, if the number of clusters is large, simple randomisation may often be sufficient.[8] This is not usually the case for these designs, however, because the number of clusters to be randomised is often small. Even if cluster specific characteristics are balanced (that is, characteristics of the randomly allocated clusters), researchers have little control over the participants within each cluster (this is the case whether the number of clusters is large or small).[8] As a result, some form of constraint (matching or stratification) is often imposed on randomisation in a cluster randomised design in an attempt to increase precision and minimise imbalance across treatment groups (see also item 8b). Any constraint imposed on the cluster randomised trial affects the sample size and the analysis and thus should be reported.

Item 3b

Standard CONSORT item: important changes to methods after trial commencement (such as eligibility criteria), with reasons

---

BOX 3 EXAMPLE OF PRECISE DETAILS OF INTERVENTION AT CLUSTER AND INDIVIDUAL LEVEL FROM MURPHY ET AL[60]

Tailored practice care

- An action plan for each practice was agreed with the practice and regularly reviewed by the study research nurse and practice
- The study nurse maintained regular contact with the practices
- The practice received a two page study newsletter every four months

Academic detailing

- An academic general practitioner (one per centre) made one 90 minute educational outreach visit to each intervention practice to promote drug prescribing guidelines for secondary prevention through interactive case based scenarios
- A study research nurse (one per centre) delivered another 90 minute session on behaviour change, which was intended to facilitate reflection on change to patient lifestyle and, through role play, new techniques to be used by the practice

Tailored patient care

- At the first intervention consultation, the patient and practitioner together identified areas of management that could be improved and the patient was invited to prioritise one particular aspect of his or her lifestyle for change
- Possible ways of achieving targets reflecting optimal management were identified and action plans individualised so that small, realistic goals for change were agreed
- A booklet containing information on all the key risk factors for coronary heart disease was used by practitioners in discussions on initial target setting and then given to the patients

Regular consultations

- Patients were invited for an appointment with the general practitioner or nurse every four months; targets and goals for optimal secondary prevention were reviewed at each visit

---

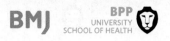

Example

Concerns that lower than expected pneumonia incidence rates would affect the trial's ability to detect an effect of nutritional supplementation on pneumonia incidence resulted in a protocol amendment 4 months into the study. A further 12 health centers were approached to join the study, eight of which were subsequently randomly assigned ... to either the nutritional supplement intervention alone arm (n=4) or the control arm (n=4)[54]

Explanation

In cluster randomised controlled trials, as in any trial, important changes may have occurred to the study methods after the original protocol was written. Knowing about these changes and the reasons for them can aid interpretation, especially if there may be suspicions of bias. Changes that affect the number of clusters will be particularly important in cluster randomised controlled trials.

Participants

Item 4a

Standard CONSORT item: eligibility criteria for participants

Extension for cluster trials: eligibility criteria for clusters

Example

The study comprised 41 practices in Wessex . . . Inclusion criteria were .4 medical partners; list size >7000; a diabetes register with >1% of practice population; and a diabetes service registered with the health authority . . . Nurses reported all new cases of diabetes to the trial office. Willing patients aged 30-70 were included in the trial. Patients were excluded if they were private patients, housebound, mentally ill, had severe learning difficulties, or were subsequently found to have been diagnosed previously with, or not to have, diabetes, or were found to have type 1 diabetes[58]

Explanation

In cluster randomised trials two sets of eligibility criteria are considered—the eligibility of the clusters (for example, the general practices) to be included in the trial and the eligibility of individual participants (for example, the eligible patients within each general practice) to be included in clusters. As such, both sets of eligibility criteria need to be reported.

Interventions

Item 5

Standard CONSORT item: the interventions for each group with sufficient details to allow replication, including how and when they were actually administered

Extension for cluster trials: whether interventions pertain to cluster level, individual participant level, or both

Example 1 (intervention at individual participant level)

In the intervention group [consisting of seven sectors or clusters] the windows of all 241 houses [units of observation within sectors] (with a total of 1336 inhabitants) were covered with loosely hanging polyester curtains impregnated with the pyrethroid insecticide . . . In the 222 houses in six of the control sectors [clusters] the windows were covered with non-impregnated curtains and in one randomly selected control sector [cluster] with 106 houses no curtains were provided[59]

Example 2 (intervention at cluster and individual participant level)

See example in box 3.[60]

Example 3 (intervention at cluster level)

The purpose of this study is to evaluate the effect of randomizing GP practices to prescribing feedback using academic detailing (postal bulletin plus an educational outreach visit) compared to postal bulletin alone on prescribing of cardiovascular preventive therapies in patients with CVD or diabetes . . . The postal bulletins contained individualized GP prescribing feedback and educational information based on the 2003 European guidelines on CVD prevention. . . . The feedback was displayed using graphs and included the actual number of GP-registered patients not receiving recommended therapy[61]

Explanation

It is important to describe whether the intervention was targeted at the cluster level or the individual participant level. The level of inference is not necessarily the same as the level at which the intervention is applied, although inference at the cluster level is usually appropriate for interventions applied at the cluster level.

Outcomes

Item 6a

Standard CONSORT item: completely defined pre-specified primary and secondary outcome measures, including how and when they were assessed

Extension for cluster trials: whether outcome measures pertain to cluster level, individual participant level, or both

Example 1 (outcome at level of cluster)

The purpose of this study is to evaluate the effect of randomizing GP practices to prescribing feedback using academic detailing (postal bulletin plus an educational outreach visit) compared to postal bulletin alone on prescribing [at the cluster level] of cardiovascular preventive therapies in patients with CVD or diabetes[61]

Example 2 (outcome at level of individual participant rather than cluster)

We evaluated the effect of a computer based clinical decision support system and cardiovascular risk chart [both targeted at physicians—at the cluster level] on patient centred outcomes of absolute cardiovascular risk and blood pressure[62]

Example 3 (outcomes at cluster level and individual participant level)

Primary outcomes were chosen for their ability to assess effectiveness and quality of service and included number of visits, referrals from RHC [rural health centres] for antenatal, intrapartum or postpartum problems [cluster level outcomes], place of delivery and low birthweight infant (<2500 g) [individual level outcomes]. The secondary outcomes were antenatal diagnosis of hypertension and twin pregnancy, perinatal mortality, operative delivery, preterm delivery (<37 weeks) [individual level outcomes] and the proportion of visits at which fundal height measurement was recorded and plotted on the antenatal record in the new model [cluster level outcome][63]

Explanation

Whether an intervention is evaluated at the cluster level or individual participant level has implications for the appropriate analysis of the outcome data. It is therefore important that the trial report is explicit about the level at which outcomes are measured.

Sample size

Item 7a

Standard CONSORT item: how sample size was determined

Extension for cluster trials: method of calculation, number of clusters, cluster size(s) (and whether equal or unequal cluster sizes are assumed), a coefficient of intracluster correlation (ICC or *k*), and an indication of its uncertainty

Example 1

We calculated sample size with a method that takes into account the intracluster correlation coefficient, the number of events, the expected effect, and the power of the study. We assumed an intracluster correlation of $\rho=0.2$, a minimum of 25 patients for each practice, and a worst case control rate of 50%. Under these assumptions we anticipated a power of 87% to detect a difference of 15% in rates between the two groups with $\alpha=0.05$ with 60 practices for each intervention group[64]

Example 2

The calculation of the sample size . . . was based on 0.6% detection of CIN grade 2+ using the conventional Pap test and an expected 33% increase using liquid-based cytology with an α of 0.05 and β of 0.20, an intraclass correlation coefficient of 0.05, an average cluster size of 250, and a standard deviation of 200. This resulted in a coefficient of variation [k] of 0.8 and design effect of 1.59. By multiplication of the design effect by sample size without cluster effect, a sample size of 44 947 women in each group was obtained[47]

Explanation

A principal difference between the planning of a cluster randomised trial and that of an individually randomised trial is the calculation of the sample size. To retain equivalent power to an individually randomised trial, the number of individuals in a cluster randomised trial needs to be increased. When clusters are of similar size, the key determinants of the increase required (which can be substantial) are the intracluster correlation coefficient and the average cluster size (see for formula). Sample size calculations when cluster sizes are unequal are discussed elsewhere[65]. Reports of cluster randomised trials should state the assumptions used when calculating the number of clusters and the cluster sample size.

The power of the trial can also be decreased by imbalances in cluster sizes at recruitment and by differences in the intracluster correlation coefficient across clusters[66]. Differences in expected recruitment across clusters should be reported, since sample size calculations usually assume equal cluster sizes.

Item 7b

Standard CONSORT item: when applicable, explanation of any interim analyses and stopping guidelines

Example

These calculations conservatively included a 10% design effect, which was expected to be negligible in view of the small cluster size and rare outcome. The data monitoring and ethics committee did conditional power calculations in 2003 and recommended that the trial be continued until October 2008[67]

Explanation

As in many individually randomised trials, there may be a need for an independent body, such as a data monitoring committee,[68] [69] to monitor accumulating data to protect patients in the trial and future patients. The main principles of interim analysis remain the same for cluster randomisation as for individual randomisation,[70] and the interim analysis would probably use the same statistical methods that were planned for the final analysis of a cluster randomised trial. Few cluster randomised trials seem to have explicit stopping boundaries, however, and cluster randomised controlled trials may need some additional considerations. For instance, if more information becomes available about the assumptions on which the original power calculations were based, or if clusters are recruited over a period of time, an interim analysis after, for example, 25% of the person time has been completed, may not provide as much as 25% of the information due to the expected variation between clusters[17]; a particular amount of person time is more informative if it comes from more, rather than fewer, clusters.[71]

Randomisation

Sequence generation

Item 8b

Standard CONSORT item: type of randomisation; details of any restriction (such as blocking and block size)

Extension for cluster trials: details of stratification or matching if used

Example 1 (stratification)

Neonatal units were stratified by designation of level of care within the managed Clinical Neonatal Networks (n=25) and by level of care delivered (level I, II or III), and then ordered alphabetically by name of hospital and imported into statistical computer software Stata V.9 at the London School of Hygiene and Tropical Medicine. The programme generated a series of blocks of varying size (two, four or six) for each stratum and allocated units to control or active intervention randomly within each block[52]

Example 2 (stratification)

The allocation schedule for random assignment of care models to clinics was computer generated, including stratification by study site and clinic characteristics, at a central location (WHO, Geneva, Switzerland) by the Statistical Unit of the UNDP/UNFPA/WHO/World Bank Special Programme of Research, Development, and Research Training in Human Reproduction[72]

Example 3 (matching)

We . . . paired the 14 [urban sectors of Trujillo, Venezuela] according to the incidence of cutaneous leishmaniasis in the 12 months before the baseline household survey. For each of the seven pairs we randomly allocated one sector (using computer created random numbers) . . . to the intervention group and the other to the control group[59]

Explanation

The way in which the randomisation sequence is generated depends on the design: if the number of clusters is large, a completely (cluster) randomised design may be a convenient option and then simple randomisation might be sufficient.[8] Otherwise, restricted randomisation may be useful. For a stratified design (for example, stratification by centre), the sequence is generated independently within each stratum. In addition, to control the probability of obtaining an allocation sequence with an undesirable sample size imbalance in the intervention groups, the randomisation within strata can be restricted. Common techniques for restricted randomisation include permuted blocks and the random allocation rule (that is, a single permuted block).[73] The random allocation rule is useful when all clusters are available at the time of generating the sequence, which is often the case. Using (more than one) random permuted blocks is more common for individually randomised designs, in which participants arrive sequentially. For the specific form of stratification of two clusters per stratum (a matched paired design), the sequence should allocate the two interventions at random to the clusters within pairs.

Allocation concealment mechanism

Item 9

Standard CONSORT item: mechanism used to implement the random allocation sequence (such as sequentially numbered containers), describing any steps taken to conceal sequence until interventions were assigned

Extension for cluster trials: specification that allocation was based on clusters rather than individuals and whether allocation concealment (if any) was at cluster level, individual participant level, or both

Example (allocation was based on clusters and concealed at cluster level)

The treatment allocation for each site was kept in Geneva until the site had completed the basic introductory training of study personnel (both in standard-model and control-model clinics [clusters]). When local investigators were ready to implement the training workshops for the staff if the clinic were assigned the new model, the study statistician sent the treatment allocation by facsimile directly to the principal investigator of the selected site[72]

Explanation

In individually randomised trials, adequate concealment of the treatment allocation is crucial for minimising potential bias. If the person recruiting participants has foreknowledge of the allocation, bias can result.[74] In a cluster randomised trial, allocation of treatment is predetermined for each member of the cluster. Hence the potential for selection bias (selective inclusion of patients into the trial) within clusters is particularly high.[5][6] It is therefore important that authors outline any strategies that were implemented to minimise the possibility of selection bias—for example, whether clusters were identified and recruited before randomisation, whether allocation was concealed from the person or people who provided access to the cluster or provided permission for the cluster to be included in the trial (for example, the cluster "guardian" or "gatekeeper")[75], whether all patients within a cluster were included or, if not, whether recruitment of patients was by a person masked to the cluster allocation. Allocation concealment for participants might be achieved by selecting participants before randomising clusters.[5]

Implementation

Item 10

Standard CONSORT item: who generated the random allocation sequence, who enrolled participants, and who assigned participants to interventions

Extension to cluster trials: replaced by items 10a, 10b, and 10c

Item 10a

Extension for cluster trials: who generated the random allocation sequence, who enrolled clusters, and who assigned clusters to interventions

Example 1 (enrolment of clusters and method of assignment)

Rural primary schools with 150 children or more, and over 15 children per class were eligible for inclusion. . . .Meetings were held in participating schools to explain the nature

and purpose of the trial to parents or legal guardians, and written informed consent was obtained. Schoolchildren with parental consent and no history of adverse reaction to sulfa-based drugs were eligible for recruitment. . . . We stratified schools into three groups according to school examination performance in previous years . . . Ten schools were randomly selected from each school-performance stratum, and within each stratum schools were randomly allocated to one of six coded drug groups by use of block randomisation .. . according to a computer-generated random number list by an investigator . . . blind to drug group[76]

Example 2 (who generated sequence and who assigned clusters to interventions)

We conducted the trial in a contiguous area encompassing most of Ward 29 and all of Ward 30 in Eastern Kolkata, a legally registered urban slum with a population of about 60,000 residents. Before vaccination, a census of the population enumerated all households and persons in the study area and characterized the socioeconomic status, water source, and hygiene status of each household. Each household and person in the census were assigned a unique study identification number. The census, together with geographic mapping, was used to define 80 contiguous geographic clusters that served as the units of randomization. . . . The clusters were stratified according to ward and the number of residents who were 18 years of age or younger (<200 vs. .200 persons) and the number of residents who were older than 18 years (<500 vs. .500 persons), resulting in eight strata. For each stratum, a statistician who was unaware of the study-group assignments used a table of random numbers to assign half the 80 clusters to each vaccine[77]

Explanation

As outlined in the original CONSORT explanatory paper[78] it is important that all the steps of the random allocation process from generation to implementation are adequately described. Within cluster randomised trials the randomisation process has the added complexity of having two levels involved in the allocation process—the inclusion and allocation of clusters and the inclusion of cluster members. As such, the implementation processes adopted for each step need to be outlined separately.

Item 10b

Extension for cluster trials: mechanism by which individual participants were included in clusters for the purposes of the trial (such as complete enumeration, random sampling)

Example 1

The family practices associated with the 2 study sites served as the units of randomization. . . . Family practices associated with the clinical study sites were randomly assigned to the liquid-based cytology or the conventional Pap test group. All women screened at 1 of the participating family practices were included in the study[47]

Example 2

All cluster residents were eligible to receive a study vaccine if they were 24 months of age or older, had no reported fever or had an axillary temperature of no more than 37.5°C at the time of administration, and were not pregnant or lactating. All subjects or their guardians provided written informed consent[77]

Example 3

Twenty seven practices agreed to participate in the trial: 10 were therefore randomly allocated to each of the two intervention arms and seven to the usual care arm. To ensure sufficient numbers of patients with adequate follow

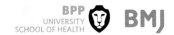

up data, 30 patients were randomly sampled from each practice[62]

Explanation

A previous study[5] showed that selection bias can arise in cluster randomised controlled trials, especially at the point when participants are selected from within clusters. This bias can be reduced by complete enumeration and inclusion of all participants identified as eligible or, if a sample from the cluster is required, by having a third party make the selection or blinding the person identifying participants until after assessment of eligibility.

Item 10c

Extension for cluster trial: from whom consent was sought (representatives of cluster, or individual participants, or both), and whether consent was sought before or after randomisation

Example 1 (who provided consent)

Because outcome data were routinely collected at hospitals and no personal identifiers were transmitted, all the institutional review boards waived the requirement for individual consent. Responsible authorities from all the hospitals provided written consent, and birth attendants also provided written consent[56]

Example 2 (consent process and when consent sought)

There were 12 antenatal-care clinics in each of three study sites and 17 in the fourth site that were eligible for the study and where the health authorities agreed to let the clinics be included in the trial . . . [cluster-level consent]. The [individual level] informed consent procedure was based on the single-consent design proposed by Zelen. Thus, informed consent was requested only from women attending the antenatal clinics assigned to the new model; women who refused were cared for according to the standard practice in their clinic. However, such women were counted in the intention-to-treat analysis as being assigned to the new-model group. Women attending the standard-model clinics received the protocols recommended in each country, in the best format offered in these clinics . . . [72]

Explanation

Many reports of cluster trials do not indicate at which level consent was sought or its timing in relation to randomisation, which can lead to bias.[79] For example, if consent is sought at the cluster level post-randomisation but from the active arm only, there may be differential attrition of whole clusters. Even if consent is sought from all clusters, attrition bias can arise if consent to treatment or provision of data is sought from individual cluster members in the active arm only (see also item 5 and box 2). This reinforces the need to be able to report flow of patients within clusters over the course of the trial (see item 13).

Specific details of how interventions were administered should be described, because there are implications for consent and for adherence. When the intervention is applied at the cluster level (such as mass media advertising), it may not be feasible to obtain consent pre-randomisation from individual cluster members—that is, consent to randomise may have to be sought at cluster level only. Likewise, consent to intervention may have to be sought at the cluster level as individual cluster members may not be able to decline the intervention. Consent will often be sought at both the cluster level (for example, from the "gatekeeper") and from individual cluster members to contribute data. The specific issues around informed consent in cluster trials have been considered elsewhere.[80] (See also item 10b.)

Blinding

Item 11a

Standard CONSORT item: if done, who was blinded after assignment to interventions (for example, participants, care providers, those assessing outcomes) and how

Example

To prevent selective assessment bias, study personnel—gynecologists, pathologists, cytotechnologists, and others—involved in the follow-up and review of histology and cytology were blinded to the cytology screening system used. . . . A panel of 4 experienced pathologists who were blinded to the cytological system, the original cytological and histological findings, and all follow-up data reviewed the histology[47]

Explanation

In individually randomised trials the importance of blinding is well recognised, as a lack of blinding can lead to the inflation of study effects.[74 78] For individually randomised trials it is therefore recommended that participants and outcome assessors should be blinded wherever possible to the intervention received. In cluster trials, however, the concept of blinding is more complicated. Often the delivery of interventions in cluster trials involves a range of different people (for example, trainers training health professionals in the use of guidelines; health professionals implementing the guidelines for individual patients; outcome assessors who could be trainers; health professionals, patients, or a completely different group) at the different cluster levels and it is often unclear from trial reports who was and was not blinded within the trial.[36 42] It is further recognised that many cluster trials are pragmatic by nature, as they are often designed to evaluate changes in service provision or interventions to change practitioners' or patients' behaviour in real world settings. In such circumstances it is widely acknowledged that blinding of the intervention is often not possible (although blinding of those assessing outcome may still be possible). If this is the case, however, it is important that it is explicitly acknowledged in the trial report—the CONSORT statement for pragmatic trials recommends that if blinding was not done, or was not possible, an explanation as to why should be included in the text.[23]

Statistical methods

Item 12a

Standard CONSORT item: statistical methods used to compare groups for primary and secondary outcomes

Extension for cluster trials: how clustering was taken into account

Example 1

Because we randomised obstetric units . . . we analysed rates of marker clinical practices by obstetric units[46]

Example 2

The primary outcome was expressed as the mean rate difference between groups (with 95% CI). This value was measured as the difference between matched hospitals (intervention hospital minus control hospital) in caesarean section rate change (caesarean section rate in the intervention period minus caesarean section rate in the baseline period) . . . A one-sample two sided t test was used to assess whether the mean rate difference between groups was statistically different from zero[56]

Example 3

We used cluster specific methods because practices rather than patients were randomised, and we expected that variance in how patients were managed would be partly explained by the practice. Because some patients had more than one consultation, we added a third level to the analysis to account for the likelihood that variance in what was done at each consultation would be partly explained by the patient . . . [81] [This article also included a box to explain the three level logistical hierarchical model used.]

Explanation

Identification of the level of inference allows readers to evaluate the methods of analysis. For example, if the inference was targeted at the cluster level (at general practitioners rather than patients, for example) and outcomes were aggregated at the cluster level, sophisticated cluster adjusted analyses are not needed (as in examples 1 and 2). However, if the cluster sizes are unequal, weighting may be recommended because the variance of the cluster summary statistics is not constant. If the inference was targeted at the individual patient level, the analysis would need to adjust for potential clustering in the data.

Results

Participant flow
Item 13a

Standard CONSORT item: for each group, the numbers of participants who were randomly assigned, received intended treatment, and were analysed for primary outcome

Extension for cluster trials: for each group, the numbers of clusters that were randomly assigned, received intended treatment, and were analysed for primary outcome

Item 13b

Standard CONSORT item: for each group, losses and exclusions after randomisation, together with reasons

Extension for cluster trials: for each group, losses and exclusions for both clusters and individual participants

Examples: presented in figures 2 and 3

Explanation

The flow diagram is a key element of the CONSORT statement and has been widely adopted. For cluster trials it is important to understand the flow of clusters as well as the flow of participants (fig 2). The potential for differential adherence and follow up is exacerbated in the cluster randomised design because there are two levels at which drop-outs can occur—whole clusters or individual participants in a cluster. It is therefore important to describe the flow of both clusters and participants when reporting a cluster randomised trial; this information is essential to interpret the study appropriately.

Although we recommend a flow diagram for communicating the flow of clusters and participants throughout the study (fig 2), the exact form and content should vary in relation to the specific features of a trial. We previously presented three options for modifying the CONSORT flow diagram for presenting clustered data—presenting the flow of data based only on clusters, only on individual participants, or on both.[9] Further experience suggests that the type of diagram should depend on the type of analysis because different approaches to analysis require information at different levels of the clustered design.

For example, if the analysis is aggregated at the level of the cluster, the flow diagram should relate to the data at cluster level. To allow meaningful interpretation, the diagram also needs to include a measure of the cluster size (and an indication of how variable cluster sizes are). If, however, the analysis is multilevel or hierarchical, the flow diagram should present data flow for both clusters and individual participants.

Baseline data
Item 15

Standard CONSORT item: a table showing baseline demographic and clinical characteristics for each group

Extension for cluster trials: baseline characteristics for cluster and individual participant levels as applicable for each group

Example: presented in table 3

Explanation

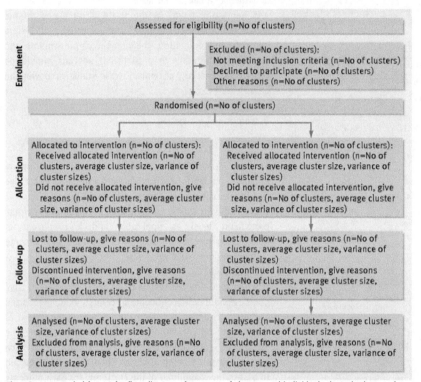

Fig 2 Recommended format for flow diagram of progress of clusters and individuals through phases of randomised trial

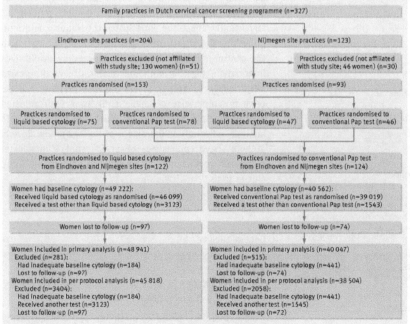

Fig 3 Example of flow diagram for cluster trial (adapted from Siebers et al[47])

Random assignment by individual ensures that any differences in group characteristics at baseline are the result of chance rather than some systematic bias.[74] For cluster randomised trials, however, the risk of chance imbalance is greater as clusters rather than individuals are randomised and the number of clusters is often small (although imbalances can occur even when the number of clusters is not limited).[66] It is therefore important to present summary baseline information for both clusters and individuals, most simply as tables of summary data (table 3).

Table 3 Example of baseline information for each group given at individual and cluster levels (adapted from Sur et al).[77] Values at individual level are numbers (percentages) and at cluster level are means (standard deviations) unless stated otherwise

Variables	Vi vaccine (n=18 869)	Hepatitis A vaccine (n=18 804)
Individual level		
Mean (SD) age (years)	28.5 (18.0)	27.9 (17.8)
Male	9876 (52)	9920 (53)
Hindu	12 335 (65)	10 825 (58)
Mean (SD) No of members of household	7.1(3.9)	7.0(3.7)
Head of household able to read and write	13 980 (74)	13 099 (70)
Monthly household per capita expenditure above median of 500 rupees	7795 (41)	7636 (41)
At least one luxury item owned in household	4131 (22)	3918 (21)
Tube-well or faucet as source of drinking water in household	2711 (14)	1824 (10)
Flush toilet in household	905 (5)	577 (3)
Access to specific place for waste disposal in household	18 547 (98)	18 429 (98)
Household farther from treatment centre than median distance	8900 (47)	9935 (53)
Cluster level		
Age groups (No/cluster):		
2-18 years	256 (118)	273 (115)
>18 years	503 (84)	500 (93)
All residents per cluster (years)	29.0 (5.0)	28.5 (4.6)
Households (No/cluster)	142 (27)	146 (36)
Vaccinated participants (No/cluster)	472 (103)	470 (104)
Cases of typhoid fever during year before study (No/1000 cluster residents)	1.54 (1.40)	1.38 (1.38)
Population density (No of residents/100m²/cluster)	18.4 (17.8)	22.2 (20.1)
Percent vaccine coverage of people .2 year of age	61 (11)	60 (12)

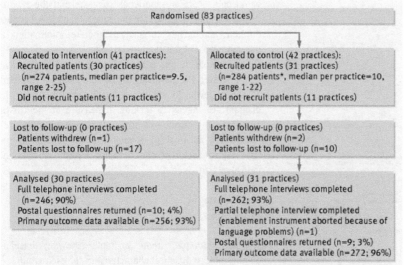

* One patient from the control group was subsequently found to have long standing asthma and was therefore determined (after consultation with the trial steering committee) to have been "recruited in error" and has not been included as a randomised patient

Fig 4 Example of flow of clusters from recruitment to analysis (reproduced from Francis et al)[108]

Numbers analysed

Item 16

Standard CONSORT item: for each group, number of participants (denominator) included in each analysis and whether the analysis was by original assigned groups

Extension for cluster trials: for each group, number of clusters included in each analysis

Example: presented in figure 4

Explanation

The number of participants who contribute to the analysis of a trial is essential to interpreting the results. However, not all participants may contribute to the analysis of each outcome. In a cluster trial this fact is compounded by the possibility that not all clusters may contribute to a particular analysis. Because the sample size calculation and hence the power of the study is calculated on the assumption that all participants and (especially) all clusters will provide information, the number of participants and clusters contributing to a particular analysis should be reported so that any potential drop in statistical power can be assessed (fig 4).

Outcomes and estimation

Item 17a

Standard CONSORT item: for each primary and secondary outcome, results for each group, and estimated effect size and its precision (such as 95% confidence interval)

Extension for cluster trials: results at cluster or individual participant level as applicable and a coefficient of intracluster correlation (ICC or k) for each primary outcome

Example: presented in table 4

Explanation

When reporting the results of a cluster randomised trial, point estimates with confidence intervals should be reported for primary outcomes. Given the impact of the extent of the intracluster correlation on the power of the study, the intracluster correlation coefficient or k statistic for each primary outcome being analysed should also be provided to assess the magnitude of the clustering for each outcome (however, if a cluster level analysis is being undertaken, the concept of the intracluster correlation is less relevant as each cluster provides a single data point). In some situations, especially if it is believed the intervention will significantly affect the intracluster correlation coefficient, publishing the intracluster correlation coefficient from both the control and the intervention arm may be useful. This information, together with the cluster size or the design effect, allows readers to assess the appropriateness of the original sample size calculations. Showing both adjusted and unadjusted estimates for clustering would provide another indication of the extent of the clustering. Several authors have published observed study intracluster correlation coefficients to help with the planning of future cluster trials.[82 83 84 85 86]

Discussion

Generalisability

Item 21

Standard CONSORT item: generalisability (external validity, applicability) of trial findings

Extension for cluster trials: generalisability to clusters or individual participants (as relevant)

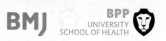

Table 4 Example of study including data on numbers analysed by cluster and intracluster correlation coefficients (adapted from Feder et al)[107]

Variable	No (%) in intervention group	No (%) in control group	Intracluster correlation coefficient	Adjusted odds ratio (95% CI)	Adjusted χ^2 statistic	P value
No of practices	25	27	—	—	—	—
No of patients	172	156	—	—	—	—
Advice given:						
Cholesterol	54/81 (67)	32/83 (39)	0.013	4.0 (1.9 to 8.2)	12.2	<0.001
Weight	74/169 (44)	32/154 (21)	0.098	3.0 (1.5 to 35.8)	10.5	<0.01
Diet	46/169 (27)	22/154 (14)	0.053	2.4 (1.2 to 4.7)	6.2	<0.05

Example (at the cluster level)

Although our trial was completed successfully from both a methodological and practical point of view, our results may not be generalisable. The 21 participating practices tended to be large, with good nursing support, and may have been particularly committed to improving their quality of care . . . Furthermore, the observed intervention effect would probably have been greater if the trial had not taken place in the context of a health authority audit initiative relating to patients with coronary heart disease, backed by a financial incentive[87]

Explanation

In the discussion section of any trial report, the external validity of the results should be considered. External validity is more complicated for cluster randomised trials because the results may be generalisable to the clusters, to the participants in those clusters, or to both, and thus the level at which external validity is addressed should be identified.

Comment

Reports of randomised controlled trials should include key information on the methods and findings to allow readers to accurately interpret the results. This information is particularly important for meta-analysts attempting to extract data from such reports. The CONSORT 2010 statement provides the latest recommendations from the CONSORT Group on essential items to be included in the report of a randomised controlled trial. In this paper we introduce and explain corresponding updates in an extension of the CONSORT checklist specific to reporting cluster randomised trials.

Use of the CONSORT statement for the reporting of two group parallel trials is associated with improved reporting quality.[88] We believe that the routine use of this proposed extension to the CONSORT statement will eventually result in similar improvements to cluster trials.

When reporting a cluster randomised trial, authors should address all 25 items on the CONSORT checklist using this document in conjunction with the main CONSORT guidelines.[3] Depending on the type of trial done, authors may also find it useful to consult the CONSORT extensions for non-pharmacological treatments[15] and non-inferiority trials.[89]

The CONSORT statement can help researchers designing trials in the future and can guide peer reviewers and editors in their evaluation of manuscripts. Many journals recommend adherence to the CONSORT recommendations in their instructions to authors. We encourage them to direct authors to this and to other extensions of CONSORT for specific trial designs. The most up to date versions of all CONSORT recommendations can be found at www.consort-statement.org.

We thank Cynthia Fraser for undertaking the electronic searches, the members of the CONSORT Group for comments on drafts, and Monica Taljaard for comments on consent issues.

Contributors: MKC, DRE, DGA, and GP each took lead responsibility for the writing of different components of the manuscript. All authors then input to, and commented on, the overall draft and subsequent revisions. MKC is guarantor.

Funding: The Health Services Research Unit is core funded by the Chief Scientist Office of the Scottish Government Health Directorates. DGA is supported by a Cancer Research UK programme grant (C5529). The views expressed in this paper are those of the authors alone.

Competing interests: All authors have completed the ICMJE uniform disclosure form at www.icmje.org/coi_disclosure.pdf (available on request from the corresponding author) and declare: no support from any organisation for the submitted work; no financial relationships with any organisations that might have an interest in the submitted work in the previous three years; no other relationships or activities that could appear to have influenced the submitted work.

Provenance and peer review: Not commissioned; externally peer reviewed.

1 Begg C, Cho M, Eastwood S, Horton R, Moher D, Olkin I, et al. Improving the quality of reporting of randomised controlled trials. The CONSORT statement. JAMA 1996;276:637-9.

2 Moher D, Schulz KF, Altman DG, CONSORT Group. The CONSORT statement: revised recommendations for improving the quality of reports of parallel-group randomised trials. Lancet 2001;357:1191-4.

3 Schulz KF, Altman DG, Moher D. CONSORT 2010 statement: updated guidelines for reporting parallel group randomised trials. BMJ 2010;340:c332.

4 Moher D, Hopewell S, Schulz KF, Montori V, Gøtzsche PC, Devereaux PJ, et al. CONSORT 2010 explanation and elaboration: updated guidelines for reporting parallel group randomised trials. BMJ 2010;340:c869.

5 Puffer S, Torgerson D, Watson J. Evidence for risk of bias in cluster randomised trials: review of recent trials published in three general medical journals. BMJ 2003;327:785-9.

6 Fayers PM, Jordhøy MS, Kaasa S. Cluster-randomized trials. Palliat Med 2002;26:69-70.

7 Grimshaw JM, Campbell MK, Eccles M, Steen IN. Experimental and quasi-experimental designs for evaluating guideline implementation strategies. Fam Pract 2000;17:S11-8.

8 Donner A, Klar N. Design and analysis of cluster randomization trials in health research . Arnold, 2000.

9 Elbourne DR, Campbell MK. Extending the CONSORT statement to cluster randomised trials: for discussion. Stat Med 2001;20:489-96.

10 Campbell MK, Elbourne DR, Altman DG. CONSORT statement: extension to cluster randomised trials. BMJ 2004;328:702-8.

11 Hopewell S, Clarke M, Moher D, Wager E, Middleton P, Altman DG, et al. CONSORT for reporting randomised trials in journal and conference abstracts. Lancet 2008;371:281-3.

12 Hopewell S, Clarke M, Moher D, Wager E, Middleton P, Altman DG, at al. CONSORT for reporting randomized controlled trials in journal and conference abstracts: explanation and elaboration. PLoS Med 2008;5:e20.

13 Lesaffre E, Garcia Zattera MJ, Redmond C, Huber H, Needleman I. Reported methodological quality of split-mouth studies. J Clin Periodontol 2007;34:756-61.

14 Roberts C, Roberts SA. Design and analysis of clinical trials with clustering effects due to treatment. Clin Trials 2002;2:152-62.

15 Boutron I, Moher D, Altman DG, Schulz KF, Ravaud P. Extending the CONSORT statement to randomized trials of nonpharmacologic treatment: explanation and elaboration. Ann Intern Med 2008;148:295-309.

16 Varnell SP, Murray DM, Baker WL. An evaluation of analysis options for the one-group-per-condition design. Can any of the alternatives overcome the problems inherent in this design? Eval Review 2001;25:440-53.

17 Hayes RJ, Moulton LH. Cluster randomised trials . Chapman and Hall/CRC, 2008.

18 Fagevik Olsén M, Hahn I, Nordgren S, Lönroth H, Lundholm K. Randomized controlled trial of prophylactic chest physiotherapy in major abdominal surgery. Br J Surg 1997;84:1535-8.

19 Turner RM, White IR, Croudace T, for the PIP Study Group. Analysis of cluster randomized cross-over trial data: a comparison of methods. Stat Med 2007;26:274-89.

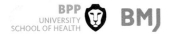

20 Mdege ND, Man M-S, Taylor (nee Brown) CA, Torgerson DJ. Systematic review of stepped wedge cluster randomized trials shows that design is particularly used to evaluate interventions during routine implementation, *J Clin Epidemiol* , 2011;64:936-48.

21 Brown CA, Lilford RJ. The stepped wedge trial design: a systematic review. *BMC Med Res Methodol* 2006;6:54.

22 Muckelbauer R, Libuda L, Clausen K, Toschke AM, Reinehr T, Kersting M. Promotion and provision of drinking water in schools for overweight prevention: randomized, controlled cluster trial. *Pediatrics* 2009;123:e661-7.

23 Zwarenstein M, Treweek S, Altman DG, Gagnier J, Tunis S, Haynes RB, et al. Improving the reporting of pragmatic trials: an extension of the CONSORT statement. *BMJ* 2008;337:a2390.

24 Campbell MJ, Donner A, Klar N. Developments in cluster randomized trials. *Stat Med* 2007;26:2-19.

25 Murray DM, Varnell SP, Blitstein JL. Design and analysis of group-randomized trials: a review of recent methodological developments. *Am J Public Health* 2004;94:423-32.

26 Eldridge S, Kerry S. *A practical guide to cluster randomised trials in health services research.* Wiley, 2012.

27 Simpson JM, Klar N, Donner A. Accounting for cluster randomization: a review of primary prevention trials, 1990 through 1993. *Am J Public Health* 1995;85:1378-83.

28 Divine GW, Brown JT, Frazier LM. The unit of analysis error in studies about physicians' patient care behaviour. *J Gen Intern Med* 1992;7:623-9.

29 Donner A, Brown KS, Brasher P. A methodological review of non-therapeutic intervention trials employing cluster randomization, 1979-1989. *Int J Epidemiol* 1990;19:795-800.

30 Chuang JH, Hripcsak G, Jenders RA. Considering clustering: a methodological review of clinical decision support system studies. *Proc AMIA Symp* 2000;146-50.

31 Maclennan GS, Ramsay CR, Thomas RE, Grimshaw JM. Unit of analysis errors in cluster randomised trials to evaluate the effectiveness of the introduction of clinical guidelines into medical practice. *Proc Int Soc Clin Biostat* 2001;186.

32 Isaakidis P, Ioannidis JPA. Evaluation of cluster randomized controlled trials in sub-Saharan Africa. *Am J Epidemiol* 2003;158:921-6.

33 Varnell SP, Murray DM, Janega JB, Blitstein JL. Design and analysis of group-randomized trials: a review of recent practices. *Am J Public Health* 2004;94:393-9.

34 Bland JM. Cluster randomised trials in the medical literature: two bibliometric surveys. *BMC Med Res Methodol* 2004;4:21.

35 Calhoun AW, Guyatt GH, Cabana MD, Lu D, Turner DA, Valentine S, et al. Addressing the unit of analysis in medical care studies: a systematic review. *Med Care* 2008;46:635-43.

36 Eldridge S, Ashby D, Bennett C, Wakelin M, Feder G. Internal and external validity of cluster randomised trials: systematic review of recent trials. *BMJ* 2008;336:876-80.

37 Murray DM, Pals SL, Blitstein JL, Alfano CM, Lehman J. Design and analysis of group-randomized trials in cancer: a review of current practices. *J Natl Cancer Inst* 2008;100:483-91.

38 Bowater RJ, Abdelmalik SM, Lilford RJ. The methodological quality of cluster randomised controlled trials for managing tropical parasitic disease: a review of trials published from 1998 to 2007. *Trans R Soc Trop Med Hyg* 2009;103:429-36.

39 Handlos LN, Chakraborty H, Sen PK. Evaluation of cluster-randomized trials on maternal and child health research in developing countries. *Trop Med Int Health* 2009;14:947-56.

40 Crespi CM, Maxwell AE, Wu S. Cluster randomized trials of cancer screening interventions: are appropriate statistical methods being used? *Contemp Clin Trials* 2011;32:477-84.

41 Walleser S, Hill SR, Bero LA. Characteristics and quality of reporting of cluster randomized trials in children: reporting needs improvement. *J Clin Epidemiol* 2011;64:1331-40.

42 Ivers NM, Taljaard M, Dixon S, Bennett C, McRae A, Taleban J, et al. Impact of the CONSORT extension for cluster randomised trials on quality of reporting and study methodology: review of a random sample of 300 trials from 2000 to 2008. *BMJ* 2011;343:d5886.

43 Cumming RG, Sherrington C, Lord SR, Simpson JM, Vogler C, Cameron ID, et al; Prevention of Older People's Injury Falls Prevention in Hospitals Research Group. Cluster randomised trial of a targeted multifactorial intervention to prevent falls among older people in hospital. *BMJ* 2008;336:758-60.

44 Cavalcante SC, Durovni B, Barnes GL, Souza FBA, Silva RF, Barroso PF, et al. Community-randomized trial of enhanced DOTS for tuberculosis control in Rio de Janeiro, Brazil. *Int J Tuberc Lung Dis* 2010;14:203-9.

45 Taljaard M, McGowan J, Grimshaw JM, Brehaut JC, McRae A, Eccles MP, et al. Electronic search strategies to identify reports of cluster randomized trials in MEDLINE: low precision will improve with adherence to reporting standards. *BMC Med Res Methodol* 2010;10:15.

46 Wyatt JC, Paterson-Brown S, Johanson R, Altman DG, Bradburn MJ, Fisk NM. Randomised trial of educational visits to enhance use of systematic reviews in 25 obstetric units. *BMJ* 1998;317:1041-6.

47 Siebers AG, Klinkhamer PJJM, Grefte JMM, Massuger LFAG, Vedder JEM, Beijers-Broos A, et al. Comparison of liquid-based cytology with conventional cytology for detection of cervical cancer precursors: a randomized controlled trial. *JAMA* 2009;302:1757-64.

48 World Medical Association. Recommendations guiding physicians in biomedical research involving human subjects. World Medical Association Declaration of Helsinki. *JAMA* 1997;277:925-6.

49 Donner A, Brown KS, Brasher P. A methodological review of non-therapeutic intervention trials employing cluster randomization, 1979-1989. *Int J Epidemiol* 1990;19:795-800.

50 Brierley G, Brabyn S, Torgerson D, Watson J. Bias in recruitment to cluster randomized trials: a review of recent publications. *J Eval Clin Pract* 2012;18:878-86.

51 Puffer S, Torgerson DJ, Watson J. Cluster randomized controlled trials. *J Eval Clin Pract* 2005;11:479-83.

52 Acolet D, Allen E, Houston R, Wilkinson AR, Costeloe K, Elbourne D. Improvement in neonatal intensive care unit care: a cluster randomised controlled trial of active dissemination of information. *Arch Dis Child Fetal Neonatal Ed* 2011;96:F434-9.

53 Atienza AA, King AC. Community-based health intervention trials: an overview of methodological issues. *Epidemiol Rev* 2002;24:72-9.

54 Dangour AD, Albala C, Allen E, Grundy E, Walker D, Aedo C, et al. Effect of a nutrition supplement and physical activity program on pneumonia and walking capacity in Chilean older people: a factorial cluster randomized trial. *PLoS Med* 2011;8:e1001023.

55 Cals JWL, Butler CC, Hopstaken RM, Hood K, Dinant GJ. Effect of point of care testing for C reactive protein and training in communication skills on antibiotic use in lower respiratory tract infections: cluster randomised trial. *BMJ* 2009;338:b1374.

56 Althabe F, Belizán JM, Villar J, Alexander S, Bergel E, Ramos S, et al. Mandatory second opinion to reduce rates of unnecessary caesarean sections in Latin America: a cluster randomised controlled trial. *Lancet* 2004;363:1934-40.

57 Altman DG, Doré CJ. Randomisation and baseline comparisons in clinical trials. *Lancet* 1990;335:149-53.

58 Kinmonth AL, Woodcock A, Griffin S, Spiegal N, Campbell MJ, Diabetes Care from Diagnosis Research Team. Randomised controlled trial of patient centred care of diabetes in general practice: impact of current wellbeing and future disease risk. *BMJ* 1998;317:1202-8.

59 Kroeger A, Avilla EC, Morison L. Insecticide impregnated curtains to control domestic transmission of cutaneous leishmaniasis in Venezuela: cluster randomised trial. *BMJ* 2002;325:810-3.

60 Murphy AW, Cupples ME, Smith SM, Byrne M, Byrne MC, Newell J. Effect of tailored practice and patient care plans on secondary prevention of heart disease in general practice: cluster randomised controlled trial. *BMJ* 2009;339:b4220.

61 Naughton C, Feely J, Bennett KA. Clustered randomized trial of the effects of feedback using academic detailing compared to postal bulletin on prescribing of preventative cardiovascular therapy. *Fam Pract* 2007;24:475-80.

62 Montgomery AA, Fahey T, Peters TJ, MacIntosh C, Sharp DJ. Evaluation of computer based clinical decision support system and risk chart for management of hypertension in primary care: randomised controlled trial. *BMJ* 2000;320:686-90.

63 Majoko F, Munjanja SP, Nyström L, Mason E, Lindmark G. Randomised controlled trial of two antenatal care models in rural Zimbabwe. *BJOG* 2007;114:802-11.

64 Grosskurth H, Mosha F, Todd J, Mwijarubi E, Klokke A, Senkoro K, et al. Impact of improved treatment of sexually transmitted diseases on HIV infection in rural Tanzania: randomised controlled trial. *Lancet* 1995;346:530-6.

65 Eldridge S, Kerry S, Ashby D. Sample size for cluster randomized trials: effect of coefficient of variation of cluster size and analysis method. *Int J Epidemiol* 2006;35:1292-300.

66 Carter B. Cluster size variability and imbalance in cluster randomized controlled trials. *Stat Med* 2010;29:2984-93.

67 Kirkwood BR, Hurt L, Amenga-Etego S, Tawiah C, Zandoh C, Danso S, et al. Effect of vitamin A supplementation in women of reproductive age on maternal survival in Ghana (ObaapaVitA): a cluster-randomised, placebo-controlled trial. *Lancet* 2010;375:1640-9.

68 Ellenberg SS, Fleming TR, De Mets DL. *Data monitoring committees in clinical trials: a practical perspective.* Wiley, 2002.

69 Grant AM, Altman DG, Babiker AB, Campbell MK, Clemens FJ, Darbyshire JH, et al. Issues in data monitoring and interim analysis of trials. *Health Technol Assess* 2005;9:1-238.

70 Zou GY, Donner A, Klar N. Group sequential methods for cluster randomization trials with binary outcomes. *Clin Trials* 2005;2:479-87.

71 Flynn TN, Whitley E, Peters TJ. Recruitment strategies in a cluster randomize trial—cost implications. *Stat Med* 2002;21:397-405.

72 Villar J, Ba'aqeel H, Piaggio G, Lumbiganon P, Miguel Belizán J, Farnot U, et al. WHO antenatal care randomised trial for the evaluation of a new model of routine antenatal care. *Lancet* 2001;357:1551-64.

73 Schulz K, Grimes D. Generation of allocation sequences in randomised trials: chance, not choice. *Lancet* 2002;359:515-9.

74 Schulz K, Chalmers I, Hayes R, Altman DG. Empirical evidence of bias: dimensions of methodological quality associated with estimates of treatment effects in controlled trials. *JAMA* 1995;273:408-12.

75 Weijer C, Grimshaw JM, Eccles MP, McRae AD, White A, Brehaut JC, et al. The Ottawa Consensus Statement on the ethical design and conduct of CRTs. *PLoS Med* (in press).

76 Clarke SE, Jukes MC, Njagi JK, Khasakhala L, Cundill B, Otido J, et al. Effect of intermittent preventive treatment of malaria on health and education in schoolchildren: a cluster randomised double-blind, placebo-controlled trial. *Lancet* 2008;372:127-38.

77 Sur D, Ochiai RL, Bhattacharya SK, Ganguly NK, Ali M, Manna B, et al. Cluster-randomized effectiveness trial of Vi typhoid vaccine in India. *N Engl J Med* 2009;361:335-44.

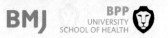

78 Altman DG, Schulz KF, Moher D, Egger M, Davidoff F, Elbourne D, et al. The revised CONSORT statement for reporting randomised trials: explanation and elaboration. *Ann Intern Med* 2001;134:663-94.

79 Taljaard M, McRae A, Weijer C, Bennett C, Dixon S, Taleban J, et al. Inadequate reporting of research ethics review and informed consent in cluster randomized trials: review of a representative sample of published trials. *BMJ* 2011;342:d2496.

80 Weijer C, Grimshaw JM, Taljaard M, Binik A, Boruch R, Brehaut JC, et al. Ethical issues posed by cluster randomized trials in health research. *Trials* 2011;12:100.

81 Flottorp S, Oxman AD, Havelsrud K, Treweek S, Herrin J. Cluster randomised trial of tailored interventions to improve the management of urinary tract infections in women and sore throat. *BMJ* 2002;325:367-72.

82 Campbell MK, Fayers PM, Grimshaw JM. Determinants of the intracluster correlation coefficient in cluster randomized trials: the case of implementation research. *Clin Trials* 2005;2:99-107.

83 Turner RM, Thompson SG, Spiegelhalter DJ. Prior distributions for the intracluster correlation coefficient, based on multiple previous estimates, and their application in cluster randomized trials. *Clin Trials* 2005;2:108-18.

84 Adams G, Gulliford MC, Ukoumunne OC, Eldridge S, Chinn S, Campbell MJ. Patterns of intra-cluster correlation from primary care research to inform study design and analysis. *J Clin Epidemiol* 2004;57:785-94.

85 Taljaard M. Intracluster correlation coefficients from the 2005 WHO Global Survey on Maternal and Perinatal Health: implications for implementation research. *Paediatr Perinat Epidemiol* 2008;22:117-25.

86 Pagel C, Prost A, Lewycka S, Das S, Colbourn T, Mahapatra R, et al. Intracluster correlation coefficients and coefficients of variation for perinatal outcomes from five cluster-randomised controlled trials in low and middle-income countries: results and methodological implications. *Trials* 2011;12:151.

87 Moher M, Yudkin P, Wright L, Turner R, Fuller A, Schofield T, et al. Cluster randomised trial to compare three methods of promoting secondary prevention of coronary heart disease in primary care. *BMJ* 2001;322:1338-42.

88 Moher D, Turner L, Shamseer L, Plint A, Weeks L, Peters J, et al. The influence on CONSORT on the quality of RCTs: an updated review. *Clin Trials* 2011;8:485.

89 Piaggio G, Elbourne DR, Altman DG, Pocock SJ, Evans SJW. Reporting of noninferiority and equivalence randomized trials: an extension of the CONSORT statement. *JAMA* 2006;295:1152-60.

90 Hayes RJ, Bennett S. Simple sample size calculation for cluster-randomized trials. *Int J Epidemiol* 1999;28:319-26.

91 Thomson A, Hayes R, Cousens S. Measures of between-cluster variability in cluster randomized trials with binary outcomes. *Stat Med* 2009;28:1739-51.

92 Klar N, Donner A. The merits of matching in community intervention trials. *Stat Med* 1997;16:1753-64.

93 Eldridge SM, Ashby D, Feder GS. Informed patient consent to participation in cluster randomized trials: an empirical exploration of trials in primary care. *Clin Trials* 2005;2:91-8.

94 Farrin A, Russell I, Torgerson D, Underwood M. Differential recruitment in a cluster randomized trial in primary care: the experience of the UK back pain, exercise, active management and manipulation (UK BEAM) feasibility study. *Clin Trials* 2005;2:119-24.

95 Hutton J. Are distinctive ethical principles required for cluster randomised trials? In: Campbell MJ, Donner A, Elbourne D, eds. Design and analysis of cluster randomized trials. *Stat Med* 2001;20:473-88.

96 Hutton JL, Eccles MP, Grimshaw JM. Ethical issues in implementation research: a discussion of the problems in achieving informed consent. *Implement Sci* 2008;3:52.

97 Edwards SJ, Braunholtz DA, Lilford RJ, Stevens AJ. Ethical issues in the design and conduct of cluster randomised trials. *BMJ* 1999;318:1407-9.

98 Mazor KM, Sabin JE, Boudreau D, Goodman MJ, Gurwitz JH, Herrinton LJ, et al. Cluster randomized trials: opportunities and barriers identified by leaders of eight health plans. *Med Care* 2007;45(suppl 2):S29-37.

99 Zelen M. A new design for randomized clinical trials. *N Engl J Med* 1979;300:1242-5.

100 Zelen M. Randomized consent designs for clinical trials: an update. *Stat Med* 1990;9:645-56.

101 Snowdon C, Elbourne D, Garcia J. Zelen randomization: attitudes of parents participating in a neonatal clinical trial. *Control Clin Trials* 1999;20:149-71.

102 Mollison J, Simpson JA, Campbell MK, Grimshaw JM. Comparison of analytical methods for cluster randomised trials: an example from a primary care setting. *J Epidemiol Biostat* 2000;5:339-48.

103 Spiegelhalter DJ. Bayesian methods for cluster randomized trials with continuous response. *Stat Med* 2001;20:435-52.

104 Turner RM, Omar RZ, Thompson SG. Bayesian methods of analysis for cluster randomized trials with binary outcome data. *Stat Med* 2001;20:453-72.

105 Thompson SG, Warn DE, Turner RM. Bayesian methods for analysis of binary outcome data in cluster randomized trials on the absolute risk scale. *Stat Med* 2004;23:389-410.

106 Ioannidis JP, Evans SJ, Gotzsche PC, O'Neill RT, Altman DG, Schulz K, et al. Better reporting of harms in randomized trials: an extension of the CONSORT statement. *Ann Intern Med* 2004;141:781-8.

107 Feder G, Griffiths C, Eldridge S, Spence M. Effect of postal prompts to patients and general practitioners on the quality of primary care after a coronary event (POST): a randomised trial. *BMJ* 1999;318:1522-6.

108 Francis NA, Butler CC, Hood K, Simpson S, Wood F, Nuttall J. Effect of using an interactive booklet about childhood respiratory tract infections in primary care consultations on reconsulting and antibiotic prescribing: a cluster randomised controlled trial. *BMJ* 2009;339:b2885.

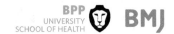

IDEAL framework for surgical innovation 1: the idea and development stages

Peter McCulloch, clinical reader in surgery[1], Jonathan A Cook, methodologist[2], Douglas G Altman, director[3], Carl Heneghan, reader in evidence based medicine[4], Markus K Diener, attending surgeon and director[5], On behalf of the IDEAL group

[1]Nuffield Department of Surgical Science, University of Oxford, Oxford, UK

[2]Health Services Research Unit, University of Aberdeen, Aberdeen, UK

[3]Centre for Statistics in Medicine, University of Oxford, UK

[4]Department of Public Health and Primary Care, University of Oxford, UK

[5]Study Centre of the German Surgical Society, Department of General, Visceral, and Transplantation Surgery, Heidelberg University, D-69120 Heidelberg, Germany

Correspondence to: M K Diener Markus.Diener@med.uni-heidelberg.de

Cite this as: *BMJ* 2013;346:f3012

http://www.bmj.com/content/346/bmj.f3012

ABSTRACT

IDEAL is a framework for evaluations of surgical innovations, which follow a distinct development pathway differing from the approach developed for pharmacological interventions. Many pathway and evaluation challenges are shared by other interventional therapies, requiring individual therapist skills and customisation of treatment to the individual, partly through medical devices. This paper provides an overview of the IDEAL framework and recommendations, and focuses on the first two stages: idea and development.

Introduction

Surgical innovations comprise new techniques, modified strategies, or innovative instruments. The evidence base for many of these approaches—and therefore for much of current surgical practice—is vastly weaker than for most modern drug treatments. Randomised trials of surgical techniques (versus placebo surgery)[1] were conducted within 10 years of the publication of the epochal streptomycin drug trial.[2] Yet, despite rapid growth in recent years, the overall number of randomised controlled trials and systematic reviews in surgical innovations remains small compared with the number of studies evaluating drug treatments. Randomised trials have also been few in number and of poor quality in some other therapeutic specialities, where the success of the intervention depends on the skill and judgment of the individual operator.[3]

The IDEAL Collaboration was born out of a series of conferences between surgeons and methodologists at Balliol College, Oxford,[4 5 6] which was convened to study why high quality trials in surgery were genuinely difficult to conduct, and what could be done to improve the evidence base for surgery. The conclusion was that innovation in surgery inevitably follows a pathway with important differences from that followed by pharmacological developments, and that a different approach to evaluation is therefore needed. It was noted that many non-surgical disciplines had similar problems with evaluation of such treatments (termed as "interventional therapies"), which rely on operator skill and tailoring of the intervention to the patient (for example, cardiac catheterisation, endoscopic techniques, or physiotherapy).

The IDEAL Collaboration developed a framework for the stages in surgical innovation (idea, development, exploration, assessment, and long term study; table) and a set of recommendations on how evaluation should be conducted at each stage (box 1). The collaboration also proposed how the environment for surgical research could be improved by editors, regulators, funders, and professional societies. An open international collaborative group has been developed to explore these issues further.[7] Recent concerns over hip resurfacing techniques[8] and breast implants[9] have raised serious questions about how medical devices are evaluated, and there has been considerable interest in applying the IDEAL framework to this problem, since many difficulties in evaluating device innovation mirror those in surgery innovation. In this series of three articles, we explain the problems and discuss proposed solutions put forward in the IDEAL recommendations, using current examples. This first article in the series focuses on the first two stages of the IDEAL framework: idea and development.

Idea (IDEAL stage 1)

Surgical innovations can arise from careful planning and laboratory studies, from necessity created by an emergency, or even by accident. Advances in technology and related devices may make new or substantially different procedures feasible (such as robotic surgery). Planned and unplanned innovations can also occur out of desperation, in situations where the prognosis seems otherwise hopeless (for example, abbreviated "damage control" surgery for major combined vascular and visceral injury[10]). More measured innovation could represent an incremental advance, where the new procedure is a small variant on an older one. Innovations can also be completely novel, and be taken through to clinical trials via a carefully planned research programme, such as the recent successful advances in transplant surgery.[11]

What should a surgeon do if they believe that they have invented or developed something new and different, or if—in the case of industry driven research—they have used a new device in humans for the first time? The answer has two parts: surgeons can report what they have done, and then evaluate the intervention. Because first-in-man studies, by their nature, deal with single cases or a small number of cases, study design considerations might be largely irrelevant; but how they are reported is important. We can develop basic principles using the three

SUMMARY POINTS

- Innovations in surgery have several features that make scientific evaluation challenging, such as an early phase of rapid modification, learning curve, and strong therapist preferences

- The IDEAL framework describes five stages of development and evaluation for surgical and interventional innovations: idea, development, exploration, assessment, and long term study

- The IDEAL recommendations identify design and reporting ideas that could help in dealing with specific problems at each stage in the framework

- At stage 1 (idea), accuracy, transparency, and completeness of reporting are key elements. Recommendations include standardisation of reports and development of an open access database for lodging reports of first-in-man procedures

- At stage 2a (development), innovations are in a state of flux, undergoing modifications and changes in indication. Prospective studies with comprehensive sequential reporting of changes to technique and indication are recommended, together with standardisation of terminology

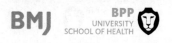

pillars of the modern framework of medical ethics: utility, beneficence, and non-maleficence.[12] Surgeons should have the opportunity of learning from each other's experiences, particularly if this helps their patients or avoids them being harmed. Therefore, surgeons have an ethical obligation to share experiences with colleagues. Further, they need to convey sufficient information about what was done and what the consequences were, so that specialist colleagues can understand how to reproduce their success or avoid their failure.

All first-in-man interventions (whether a new procedure or new use of a device) should be included in an open access registry recording key details of the innovation. This registry would facilitate information searches in the published literature, which surgeons should carry out before embarking on a planned first-in-man intervention.[13] Box 2 provides an example of a study at the idea stage. The use of a new innovation, particularly if it is the first use of the innovation at the surgeon's institution, should have some form of independent oversight by those responsible for local clinical governance. Consent for new procedures is important: patients contemplating whether to undergo such procedures must fully understand their experimental nature, and the uncertainty that therefore surrounds any estimates of risk. If patient incapacity or time urgency prevents informed consent, governance authorities and patients' relatives or advocates may need to reach an agreement by discussion, even for retrospective cases. Therefore, hospitals would need systems that allow the right mix of clinical and ethical expertise to be bought to bear rapidly, and outside of normal hours if necessary.

Although surgeons may not need much incentive to report their successful innovations, it is arguably just as important to formally record their unsuccessful ideas or initial failures, to avoid unnecessary repetition by others. For this reason, the IDEAL recommendations include registration of all first-in-man procedures, with the suggestion that anonymous reporting might be permitted. In principle, anonymous reporting of harms or "near misses" might be desirable, but it has serious ethical, practical, and legal difficulties. If reporting is truly anonymous, how can spam or deliberately misleading reports be screened out? On the other hand, if identification of the author is possible in principle, legal discovery attempts and claims for compensation are a near certainty. The unique nature of new procedures might also make it difficult to maintain patient confidentiality. To allow surgeons to report their unsuccessful first-in-man efforts with confidence, a legal framework may be required, supported by the relevant governance and professional bodies to protect surgeons from compensation claims, provided that oversight and informed consent have been satisfactory.

Development (IDEAL stage 2a)

The IDEAL development stage begins once surgeons start to plan a series of procedures using a new technique or device (table). Innovations are especially fluid in this phase; innovations undergo rapid iterative change in the light of experience. Therefore, it is the development stage that most clearly differentiates the pathway for surgery innovation from that for pharmaceutical innovations. In both a scientific and ethical sense, development is the most problematic of the stages, and as a result is often poorly reported.

Experience often makes the need for modification obvious after only a few repetitions, although surgeons are insecure about the logical and ethical justification for making changes on the basis of scarce data that are not definitive. It is therefore tempting for authors to wait until the development stage has ended, and then report the initial results as if the final version of the technique had been used in all cases. This strategy is adopted in the classic retrospective surgical case series, and is deeply problematic. Obscuring details

TABLE IDEAL framework

Stage 1: Idea	Stage 2a: Development	Stage 2b: Exploration	Stage 3: Assessment	Stage 4: Long term study
Question				
Can the procedure or device achieve a specific physical or physiological goal?	What is the optimal technique or design, and for which patients does it work best?	What are the outcomes of more widespread use? Can consensus equipoise be reached on a trial question?	How well does the procedure work compared with current standards of care?	What are the long term effects and outcomes of the procedure?
Aim				
Proof of concept	Safety, efficacy	Efficacy	Comparative effectiveness	Quality assurance
Patient base				
Single to few	10s	100s	100s+	100s+
Optimal study design(s)				
First-in-man study; structured case report	Prospective development study	Prospective collaborative observational study (Phase IIS) or feasibility randomised controlled trial (or both)	Randomised controlled trial	Observational study or randomised trial nested within a comprehensive disease based registry
Example of procedure at this stage				
Stem cell based tracheal transplant for tracheal stenosis[2]	Peroral endoscopic myotomy for oesophageal achalasia	Single incision laparoscopy for abdominal surgery	Minimally invasive oesophagectomy	Banding and bypass surgery for morbid obesity

---

BOX 1 RECOMMENDATIONS FOR STUDIES IN STAGES 1 (IDEA) AND 2 (DEVELOPMENT)

Idea

- Mandatory registry for interventions thought to be first in man, with anonymous reporting option
- Protocols pre-registered on the above mandatory registry, for planned research programmes on a first-in-man intervention
- Development and use of agreed reporting standards and definitions for key outcomes and modifying factors

Development

- Prospective development studies, with pre-published protocol and consecutive cases
- Publication of findings, including transparent reporting of changes in technique or device design and indication

---

BOX 2 EXAMPLE OF STUDY AT IDEA STAGE 1

Stem cell tracheal transplant (based on reference 11)

Clinical background at the time of conduct

- Loss of an airway is debilitating and replacement is difficult
- A stem cell graft embedded in a framework constructed using a de-antigenised collagen matrix may overcome current limitations

Design

- Staged programme of multidisciplinary research beginning with detailed preclinical studies
- Explicit clinical and data collection protocol written in advance and submitted for ethical review
- Detailed informed consent process
- Oversight provided by multiple agencies

Findings

- Replacement using stem cell tracheal graft is feasible and a good early outcome is achievable
- No sign of rejection was achieved without the need for immunosuppressive drugs

that authors may not wish to report deprives others of the opportunity to learn from the development process, and can provide a misleading picture of the use of a procedure or device. Authors obscuring changes in eligibility, which naturally occur during development, in order to make it appear predetermined is similarly unhelpful. If the patients undergoing a technique are different at the beginning and end of a reported series, the aggregate outcome might not indicate much about what can be expected from using the final version of the technique in the patient group that trial and error has shown to be most suited to it.

Judgments about success or failure at this stage may be made on the basis of short term outcome measures that might not reflect the most important effects of the procedure, and frequently the data are insufficient to allow any meaningful statistical analysis (even if available data are maximised[14]). A cancer operation or a new artificial joint might seem successful at this stage because recovery from the surgery is quick or complications few, but subsequent data about survival rates or function in the long term may reverse these impressions. One may reasonably question the value of reporting such unreliable figures, but the alternative may be waiting many years for the results of definitive trials—which are unlikely to be undertaken without some pilot data. The pressure to innovate and improve is such that funders, patients, and clinical colleagues expect to be updated on the promise of innovations as rapidly as possible, in order to make decisions about funding, treatment, or use. If such decisions are to be made regardless (which seems a reasonable assumption barring a radical change in how health provision is organised internationally), they should at least be made using the most complete and accurate information available. The key principle, therefore, is transparency.

The IDEAL recommendations recognise that at the development stage, a randomised trial is often operationally undesirable and scientifically of limited use, owing to procedural modifications and varying eligibility. IDEAL supports prospective rather than retrospective studies at this stage, with sequential reporting of all cases and outcomes without omissions, and with clear explanations of when and how technique, design, or indications were changed. Sequential presentation of results might also reveal the effects of operator learning curves, which have an even more important role in the next stage of exploration. To ensure full reporting of relevant outcomes, the prior publication of a protocol at the outset of this type of study would be helpful. The United States Food and Drug Administration, which has been re-evaluating the regulatory framework for implantable devices since the Institute of Medicine report of 2011,[15] has put forward proposals for early studies of innovative devices that closely follow this model, which is encouraging.

The prospective development studies recommended by the IDEAL Collaboration represent a new type of observational study, which will no doubt change and evolve, but examples of this kind of study are now beginning to appear.[16 17] Key elements are a prior protocol, clearly defined objective outcomes, and transparent sequential reporting of cases, showing when changes in indication or technique are made. Data from this type of study will be more reliable and valid than information obtained from retrospective series, although retrospective data require much less effort and planning. We therefore suggest that for techniques and devices in the development stage, journals positively discriminate in favour of prospective studies, and should cease to accept studies based on retrospective data except when it can convincingly be shown that no viable alternative exists.

A much needed, important parallel improvement is the development of international standards for reporting surgical outcomes and contextual factors. Reports that use a common terminology and taxonomy are much more useful than those in which a plethora of definitions of the key data sow confusion and doubt. Groups such as COMET[18] and the Zurich group responsible for the Dindo-Clavien classification of complications[19] have made an important contribution to standardising this language, but further work is still needed. Many specialist endpoints will be best defined by consensus among the specialist community, and specialist societies and journals should work together to standardise terminology in their area of interest. Box 3 shows key outcomes and contextual factors that will need general agreement across the international surgical community. This agreement will need a concerted effort from international societies, national professional bodies, and leading journals, but research funders could also help by insisting on the use of standardised terms in funding applications.

Discussion

Early evaluations of a surgical innovation face common challenges; however, these difficulties must not prevent such studies being conducted. Current practices of study design and reporting are suboptimal and need upgrading. In particular, meaningful reporting of first-in-man cases should become routine (irrespective of the findings). Studies in the development stage need to be prospective, based on consecutive case reporting, and need to be open about the changes in indication, technique, and use of equipment that occur as experience is gained. Studies in the development stage also need a rapid, flexible, and expert system of governance to make decisions about whether to permit new procedures or devices to go ahead, and particularly about whether these new interventions can be modified, as is typical during this stage. Research ethics committees and device regulatory bodies could help by requiring a declaration of the IDEAL stage that the investigators feel the device or procedure has reached, with supporting evidence. Innovations in the idea stage would then be expected to lead to proposals for a prospective development study.

Modifications of interventions are a problem because of their likely frequency and the need for a rapid and ethical response. This task could be delegated to hospitals and universities, because more centralised bodies would be unable to gather information and respond appropriately in a realistic timescale. It would be sensible for existing structures to take on this role, in addition to their other functions, rather than to set up a new infrastructure. In the United Kingdom, trusts each have a committee to review

---

BOX 3 COMMON ITEMS FOR WHICH AGREED STANDARD DEFINITIONS ARE NEEDED

Contextual factors
- Grading of patient risk factors
- Severity grading of comorbid pathology or general health
- Scale of surgical insult
- Urgency status of procedure
- Environment for surgery (hospital or unit type)

Outcomes
- Grading of functional performance
- Scope and severity of complications

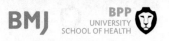

proposals for procedures that are new to the trust, which would be the obvious body to prepare such a response. It is essential that the body responsible for providing an ethical opinion abides by certain principles to maintain an appropriate balance between fostering innovation and protecting current patients. Such considerations include developing sensible standards for documentation, reporting, and patient consent procedures; ensuring oversight of the committee itself; and ensuring access to suitable expert advice. Professional societies and bodies, healthcare institutions, and national regulatory agencies can all contribute towards better surgical research.

Summary

Early evaluations of a surgical innovation (whether an operation, invasive procedure, or use of a medical device) face a common set of difficulties, related principally to the need to modify and redefine the intervention and indication during evaluation. The IDEAL recommendations propose abandonment of retrospective case series, and instead recommend adoption of mandatory registration of first-in-man reporting, standardisation of reporting, and use of prospective study designs. Current regulatory and ethical governance structures need to be refined to facilitate an appropriate balance between fostering innovation and protecting patients.

Contributors: JAC and PM formulated the IDEAL series to which this paper belongs. PM wrote the first draft of this paper and MKD, JAC, CH, and DGA all commented on the draft. All authors approved the final version, and PM is the guarantor. The papers were informed by discussions during the IDEAL group in December 2010.

IDEAL workshop participants (December 2010): Doug Altman, Jeff Aronson, David Beard, Jane Blazeby, Bruce Campbell, Andrew Carr, Tammy Clifford, Jonathan Cook, Pierre Dagenais, Philipp Dahm, Peter Davidson, Hugh Davies, Markus K Diener, Jonothan Earnshaw, Patrick Ergina, Shamiram Feinglass, Trish Groves, Sion Glyn-Jones, Muir Gray, Alison Halliday, Judith Hargreaves, Carl Heneghan, Jo Carol Hiatt, Sean Kehoe, Nicola Lennard, Georgios Lyratzopoulos, Guy Maddern, Danica Marinac-Dabic, Peter McCulloch, Jon Nicholl, Markus Ott, Art Sedrakyan, Dan Schaber, Frank Schuller, Bill Summerskill.

Funding: The IDEAL group meeting in December 2010 was funded by the National Institute for Health Research's Health Technology Assessment programme, Johnson & Johnson, Medtronic, and Zimmer (all unrestricted grants). JAC holds a Medical Research Council Methodology Fellowship (G1002292).

Competing interests: All authors have completed the ICMJE uniform disclosure form at www.icmje.org/coi_disclosure.pdf and declare: PM received financial support from the National Institute for Health Research's Health Technology Assessment programme, Johnson & Johnson, Medtronic, and Zimmer for the IDEAL collaboration and for a workshop; PM and JC received support for travel to the US from the FDA to attend a seminar on IDEAL; no other financial relationships with any organisations that might have an interest in the submitted work in the previous three years; no other relationships or activities that could appear to have influenced the submitted work.

Peer review and provenance: Not commissioned; externally peer reviewed.

1 Cobb LA, Thomas GI, Dillard DH, Meredino KA, Bruce RA. An evaluation of internal mammary artery ligation by a double-blind technic. N Engl J Med 1959;260:1115-8.

2 Streptomycin in Tuberculosis Trials Committee. Streptomycin treatment of pulmonary tuberculosis. A Medical Research Council investigation. BMJ 1948;2:769-82.

3 Wente MN, Seiler CM, Uhl W, Büchler MW. Perspectives of evidence-based surgery. Dig Surg 2003;20:263-9.

4 Barkun JS, Aronson JK, Feldman LS, Maddern GJ, Strasberg SM; Balliol Collaboration, et al. Evaluation and stages of surgical innovations. Lancet 2009;374:1089-96.

5 Ergina PL, Cook JA, Blazeby JM, Boutron I, Clavien PA, Reeves BC, et al. Challenges in evaluating surgical innovation. Lancet 2009;374:1097-104.

6 McCulloch P, Altman DG, Campbell WB, Flum DR, Glasziou P, Marshall JC, et al. No surgical innovation without evaluation: the IDEAL recommendations. Lancet 2009;374:1105-12.

7 IDEAL Collaboration. Home page. 2013. www.ideal-collaboration.net/.

8 Graves SE, Rothwell A, Tucker K, Jacobs JJ, Sedrakyan A. A multinational assessment of metal-on metal bearings in hip replacement. J Bone Joint Surg Am 2011;93(suppl 3):43-7.

9 O'Dowd A. French women to have PIP breast implants removed for free. BMJ 2011;343:d8329.

10 Rotondo MF, Schwab CW, McGonigal MD, Phillips GR 3rd, Fruchterman TM, Kauder DR, et al. 'Damage control': an approach for improved survival in exsanguinating penetrating abdominal injury. J Trauma 1993;35:375-82.

11 Macchiarini P, Jungebluth P, Go T, Asnaghi MA, Rees LE, Cogan TA, et al. Clinical transplantation of a tissue-engineered airway. Lancet 2008;372:2023-30.

12 Gillon R. Doctors and patients. Br Med J (Clin Res Ed) 1986;292:466-9.

13 Clarke M, Hopewell S, Chalmers I. Reports of clinical trials should begin and end with up-to-date systematic reviews of other relevant evidence: a status report. J R Soc Med 2007;100:187-90.

14 Lilford RJ, Thornton JG, Braunholtz D. Clinical trials and rare diseases: a way out of a conundrum. BMJ 1995;311:1621-5.

15 Institute of Medicine. Medical devices and the public's health: the FDA's 510(k) clearance process at 35 years. National Academies Press, 2011.

16 Blazeby JM, Blencowe NS, Titcomb DR, Metcalfe C, Hollowood AD, Barham CP. Demonstration of the IDEAL recommendations for evaluating and reporting surgical innovation in minimally invasive oesophagectomy. Br J Surg 2011;98:544-51.

17 Ahmed HU, Hindley RG, Dickinson L, Freeman A, Kirkham AP, Sahu M, et al. Focal therapy for localised unifocal and multifocal prostate cancer: a prospective development study. Lancet Oncol 2012;13:622-32.

18 Comet Initiative. Home page. 2013. www.comet-initiative.org/.

19 Dindo D, Demartines N, Clavien PA. Classification of surgical complications: a new proposal with evaluation in a cohort of 6336 patients and results of a survey. Ann Surg 2004;240:205-13.

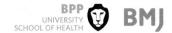

Developing and evaluating complex interventions: the new Medical Research Council guidance

Peter Craig, programme manager[1], Paul Dieppe, professor[2], Sally Macintyre, director[3], Susan Michie, professor[4], Irwin Nazareth, director[5], Mark Petticrew, professor[6]

[1]MRC Population Health Sciences Research Network, Glasgow G12 8RZ

[2]Nuffield Department of Orthopaedic Surgery, University of Oxford, Nuffield Orthopaedic Centre, Oxford OX3 7LD

[3]MRC Social and Public Health Sciences Unit, Glasgow G12 8RZ

[4]Centre for Outcomes Research and Effectiveness, University College London, London WC1E 7HB

[5]MRC General Practice Research Framework, London NW1 2ND

[6]Public and Environmental Health Research Unit, Department of Public Health and Policy, London School of Hygiene and Tropical Medicine, London WC1E 7HT

Cite this as: BMJ 2008;337:a1655

http://www.bmj.com/content/337/bmj.a1655

ABSTRACT

Evaluating complex interventions is complicated. The Medical Research Council's evaluation framework (2000) brought welcome clarity to the task. Now the council has updated its guidance

Complex interventions are widely used in the health service, in public health practice, and in areas of social policy that have important health consequences, such as education, transport, and housing. They present various problems for evaluators, in addition to the practical and methodological difficulties that any successful evaluation must overcome. In 2000, the Medical Research Council (MRC) published a framework[1] to help researchers and research funders to recognise and adopt appropriate methods. The framework has been highly influential, and the accompanying *BMJ* paper is widely cited.[2] However, much valuable experience has since accumulated of both conventional and more innovative methods. This has now been incorporated in comprehensively revised and updated guidance recently released by the MRC (www.mrc.ac.uk/complexinterventionsguidance). In this article we summarise the issues that prompted the revision and the key messages of the new guidance.

Revisiting the 2000 MRC framework

As experience of evaluating complex interventions has accumulated since the 2000 framework was published, interest in the methodology has also grown. Several recent papers have identified limitations in the framework, recommending, for example, greater attention to early phase piloting and development work,[3] a less linear model of evaluation process,[4] integration of process and outcome evaluation,[5] recognition that complex interventions may work best if they are tailored to local contexts rather than completely standardised,[6] and greater use of the insights provided by the theory of complex adaptive systems.[7]

A workshop held by the MRC Population Health Sciences Research Network to consider whether and how the framework should be updated likewise recommended the inclusion of a model of the evaluation process less closely to tied to the phases of drug development; more guidance on how to approach the development, reporting, and implementation of complex interventions; and greater attention to the contexts in which interventions take place. It further recommended consideration of alternatives to randomised trials, and of highly complex or non-health sector interventions to which biomedical methods may not be applicable, and more evidence and examples to back up and illustrate the recommendations. The new guidance addresses these issues in depth, and here we set out the key messages.

What are complex interventions?

Complex interventions are usually described as interventions that contain several interacting components, but they have other characteristics that evaluators should take into account (box 1). There is no sharp boundary between simple and complex interventions. Few interventions are truly simple, but the number of components and range of effects may vary widely. Some highly complex interventions, such as the Sure Start intervention to support families with young children in deprived communities,[8] may comprise a set of individually complex interventions.

How these characteristics are dealt with will depend on the aims of the evaluation. A key question in evaluating complex interventions is whether they are effective in everyday practice (box 2).[9] It is therefore important to understand the whole range of effects and how they vary, for example, among recipients or between sites. A second key question in evaluating complex interventions is how the intervention works: what are the active ingredients and how are they exerting their effect? Answers to this kind of question are needed to design more effective interventions and apply them appropriately across group and setting.[10]

Development, evaluation, and implementation

The 2000 framework characterised the process of development through to implementation of a complex intervention in terms of the phases of drug development. Although it is useful to think in terms of phases, in practice these may not follow a linear or even a cyclical sequence (figure 1).[4]

Best practice is to develop interventions systematically, using the best available evidence and appropriate theory, then to test them using a carefully phased approach, starting with a series of pilot studies targeted at each of the key uncertainties in the design, and moving on to an exploratory and then a definitive evaluation. The results

SUMMARY POINTS

- The Medical Research Council guidance for the evaluation of complex interventions has been revised and updated
- The process of developing and evaluating a complex intervention has several phases, although they may not follow a linear sequence
- Experimental designs are preferred to observational designs in most circumstances, but are not always practicable
- Understanding processes is important but does not replace evaluation of outcomes
- Complex interventions may work best if tailored to local circumstances rather than being completely standardised
- Reports of studies should include a detailed description of the intervention to enable replication, evidence synthesis, and wider implementation

should be disseminated as widely and persuasively as possible, with further research to assist and monitor the process of implementation.

In practice, evaluation takes place in a wide range of settings that constrain researchers' choice of interventions to evaluate and their choice of evaluation methods. Ideas for complex interventions emerge from various sources, which may greatly affect how much leeway the researcher has to modify the intervention, to influence the way it is implemented, or to adopt an ideal evaluation design.[8] Evaluation may take place alongside large scale implementation, rather than starting beforehand. Strong evidence may be ignored or weak evidence taken up, depending on its political acceptability or fit with other ideas about what works.[11]

Researchers need to consider carefully the trade-off between the importance of the intervention and the value of the evidence that can be gathered given these constraints. In an evaluation of the health impact of a social intervention, such as a programme of housing improvement, the researcher may have no say in what the intervention consists of and little influence over how or when the programme is implemented, limiting the scope to undertake development work or to determine allocation. Experimental methods are becoming more widely accepted as methods to evaluate policy,[12] but there may be political or ethical objections to using them to assess health effects, especially if the intervention provides important non-health benefits.[13] Given the cost of such interventions, evaluation should still be considered—the best available methods, even if they are not optimal in terms of internal validity, may yield useful results.[14]

If non-experimental methods are used, researchers should be aware of their limitations and interpret and present the findings with due caution. Wherever possible, evidence should be combined from different sources that do not share the same weaknesses.[15] Researchers should be prepared to explain to decision makers the need for adequate development work, the pros and cons of experimental and non-experimental approaches, and the trade-offs involved in settling for weaker methods. They should be prepared to challenge decision makers when interventions of uncertain effectiveness are being implemented in a way that would make strengthening the evidence through a rigorous evaluation difficult, or when a modification of the implementation strategy would open up the possibility of a much more informative evaluation.

Developing a complex intervention

Identifying existing evidence—Before a substantial evaluation is undertaken, the intervention must be developed to the point where it can reasonably be expected to have a worthwhile effect. The first step is to identify what is already known about similar interventions and the methods that have been used to evaluate them. If there is no recent, high quality systematic review of the relevant evidence, one should be conducted and updated as the evaluation proceeds.

Identifying and developing theory—The rationale for a complex intervention, the changes that are expected, and how change is to be achieved may not be clear at the outset. A key early task is to develop a theoretical understanding of the likely process of change by drawing on existing evidence and theory, supplemented if necessary by new primary research. This should be done whether the researcher is developing the intervention or evaluating one that has already been developed.

Modelling process and outcomes—Modelling a complex intervention before a full scale evaluation can provide important information about the design of both the intervention and the evaluation. A series of studies may be required to progressively refine the design before embarking on a full scale evaluation. Developers of a trial of physical activity to prevent type 2 diabetes adopted a causal modelling approach that included a range of primary and desk based studies to design the intervention, identify suitable measures, and predict long term outcomes.[3] Another useful approach is a prior economic evaluation.[16] This may identify weaknesses and lead to refinements, or even show that a full scale evaluation is unwarranted. A modelling exercise to prepare for a trial of falls prevention in elderly people showed that the proposed system of screening and referral was highly unlikely to be cost effective and informed the decision not to proceed with the trial.[17]

Assessing feasibility

Evaluations are often undermined by problems of acceptability, compliance, delivery of the intervention, recruitment and retention, and smaller than expected effect sizes that could have been predicted by thorough piloting.[18] A feasibility study for an evaluation of an adolescent sexual health intervention in rural Zimbabwe found that the planned classroom based programme was inappropriate, given cultural norms, teaching styles, and relationships between teachers and pupils in the country, and it was replaced by a community based programme.[19] As well as

---

BOX 1 WHAT MAKES AN INTERVENTION COMPLEX?

- Number of interacting components within the experimental and control interventions
- Number and difficulty of behaviours required by those delivering or receiving the intervention
- Number of groups or organisational levels targeted by the intervention
- Number and variability of outcomes
- Degree of flexibility or tailoring of the intervention permitted

---

BOX 2 DEVELOPING AND EVALUATING COMPLEX STUDIES

- A good theoretical understanding is needed of how the intervention causes change, so that weak links in the causal chain can be identified and strengthened
- Lack of effect may reflect implementation failure (or teething problems) rather than genuine ineffectiveness; a thorough process evaluation is needed to identify implementation problems
- Variability in individual level outcomes may reflect higher level processes; sample sizes may need to be larger to take account of the extra variability and cluster randomised designs considered
- A single primary outcome may not make best use of the data; a range of measures will be needed and unintended consequences picked up where possible
- Ensuring strict standardisation may be inappropriate; the intervention may work better if a specified degree of adaptation to local settings is allowed for in the protocol

---

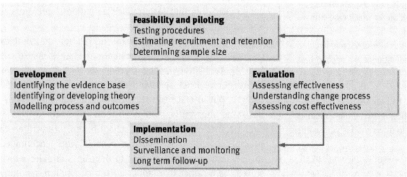

Fig 1 Key elements of the development and evaluation process

illustrating the value of feasibility testing, the example shows the importance of understanding the context in which interventions take place.

A pilot study need not be a scale model of the planned evaluation but should examine the key uncertainties that have been identified during development. Pilot studies for a trial of free home insulation suggested that attrition might be high, so the design was amended such that participants in the control group received the intervention after the study.[20] Pilot study results should be interpreted cautiously when making assumptions about the numbers required when the evaluation is scaled up. Effects may be smaller or more variable and response rates lower when the intervention is rolled out across a wider range of settings.

Evaluating a complex intervention

There are many study designs to choose from, and different designs suit different questions and circumstances. Researchers should beware of blanket statements about what designs are suitable for what kind of intervention and choose on the basis of specific characteristics of the study, such as expected effect size and likelihood of selection or allocation bias. Awareness of the whole range of experimental and non-experimental approaches should lead to more appropriate methodological choices.

BOX 3 EXPERIMENTAL DESIGNS FOR EVALUATING COMPLEX INTERVENTIONS

Individually randomised trials—Individuals are randomly allocated to receive either an experimental intervention or an alternative such as standard treatment, a placebo, or remaining on a waiting list. Such trials are sometimes dismissed as inapplicable to complex interventions, but there are many variants, and often solutions can be found to the technical and ethical problems associated with randomisation

Cluster randomised trials are one solution to the problem of contamination of the control group, leading to biased estimates of effect size, in trials of population level interventions. Groups such as patients in a general practice or tenants in a housing scheme are randomly allocated to the experimental or control intervention

Stepped wedge designs may be used to overcome practical or ethical objections to experimentally evaluating an intervention for which there is some evidence of effectiveness or which cannot be made available to the whole population at once. It allows a trial to be conducted without delaying roll-out of the intervention. Eventually, the whole population receives the intervention, but with randomisation built into the phasing of implementation

Preference trials and randomised consent designs—Practical or ethical obstacles to randomisation can sometimes be overcome by using non-standard designs. When patients have strong preferences among treatments, basing treatment allocation on patients' preferences or randomising patients before seeking consent may be appropriate.

N of 1 designs—Conventional trials aim to estimate the average effect of an intervention in a population. N of 1 trials, in which individuals undergo interventions with the order or scheduling decided at random, can be used to assess between and within person change and to investigate theoretically predicted mediators of that change

---

BOX 4 CHOOSING BETWEEN RANDOMISED AND NON-RANDOMISED DESIGNS

Size and timing of effects—Randomisation may be unnecessary if the effects of the intervention are so large or immediate that confounding or underlying trends are unlikely to explain differences in outcomes before and after exposure. It may be inappropriate—for example, on grounds of cost or delay—if the changes are very small or take a long time to appear. In these circumstances a non-randomised design may be the only feasible option, in which case firm conclusions about the impact of the intervention may be unattainable

Likelihood of selection bias—Randomisation is needed if exposure to the intervention is likely to be associated with other factors that influence outcomes. Post-hoc adjustment is a second best solution; its effectiveness is limited by errors in the measurement of the confounding variables and the difficulty of dealing with unknown or unmeasured confounders

Feasibility and acceptability of experimentation—Randomisation may be impractical if the intervention is already in widespread use, or if key decisions about how it will be implemented have already been taken, as is often the case with policy changes and interventions whose effect on health is secondary to their main purpose

Cost—If an experimental study is feasible and would provide more reliable information than an observational study but would also cost more, the additional cost should be weighed against the value of having better information

---

Assessing effectiveness

Randomisation should always be considered because it is the most robust method of preventing selection bias. If a conventional parallel group randomised trial is not appropriate, other randomised designs should be considered (box 3).

If an experimental approach is not feasible, because the intervention is irreversible, necessarily applies to the whole population, or because large scale implementation is already under way, a quasi-experimental or an observational design may be considered. In some circumstances, randomisation may be unnecessary and other designs preferable,[21] [22] but the conditions under which observational methods can yield reliable estimates of effect are limited (box 4).[23] Successful examples, such as the evaluation of legislation to restrict access to means of suicide,[24] reduce air pollution,[25] or ban smoking in public places,[26] tend to occur where interventions have rapid, large effects.

Measuring outcomes

Researchers need to decide which outcomes are most important, which are secondary, and how they will deal with multiple outcomes in the analysis. A single primary outcome and a small number of secondary outcomes are the most straightforward for statistical analysis but may not represent the best use of the data or provide an adequate assessment of the success or otherwise of an intervention that has effects across a range of domains. It is important also to consider which sources of variation in outcomes matter and to plan appropriate subgroup analyses.

Long term follow-up may be needed to determine whether outcomes predicted by interim or surrogate measures do occur or whether short term changes persist. Although uncommon, such studies can be highly informative. Evaluation of a preschool programme for disadvantaged children showed that, as well as improved educational attainment, there was a range of economic and social benefits at ages 27 and 40.[27]

Understanding processes

Process evaluations, which explore the way in which the intervention under study is implemented, can provide valuable insight into why an intervention fails or has unexpected consequences, or why a successful intervention works and how it can be optimised. A process evaluation nested inside a trial can be used to assess fidelity and quality of implementation, clarify causal mechanisms, and identify contextual factors associated with variation in outcomes.[5] However, it is not a substitute for evaluation of outcomes. A process evaluation[28] carried out in connection with a trial of educational visits to encourage general practitioners to follow prescribing guidelines[29] found that the visits were well received and recall of the guidelines was good, yet there was little change in prescribing behaviour, which was constrained by other factors such as patients' preferences and local hospital policy.

Fidelity is not straightforward in relation to complex interventions.[30] In some evaluations, such as those seeking to identify active ingredients within a complex intervention, strict standardisation may be required and controls put in place to limit variation in implementation.[31] But some interventions are designed to be adapted to local circumstances. In a trial of a school based intervention to promote health and wellbeing, schools were encouraged to use a standardised process to develop strategies which suited them rather than adopt a fixed curriculum, resulting in widely varied practice between schools.[32] The key is to be clear about how much change or adaptation is permissible and to record variations in implementation so that fidelity can be assessed in relation the degree of standardisation required by the study protocol.

Variability in implementation, preplanned or otherwise, makes it important that both process and outcome evaluations are reported fully and that a clear description of the intervention is provided to enable replication and synthesis of evidence.[33] This has been a weakness of the reporting of complex intervention studies in the past,[34] but the availability of a comprehensive range of reporting guidelines, now covering non-drug trials[35] and observational studies[36] and accessible through a single website (www. equator-network.org) should lead to improvement.

Conclusions

We recognise that many issues surrounding evaluation of complex interventions are still debated, that methods will continue to develop, and that practical applications will be found for some of the newer theories. We do not intend the revised guidance to be prescriptive but to help researchers, funders, and other decision makers to make appropriate methodological and practical choices. We have primarily aimed our messages at researchers, but publishers, funders, and commissioners of research also have an important part to play. Journal editors should insist on high and consistent standards of reporting. Research funders should be prepared to support developmental studies before large scale evaluations. The key message for policy makers is the need to consider evaluation requirements in the planning of new initiatives, and wherever possible to allow for an experimental or a high quality non-experimental approach to the evaluation of initiatives when there is uncertainty about their effectiveness.

Contributors: PD had the idea of revising and updating the MRC framework. It was further developed at a workshop co-convened with Sally Macintyre and Janet Darbyshire, and organised with the help of Linda Morris on 15-16 May 2006. Workshop participants and others with an interest in the evaluation of complex interventions were invited to comment on a draft of the revised guidance, which was also reviewed by members of the MRC Health Services and Public Health Research Board and MRC Methodology Research Panel. A full list of all those who contributed suggestions is provided in the full guidance document.

Funding: MRC Health Services and Public Health Research Board and the MRC Population Health Sciences Research Network.

Competing interests: None declared.

Provenance and peer review: Not commissioned; externally peer reviewed.

1 Medical Research Council. *A framework for the development and evaluation of RCTs for complex interventions to improve health.* London: MRC, 2000.

2 Campbell M, Fitzpatrick R, Haines A, Kinmonth AL, Sandercock P, Spiegelhalter D, et al. Framework for the design and evaluation of complex interventions to improve health. *BMJ* 2000;321:694-6.

3 Hardeman W, Sutton S, Griffin S, Johnston M, White A, Wareham NJ, et al. A causal modelling approach to the development of theory-based behaviour change programmes for trial evaluation. *Health Educ Res* 2005;20:676-87.

4 Campbell NC, Murray E, Darbyshire J, Emery J, Farmer A, Griffiths F, et al. Designing and evaluating complex interventions to improve health care. *BMJ* 2007;334:455-9.

5 Oakley A, Strange V, Bonell C, Allen E, Stephenson J, Ripple Study Team. Process evaluation in randomised controlled trials of complex interventions. *BMJ* 2006;332:413-6.

6 Campbell M, Donner A, Klar N. Developments in cluster randomised trials and Statistics in Medicine. *Stat Med* 2007;26:2-19.

7 Shiell A, Hawe P, Gold L. Complex interventions or complex systems? Implications for health economic evaluation. *BMJ* 2008;336:1281-3.

8 Belsky J, Melhuish E, Barnes J, Leyland AH, Romaniuk H, National Evaluation of Sure Start Research Team. Effects of Sure Start local programmes on children and families: early findings from a quasi-experimental, cross sectional study. *BMJ* 2006;332:1476-81.

9 Haynes B. Can it work? Does it work? Is it worth it? The testing of healthcare interventions is evolving. *BMJ* 1999;319:652-3.

10 Michie S, Abraham C. Interventions to change health behaviours: evidence-based or evidence-inspired? *Psychol Health* 2004;19:29-49.

11 Muir H. Let science rule: the rational way to run societies. *New Scientist* 2008;198:40-3.

12 Creegan C, Hedges A. *Towards a policy evaluation service: developing infrastructure to support the use of experimental and quasi-experimental methods* . London: Ministry of Justice, 2007.

13 Thomson H, Hoskins R, Petticrew M, Ogilvie D, Craig N, Quinn T, et al. Evaluating the health effects of social interventions. *BMJ* 2004;328:282-5.

14 Ogilvie D, Mitchell R, Mutrie N, Petticrew M, Platt S. Evaluating health effects of transport interventions: methodologic case study. *Am J Prev Med* 2006;31:118-26.

15 Academy of Medical Sciences. *Identifying the environmental causes of disease: how should we decide what to believe and when to take action* ? London: Academy of Medical Sciences, 2007.

16 Torgerson D, Byford S. Economic modelling before clinical trials. *BMJ* 2002;325:98.

17 Eldridge S, Spencer A, Cryer C, Pearsons S, Underwood M, Feder G. Why modelling a complex intervention is an important precursor to trial design: lessons from studying an intervention to reduce falls-related injuries in elderly people. *J Health Services Res Policy* 2005;10:133-42.

18 Eldridge S, Ashby D, Feder G, Rudnicka AR, Ukoumunne OC. Lessons for cluster randomized trials in the twenty-first century: a systematic review of trials in primary care. *Clin Trials* 2004;1:80-90.

19 Power R, Langhaug L, Nyamurera T, Wilson D, Bassett M, Cowan F. Developing complex interventions for rigorous evaluation—a case study from rural Zimbabwe. *Health Educ Res* 2004;19:570-5.

20 Howden-Chapman P, Crane J, Matheson A, Viggers H, Cunningham M, Blakely T, et al. Retrofitting houses with insulation to reduce health inequalities: aims and methods of a clustered community-based trial. *Soc Sci Med* 2005;61:2600-10.

21 Black N. Why we need observational studies to evaluate the effectiveness of health care. *BMJ* 1996;312:1215-8.

22 Glasziou P, Chalmers I, Rawlins M, McCulloch P. When are randomised trials unnecessary? Picking signal from noise. *BMJ* 2007;334:349-51.

23 MacMahon S, Collins R. Reliable assessment of the effects of treatment on mortality and major morbidity. II. observational studies. *Lancet* 2001;357:455-62.

24 Gunnell D, Fernando R, Hewagama M, Priyangika W, Konradsen F, Eddleston M. The impact of pesticide regulations on suicide in Sri Lanka. *Int J Epidemiol* 2007;36:1235-42.

25 Clancy L, Goodman P, Sinclair H, Dockery DW. Effect of air pollution control on death rates in Dublin, Ireland: an intervention study. *Lancet* 2002;360:1210-4.

26 Haw SJ, Gruer L. Changes in exposure of adult non-smokers to secondhand smoke after implementation of smoke-free legislation in Scotland: national cross sectional survey. *BMJ* 2007;335:549-52.

27 Wortman PM. An exemplary evaluation of a program that worked: the High/Scope Perry preschool project. *Am J Eval* 1995;16:257-65.

28 Nazareth I, Freemantle N, Duggan C, Mason J, Haines A. Evaluation of a complex intervention for changing professional behaviour: the evidence based out reach (EBOR) trial. *J Health Services Res Policy* 2002;7:230-8.

29 Freemantle N, Nazareth I, Eccles M, Wood J, Haines A, EBOR Triallists. A randomised controlled trial of the effect of educational outreach by community pharmacists on prescribing in UK general practice. *Br J Gen Pract* 2002;52:290-5.

30 Hawe P, Shiell A, Riley T. Complex interventions: how "out of control" can a randomised trial be? *BMJ* 2004;328:1561-3.

31 Farmer A, Wade A, Goyder E, Yudkin P, French D, Craven A, et al. Impact of self-monitoring of blood glucose in the management of patients with non-insulin treated diabetes: open parallel group randomised trial. *BMJ* 2007;335:132-9.

32 Patton G, Bond L, Butler H, Glover S. Changing schools, changing health? Design and implementation of the Gatehouse Project. *J Adolesc Health* 2003;33:231-9.

33 Abraham C, Michie S. A taxonomy of behavior change techniques used in interventions. *Health Psychol* 2008;27:379-87.

34 Glasziou P, Meats E, Heneghan C, Shepperd S. What is missing from descriptions of treatments in trials and reviews? *BMJ* 2008;336:1472-4.

35 Boutron I, Moher D, Altman D, Scultz K, Ravaud P. Extending the CONSORT statement to randomized trials of non-pharmacologic treatment: explanation and elaboration. *Ann Int Med* 2008;148:295-309.

36 Von Elm E, Altman D, Egger M, Pocock SJ, Gotzsche P, Vandenbroucke JP, et al. Strengthening the reporting of observational studies in epidemiology (STROBE) statement: guidelines for reporting observational studies. *BMJ* 2007;335:806-8.

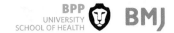

The PRISMA statement for reporting systematic reviews and meta-analyses of studies that evaluate healthcare interventions: explanation and elaboration

Alessandro Liberati[1] [2], Douglas G Altman[3], Jennifer Tetzlaff[4], Cynthia Mulrow[5], Peter C Gøtzsche[6], John P A Ioannidis[7], Mike Clarke[8] [9], P J Devereaux[10], Jos Kleijnen[11] [12], David Moher[4] [13]

[1]Università di Modena e Reggio Emilia, Modena, Italy

[2]Centro Cochrane Italiano, Istituto Ricerche Farmacologiche Mario Negri, Milan, Italy

[3]Centre for Statistics in Medicine, University of Oxford, Oxford

[4]Ottawa Methods Centre, Ottawa Hospital Research Institute, Ottawa, Ontario, Canada

[6]Nordic Cochrane Centre, Copenhagen, Denmark

[7]Department of Hygiene and Epidemiology, University of Ioannina School of Medicine, Ioannina, Greece

[8]UK Cochrane Centre, Oxford

[9]School of Nursing and Midwifery, Trinity College, Dublin, Republic of Ireland

[10]Departments of Medicine, Clinical Epidemiology and Biostatistics, McMaster University, Hamilton, Ontario, Canada

[11]Kleijnen Systematic Reviews, York

[12]School for Public Health and Primary Care (CAPHRI), University of Maastricht, Maastricht, Netherlands

[13]Department of Epidemiology and Community Medicine, Faculty of Medicine, Ottawa, Ontario, Canada

Correspondence to: alesslib@mailbase.it

Cite this as: BMJ 2009;339:b2700

DOI: 10.1136/bmj.b2700

http://www.bmj.com/content/339/bmj.b2700

ABSTRACT

Systematic reviews and meta-analyses are essential to summarise evidence relating to efficacy and safety of healthcare interventions accurately and reliably. The clarity and transparency of these reports, however, are not optimal. Poor reporting of systematic reviews diminishes their value to clinicians, policy makers, and other users.

Since the development of the QUOROM (quality of reporting of meta-analysis) statement—a reporting guideline published in 1999—there have been several conceptual, methodological, and practical advances regarding the conduct and reporting of systematic reviews and meta-analyses. Also, reviews of published systematic reviews have found that key information about these studies is often poorly reported. Realising these issues, an international group that included experienced authors and methodologists developed PRISMA (preferred reporting items for systematic reviews and meta-analyses) as an evolution of the original QUOROM guideline for systematic reviews and meta-analyses of evaluations of health care interventions.

The PRISMA statement consists of a 27-item checklist and a four-phase flow diagram. The checklist includes items deemed essential for transparent reporting of a systematic review. In this explanation and elaboration document, we explain the meaning and rationale for each checklist item. For each item, we include an example of good reporting and, where possible, references to relevant empirical studies and methodological literature. The PRISMA statement, this document, and the associated website (www.prisma-statement.org/) should be helpful resources to improve reporting of systematic reviews and meta-analyses.

Introduction

Systematic reviews and meta-analyses are essential tools for summarising evidence accurately and reliably. They help clinicians keep up to date; provide evidence for policy makers to judge risks, benefits, and harms of healthcare behaviours and interventions; gather together and summarise related research for patients and their carers; provide a starting point for clinical practice guideline developers; provide summaries of previous research for funders wishing to support new research;[1] and help editors judge the merits of publishing reports of new studies.[2] Recent data suggest that at least 2500 new systematic reviews reported in English are indexed in Medline annually.[3]

Unfortunately, there is considerable evidence that key information is often poorly reported in systematic reviews, thus diminishing their potential usefulness.[3] [4] [5] [6] As is true for all research, systematic reviews should be reported fully and transparently to allow readers to assess the strengths and weaknesses of the investigation.[7] That rationale led to the development of the QUOROM (quality of reporting of meta-analysis) statement; those detailed reporting recommendations were published in 1999.[8] In this paper we describe the updating of that guidance. Our aim is to ensure clear presentation of what was planned, done, and found in a systematic review.

Terminology used to describe systematic reviews and meta-analyses has evolved over time and varies across different groups of researchers and authors (see box 1 at end of document). In this document we adopt the definitions used by the Cochrane Collaboration.[9] A systematic review attempts to collate all empirical evidence that fits pre-specified eligibility criteria to answer a specific research question. It uses explicit, systematic methods that are selected to minimise bias, thus providing reliable findings from which conclusions can be drawn and decisions made. Meta-analysis is the use of statistical methods to summarise and combine the results of independent studies. Many systematic reviews contain meta-analyses, but not all.

The QUOROM statement and its evolution into PRISMA

The QUOROM statement, developed in 1996 and published in 1999,[8] was conceived as a reporting guidance for authors reporting a meta-analysis of randomised trials. Since then, much has happened. First, knowledge about the conduct and reporting of systematic reviews has expanded considerably. For example, the Cochrane Library's Methodology Register (which includes reports of studies relevant to the methods for systematic reviews) now contains more than 11000 entries (March 2009). Second, there have been many conceptual advances, such as "outcome-level" assessments of the risk of bias,[10] [11] that apply to systematic reviews. Third, authors have increasingly used systematic reviews to summarise evidence other than that provided by randomised trials.

However, despite advances, the quality of the conduct and reporting of systematic reviews remains well short of ideal.[3] [4] [5] [6] All of these issues prompted the need for an update and expansion of the QUOROM statement. Of note, recognising that the updated statement now addresses the above conceptual and methodological issues and may also have broader applicability than the original QUOROM statement, we changed the name of the reporting guidance to PRISMA (preferred reporting items for systematic reviews and meta-analyses).

Development of PRISMA

The PRISMA statement was developed by a group of 29 review authors, methodologists, clinicians, medical editors, and consumers.[12] They attended a three day meeting in 2005 and participated in extensive post-meeting electronic correspondence. A consensus process that was informed by evidence, whenever possible, was used to develop a 27-item checklist (table 1) and a four-phase flow diagram (fig 1) (also available as extra items on bmj.com for researchers to download and re-use). Items deemed essential for transparent reporting of a systematic review were included in the checklist. The flow diagram originally proposed by QUOROM was also modified to show numbers of identified records, excluded articles, and included studies. After 11 revisions the group approved the checklist, flow diagram, and this explanatory paper.

The PRISMA statement itself provides further details regarding its background and development.[12] This accompanying explanation and elaboration document explains the meaning and rationale for each checklist item. A few PRISMA Group participants volunteered to help draft specific items for this document, and four of these (DGA, AL, DM, and JT) met on several occasions to further refine the document, which was circulated and ultimately approved by the larger PRISMA Group.

Scope of PRISMA

PRISMA focuses on ways in which authors can ensure the transparent and complete reporting of systematic reviews and meta-analyses. It does not address directly or in a detailed manner the conduct of systematic reviews, for which other guides are available.[13] [14] [15] [16]

We developed the PRISMA statement and this explanatory document to help authors report a wide array of systematic reviews to assess the benefits and harms of a healthcare intervention. We consider most of the checklist items relevant when reporting systematic reviews of non-randomised studies assessing the benefits and harms of interventions. However, we recognise that authors who address questions relating to aetiology, diagnosis, or prognosis, for example, and who review epidemiological or diagnostic accuracy studies may need to modify or incorporate additional items for their systematic reviews.

How to use this paper

We modeled this explanation and elaboration document after those prepared for other reporting guidelines.[17] [18] [19] To maximise the benefit of this document, we encourage people to read it in conjunction with the PRISMA statement.[11]

We present each checklist item and follow it with a published exemplar of good reporting for that item. (We edited some examples by removing citations or web addresses, or by spelling out abbreviations.) We then explain the pertinent issue, the rationale for including the item, and relevant evidence from the literature, whenever possible. No systematic search was carried out to identify exemplars and evidence. We also include seven boxes at the end of the document that provide a more comprehensive explanation of certain thematic aspects of the methodology and conduct of systematic reviews.

Although we focus on a minimal list of items to consider when reporting a systematic review, we indicate places where additional information is desirable to improve transparency of the review process. We present the items numerically from 1 to 27; however, authors need not address items in this particular order in their reports. Rather, what is important is that the information for each item is given somewhere within the report.

The PRISMA checklist

Title and abstract

Item 1: Title

Identify the report as a systematic review, meta-analysis, or both.

Examples "Recurrence rates of video-assisted thoracoscopic versus open surgery in the prevention of recurrent pneumothoraces: a systematic review of randomised and non-randomised trials"[20]

"Mortality in randomised trials of antioxidant supplements for primary and secondary prevention: systematic review and meta-analysis"[21]

Explanation Authors should identify their report as a systematic review or meta-analysis. Terms such as "review" or "overview" do not describe for readers whether the review was systematic or whether a meta-analysis was performed. A recent survey found that 50% of 300 authors did not mention the terms "systematic review" or "meta-analysis" in the title or abstract of their systematic review.[3] Although sensitive search strategies have been developed to identify systematic reviews,[22] inclusion of the terms systematic review or meta-analysis in the title may improve indexing and identification.

We advise authors to use informative titles that make key information easily accessible to readers. Ideally, a title reflecting the PICOS approach (participants, interventions, comparators, outcomes, and study design) (see item 11 and box 2) may help readers as it provides key information about the scope of the review. Specifying the design(s) of the studies included, as shown in the examples, may also help some readers and those searching databases.

Some journals recommend "indicative titles" that indicate the topic matter of the review, while others require declarative titles that give the review's main conclusion. Busy practitioners may prefer to see the conclusion of the review in the title, but declarative titles can oversimplify or

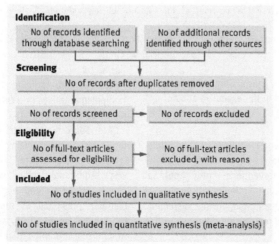

Identification

| No of records identified through database searching | No of additional records identified through other sources |

Screening

No of records after duplicates removed

| No of records screened | → | No of records excluded |

Eligibility

| No of full-text articles assessed for eligibility | → | No of full-text articles excluded, with reasons |

Included

No of studies included in qualitative synthesis

No of studies included in quantitative synthesis (meta-analysis)

Fig 1 Flow of information through the different phases of a systematic review.

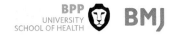

Table 1 Checklist of items to include when reporting a systematic review or meta-analysis

Section/topic	Item No	Checklist item	Reported on page No
Title			
Title	1	Identify the report as a systematic review, meta-analysis, or both	
Abstract			
Structured summary	2	Provide a structured summary including, as applicable, background, objectives, data sources, study eligibility criteria, participants, interventions, study appraisal and synthesis methods, results, limitations, conclusions and implications of key findings, systematic review registration number	
Introduction			
Rationale	3	Describe the rationale for the review in the context of what is already known	
Objectives	4	Provide an explicit statement of questions being addressed with reference to participants, interventions, comparisons, outcomes, and study design (PICOS)	
Methods			
Protocol and registration	5	Indicate if a review protocol exists, if and where it can be accessed (such as web address), and, if available, provide registration information including registration number	
Eligibility criteria	6	Specify study characteristics (such as PICOS, length of follow-up) and report characteristics (such as years considered, language, publication status) used as criteria for eligibility, giving rationale	
Information sources	7	Describe all information sources (such as databases with dates of coverage, contact with study authors to identify additional studies) in the search and date last searched	
Search	8	Present full electronic search strategy for at least one database, including any limits used, such that it could be repeated	
Study selection	9	State the process for selecting studies (that is, screening, eligibility, included in systematic review, and, if applicable, included in the meta-analysis)	
Data collection process	10	Describe method of data extraction from reports (such as piloted forms, independently, in duplicate) and any processes for obtaining and confirming data from investigators	
Data items	11	List and define all variables for which data were sought (such as PICOS, funding sources) and any assumptions and simplifications made	
Risk of bias in individual studies	12	Describe methods used for assessing risk of bias of individual studies (including specification of whether this was done at the study or outcome level), and how this information is to be used in any data synthesis	
Summary measures	13	State the principal summary measures (such as risk ratio, difference in means).	
Synthesis of results	14	Describe the methods of handling data and combining results of studies, if done, including measures of consistency (such as I2) for each meta-analysis	
Risk of bias across studies	15	Specify any assessment of risk of bias that may affect the cumulative evidence (such as publication bias, selective reporting within studies)	
Additional analyses	16	Describe methods of additional analyses (such as sensitivity or subgroup analyses, meta-regression), if done, indicating which were pre-specified	
Results			
Study selection	17	Give numbers of studies screened, assessed for eligibility, and included in the review, with reasons for exclusions at each stage, ideally with a flow diagram	
Study characteristics	18	For each study, present characteristics for which data were extracted (such as study size, PICOS, follow-up period) and provide the citations	
Risk of bias within studies	19	Present data on risk of bias of each study and, if available, any outcome-level assessment (see item 12).	
Results of individual studies	20	For all outcomes considered (benefits or harms), present for each study (a) simple summary data for each intervention group and (b) effect estimates and confidence intervals, ideally with a forest plot	
Synthesis of results	21	Present results of each meta-analysis done, including confidence intervals and measures of consistency	
Risk of bias across studies	22	Present results of any assessment of risk of bias across studies (see item 15)	
Additional analysis	23	Give results of additional analyses, if done (such as sensitivity or subgroup analyses, meta-regression [see item 16])	
Discussion			
Summary of evidence	24	Summarise the main findings including the strength of evidence for each main outcome; consider their relevance to key groups (such as health care providers, users, and policy makers)	
Limitations	25	Discuss limitations at study and outcome level (such as risk of bias), and at review level (such as incomplete retrieval of identified research, reporting bias)	
Conclusions	26	Provide a general interpretation of the results in the context of other evidence, and implications for future research	
Funding			
Funding	27	Describe sources of funding for the systematic review and other support (such as supply of data) and role of funders for the systematic review	

exaggerate findings. Thus, many journals and methodologists prefer indicative titles as used in the examples above.

Item 2: Structured summary

Provide a structured summary including, as applicable, background; objectives; data sources; study eligibility criteria, participants, and interventions; study appraisal and synthesis methods; results; limitations; conclusions and implications of key findings; funding for the systematic review; and systematic review registration number.

Example "*Context*: The role and dose of oral vitamin D supplementation in nonvertebral fracture prevention have not been well established.

Objective: To estimate the effectiveness of vitamin D supplementation in preventing hip and nonvertebral fractures in older persons.

Data Sources: A systematic review of English and non-English articles using MEDLINE and the Cochrane Controlled Trials Register (1960-2005), and EMBASE (1991-2005). Additional studies were identified by contacting clinical experts and searching bibliographies and abstracts presented at the American Society for Bone and Mineral Research (1995-2004). Search terms included randomised controlled trial (RCT), controlled clinical trial, random allocation, double-blind method, cholecalciferol, ergocalciferol, 25-hydroxyvitamin D, fractures, humans, elderly, falls, and bone density.

Study Selection: Only double-blind RCTs of oral vitamin D supplementation (cholecalciferol, ergocalciferol) with or without calcium supplementation vs calcium supplementation or placebo in older persons (>60 years) that examined hip or nonvertebral fractures were included.

Data Extraction: Independent extraction of articles by 2 authors using predefined data fields, including study quality indicators.

Data Synthesis: All pooled analyses were based on random-effects models. Five RCTs for hip fracture (n=9294) and 7 RCTs for nonvertebral fracture risk (n=9820) met our inclusion criteria. All trials used cholecalciferol. Heterogeneity among studies for both hip and nonvertebral fracture prevention was observed, which disappeared after pooling RCTs with low-dose (400 IU/d) and higher-dose vitamin D (700-800 IU/d), separately. A vitamin D dose of 700 to 800 IU/d reduced the relative risk (RR) of hip fracture by 26% (3 RCTs with 5572 persons; pooled RR, 0.74; 95% confidence interval [CI], 0.61-0.88) and any nonvertebral fracture by 23% (5 RCTs with 6098 persons; pooled RR, 0.77; 95% CI, 0.68-0.87) vs calcium or placebo. No significant benefit was observed for RCTs with 400 IU/d vitamin D (2 RCTs with 3722 persons; pooled RR for hip fracture, 1.15; 95% CI, 0.88-1.50; and pooled RR for any nonvertebral fracture, 1.03; 95% CI, 0.86-1.24).

Conclusions: Oral vitamin D supplementation between 700 to 800 IU/d appears to reduce the risk of hip and any nonvertebral fractures in ambulatory or institutionalised elderly persons. An oral vitamin D dose of 400 IU/d is not sufficient for fracture prevention."[23]

Explanation Abstracts provide key information that enables readers to understand the scope, processes, and findings of a review and to decide whether to read the full report. The abstract may be all that is readily available to a reader, for example, in a bibliographic database. The abstract should present a balanced and realistic assessment of the review's findings that mirrors, albeit briefly, the main text of the report.

We agree with others that the quality of reporting in abstracts presented at conferences and in journal publications needs improvement.[24] [25] While we do not uniformly favour a specific format over another, we generally recommend structured abstracts. Structured abstracts provide readers with a series of headings pertaining to the purpose, conduct, findings, and conclusions of the systematic review being reported.[26] [27] They give readers more complete information and facilitate finding information more easily than unstructured abstracts.[28] [29] [30] [31] [32]

A highly structured abstract of a systematic review could include the following headings: *Context* (or *Background*); *Objective* (or *Purpose*); *Data sources*; *Study selection* (or *Eligibility criteria*); *Study appraisal* and *Synthesis methods* (or *Data extraction* and *Data synthesis*); *Results*; *Limitations*; and *Conclusions* (or *Implications*). Alternatively, a simpler structure could cover but collapse some of the above headings (such as label *Study selection* and *Study appraisal* as *Review methods*) or omit some headings such as *Background* and *Limitations*.

In the highly structured abstract mentioned above, authors use the *Background* heading to set the context for readers and explain the importance of the review question. Under the *Objectives* heading, they ideally use elements of PICOS (see box 2) to state the primary objective of the review. Under a *Data sources* heading, they summarise sources that were searched, any language or publication type restrictions, and the start and end dates of searches. *Study selection* statements then ideally describe who selected studies using what inclusion criteria. *Data extraction methods* statements describe appraisal methods during data abstraction and the methods used to integrate or summarise the data. The *Data synthesis* section is where the main results of the review are reported. If the review includes meta-analyses, authors should provide numerical results with confidence intervals for the most important outcomes. Ideally, they should specify the amount of evidence in these analyses (numbers of studies and numbers of participants). Under a *Limitations* heading, authors might describe the most important weaknesses of included studies as well as limitations of the review process. Then authors should provide clear and balanced *Conclusions* that are closely linked to the objective and findings of the review. Additionally, it would be helpful if authors included some information about funding for the review. Finally, although protocol registration for systematic reviews is still not common practice, if authors have registered their review or received a registration number, we recommend providing the registration information at the end of the abstract.

Taking all the above considerations into account, the intrinsic tension between the goal of completeness of the abstract and its keeping into the space limit often set by journal editors is recognised as a major challenge.

Introduction

Item 3: Rationale
Describe the rationale for the review in the context of what is already known.

Example "Reversing the trend of increasing weight for height in children has proven difficult. It is widely accepted that increasing energy expenditure and reducing energy intake form the theoretical basis for management. Therefore, interventions aiming to increase physical activity and improve diet are the foundation of efforts to prevent and treat childhood obesity. Such lifestyle interventions have been supported by recent systematic reviews, as well as by the Canadian Paediatric Society, the Royal College of Paediatrics and Child Health, and the American Academy of Pediatrics. However, these interventions are fraught with poor adherence. Thus, school-based interventions are theoretically appealing because adherence with interventions can be improved. Consequently, many local governments have enacted or are considering policies that mandate increased physical activity in schools, although the effect of such interventions on body composition has not been assessed."[33]

Explanation Readers need to understand the rationale behind the study and what the systematic review may add to what is already known. Authors should tell readers whether their report is a new systematic review or an update of an existing one. If the review is an update, authors should state reasons for the update, including what has been added to the evidence base since the previous version of the review.

An ideal background or introduction that sets context for readers might include the following. First, authors might define the importance of the review question from different perspectives (such as public health, individual patient, or health policy). Second, authors might briefly mention the current state of knowledge and its limitations. As in the above example, information about the effects of several different interventions may be available that helps readers understand why potential relative benefits or harms of particular interventions need review. Third, authors might whet readers' appetites by clearly stating what the review aims to add. They also could discuss the extent to which the limitations of the existing evidence base may be overcome by the review.

Item 4: Objectives

Provide an explicit statement of questions being addressed with reference to participants, interventions, comparisons, outcomes, and study design (PICOS).

Example "To examine whether topical or intraluminal antibiotics reduce catheter-related bloodstream infection, we reviewed randomised, controlled trials that assessed the efficacy of these antibiotics for primary prophylaxis against catheter-related bloodstream infection and mortality compared with no antibiotic therapy in adults undergoing hemodialysis."[34]

Explanation The questions being addressed, and the rationale for them, are one of the most critical parts of a systematic review. They should be stated precisely and explicitly so that readers can understand quickly the review's scope and the potential applicability of the review to their interests.[35] Framing questions so that they include the following five "PICOS" components may improve the explicitness of review questions: (1) the patient population or disease being addressed (P), (2) the interventions or exposure of interest (I), (3) the comparators (C), (4) the main outcome or endpoint of interest (O), and (5) the study designs chosen (S). For more detail regarding PICOS, see box 2.

Good review questions may be narrowly focused or broad, depending on the overall objectives of the review. Sometimes broad questions might increase the applicability of the results and facilitate detection of bias, exploratory analyses, and sensitivity analyses.[35 36] Whether narrowly focused or broad, precisely stated review objectives are critical as they help define other components of the review process such as the eligibility criteria (item 6) and the search for relevant literature (items 7 and 8).

Methods

Item 5: Protocol and registration

Indicate if a review protocol exists, if and where it can be accessed (such as a web address), and, if available, provide registration information including the registration number.

Example "Methods of the analysis and inclusion criteria were specified in advance and documented in a protocol."[37]

Explanation A protocol is important because it pre-specifies the objectives and methods of the systematic review. For instance, a protocol specifies outcomes of primary interest, how reviewers will extract information about those outcomes, and methods that reviewers might use to quantitatively summarise the outcome data (see item 13). Having a protocol can help restrict the likelihood of biased post hoc decisions in review methods, such as selective outcome reporting. Several sources provide guidance about elements to include in the protocol for a systematic review.[16 38 39] For meta-analyses of individual patient-level data, we advise authors to describe whether a protocol was explicitly designed and whether, when, and how participating collaborators endorsed it.[40 41]

Authors may modify protocols during the research, and readers should not automatically consider such modifications inappropriate. For example, legitimate modifications may extend the period of searches to include older or newer studies, broaden eligibility criteria that proved too narrow, or add analyses if the primary analyses

suggest that additional ones are warranted. Authors should, however, describe the modifications and explain their rationale.

Although worthwhile protocol amendments are common, one must consider the effects that protocol modifications may have on the results of a systematic review, especially if the primary outcome is changed. Bias from selective outcome reporting in randomised trials has been well documented.[42 43] An examination of 47 Cochrane reviews revealed indirect evidence for possible selective reporting bias for systematic reviews. Almost all (n=43) contained a major change, such as the addition or deletion of outcomes, between the protocol and the full publication.[44] Whether (or to what extent) the changes reflected bias, however, was not clear. For example, it has been rather common not to describe outcomes that were not presented in any of the included studies.

Registration of a systematic review, typically with a protocol and registration number, is not yet common, but some opportunities exist.[45 46] Registration may possibly reduce the risk of multiple reviews addressing the same question,[45 46 47 48] reduce publication bias, and provide greater transparency when updating systematic reviews. Of note, a survey of systematic reviews indexed in Medline in November 2004 found that reports of protocol use had increased to about 46%[3] from 8% noted in previous surveys.[49] The improvement was due mostly to Cochrane reviews, which, by requirement, have a published protocol.[3]

Item 6: Eligibility criteria

Specify study characteristics (such as PICOS, length of follow-up) and report characteristics (such as years considered, language, publication status) used as criteria for eligibility, giving rationale.

Examples Types of studies: "Randomised clinical trials studying the administration of hepatitis B vaccine to CRF [chronic renal failure] patients, with or without dialysis. No language, publication date, or publication status restrictions were imposed…"

Types of participants: "Participants of any age with CRF or receiving dialysis (haemodialysis or peritoneal dialysis) were considered. CRF was defined as serum creatinine greater than 200 µmol/L for a period of more than six months or individuals receiving dialysis (haemodialysis or peritoneal dialysis)…Renal transplant patients were excluded from this review as these individuals are immunosuppressed and are receiving immunosuppressant agents to prevent rejection of their transplanted organs, and they have essentially normal renal function…"

Types of intervention: "Trials comparing the beneficial and harmful effects of hepatitis B vaccines with adjuvant or cytokine co-interventions [and] trials comparing the beneficial and harmful effects of immunoglobulin prophylaxis. This review was limited to studies looking at active immunisation. Hepatitis B vaccines (plasma or recombinant (yeast) derived) of all types, dose, and regimens versus placebo, control vaccine, or no vaccine…"

Types of outcome measures: "Primary outcome measures: Seroconversion, ie, proportion of patients with adequate anti-HBs response (>10 IU/L or Sample Ratio Units). Hepatitis B infections (as measured by hepatitis B core antigen (HBcAg) positivity or persistent HBsAg positivity), both acute and chronic. Acute (primary) HBV [hepatitis B virus] infections were defined as seroconversion to HBsAg positivity or development of IgM anti-HBc. Chronic HBV infections were defined as the persistence of HBsAg for more than six months or HBsAg positivity and liver biopsy compatible with a diagnosis or chronic hepatitis B. Secondary outcome measures: Adverse events of hepatitis B vaccinations...[and]...mortality."[50]

Explanation Knowledge of the eligibility criteria is essential in appraising the validity, applicability, and comprehensiveness of a review. Thus, authors should unambiguously specify eligibility criteria used in the review. Carefully defined eligibility criteria inform various steps of the review methodology. They influence the development of the search strategy and serve to ensure that studies are selected in a systematic and unbiased manner.

A study may be described in multiple reports, and one report may describe multiple studies. Therefore, we separate eligibility criteria into the following two components: study characteristics and report characteristics. Both need to be reported. Study eligibility criteria are likely to include the populations, interventions, comparators, outcomes, and study designs of interest (PICOS, see box 2), as well as other study-specific elements, such as specifying a minimum length of follow-up. Authors should state whether studies will be excluded because they do not include (or report) specific outcomes to help readers ascertain whether the systematic review may be biased as a consequence of selective reporting.[42][43]

Report eligibility criteria are likely to include language of publication, publication status (such as inclusion of unpublished material and abstracts), and year of publication. Inclusion or not of non-English language literature,[51][52][53][54][55] unpublished data, or older data can influence the effect estimates in meta-analyses.[56][57][58][59] Caution may need to be exercised in including all identified studies due to potential differences in the risk of bias such as, for example, selective reporting in abstracts.[60][61][62]

Item 7: Information sources
Describe all information sources in the search (such as databases with dates of coverage, contact with study authors to identify additional studies) and date last searched.

Example "Studies were identified by searching electronic databases, scanning reference lists of articles and consultation with experts in the field and drug companies... No limits were applied for language and foreign papers were translated. This search was applied to Medline (1966 - Present), CancerLit (1975 - Present), and adapted for Embase (1980 - Present), Science Citation Index Expanded (1981 - Present) and Pre-Medline electronic databases. Cochrane and DARE (Database of Abstracts of Reviews of Effectiveness) databases were reviewed...The last search was run on 19 June 2001. In addition, we handsearched contents pages of Journal of Clinical Oncology 2001, European Journal of Cancer 2001 and Bone 2001, together with abstracts printed in these journals 1999 - 2001. A limited update literature search was performed from 19 June 2001 to 31 December 2003."[63]

Explanation The National Library of Medicine's Medline database is one of the most comprehensive sources of healthcare information in the world. Like any database, however, its coverage is not complete and varies according to the field. Retrieval from any single database, even by an experienced searcher, may be imperfect, which is why detailed reporting is important within the systematic review.

At a minimum, for each database searched, authors should report the database, platform, or provider (such as Ovid, Dialog, PubMed) and the start and end dates for the search of each database. This information lets readers assess the currency of the review, which is important

because the publication time-lag outdates the results of some reviews.[64] This information should also make updating more efficient.[65] Authors should also report who developed and conducted the search.[66]

In addition to searching databases, authors should report the use of supplementary approaches to identify studies, such as hand searching of journals, checking reference lists, searching trials registries or regulatory agency websites,[67] contacting manufacturers, or contacting authors. Authors should also report if they attempted to acquire any missing information (such as on study methods or results) from investigators or sponsors; it is useful to describe briefly who was contacted and what unpublished information was obtained.

Item 8: Search
Present the full electronic search strategy for at least one major database, including any limits used, such that it could be repeated.

Examples In text: "We used the following search terms to search all trials registers and databases: immunoglobulin*; IVIG; sepsis; septic shock; septicaemia; and septicemia..."[68]

In appendix: "Search strategy: MEDLINE (OVID)

01. immunoglobulins/
02. immunoglobulin$.tw.
03. ivig.tw.
04. 1 or 2 or 3
05. sepsis/
06. sepsis.tw.
07. septic shock/
08. septic shock.tw.
09. septicemia/
10. septicaemia.tw.
11. septicemia.tw.
12. 5 or 6 or 7 or 8 or 9 or 10 or 11
13. 4 and 12
14. randomised controlled trials/
15. randomised-controlled-trial.pt.
16. controlled-clinical-trial.pt.
17. random allocation/
18. double-blind method/
19. single-blind method/
20. 14 or 15 or 16 or 17 or 18 or 19
21. exp clinical trials/
22. clinical-trial.pt.
23. (clin$ adj trial$).ti,ab.
24. ((singl$ or doubl$ or trebl$ or tripl$) adj (blind$)).ti,ab.
25. placebos/
26. placebo$.ti,ab.
27. random$.ti,ab.
28. 21 or 22 or 23 or 24 or 25 or 26 or 27
29. research design/
30. comparative study/
31. exp evaluation studies/
32. follow-up studies/
33. prospective studies/
34. (control$ or prospective$ or volunteer$).ti,ab.
35. 30 or 31 or 32 or 33 or 34
36. 20 or 28 or 29 or 35
37. 13 and 36"[68]

Explanation The search strategy is an essential part of the report of any systematic review. Searches may be complicated and iterative, particularly when reviewers search unfamiliar databases or their review is addressing a broad or new topic. Perusing the search strategy allows interested readers to assess the comprehensiveness and completeness of the search, and to replicate it. Thus, we advise authors to report their full electronic search strategy for at least one major database. As an alternative to presenting search strategies for all databases, authors could indicate how the search took into account other databases searched, as index terms vary across databases. If different searches are used for different parts of a wider question (such as questions relating to benefits and questions relating to harms), we recommend authors provide at least one example of a strategy for each part of the objective.[69] We also encourage authors to state whether search strategies were peer reviewed as part of the systematic review process.[70]

We realise that journal restrictions vary and that having the search strategy in the text of the report is not always feasible. We strongly encourage all journals, however, to find ways—such as a "web extra," appendix, or electronic link to an archive—to make search strategies accessible to readers. We also advise all authors to archive their searches so that (1) others may access and review them (such as replicate them or understand why their review of a similar topic did not identify the same reports), and (2) future updates of their review are facilitated.

Several sources provide guidance on developing search strategies.[71] [72] [73] Most searches have constraints, such as relating to limited time or financial resources, inaccessible or inadequately indexed reports and databases, unavailability of experts with particular language or database searching skills, or review questions for which pertinent evidence is not easy to find. Authors should be straightforward in describing their search constraints. Apart from the keywords used to identify or exclude records, they should report any additional limitations relevant to the search, such as language and date restrictions (see also eligibility criteria, item 6).[51]

Item 9: Study selection
State the process for selecting studies (that is, for screening, for determining eligibility, for inclusion in the systematic review, and, if applicable, for inclusion in the meta-analysis).

Example "Eligibility assessment…[was] performed independently in an unblinded standardized manner by 2 reviewers…Disagreements between reviewers were resolved by consensus."[74]

Explanation There is no standard process for selecting studies to include in a systematic review. Authors usually start with a large number of identified records from their search and sequentially exclude records according to eligibility criteria. We advise authors to report how they screened the retrieved records (typically a title and abstract), how often it was necessary to review the full text publication, and if any types of record (such as letters to the editor) were excluded. We also advise using the PRISMA flow diagram to summarise study selection processes (see item 17 and box 3).

Efforts to enhance objectivity and avoid mistakes in study selection are important. Thus authors should report whether each stage was carried out by one or several people, who these people were, and, whenever multiple independent investigators performed the selection, what the process was for resolving disagreements. The use of at least two investigators may reduce the possibility of rejecting relevant reports.[75] The benefit may be greatest for topics where selection or rejection of an article requires difficult judgments.[76] For these topics, authors should ideally tell readers the level of inter-rater agreement, how commonly arbitration about selection was required, and what efforts were made to resolve disagreements (such as by contact with the authors of the original studies).

Item 10: Data collection process
Describe the method of data extraction from reports (such as piloted forms, independently by two reviewers) and any processes for obtaining and confirming data from investigators.

Example "We developed a data extraction sheet (based on the Cochrane Consumers and Communication Review Group's data extraction template), pilot-tested it on ten randomly-selected included studies, and refined it accordingly. One review author extracted the following data from included studies and the second author checked the extracted data…Disagreements were resolved by discussion between the two review authors; if no agreement could be reached, it was planned a third author would decide. We contacted five authors for further information. All responded and one provided numerical data that had only been presented graphically in the published paper."[77]

Explanation Reviewers extract information from each included study so that they can critique, present, and summarise evidence in a systematic review. They might also contact authors of included studies for information that has not been, or is unclearly, reported. In meta-analysis of individual patient data, this phase involves collection and scrutiny of detailed raw databases. The authors should describe these methods, including any steps taken to reduce bias and mistakes during data collection and data extraction.[78] (See box 3)

Some systematic reviewers use a data extraction form that could be reported as an appendix or "Web extra" to their report. These forms could show the reader what information reviewers sought (see item 11) and how they extracted it. Authors could tell readers if the form was piloted. Regardless, we advise authors to tell readers who extracted what data, whether any extractions were completed in duplicate, and, if so, whether duplicate abstraction was done independently and how disagreements were resolved.

Published reports of the included studies may not provide all the information required for the review. Reviewers should describe any actions they took to seek additional information from the original researchers (see item 7). The description might include how they attempted to contact researchers, what they asked for, and their success in obtaining the necessary information. Authors should also tell readers when individual patient data were sought from the original researchers.[41] (see item 11) and indicate the studies for which such data were used in the analyses. The reviewers ideally should also state whether they confirmed the accuracy of the information included in their review with the original researchers, for example, by sending them a copy of the draft review.[79]

Some studies are published more than once. Duplicate publications may be difficult to ascertain, and their inclusion may introduce bias.[80] [81] We advise authors to describe any steps they used to avoid double counting and piece together data from multiple reports of the same study (such as juxtaposing author names, treatment comparisons, sample sizes, or outcomes). We also advise authors to indicate whether all reports on a study were considered, as inconsistencies may reveal important limitations. For example, a review of multiple publications of drug trials showed that reported study characteristics may differ from report to report, including the description of the design, number of patients analysed, chosen significance level, and outcomes.[82] Authors ideally should present any algorithm that they used to select data from overlapping reports and any efforts they used to solve logical inconsistencies across reports.

Item 11: Data items
List and define all variables for which data were sought (such as PICOS, funding sources) and any assumptions and simplifications made.

Examples "Information was extracted from each included trial on: (1) characteristics of trial participants (including age, stage and severity of disease, and method of diagnosis), and the trial's inclusion and exclusion criteria; (2) type of intervention (including type, dose, duration and frequency of the NSAID [non-steroidal anti-inflammatory drug]; versus placebo or versus the type, dose, duration and frequency of another NSAID; or versus another pain management drug; or versus no treatment); (3) type of outcome measure (including the level of pain reduction, improvement in quality of life score (using a validated scale), effect on daily activities, absence from work or school, length of follow up, unintended effects of treatment, number of women requiring more invasive treatment)."[83]

Explanation It is important for readers to know what information review authors sought, even if some of this information was not available.[84] If the review is limited to reporting only those variables that were obtained, rather than those that were deemed important but could not be obtained, bias might be introduced and the reader might be misled. It is therefore helpful if authors can refer readers to the protocol (see item 5) and archive their extraction forms (see item 10), including definitions of variables. The published systematic review should include a description of the processes used with, if relevant, specification of how readers can get access to additional materials.

We encourage authors to report whether some variables were added after the review started. Such variables might include those found in the studies that the reviewers identified (such as important outcome measures that the reviewers initially overlooked). Authors should describe the reasons for adding any variables to those already pre-specified in the protocol so that readers can understand the review process.

We advise authors to report any assumptions they made about missing or unclear information and to explain those processes. For example, in studies of women aged 50 or older it is reasonable to assume that none were pregnant, even if this is not reported. Likewise, review authors might make assumptions about the route of administration of drugs assessed. However, special care should be taken in making assumptions about qualitative information. For example, the upper age limit for "children" can vary from 15 years to 21 years, "intense" physiotherapy might mean very different things to different researchers at different times and for different patients, and the volume of blood associated with "heavy" blood loss might vary widely depending on the setting.

Item 12: Risk of bias in individual studies
Describe methods used for assessing risk of bias in individual studies (including specification of whether this was done at the study or outcome level, or both), and how this information is to be used in any data synthesis.

Example "To ascertain the validity of eligible randomized trials, pairs of reviewers working independently and with adequate reliability determined the adequacy of randomization and concealment of allocation, blinding of patients, health care providers, data collectors, and outcome assessors; and extent of loss to follow-up (i.e. proportion of patients in whom the investigators were not able to ascertain outcomes)."[85]

"To explore variability in study results (heterogeneity) we specified the following hypotheses before conducting the analysis. We hypothesised that effect size may differ according to the methodological quality of the studies."[86]

Explanation The likelihood that the treatment effect reported in a systematic review approximates the truth depends on the validity of the included studies, as certain methodological characteristics may be associated with effect sizes.[87][88] For example, trials without reported adequate allocation concealment exaggerate treatment effects on average compared with those with adequate concealment.[88] Therefore, it is important for authors to describe any methods that they used to gauge the risk of bias in the included studies and how that information was used.[89] Additionally, authors should provide a rationale if no assessment of risk of bias was undertaken. The most popular term to describe the issues relevant to this item is "quality," but for the reasons that are elaborated in box 4 we prefer to name this item as "assessment of risk of bias."

Many methods exist to assess the overall risk of bias in included studies, including scales, checklists, and individual components.[90][91] As discussed in box 4, scales that numerically summarise multiple components into a single number are misleading and unhelpful.[92][93] Rather, authors should specify the methodological components that they assessed. Common markers of validity for randomised trials include the following: appropriate generation of random allocation sequence;[94] concealment of the allocation sequence;[93] blinding of participants, health care providers, data collectors, and outcome adjudicators;[95][96][97][98] proportion of patients lost to follow-up;[99][100] stopping of trials early for benefit;[101] and whether the analysis followed the intention-to-treat principle.[100][102] The ultimate decision regarding which methodological features to evaluate requires consideration of the strength of the empiric data, theoretical rationale, and the unique circumstances of the included studies.

Authors should report how they assessed risk of bias; whether it was in a blind manner; and if assessments were completed by more than one person, and if so, whether they were completed independently.[103][104] Similarly, we encourage authors to report any calibration exercises among review team members that were done. Finally, authors need to report how their assessments of risk of bias are used subsequently in the data synthesis (see item 16). Despite the often difficult task of assessing the risk of bias in included studies, authors are sometimes silent on what they did with the resultant assessments.[89] If authors exclude studies from the review or any subsequent analyses on the basis of the risk of bias, they should tell readers which studies they excluded and explain the reasons for those exclusions (see item 6). Authors should also describe any planned sensitivity or subgroup analyses related to bias assessments (see item 16).

Item 13: Summary measures
State the principal summary measures (such as risk ratio, difference in means).

Examples "Relative risk of mortality reduction was the primary measure of treatment effect."[105]

"The meta-analyses were performed by computing relative risks (RRs) using random-effects model. Quantitative analyses were performed on an intention-to-treat basis and were confined to data derived from the period of follow-up. RR and 95% confidence intervals for each side effect (and all side effects) were calculated."[106]

"The primary outcome measure was the mean difference in log10 HIV-1 viral load comparing zinc supplementation to placebo..."[107]

Explanation When planning a systematic review, it is generally desirable that authors pre-specify the outcomes of primary interest (see item 5) as well as the intended summary effect measure for each outcome. The chosen summary effect measure may differ from that used in some of the included studies. If possible the choice of effect measures should be explained, though it is not always easy to judge in advance which measure is the most appropriate.

For binary outcomes, the most common summary measures are the risk ratio, odds ratio, and risk difference.[108] Relative effects are more consistent across studies than absolute effects,[109] [110] although absolute differences are important when interpreting findings (see item 24).

For continuous outcomes, the natural effect measure is the difference in means.[108] Its use is appropriate when outcome measurements in all studies are made on the same scale. The standardised difference in means is used when the studies do not yield directly comparable data. Usually this occurs when all studies assess the same outcome but measure it in a variety of ways (such as different scales to measure depression).

For time-to-event outcomes, the hazard ratio is the most common summary measure. Reviewers need the log hazard ratio and its standard error for a study to be included in a meta-analysis.[111] This information may not be given for all studies, but methods are available for estimating the desired quantities from other reported information.[111] Risk ratio and odds ratio (in relation to events occurring by a fixed time) are not equivalent to the hazard ratio, and median survival times are not a reliable basis for meta-analysis.[112] If authors have used these measures they should describe their methods in the report.

Item 14: Planned methods of analysis

Describe the methods of handling data and combining results of studies, if done, including measures of consistency (such as I[2]) for each meta-analysis.

Examples "We tested for heterogeneity with the Breslow-Day test, and used the method proposed by Higgins et al. to measure inconsistency (the percentage of total variation across studies due to heterogeneity) of effects across lipid-lowering interventions. The advantages of this measure of inconsistency (termed I[2]) are that it does not inherently depend on the number of studies and is accompanied by an uncertainty interval."[113]

"In very few instances, estimates of baseline mean or mean QOL [Quality of life] responses were obtained without corresponding estimates of variance (standard deviation [SD] or standard error). In these instances, an SD was imputed from the mean of the known SDs. In a number of cases, the response data available were the mean and variance in a pre study condition and after therapy. The within-patient variance in these cases could not be calculated directly and was approximated by assuming independence."[114]

Explanation The data extracted from the studies in the review may need some transformation (processing) before they are suitable for analysis or for presentation in an evidence table. Although such data handling may facilitate meta-analyses, it is sometimes needed even when meta-analyses are not done. For example, in trials with more than two intervention groups it may be necessary to combine results for two or more groups (such as receiving similar but non-identical interventions), or it may be desirable to include only a subset of the data to match the review's inclusion criteria. When several different scales (such as for depression) are used across studies, the sign of some scores may need to be reversed to ensure that all scales are aligned (such as so low values represent good health on all scales). Standard deviations may have to be reconstructed from other statistics such as P values and t statistics,[115] [116] or occasionally they may be imputed from the standard deviations observed in other studies.[117] Time-to-event data also usually need careful conversions to a consistent format.[111] Authors should report details of any such data processing.

Statistical combination of data from two or more separate studies in a meta-analysis may be neither necessary nor desirable (see box 5 and item 21). Regardless of the decision to combine individual study results, authors should report how they planned to evaluate between-study variability (heterogeneity or inconsistency) (box 6). The consistency of results across trials may influence the decision of whether to combine trial results in a meta-analysis.

When meta-analysis is done, authors should specify the effect measure (such as relative risk or mean difference) (see item 13), the statistical method (such as inverse variance), and whether a fixed-effects or random-effects approach, or some other method (such as Bayesian) was used (see box 6). If possible, authors should explain the reasons for those choices.

Item 15: Risk of bias across studies

Specify any assessment of risk of bias that may affect the cumulative evidence (such as publication bias, selective reporting within studies).

Examples "For each trial we plotted the effect by the inverse of its standard error. The symmetry of such 'funnel plots' was assessed both visually, and formally with Egger's test, to see if the effect decreased with increasing sample size."[118]

"We assessed the possibility of publication bias by evaluating a funnel plot of the trial mean differences for asymmetry, which can result from the non publication of small trials with negative results...Because graphical evaluation can be subjective, we also conducted an adjusted rank correlation test and a regression asymmetry test as formal statistical tests for publication bias...We acknowledge that other factors, such as differences in trial quality or true study heterogeneity, could produce asymmetry in funnel plots."[119]

Explanation Reviewers should explore the possibility that the available data are biased. They may examine results from the available studies for clues that suggest there may be missing studies (publication bias) or missing data from the included studies (selective reporting bias) (see box 7). Authors should report in detail any methods used to investigate possible bias across studies.

It is difficult to assess whether within-study selective reporting is present in a systematic review. If a protocol of an individual study is available, the outcomes in the protocol and the published report can be compared. Even in the absence of a protocol, outcomes listed in the methods section of the published report can be compared with those for which results are presented.[120] In only half of 196 trial reports describing comparisons of two drugs in arthritis were all the effect variables in the methods and results sections the same.[82] In other cases, knowledge of the clinical area may suggest that it is likely that the outcome was measured even if it was not reported. For example, in a particular disease, if one of two linked outcomes is reported but the other is not, then one should question whether the latter has been selectively omitted.[121][122]

Only 36% (76 of 212) of therapeutic systematic reviews published in November 2004 reported that study publication bias was considered, and only a quarter of those intended to carry out a formal assessment for that bias.[3] Of 60 meta-analyses in 24 articles published in 2005 in which formal assessments were reported, most were based on fewer than 10 studies; most displayed statistically significant heterogeneity; and many reviewers misinterpreted the results of the tests employed.[123] A review of trials of antidepressants found that meta-analysis of only the published trials gave effect estimates 32% larger on average than when all trials sent to the drug agency were analysed.[67]

Item 16: Additional analyses
Describe methods of additional analyses (such as sensitivity or subgroup analyses, meta-regression), if done, indicating which were pre-specified.

Example "Sensitivity analyses were pre-specified. The treatment effects were examined according to quality components (concealed treatment allocation, blinding of patients and caregivers, blinded outcome assessment), time to initiation of statins, and the type of statin. One post-hoc sensitivity analysis was conducted including unpublished data from a trial using cerivastatin."[124]

Explanation Authors may perform additional analyses to help understand whether the results of their review are robust, all of which should be reported. Such analyses include sensitivity analysis, subgroup analysis, and meta-regression.[125]

Sensitivity analyses are used to explore the degree to which the main findings of a systematic review are affected by changes in its methods or in the data used from individual studies (such as study inclusion criteria, results of risk of bias assessment). Subgroup analyses address whether the summary effects vary in relation to specific (usually clinical) characteristics of the included studies or their participants. Meta-regression extends the idea of subgroup analysis to the examination of the quantitative influence of study characteristics on the effect size.[126] Meta-regression also allows authors to examine the contribution of different variables to the heterogeneity in study findings. Readers of systematic reviews should be aware that meta-regression has many limitations, including a danger of over-interpretation of findings.[127][128]

Even with limited data, many additional analyses can be undertaken. The choice of which analysis to undertake will depend on the aims of the review. None of these analyses, however, is exempt from producing potentially misleading results. It is important to inform readers whether these analyses were performed, their rationale, and which were pre-specified.

Results
Item 17: Study selection
Give numbers of studies screened, assessed for eligibility, and included in the review, with reasons for exclusions at each stage, ideally with a flow diagram.

Examples In text: "A total of 10 studies involving 13 trials were identified for inclusion in the review. The search of Medline, PsycInfo and Cinahl databases provided a total of 584 citations. After adjusting for duplicates 509 remained. Of these, 479 studies were discarded because after reviewing the abstracts it appeared that these papers clearly did not meet the criteria. Three additional studies...were discarded because full text of the study was not available or the paper could not be feasibly translated into English. The full text of the remaining 27 citations was examined in more detail. It appeared that 22 studies did not meet the inclusion criteria as described. Five studies...met the inclusion criteria and were included in the systematic review. An additional five studies...that met the criteria for inclusion were identified by checking the references of located, relevant papers and searching for studies that have cited these papers. No unpublished relevant studies were obtained."[129]

See flow diagram in fig 2.

Explanation Authors should report, ideally with a flow diagram, the total number of records identified from electronic bibliographic sources (including specialised database or registry searches), hand searches of various sources, reference lists, citation indices, and experts. It is useful if authors delineate for readers the number of selected articles that were identified from the different sources so that they can see, for example, whether most articles were identified through electronic bibliographic sources or from references or experts. Literature identified primarily from references or experts may be prone to citation or publication bias.[131][132]

The flow diagram and text should describe clearly the process of report selection throughout the review. Authors should report unique records identified in searches, records excluded after preliminary screening (such as screening of titles and abstracts), reports retrieved for detailed evaluation, potentially eligible reports that were not retrievable, retrieved reports that did not meet inclusion criteria and the primary reasons for exclusion, and the studies included in the review. Indeed, the most appropriate layout may vary for different reviews.

Authors should also note the presence of duplicate or supplementary reports so that readers understand the number of individual studies compared with the number of reports that were included in the review. Authors should be consistent in their use of terms, such as whether they are reporting on counts of citations, records, publications, or studies. We believe that reporting the number of studies is the most important.

A flow diagram can be very useful; it should depict all the studies included based on fulfilling the eligibility criteria, and whether data have been combined for statistical analysis. A recent review of 87 systematic reviews found that about half included a QUOROM flow diagram.[133] The authors of this research recommended some important ways that reviewers can improve the use of a flow diagram when describing the flow of information throughout the review process, including a separate flow diagram for each important outcome reported.[133]

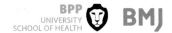

Item 18: Study characteristics

For each study, present characteristics for which data were extracted (such as study size, PICOS, follow-up period) and provide the citation.

Examples In text: "*Characteristics of included studies*
Methods

All four studies finally selected for the review were randomised controlled trials published in English. The duration of the intervention was 24 months for the RIO-North America and 12 months for the RIO-Diabetes, RIO-Lipids and RIO-Europe study. Although the last two described a period of 24 months during which they were conducted, only the first 12-months results are provided. All trials had a run-in, as a single blind period before the randomisation.

Participants

The included studies involved 6625 participants. The main inclusion criteria entailed adults (18 years or older), with a body mass index greater than 27 kg/m² and less than 5 kg variation in body weight within the three months before study entry.

Intervention

All trials were multicentric. The RIO-North America was conducted in the USA and Canada, RIO-Europe in Europe and the USA, RIO-Diabetes in the USA and 10 other different countries not specified, and RIO-Lipids in eight unspecified different countries.

The intervention received was placebo, 5 mg of rimonabant or 20 mg of rimonabant once daily in addition to a mild hypocaloric diet (600 kcal/day deficit).

Outcomes
Primary

In all studies the primary outcome assessed was weight change from baseline after one year of treatment and the RIO-North America study also evaluated the prevention of weight regain between the first and second year. All studies evaluated adverse effects, including those of any kind and serious events. Quality of life was measured in only one study, but the results were not described (RIO-Europe).

Secondary and additional outcomes

These included prevalence of metabolic syndrome after one year and change in cardiometabolic risk factors such as blood pressure, lipid profile, etc.

No study included mortality and costs as outcome.

The timing of outcome measures was variable and could include monthly investigations, evaluations every three months or a single final evaluation after one year."[134] See table 2.

Explanation For readers to gauge the validity and applicability of a systematic review's results, they need to know something about the included studies. Such information includes PICOS (box 2) and specific information relevant to the review question. For example, if the review is examining the long term effects of antidepressants for moderate depressive disorder, authors should report the follow-up periods of the included studies. For each included study, authors should provide a citation for the source of their information regardless of whether or not the study is published. This information makes it easier for interested readers to retrieve the relevant publications or documents.

Reporting study-level data also allows the comparison of the main characteristics of the studies included in the review. Authors should present enough detail to allow readers to make their own judgments about the relevance of included studies. Such information also makes it possible for readers to conduct their own subgroup analyses and interpret subgroups, based on study characteristics.

Authors should avoid, whenever possible, assuming information when it is missing from a study report (such as sample size, method of randomisation). Reviewers may contact the original investigators to try to obtain missing information or confirm the data extracted for the systematic review. If this information is not obtained, this should be noted in the report. If information is imputed, the reader should be told how this was done and for which items. Presenting study-level data makes it possible to clearly identify unpublished information obtained from the original researchers and make it available for the public record.

Typically, study-level characteristics are presented as a table as in the example (table 2). Such presentation ensures that all pertinent items are addressed and that missing or unclear information is clearly indicated. Although paper based journals do not generally allow for the quantity of information available in electronic journals or Cochrane reviews, this should not be accepted as an excuse for omission of important aspects of the methods or results of included studies, since these can, if necessary, be shown on a website.

Following the presentation and description of each included study, as discussed above, reviewers usually provide a narrative summary of the studies. Such a summary provides readers with an overview of the included studies. It may, for example, address the languages of the published papers, years of publication, and geographic origins of the included studies.

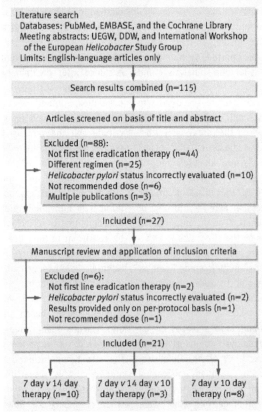

Fig 2 Example flow diagram of study selection. DDW = Digestive Disease Week; UEGW = United European Gastroenterology Week. Adapted from Fuccio et al[130]

The PICOS framework is often helpful in reporting the narrative summary indicating, for example, the clinical characteristics and disease severity of the participants and the main features of the intervention and of the comparison group. For non-pharmacological interventions, it may be helpful to specify for each study the key elements of the intervention received by each group. Full details of the interventions in included studies were reported in only three of 25 systematic reviews relevant to general practice.[84]

Item 19: Risk of bias within studies
Present data on risk of bias of each study and, if available, any outcome-level assessment (see item 12).

Example See table 3.

Explanation We recommend that reviewers assess the risk of bias in the included studies using a standard approach with defined criteria (see item 12). They should report the results of any such assessments.[89]

Reporting only summary data (such as "two of eight trials adequately concealed allocation") is inadequate because it fails to inform readers which studies had the particular methodological shortcoming. A more informative approach is to explicitly report the methodological features evaluated for each study. The Cochrane Collaboration's new tool for assessing the risk of bias also requests that authors substantiate these assessments with any relevant text from the original studies.[11] It is often easiest to provide these data in a tabular format, as in the example. However, a narrative summary describing the tabular data can also be helpful for readers.

Item 20: Results of individual studies
For all outcomes considered (benefits and harms), present, for each study, simple summary data for each intervention group and effect estimates and confidence intervals, ideally with a forest plot.

Examples See table 4 and fig 3.

Explanation Publication of summary data from individual studies allows the analyses to be reproduced and other analyses and graphical displays to be investigated. Others may wish to assess the impact of excluding particular studies or consider subgroup analyses not reported by the review authors. Displaying the results of each treatment group in included studies also enables inspection of individual study features. For example, if only odds ratios are provided, readers cannot assess the variation in event rates across the studies, making the odds ratio impossible to interpret.[138] Additionally, because data extraction errors in meta-analyses are common and can be large,[139] the presentation of the results from individual studies makes it easier to identify errors. For continuous outcomes, readers may wish to examine the consistency of standard deviations across studies, for example, to be reassured that standard deviation and standard error have not been confused.[138]

For each study, the summary data for each intervention group are generally given for binary outcomes as frequencies with and without the event (or as proportions such as 12/45). It is not sufficient to report event rates per intervention group as percentages. The required summary data for continuous outcomes are the mean, standard deviation, and sample size for each group. In reviews that examine time-to-event data, the authors should report the log hazard ratio and its standard error (or confidence interval) for each included study. Sometimes, essential data are missing from the reports of the included studies and cannot be calculated from other data but may need to be imputed by the reviewers. For example, the standard deviation may be imputed using the typical standard deviations in the other trials[116] [117] (see item 14). Whenever relevant, authors should indicate which results were not reported directly and had to be estimated from other information (see item 13). In addition, the inclusion of unpublished data should be noted.

For all included studies it is important to present the estimated effect with a confidence interval. This information may be incorporated in a table showing study characteristics or may be shown in a forest plot.[140] The key elements of the forest plot are the effect estimates and confidence intervals for each study shown graphically, but it is preferable also to include, for each study, the numerical group-specific summary data, the effect size and confidence interval, and the percentage weight (see second example, fig 3). For discussion of the results of meta-analysis, see item 21.

In principle, all the above information should be provided for every outcome considered in the review, including both benefits and harms. When there are too many outcomes for full information to be included, results for the most important outcomes should be included in the main report with other information provided as a web appendix. The choice of the information to present should be justified in light of what was originally stated in the protocol. Authors should explicitly mention if the planned main outcomes cannot be presented due to lack of information. There is some evidence that information on harms is only rarely reported in systematic reviews, even when it is available in the original studies.[141] Selective omission of harms results biases a systematic review and decreases its ability to contribute to informed decision making.

Table 2 Example of summary of study characteristics: Summary of included studies evaluating the efficacy of antiemetic agents in acute gastroenteritis. Adapted from DeCamp et al[135]

Source	Setting	No of patients	Age range	Inclusion criteria	Antiemetic agent	Route	Follow-up
Freedman et al 2006	ED	214	6 months-10 years	GE with mild to moderate dehydration and vomiting in the preceding 4 hours	Ondansetron	PO	1-2 weeks
Reeves et al 2002	ED	107	1 month-22 years	GE and vomiting requiring IV rehydration	Ondansetron	IV	5-7 days
Roslund et al 2007	ED	106	1-10 years	GE with failed oral rehydration attempt in ED	Ondansetron	PO	1 week
Stork et al 2006	ED	137	6 months-12 years	GE, recurrent emesis, mild to moderate dehydration, and failed oral hydration	Ondansetron and dexamethasone	IV	1 and 2 days

ED = emergency department; GE = gastroenteritis; IV = intravenous; PO = by mouth.

Table 3 Example of assessment of the risk of bias: Quality measures of the randomised controlled trials that failed to fulfil any one of six markers of validity. Adapted from Devereaux et al[96]

Trials	Concealment of randomisation	RCT stopped early	Patients blinded	Healthcare providers blinded	Data collectors blinded	Outcome assessors blinded
Liu	No	No	Yes	Yes	Yes	Yes
Stone	Yes	No	No	Yes	Yes	Yes
Polderman	Yes	Yes	No	No	No	Yes
Zaugg	Yes	No	No	No	Yes	Yes
Urban	Yes	Yes	No	No, except anaesthesiologists	Yes	Yes

RCT = randomised controlled trial.

Item 21: Syntheses of results
Present the main results of the review. If meta-analyses are done, include for each, confidence intervals and measures of consistency.

Examples "Mortality data were available for all six trials, randomizing 311 patients and reporting data for 305 patients. There were no deaths reported in the three respiratory syncytial virus/severe bronchiolitis trials; thus our estimate is based on three trials randomizing 232 patients, 64 of whom died. In the pooled analysis, surfactant was associated with significantly lower mortality (relative risk =0.7, 95% confidence interval =0.4-0.97, P=0.04). There was no evidence of heterogeneity (I^2=0%)."[142]

"Because the study designs, participants, interventions, and reported outcome measures varied markedly, we focused on describing the studies, their results, their applicability, and their limitations and on qualitative synthesis rather than meta-analysis."[143]

"We detected significant heterogeneity within this comparison (I^2=46.6%, χ^2=13.11, df=7, P=0.07). Retrospective exploration of the heterogeneity identified one trial that seemed to differ from the others. It included only small ulcers (wound area less than 5 cm²). Exclusion of this trial removed the statistical heterogeneity and did not affect the finding of no evidence of a difference in healing rate between hydrocolloids and simple low adherent dressings (relative risk=0.98, [95% confidence interval] 0.85 to 1.12, I^2=0%)."[144]

Explanation Results of systematic reviews should be presented in an orderly manner. Initial narrative descriptions of the evidence covered in the review (see item 18) may tell readers important things about the study populations and the design and conduct of studies. These descriptions can facilitate the examination of patterns across studies. They may also provide important information about applicability of evidence, suggest the likely effects of any major biases, and allow consideration, in a systematic manner, of multiple explanations for possible differences of findings across studies.

If authors have conducted one or more meta-analyses, they should present the results as an estimated effect across studies with a confidence interval. It is often simplest to show each meta-analysis summary with the actual results of included studies in a forest plot (see item 20).[140] It should always be clear which of the included studies contributed to each meta-analysis. Authors should also provide, for each meta-analysis, a measure of the consistency of the results from the included studies such as I^2 (heterogeneity, see box 6); a confidence interval may also be given for this measure.[145] If no meta-analysis was performed, the qualitative inferences should be presented as systematically as possible with an explanation of why meta-analysis was not done, as in the second example above.[143] Readers may find a forest plot, without a summary estimate, helpful in such cases.

Authors should in general report syntheses for all the outcome measures they set out to investigate (that is, those described in the protocol, see item 4) to allow readers to draw their own conclusions about the implications of the results. Readers should be made aware of any deviations from the planned analysis. Authors should tell readers if the planned meta-analysis was not thought appropriate or possible for some of the outcomes and the reasons for that decision.

It may not always be sensible to give meta-analysis results and forest plots for each outcome. If the review addresses a broad question, there may be a very large number of outcomes. Also, some outcomes may have been reported in only one or two studies, in which case forest plots are of little value and may be seriously biased.

Of 300 systematic reviews indexed in Medline in 2004, a little more than half (54%) included meta-analyses, of which the majority (91%) reported assessing for inconsistency in results.

Item 22: Risk of bias across studies
Present results of any assessment of risk of bias across studies (see item 15).

Example "Strong evidence of heterogeneity (I^2=79%, P<0.001) was observed. To explore this heterogeneity, a funnel plot was drawn. The funnel plot [fig 4] shows evidence of considerable asymmetry."[146]

"Specifically, four sertraline trials involving 486 participants and one citalopram trial involving 274 participants were reported as having failed to achieve a statistically significant drug effect, without reporting mean HRSD [Hamilton Rating Scale for Depression] scores. We were unable to find data from these trials on pharmaceutical company Web sites or through our search of the published literature. These omissions represent 38% of patients in sertraline trials and 23% of patients in citalopram trials. Analyses with and without inclusion of these trials found no differences in the patterns of results; similarly, the revealed patterns do not interact with drug type. The purpose of using the data obtained from the FDA was to avoid publication bias, by including unpublished as well as published trials. Inclusion of only those sertraline and citalopram trials for which means were reported to the FDA would constitute a form of reporting bias similar to publication bias and would

Table 4 Example of summary results: Heterotopic ossification in trials comparing radiotherapy to non-steroidal anti-inflammatory drugs after major hip procedures and fractures. Adapted from Pakos et al[136]

Author (year)	Radiotherapy		NSAID	
Kienapfel (1999)	12/49	24.5%	20/55	36.4%
Sell (1998)	2/77	2.6%	18/77	23.4%
Kolbl (1997)	39/188	20.7%	18/113	15.9%
Kolbl (1998)	22/46	47.8%	6/54	11.1%
Moore (1998)	9/33	27.3%	18/39	46.2%
Bremen-Kuhne (1997)	9/19	47.4%	11/31	35.5%
Knelles (1997)	5/101	5.0%	46/183	25.4%

NSAID = non-steroidal anti-inflammatory drug.

Description	Tetracycline-rifampicin n/N	Tetracycline-streptomycin n/N	Relative risk (fixed) (95% CI)	Relative risk (fixed) (95% CI)
Acocella 1989[w72]	3/63	2/53		1.26 (0.22 to 7.27)
Ariza 1985[w73]	7/18	2/28		5.44 (1.27 to 23.34)
Ariza 1992[w74]	5/44	3/51		1.93 (0.49 to 7.63)
Bayindir 2003[w75]	5/20	6/41		1.71 (0.59 to 4.93)
Colmenero 1989[w76]	7/52	5/59		1.59 (0.54 to 4.70)
Colmenero 1994[w77]	2/10	0/9		4.55 (0.25 to 83.70)
Dorado 1988[w78]	8/27	4/24		1.78 (0.61 to 5.17)
Ersoy 2005[w79]	7/45	4/32		1.24 (0.40 to 3.90)
Kosmidis 1982[w80]	1/10	2/10		0.50 (0.05 to 4.67)
Montejo 1993[w81]	6/46	4/84		2.74 (0.81 to 9.21)
Rodriguez Zapata 1987[w82]	3/32	1/36		3.38 (0.37 to 30.84)
Solera 1991[w83]	12/34	3/36		4.24 (1.31 to 13.72)
Solera 1995[w84]	28/100	9/94		2.92 (1.46 to 5.87)
Total (95% CI)	501	557		2.30 (1.65 to 3.21)

Total events: 94 (tetracycline-rifampicin), 45 (tetracycline-streptomycin)

0.1 0.2 0.5 1 2 5 10
Favours tetracycline-rifampicin   Favours tetracycline-streptomycin

Test for heterogeneity: χ^2=7.64, df=12, P=0.81, I^2=0%
Test for overall effect: z=4.94, P<0.001

Fig 3 Example of summary results: Overall failure (defined as failure of assigned regimen or relapse) with tetracycline-rifampicin versus tetracycline-streptomycin. Adapted from Skalsky et al[137]

lead to overestimation of drug–placebo differences for these drug types. Therefore, we present analyses only on data for medications for which complete clinical trials' change was reported."[147]

Explanation Authors should present the results of any assessments of risk of bias across studies. If a funnel plot is reported, authors should specify the effect estimate and measure of precision used, presented typically on the x axis and y axis, respectively. Authors should describe if and how they have tested the statistical significance of any possible asymmetry (see item 15). Results of any investigations of selective reporting of outcomes within studies (as discussed in item 15) should also be reported. Also, we advise authors to tell readers if any pre-specified analyses for assessing risk of bias across studies were not completed and the reasons (such as too few included studies).

Item 23: Additional analyses
Give results of additional analyses, if done (such as sensitivity or subgroup analyses, meta-regression [see item 16]).

Example "...benefits of chondroitin were smaller in trials with adequate concealment of allocation compared with trials with unclear concealment (P for interaction =0.050), in trials with an intention-to-treat analysis compared with those that had excluded patients from the analysis (P for interaction =0.017), and in large compared with small trials (P for interaction =0.022)."[148]

"Subgroup analyses according to antibody status, antiviral medications, organ transplanted, treatment duration, use of antilymphocyte therapy, time to outcome assessment, study quality and other aspects of study design did not demonstrate any differences in treatment effects. Multivariate meta-regression showed no significant difference in CMV [cytomegalovirus] disease after allowing for potential confounding or effect-modification by prophylactic drug used, organ transplanted or recipient serostatus in CMV positive recipients and CMV negative recipients of CMV positive donors."[149]

Explanation Authors should report any subgroup or sensitivity analyses and whether they were pre-specified (see items 5 and 16). For analyses comparing subgroups of studies (such as separating studies of low and high dose aspirin), the authors should report any tests for interactions, as well as estimates and confidence intervals from meta-analyses within each subgroup. Similarly, meta-regression results (see item 16) should not be limited to P values but should include effect sizes and confidence intervals,[150] as the first example reported above does in a table. The amount of data included in each additional analysis should be specified if different from that considered in the

main analyses. This information is especially relevant for sensitivity analyses that exclude some studies; for example, those with high risk of bias.

Importantly, all additional analyses conducted should be reported, not just those that were statistically significant. This information will help avoid selective outcome reporting bias within the review as has been demonstrated in reports of randomised controlled trials.[42 44 121 151 152] Results from exploratory subgroup or sensitivity analyses should be interpreted cautiously, bearing in mind the potential for multiple analyses to mislead.

Discussion

Item 24: Summary of evidence
Summarise the main findings, including the strength of evidence for each main outcome; consider their relevance to key groups (such as healthcare providers, users, and policy makers).

Example "Overall, the evidence is not sufficiently robust to determine the comparative effectiveness of angioplasty (with or without stenting) and medical treatment alone. Only 2 randomized trials with long-term outcomes and a third randomized trial that allowed substantial crossover of treatment after 3 months directly compared angioplasty and medical treatment...the randomized trials did not evaluate enough patients or did not follow patients for a sufficient duration to allow definitive conclusions to be made about clinical outcomes, such as mortality and cardiovascular or kidney failure events.

Some acceptable evidence from comparison of medical treatment and angioplasty suggested no difference in long-term kidney function but possibly better blood pressure control after angioplasty, an effect that may be limited to patients with bilateral atherosclerotic renal artery stenosis. The evidence regarding other outcomes is weak. Because the reviewed studies did not explicitly address patients with rapid clinical deterioration who may need acute intervention, our conclusions do not apply to this important subset of patients."[143]

Explanation Authors should give a brief and balanced summary of the nature and findings of the review. Sometimes, outcomes for which little or no data were found should be noted due to potential relevance for policy decisions and future research. Applicability of the review's findings—to different patients, settings, or target audiences, for example—should be mentioned. Although there is no standard way to assess applicability simultaneously to different audiences, some systems do exist.[153] Sometimes, authors formally rate or assess the overall body of evidence addressed in the review and can present the strength of their summary recommendations tied to their assessments of the quality of evidence (such as the GRADE system).[10]

Authors need to keep in mind that statistical significance of the effects does not always suggest clinical or policy relevance. Likewise, a non-significant result does not demonstrate that a treatment is ineffective. Authors should ideally clarify trade-offs and how the values attached to the main outcomes would lead different people to make different decisions. In addition, adroit authors consider factors that are important in translating the evidence to different settings and that may modify the estimates of effects reported in the review.[153] Patients and healthcare providers may be primarily interested in which intervention is most likely to provide a benefit with acceptable harms, while policy makers and administrators may value data on organisational impact and resource utilisation.

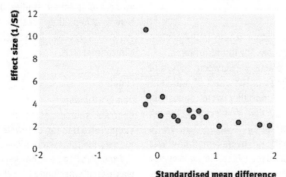

Fig 4 Example of a funnel plot showing evidence of considerable asymmetry. SE = standard error. Adapted from Appleton et al[146]

Item 25: Limitations

Discuss limitations at study and outcome level (such as risk of bias), and at review level (such as incomplete retrieval of identified research, reporting bias).

Examples Outcome level: "The meta-analysis reported here combines data across studies in order to estimate treatment effects with more precision than is possible in a single study. The main limitation of this meta-analysis, as with any overview, is that the patient population, the antibiotic regimen and the outcome definitions are not the same across studies."[154]

Study and review level: "Our study has several limitations. The quality of the studies varied. Randomization was adequate in all trials; however, 7 of the articles did not explicitly state that analysis of data adhered to the intention-to-treat principle, which could lead to overestimation of treatment effect in these trials, and we could not assess the quality of 4 of the 5 trials reported as abstracts. Analyses did not identify an association between components of quality and re-bleeding risk, and the effect size in favour of combination therapy remained statistically significant when we excluded trials that were reported as abstracts.

Publication bias might account for some of the effect we observed. Smaller trials are, in general, analyzed with less methodological rigor than larger studies, and an asymmetrical funnel plot suggests that selective reporting may have led to an overestimation of effect sizes in small trials."[155]

Explanation A discussion of limitations should address the validity (that is, risk of bias) and reporting (informativeness) of the included studies, limitations of the review process, and generalisability (applicability) of the review. Readers may find it helpful if authors discuss whether studies were threatened by serious risks of bias, whether the estimates of the effect of the intervention are too imprecise, or if there were missing data for many participants or important outcomes.

Limitations of the review process might include limitations of the search (such as restricting to English-language publications), and any difficulties in the study selection, appraisal, and meta-analysis processes. For example, poor or incomplete reporting of study designs, patient populations, and interventions may hamper interpretation and synthesis of the included studies.[84] Applicability of the review may be affected if there are limited data for certain populations or subgroups where the intervention might perform differently or few studies assessing the most important outcomes of interest; or if there is a substantial amount of data relating to an outdated intervention or comparator or heavy reliance on imputation of missing values for summary estimates (item 14).

Item 26: Conclusions

Provide a general interpretation of the results in the context of other evidence, and implications for future research.

Example Implications for practice: "Between 1995 and 1997 five different meta-analyses of the effect of antibiotic prophylaxis on infection and mortality were published. All confirmed a significant reduction in infections, though the magnitude of the effect varied from one review to another. The estimated impact on overall mortality was less evident and has generated considerable controversy on the cost effectiveness of the treatment. Only one among the five available reviews, however, suggested that a weak association between respiratory tract infections and mortality exists and lack of sufficient statistical power may have accounted for the limited effect on mortality."

Implications for research: "A logical next step for future trials would thus be the comparison of this protocol against a regimen of a systemic antibiotic agent only to see whether the topical component can be dropped. We have already identified six such trials but the total number of patients so far enrolled (n=1056) is too small for us to be confident that the two treatments are really equally effective. If the hypothesis is therefore considered worth testing more and larger randomised controlled trials are warranted. Trials of this kind, however, would not resolve the relevant issue of treatment induced resistance. To produce a satisfactory answer to this, studies with a different design would be necessary. Though a detailed discussion goes beyond the scope of this paper, studies in which the intensive care unit rather than the individual patient is the unit of randomisation and in which the occurrence of antibiotic resistance is monitored over a long period of time should be undertaken."[156]

Explanation Systematic reviewers sometimes draw conclusions that are too optimistic[157] or do not consider the harms equally as carefully as the benefits, although some evidence suggests these problems are decreasing.[158] If conclusions cannot be drawn because there are too few reliable studies, or too much uncertainty, this should be stated. Such a finding can be as important as finding consistent effects from several large studies.

Authors should try to relate the results of the review to other evidence, as this helps readers to better interpret the results. For example, there may be other systematic reviews about the same general topic that have used different methods or have addressed related but slightly different questions.[159] [160] Similarly, there may be additional information relevant to decision makers, such as the cost-effectiveness of the intervention (such as health technology assessment). Authors may discuss the results of their review in the context of existing evidence regarding other interventions.

We advise authors also to make explicit recommendations for future research. In a sample of 2535 Cochrane reviews, 82% included recommendations for research with specific interventions, 30% suggested the appropriate type of participants, and 52% suggested outcome measures for future research.[161] There is no corresponding assessment about systematic reviews published in medical journals, but we believe that such recommendations are much less common in those reviews.

Clinical research should not be planned without a thorough knowledge of similar, existing research.[162] There is evidence that this still does not occur as it should and that authors of primary studies do not consider a systematic review when they design their studies.[163] We believe systematic reviews have great potential for guiding future clinical research.

Funding

Item 27: Funding

Describe sources of funding or other support (such as supply of data) for the systematic review, and the role of funders for the systematic review.

Examples "The evidence synthesis upon which this article was based was funded by the Centers for Disease Control and Prevention for the Agency for Healthcare Research and Quality and the U.S. Prevention Services Task Force."[164]

"Role of funding source: The funders played no role in study design, collection, analysis, interpretation of data, writing of the report, or in the decision to submit the paper for publication. They accept no responsibility for the contents."[165]

Explanation Authors of systematic reviews, like those of any other research study, should disclose any funding they received to carry out the review, or state if the review was not funded. Lexchin and colleagues[166] observed that outcomes of reports of randomised trials and meta-analyses of clinical trials funded by the pharmaceutical industry are more likely to favor the sponsor's product compared with studies with other sources of funding. Similar results have been reported elsewhere.[167] [168] Analogous data suggest that similar biases may affect the conclusions of systematic reviews.[169]

Given the potential role of systematic reviews in decision making, we believe authors should be transparent about the funding and the role of funders, if any. Sometimes the funders will provide services, such as those of a librarian to complete the searches for relevant literature or access to commercial databases not available to the reviewers. Any level of funding or services provided to the systematic review team should be reported. Authors should also report whether the funder had any role in the conduct or report of the review. Beyond funding issues, authors should report any real or perceived conflicts of interest related to their role or the role of the funder in the reporting of the systematic review.[170]

In a survey of 300 systematic reviews published in November 2004, funding sources were not reported in 41% of the reviews.[3] Only a minority of reviews (2%) reported being funded by for-profit sources, but the true proportion may be higher.[171]

Additional considerations for systematic reviews of non-randomised intervention studies or for other types of systematic reviews

The PRISMA statement and this document have focused on systematic reviews of reports of randomised trials. Other study designs, including non-randomised studies, quasi-experimental studies, and interrupted time series, are included in some systematic reviews that evaluate the effects of healthcare interventions.[172] [173] The methods of these reviews may differ to varying degrees from the typical intervention review, for example regarding the literature search, data abstraction, assessment of risk of bias, and analysis methods. As such, their reporting demands might also differ from what we have described here. A useful principle is for systematic review authors to ensure that their methods are reported with adequate clarity and transparency to enable readers to critically judge the available evidence and replicate or update the research.

In some systematic reviews, the authors will seek the raw data from the original researchers to calculate the summary statistics. These systematic reviews are called individual patient (or participant) data reviews.[40] [41] Individual patient data meta-analyses may also be conducted with prospective accumulation of data rather than retrospective accumulation of existing data. Here too, extra information about the methods will need to be reported.

Other types of systematic reviews exist. Realist reviews aim to determine how complex programmes work in specific contexts and settings.[174] Meta-narrative reviews aim to explain complex bodies of evidence through mapping and comparing different overarching storylines.[175] Network meta-analyses, also known as multiple treatments meta-analyses, can be used to analyse data from comparisons of many different treatments.[176] [177] They use both direct and indirect comparisons and can be used to compare interventions that have not been directly compared.

We believe that the issues we have highlighted in this paper are relevant to ensure transparency and understanding of the processes adopted and the limitations of the information presented in systematic reviews of different types. We hope that PRISMA can be the basis for more detailed guidance on systematic reviews of other types of research, including diagnostic accuracy and epidemiological studies.

Discussion

We developed the PRISMA statement using an approach for developing reporting guidelines that has evolved over several years.[178] The overall aim of PRISMA is to help ensure the clarity and transparency of reporting of systematic reviews, and recent data indicate that this reporting guidance is much needed.[3] PRISMA is not intended to be a quality assessment tool and it should not be used as such.

This PRISMA explanation and elaboration document was developed to facilitate the understanding, uptake, and dissemination of the PRISMA statement and hopefully provide a pedagogical framework for those interested in conducting and reporting systematic reviews. It follows a format similar to that used in other explanatory documents.[17] [18] [19] Following the recommendations in the PRISMA checklist may increase the word count of a systematic review report. We believe, however, that the benefit of readers being able to critically appraise a clear, complete, and transparent systematic review report outweighs the possible slight increase in the length of the report.

While the aims of PRISMA are to reduce the risk of flawed reporting of systematic reviews and improve the clarity and transparency in how reviews are conducted, we have little data to state more definitively whether this "intervention" will achieve its intended goal. A previous effort to evaluate QUOROM was not successfully completed.[178] Publication of the QUOROM statement was delayed for two years while a research team attempted to evaluate its effectiveness by conducting a randomised controlled trial with the participation of eight major medical journals. Unfortunately that trial was not completed due to accrual problems (David Moher, personal communication). Other evaluation methods might be easier to conduct. At least one survey of 139 published systematic reviews in the critical care literature[179] suggests that their quality improved after the publication of QUOROM.

If the PRISMA statement is endorsed by and adhered to in journals, as other reporting guidelines have been,[17] [18] [19] [180] there should be evidence of improved reporting of systematic reviews. For example, there have been several evaluations of whether the use of CONSORT improves reports of randomised controlled trials. A systematic review of these studies[181] indicates that use of CONSORT is associated with improved reporting of certain items, such as allocation concealment. We aim to evaluate the benefits (that is, improved reporting) and possible adverse effects (such as increased word length) of PRISMA and we encourage others to consider doing likewise.

Even though we did not carry out a systematic literature search to produce our checklist, and this is indeed a limitation of our effort, PRISMA was developed using an evidence based approach whenever possible. Checklist items were included if there was evidence that not reporting the item was associated with increased risk of bias, or where it was clear that information was necessary to appraise the reliability of a review. To keep PRISMA up to date and as evidence based as possible requires regular vigilance of the literature, which is growing rapidly. Currently the Cochrane Methodology Register has more than 11 000 records pertaining to the conduct and reporting of systematic reviews and other evaluations of health and social care. For some checklist items, such as reporting the abstract (item 2), we have used evidence from elsewhere in the belief that the issue applies equally well to reporting of systematic reviews. Yet for other items, evidence does not exist; for example, whether a training exercise improves the accuracy and reliability of data extraction. We hope PRISMA will act as a catalyst to help generate further evidence that can be considered when further revising the checklist in the future.

More than 10 years have passed between the development of the QUOROM statement and its update, the PRISMA statement. We aim to update PRISMA more frequently. We hope that the implementation of PRISMA will be better than it has been for QUOROM. There are at least two reasons to be optimistic. First, systematic reviews are increasingly used by healthcare providers to inform "best practice" patient care. Policy analysts and managers are using systematic reviews to inform healthcare decision making and to better target future research. Second, we anticipate benefits from the development of the EQUATOR Network, described below.

Developing any reporting guideline requires considerable effort, experience, and expertise. While reporting guidelines have been successful for some individual efforts,[17] [18] [19] there are likely others who want to develop reporting guidelines who possess little time, experience, or knowledge as to how to do so appropriately. The EQUATOR (enhancing the quality and transparency of health research) Network aims to help such individuals and groups by serving as a global resource for anybody interested in developing reporting guidelines, regardless of the focus.[7] [180] [182] The overall goal of EQUATOR is to improve the quality of reporting of all health science research through the development and translation of reporting guidelines. Beyond this aim, the network plans to develop a large web presence by developing and maintaining a resource centre of reporting tools, and other information for reporting research (www.equator-network. org/).

We encourage healthcare journals and editorial groups, such as the World Association of Medical Editors and the International Committee of Medical Journal Editors, to endorse PRISMA in much the same way as they have endorsed other reporting guidelines, such as CONSORT. We also encourage editors of healthcare journals to support PRISMA by updating their "instructions to authors" and including the PRISMA web address, and by raising awareness through specific editorial actions.

The following people contributed to this paper: Doug Altman, Centre for Statistics in Medicine (Oxford, UK); Gerd Antes, University Hospital Freiburg (Freiburg, Germany); David Atkins, Health Services Research and Development Service, Veterans Health Administration (Washington DC, USA); Virginia Barbour, *PLoS Medicine* (Cambridge, UK); Nick Barrowman, Children's Hospital of Eastern Ontario (Ottawa, Canada); Jesse A Berlin, Johnson & Johnson Pharmaceutical Research and Development (Titusville NJ, USA); Jocalyn Clark, *PLoS Medicine* (at the time of writing, *BMJ*, London); Mike Clarke, UK Cochrane Centre (Oxford, UK) and School of Nursing and Midwifery, Trinity College (Dublin, Ireland); Deborah Cook, Departments of Medicine, Clinical Epidemiology and Biostatistics, McMaster University (Hamilton, Canada); Roberto D'Amico, Università di Modena e Reggio Emilia (Modena, Italy) and Centro Cochrane Italiano, Istituto Ricerche Farmacologiche Mario Negri (Milan, Italy); Jonathan J Deeks, University of Birmingham (Birmingham); P J Devereaux, Departments of Medicine, Clinical Epidemiology and Biostatistics, McMaster University (Hamilton, Canada); Kay Dickersin, Johns Hopkins Bloomberg School of Public Health (Baltimore MD, USA); Matthias Egger, Department of Social and Preventive Medicine, University of Bern (Bern, Switzerland); Edzard Ernst, Peninsula Medical School (Exeter, UK); Peter C Gøtzsche, Nordic Cochrane Centre (Copenhagen, Denmark); Jeremy Grimshaw, Ottawa Hospital Research Institute (Ottawa, Canada); Gordon Guyatt, Departments of Medicine, Clinical Epidemiology and Biostatistics, McMaster University; Julian Higgins, MRC Biostatistics Unit (Cambridge, UK); John P A Ioannidis, University of Ioannina Campus (Ioannina, Greece); Jos Kleijnen, Kleijnen Systematic Reviews (York, UK) and School for Public Health and Primary Care (CAPHRI), University of Maastricht (Maastricht, Netherlands); Tom Lang, Tom Lang Communications and Training (Davis CA, USA); Alessandro Liberati, Università di Modena e Reggio Emilia (Modena, Italy) and Centro Cochrane Italiano, Istituto Ricerche Farmacologiche Mario Negri (Milan, Italy); Nicola Magrini, NHS Centre for the Evaluation of the Effectiveness of Health Care—CeVEAS (Modena, Italy); David McNamee, *Lancet* (London, UK); David Moher, Ottawa Methods Centre, Ottawa Hospital Research Institute (Ottawa,

---

BOX 1 TERMINOLOGY

The terminology used to describe systematic reviews and meta-analyses has evolved over time and varies between fields. Different terms have been used by different groups, such as educators and psychologists. The conduct of a systematic review comprises several explicit and reproducible steps, such as identifying all likely relevant records, selecting eligible studies, assessing the risk of bias, extracting data, qualitative synthesis of the included studies, and possibly meta-analyses.

Initially this entire process was termed a meta-analysis and was so defined in the QUOROM statement.[8] More recently, especially in healthcare research, there has been a trend towards preferring the term systematic review. If quantitative synthesis is performed, this last stage alone is referred to as a meta-analysis. The Cochrane Collaboration uses this terminology,[9] under which a meta-analysis, if performed, is a component of a systematic review. Regardless of the question addressed and the complexities involved, it is always possible to complete a systematic review of existing data, but not always possible or desirable, to quantitatively synthesise results because of clinical, methodological, or statistical differences across the included studies. Conversely, with prospective accumulation of studies and datasets where the plan is eventually to combine them, the term "(prospective) meta-analysis" may make more sense than "systematic review."

For retrospective efforts, one possibility is to use the term systematic review for the whole process up to the point when one decides whether to perform a quantitative synthesis. If a quantitative synthesis is performed, some researchers refer to this as a meta-analysis. This definition is similar to that found in the current edition of the *Dictionary of Epidemiology*.[183]

While we recognise that the use of these terms is inconsistent and there is residual disagreement among the members of the panel working on PRISMA, we have adopted the definitions used by the Cochrane Collaboration.[9]

Systematic review A systematic review attempts to collate all empirical evidence that fits pre-specified eligibility criteria to answer a specific research question. It uses explicit, systematic methods that are selected with a view to minimising bias, thus providing reliable findings from which conclusions can be drawn and decisions made.[184] [185] The key characteristics of a systematic review are (a) a clearly stated set of objectives with an explicit, reproducible methodology; (b) a systematic search that attempts to identify all studies that would meet the eligibility criteria; (c) an assessment of the validity of the findings of the included studies, such as through the assessment of risk of bias; and (d) systematic presentation and synthesis of the characteristics and findings of the included studies.

Meta-analysis Meta-analysis is the use of statistical techniques to integrate and summarise the results of included studies. Many systematic reviews contain meta-analyses, but not all. By combining information from all relevant studies, meta-analyses can provide more precise estimates of the effects of health care than those derived from the individual studies included within a review.

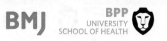

BOX 2 HELPING TO DEVELOP THE RESEARCH QUESTION(S): THE PICOS APPROACH

Formulating relevant and precise questions that can be answered in a systematic review can be complex and time consuming. A structured approach for framing questions that uses five components may help facilitate the process. This approach is commonly known by the acronym "PICOS" where each letter refers to a component: the patient population or the disease being addressed (P), the interventions or exposure (I), the comparator group (C), the outcome or endpoint (O), and the study design chosen (S).[186] Issues relating to PICOS affect several PRISMA items (items 6, 8, 9, 10, 11, and 18).

- *P*—Providing information about the population requires a precise definition of a group of participants (often patients), such as men over the age of 65 years, their defining characteristics of interest (often disease), and possibly the setting of care considered, such as an acute care hospital.

- *I*—The interventions (exposures) under consideration in the systematic review need to be transparently reported. For example, if the reviewers answer a question regarding the association between a woman's prenatal exposure to folic acid and subsequent offspring's neural tube defects, reporting the dose, frequency, and duration of folic acid used in different studies is likely to be important for readers to interpret the review's results and conclusions. Other interventions (exposures) might include diagnostic, preventive, or therapeutic treatments; arrangements of specific processes of care; lifestyle changes; psychosocial or educational interventions; or risk factors.

- *C*—Clearly reporting the comparator (control) group intervention(s)—such as usual care, drug, or placebo—is essential for readers to fully understand the selection criteria of primary studies included in the systematic review, and might be a source of heterogeneity investigators have to deal with. Comparators are often poorly described. Clearly reporting what the intervention is compared with is important and may sometimes have implications for the inclusion of studies in a review—many reviews compare with "standard care," which is otherwise undefined; this should be properly addressed by authors.

- *O*—The outcomes of the intervention being assessed—such as mortality, morbidity, symptoms, or quality of life improvements—should be clearly specified as they are required to interpret the validity and generalisability of the systematic review's results.

- *S*—Finally, the type of study design(s) included in the review should be reported. Some reviews include only reports of randomised trials, whereas others have broader design criteria and include randomised trials and certain types of observational studies. Still other reviews, such as those specifically answering questions related to harms, may include a wide variety of designs ranging from cohort studies to case reports. Whatever study designs are included in the review, these should be reported.

Independently from how difficult it is to identify the components of the research question, the important point is that a structured approach is preferable, and this extends beyond systematic reviews of effectiveness. Ideally the PICOS criteria should be formulated a priori, in the systematic review's protocol, although some revisions might be required because of the iterative nature of the review process. Authors are encouraged to report their PICOS criteria and whether any modifications were made during the review process. A useful example in this realm is the appendix of the "systematic reviews of water fluoridation" undertaken by the Centre for Reviews and Dissemination.[187]

BOX 3 IDENTIFICATION OF STUDY REPORTS AND DATA EXTRACTION

Comprehensive searches usually result in a large number of identified records, a much smaller number of studies included in the systematic review, and even fewer of these studies included in any meta-analyses. Reports of systematic reviews often provide little detail as to the methods used by the review team in this process. Readers are often left with what can be described as the "X-files" phenomenon, as it is unclear what occurs between the initial set of identified records and those finally included in the review.

Sometimes, review authors simply report the number of included studies; more often they report the initial number of identified records and the number of included studies. Rarely, although this is optimal for readers, do review authors report the number of identified records, the smaller number of potentially relevant studies, and the even smaller number of included studies, by outcome. Review authors also need to differentiate between the number of reports and studies. Often there will not be a 1:1 ratio of reports to studies and this information needs to be described in the systematic review report.

Ideally, the identification of study reports should be reported as text in combination with use of the PRISMA flow diagram. While we recommend use of the flow diagram, a small number of reviews might be particularly simple and can be sufficiently described with a few brief sentences of text. More generally, review authors will need to report the process used for each step: screening the identified records; examining the full text of potentially relevant studies (and reporting the number that could not be obtained); and applying eligibility criteria to select the included studies.

Such descriptions should also detail how potentially eligible records were promoted to the next stage of the review (such as full text screening) and to the final stage of this process, the included studies. Often review teams have three response options for excluding records or promoting them to the next stage of the winnowing process: "yes," "no," and "maybe."

Similarly, some detail should be reported on who participated and how such processes were completed. For example, a single person may screen the identified records while a second person independently examines a small sample of them. The entire winnowing process is one of "good bookkeeping" whereby interested readers should be able to work backwards from the included studies to come up with the same numbers of identified records.

There is often a paucity of information describing the data extraction processes in reports of systematic reviews. Authors may simply report that "relevant" data were extracted from each included study with little information about the processes used for data extraction. It may be useful for readers to know whether a systematic review's authors developed, a priori or not, a data extraction form, whether multiple forms were used, the number of questions, whether the form was pilot tested, and who completed the extraction. For example, it is important for readers to know whether one or more people extracted data, and if so, whether this was completed independently, whether "consensus" data were used in the analyses, and if the review team completed an informal training exercise or a more formal reliability exercise.

BOX 4 STUDY QUALITY AND RISK OF BIAS

In this paper, and elsewhere,[11] we sought to use a new term for many readers, namely, risk of bias, for evaluating each included study in a systematic review. Previous papers[89][188] tended to use the term "quality." When carrying out a systematic review we believe it is important to distinguish between quality and risk of bias and to focus on evaluating and reporting the latter. Quality is often the best the authors have been able to do. For example, authors may report the results of surgical trials in which blinding of the outcome assessors was not part of the trial's conduct. Even though this may have been the best methodology the researchers were able to do, there are still theoretical grounds for believing that the study was susceptible to (risk of) bias.

Assessing the risk of bias should be part of the conduct and reporting of any systematic review. In all situations, we encourage systematic reviewers to think ahead carefully about what risks of bias (methodological and clinical) may have a bearing on the results of their systematic reviews.

For systematic reviewers, understanding the risk of bias on the results of studies is often difficult, because the report is only a surrogate of the actual conduct of the study. There is some suggestion[189][190] that the report may not be a reasonable facsimile of the study, although this view is not shared by all.[88][191] There are three main ways to assess risk of bias—individual components, checklists, and scales. There are a great many scales available,[192] although we caution against their use based on theoretical grounds[193] and emerging empirical evidence.[194] Checklists are less frequently used and potentially have the same problems as scales. We advocate using a component approach and one that is based on domains for which there is good empirical evidence and perhaps strong clinical grounds. The new Cochrane risk of bias tool11 is one such component approach.

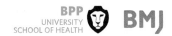

The Cochrane risk of bias tool consists of five items for which there is empirical evidence for their biasing influence on the estimates of an intervention's effectiveness in randomised trials (sequence generation, allocation concealment, blinding, incomplete outcome data, and selective outcome reporting) and a catch-all item called "other sources of bias".11 There is also some consensus that these items can be applied for evaluation of studies across diverse clinical areas.93 Other risk of bias items may be topic or even study specific—that is, they may stem from some peculiarity of the research topic or some special feature of the design of a specific study. These peculiarities need to be investigated on a case-by-case basis, based on clinical and methodological acumen, and there can be no general recipe. In all situations, systematic reviewers need to think ahead carefully about what aspects of study quality may have a bearing on the results.

BOX 5 WHETHER TO COMBINE DATA

Deciding whether to combine data involves statistical, clinical, and methodological considerations. The statistical decisions are perhaps the most technical and evidence-based. These are more thoroughly discussed in box 6. The clinical and methodological decisions are generally based on discussions within the review team and may be more subjective.

Clinical considerations will be influenced by the question the review is attempting to address. Broad questions might provide more "license" to combine more disparate studies, such as whether "Ritalin is effective in increasing focused attention in people diagnosed with attention deficit hyperactivity disorder (ADHD)." Here authors might elect to combine reports of studies involving children and adults. If the clinical question is more focused, such as whether "Ritalin is effective in increasing classroom attention in previously undiagnosed ADHD children who have no comorbid conditions," it is likely that different decisions regarding synthesis of studies are taken by authors. In any case authors should describe their clinical decisions in the systematic review report.

Deciding whether to combine data also has a methodological component. Reviewers may decide not to combine studies of low risk of bias with those of high risk of bias (see items 12 and 19). For example, for subjective outcomes, systematic review authors may not wish to combine assessments that were completed under blind conditions with those that were not.

For any particular question there may not be a "right" or "wrong" choice concerning synthesis, as such decisions are likely complex. However, as the choice may be subjective, authors should be transparent as to their key decisions and describe them for readers.

BOX 6 META-ANALYSIS AND ASSESSMENT OF CONSISTENCY (HETEROGENEITY)

Meta-analysis: statistical combination of the results of multiple studies

If it is felt that studies should have their results combined statistically, other issues must be considered because there are many ways to conduct a meta-analysis. Different effect measures can be used for both binary and continuous outcomes (see item 13). Also, there are two commonly used statistical models for combining data in a meta-analysis.[195] The fixed-effect model assumes that there is a common treatment effect for all included studies;[196] it is assumed that the observed differences in results across studies reflect random variation.[196] The random-effects model assumes that there is no common treatment effect for all included studies but rather that the variation of the effects across studies follows a particular distribution.[197] In a random-effects model it is believed that the included studies represent a random sample from a larger population of studies addressing the question of interest.[198]

There is no consensus about whether to use fixed- or random-effects models, and both are in wide use. The following differences have influenced some researchers regarding their choice between them. The random-effects model gives more weight to the results of smaller trials than does the fixed-effect analysis, which may be undesirable as small trials may be inferior and most prone to publication bias. The fixed-effect model considers only within-study variability, whereas the random-effects model considers both within- and between-study variability. This is why a fixed-effect analysis tends to give narrower confidence intervals (that is, provides greater precision) than a random-effects analysis.[110 196 199] In the absence of any between-study heterogeneity, the fixed- and random-effects estimates will coincide.

In addition, there are different methods for performing both types of meta-analysis.[200] Common fixed-effect approaches are Mantel-Haenszel and inverse variance, whereas random-effects analyses usually use the DerSimonian and Laird approach, although other methods exist, including Bayesian meta-analysis.[201]

In the presence of demonstrable between-study heterogeneity (see below), some consider that the use of a fixed-effect analysis is counterintuitive because their main assumption is violated. Others argue that it is inappropriate to conduct any meta-analysis when there is unexplained variability across trial results. If the reviewers decide not to combine the data quantitatively, a danger is that eventually they may end up using quasi-quantitative rules of poor validity (such as vote counting of how many studies have nominally significant results) for interpreting the evidence. Statistical methods to combine data exist for almost any complex situation that may arise in a systematic review, but one has to be aware of their assumptions and limitations to avoid misapplying or misinterpreting these methods.

Assessment of consistency (heterogeneity)

We expect some variation (inconsistency) in the results of different studies due to chance alone. Variability in excess of that due to chance reflects true differences in the results of the trials, and is called "heterogeneity." The conventional statistical approach to evaluating heterogeneity is a χ^2 test (Cochran's Q), but it has low power when there are few studies and excessive power when there are many studies.[202] By contrast, the I^2 statistic quantifies the amount of variation in results across studies beyond that expected by chance and so is preferable to Q.[202 203] I^2 represents the percentage of the total variation in estimated effects across studies that is due to heterogeneity rather than to chance; some authors consider an I^2 value less than 25% as low.[202] However, I^2 also suffers from large uncertainty in the common situation where only a few studies are available,[204] and reporting the uncertainty in I^2 (such as 95% confidence interval) may be helpful.[145] When there are few studies, inferences about heterogeneity should be cautious.

When considerable heterogeneity is observed, it is advisable to consider possible reasons.[205] In particular, the heterogeneity may be due to differences between subgroups of studies (see item 16). Also, data extraction errors are a common cause of substantial heterogeneity in results with continuous outcomes.[139]

BOX 7 BIAS CAUSED BY SELECTIVE PUBLICATION OF STUDIES OR RESULTS WITHIN STUDIES

Systematic reviews aim to incorporate information from all relevant studies. The absence of information from some studies may pose a serious threat to the validity of a review. Data may be incomplete because some studies were not published, or because of incomplete or inadequate reporting within a published article. These problems are often summarised as "publication bias," although the bias arises from non-publication of full studies and selective publication of results in relation to their findings. Non-publication of research findings dependent on the actual results is an important risk of bias to a systematic review and meta-analysis.

Missing studies

Several empirical investigations have shown that the findings from clinical trials are more likely to be published if the results are statistically significant (P<0.05) than if they are not.[125 206 207] For example, of 500 oncology trials with more than 200 participants for which preliminary results were presented at a conference of the American Society of Clinical Oncology, 81% with P<0.05 were published in full within five years compared with only 68% of those with P>0.05.[208]

Also, among published studies, those with statistically significant results are published sooner than those with non-significant findings.[209] When some studies are missing for these reasons, the available results will be biased towards exaggerating the effect of an intervention.

Missing outcomes

In many systematic reviews only some of the eligible studies (often a minority) can be included in a meta-analysis for a specific outcome. For some studies, the outcome may not be measured or may be measured but not reported. The former will not lead to bias, but the latter could.

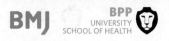

Evidence is accumulating that selective reporting bias is widespread and of considerable importance.[42 43] In addition, data for a given outcome may be analysed in multiple ways and the choice of presentation influenced by the results obtained. In a study of 102 randomised trials, comparison of published reports with trial protocols showed that a median of 38% efficacy and 50% safety outcomes per trial, respectively, were not available for meta-analysis. Statistically significant outcomes had higher odds of being fully reported in publications when compared with non-significant outcomes for both efficacy (pooled odds ratio 2.4 (95% confidence interval 1.4 to 4.0)) and safety (4.7 (1.8 to 12)) data. Several other studies have had similar findings.[210 211]

Detection of missing information

Missing studies may increasingly be identified from trials registries. Evidence of missing outcomes may come from comparison with the study protocol, if available, or by careful examination of published articles.[11] Study publication bias and selective outcome reporting are difficult to exclude or verify from the available results, especially when few studies are available.

If the available data are affected by either (or both) of the above biases, smaller studies would tend to show larger estimates of the effects of the intervention. Thus one possibility is to investigate the relation between effect size and sample size (or more specifically, precision of the effect estimate). Graphical methods, especially the funnel plot,[212] and analytic methods (such as Egger's test) are often used,[213 214 215] although their interpretation can be problematic.[216 217] Strictly speaking, such analyses investigate "small study bias"; there may be many reasons why smaller studies have systematically different effect sizes than larger studies, of which reporting bias is just one.[218] Several alternative tests for bias have also been proposed, beyond the ones testing small study bias,[215 219 220] but none can be considered a gold standard. Although evidence that smaller studies had larger estimated effects than large ones may suggest the possibility that the available evidence is biased, misinterpretation of such data is common.[123]

Canada); Lorenzo Moja, Centro Cochrane Italiano, Istituto Ricerche Farmacologiche Mario Negri; Maryann Napoli, Center for Medical Consumers (New York, USA); Cynthia Mulrow, *Annals of Internal Medicine* (Philadelphia, Pennsylvania, US); Andy Oxman, Norwegian Health Services Research Centre (Oslo, Norway); Ba' Pham, Toronto Health Economics and Technology Assessment Collaborative (Toronto, Canada) (at the time of first meeting of the group, GlaxoSmithKline Canada, Mississauga, Canada); Drummond Rennie, University of California San Francisco (San Francisco CA, USA); Margaret Sampson, Children's Hospital of Eastern Ontario (Ottawa, Canada); Kenneth F Schulz, Family Health International (Durham NC, USA); Paul G Shekelle, Southern California Evidence Based Practice Center (Santa Monica CA, USA); Jennifer Tetzlaff, Ottawa Methods Centre, Ottawa Hospital Research Institute (Ottawa, Canada); David Tovey, *Cochrane Library*, Cochrane Collaboration (Oxford, UK) (at the time of first meeting of the group, BMJ, London); Peter Tugwell, Institute of Population Health, University of Ottawa (Ottawa, Canada).

Lorenzo Moja helped with the preparation and the several updates of the manuscript and assisted with the preparation of the reference list. AL is the guarantor of the manuscript.

Competing interests: None declared.

Provenance and peer review: Not commissioned; externally peer reviewed.

In order to encourage dissemination of the PRISMA statement, this article is freely accessible on bmj.com and will also be published in *PLoS Medicine*, *Annals of Internal Medicine*, *Journal of Clinical Epidemiology*, and *Open Medicine*. The authors jointly hold the copyright of this article. For details on further use, see the PRISMA website (www.prisma-statement.org/).

1   Canadian Institutes of Health Research (2006) Randomized controlled trials registration/application checklist (12/2006). Available: http://www.cihr-irsc.gc.ca/e/documents/rct_reg_e.pdf. Accessed 26 May 2009.

2   Young C, Horton R. Putting clinical trials into context. *Lancet* 2005;366:107-108.

3   Moher D, Tetzlaff J, Tricco AC, Sampson M, Altman DG. Epidemiology and reporting characteristics of systematic reviews. *PLoS Med* 2007;4:e78. doi:10.1371/journal.pmed.0040078

4   Dixon E, Hameed M, Sutherland F, Cook DJ, Doig C. Evaluating meta-analyses in the general surgical literature: A critical appraisal. *Ann Surg* 2005;241:450-459.

5   Hemels ME, Vicente C, Sadri H, Masson MJ, Einarson TR. Quality assessment of meta-analyses of RCTs of pharmacotherapy in major depressive disorder. *Curr Med Res Opin* 2004;20:477-484.

6   Jin W, Yu R, Li W, Youping L, Ya L, et al. The reporting quality of meta-analyses improves: A random sampling study. *J Clin Epidemiol* 2008;61:770-775.

7   Moher D, Simera I, Schulz KF, Hoey J, Altman DG. Helping editors, peer reviewers and authors improve the clarity, completeness and transparency of reporting health research. *BMC Med* 2008;6:13.

8   Moher D, Cook DJ, Eastwood S, Olkin I, Rennie D, et al. Improving the quality of reports of meta-analyses of randomised controlled trials: The QUOROM statement. Quality of Reporting of Meta-analyses. *Lancet* 1999;354:1896-1900.

9   Green S, Higgins JPT, Alderson P, Clarke M, Mulrow CD, et al. Chapter 1: What is a systematic review? In: Higgins JPT, Green S, eds. Cochrane handbook for systematic reviews of interventions version 5.0.0 [updated February 2008]. The Cochrane Collaboration, 2008. Available: http://www.cochrane-handbook.org/. Accessed 26 May 2009.

10   Guyatt GH, Oxman AD, Vist GE, Kunz R, Falck-Ytter Y, et al. GRADE: An emerging consensus on rating quality of evidence and strength of recommendations. *BMJ* 2008;336:924-926.

11   Higgins JPT, Altman DG. Chapter 8: Assessing risk of bias in included studies. In: Higgins JPT, Green S, eds. Cochrane handbook for systematic reviews of interventions version 5.0.0 [updated February

2008]. The Cochrane Collaboration, 2008. Available: http://www.cochrane-handbook.org/. Accessed 26 May 2009.

12   Moher D, Liberati A, Tetzlaff J, Altman DG, The PRISMA Group. Preferred reporting items for systematic reviews and meta-analyses: The PRISMA Statement. *PLoS Med* 2008;6:e1000097. 10.1371/journal.pmed.1000097

13   Atkins D, Fink K, Slutsky J. Better information for better health care: The Evidence-based Practice Center program and the Agency for Healthcare Research and Quality. *Ann Intern Med* 2005;142:1035-1041.

14   Helfand M, Balshem H. Principles for developing guidance: AHRQ and the effective health-care program. *J Clin Epidemiol* 2009, In press.

15   Higgins JPT, Green S. Cochrane handbook for systematic reviews of interventions version 5.0.0 [updated February 2008]. The Cochrane Collaboration, 2008. Available: http://www.cochrane-handbook.org/. Accessed 26 May 2009.

16   Centre for Reviews and Dissemination. Systematic reviews: CRD's guidance for undertaking reviews in health care. York: University of York, 2009. Available: http://www.york.ac.uk/inst/crd/systematic_reviews_book.htm. Accessed 26 May 2009.

17   Altman DG, Schulz KF, Moher D, Egger M, Davidoff F, et al. The revised CONSORT statement for reporting randomized trials: Explanation and elaboration. *Ann Intern Med* 2001;134:663-694.

18   Bossuyt PM, Reitsma JB, Bruns DE, Gatsonis CA, Glasziou PP, et al. The STARD statement for reporting studies of diagnostic accuracy: Explanation and elaboration. *Clin Chem* 2003;49:7-18.

19   Vandenbroucke JP, von Elm E, Altman DG, Gøtzsche PC, Mulrow CD, et al. Strengthening the Reporting of Observational Studies in Epidemiology (STROBE): Explanation and elaboration. *PLoS Med* 2007;4:e297. doi:10.1371/journal.pmed.0040297

20   Barker A, Maratos EC, Edmonds L, Lim E. Recurrence rates of video-assisted thoracoscopic versus open surgery in the prevention of recurrent pneumothoraces: A systematic review of randomised and non-randomised trials. *Lancet* 2007;370:329-335.

21   Bjelakovic G, Nikolova D, Gluud LL, Simonetti RG, Gluud C. Mortality in randomized trials of antioxidant supplements for primary and secondary prevention: Systematic review and meta-analysis. *JAMA* 2007;297:842-857.

22   Montori VM, Wilczynski NL, Morgan D, Haynes RB. Optimal search strategies for retrieving systematic reviews from Medline: Analytical survey. *BMJ* 2005;330:68.

23   Bischoff-Ferrari HA, Willett WC, Wong JB, Giovannucci E, Dietrich T, et al. Fracture prevention with vitamin D supplementation: A meta-analysis of randomized controlled trials. *JAMA* 2005;293:2257-2264.

24   Hopewell S, Clarke M, Moher D, Wager E, Middleton P, et al. CONSORT for reporting randomised trials in journal and conference abstracts. *Lancet* 2008;371:281-283.

25   Hopewell S, Clarke M, Moher D, Wager E, Middleton P, et al. CONSORT for reporting randomized controlled trials in journal and conference abstracts: Explanation and elaboration. *PLoS Med* 2008;5:e20. doi:10.1371/journal.pmed.0050020

26   Haynes RB, Mulrow CD, Huth EJ, Altman DG, Gardner MJ. More informative abstracts revisited. *Ann Intern Med* 1990;113:69-76.

27   Mulrow CD, Thacker SB, Pugh JA. A proposal for more informative abstracts of review articles. *Ann Intern Med* 1988;108:613-615.

28   Froom P, Froom J. Deficiencies in structured medical abstracts. *J Clin Epidemiol* 1993;46:591-594.

29   Hartley J. Clarifying the abstracts of systematic literature reviews. *Bull Med Libr Assoc* 2000;88:332-337.

30   Hartley J, Sydes M, Blurton A. Obtaining information accurately and quickly: Are structured abstract more efficient? *J Infor Sci* 1996;22:349-356.

31   Pocock SJ, Hughes MD, Lee RJ. Statistical problems in the reporting of clinical trials. A survey of three medical journals. *N Engl J Med* 1987;317:426-432.

32   Taddio A, Pain T, Fassos FF, Boon H, Ilersich AL, et al. Quality of nonstructured and structured abstracts of original research articles in the British Medical Journal, the Canadian Medical Association Journal and the Journal of the American Medical Association. *CMAJ* 1994;150:1611-1615.

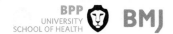

33   Harris KC, Kuramoto LK, Schulzer M, Retallack JE. Effect of school-based physical activity interventions on body mass index in children: A meta-analysis. *CMAJ* 2009;180:719-726.

34   James MT, Conley J, Tonelli M, Manns BJ, MacRae J, et al. Meta-analysis: Antibiotics for prophylaxis against hemodialysis catheter-related infections. *Ann Intern Med* 2008;148:596-605.

35   Counsell C. Formulating questions and locating primary studies for inclusion in systematic reviews. *Ann Intern Med* 1997;127:380-387.

36   Gotzsche PC. Why we need a broad perspective on meta-analysis. It may be crucially important for patients. *BMJ* 2000;321:585-586.

37   Grossman P, Niemann L, Schmidt S, Walach H. Mindfulness-based stress reduction and health benefits. A meta-analysis. *J Psychosom Res* 2004;57:35-43.

38   Brunton G, Green S, Higgins JPT, Kjeldstrøm M, Jackson N, et al. Chapter 2: Preparing a Cochrane review. In: Higgins JPT, Green S, eds. Cochrane handbook for systematic reviews of interventions version 5.0.0 [updated February 2008]. The Cochrane Collaboration, 2008. Available: http://www.cochrane-handbook.org/. Accessed 26 May 2009.

39   Sutton AJ, Abrams KR, Jones DR, Sheldon TA, Song F. Systematic reviews of trials and other studies. *Health Technol Assess* 1998;2:1-276.

40   Ioannidis JP, Rosenberg PS, Goedert JJ, O'Brien TR. Commentary: meta-analysis of individual participants' data in genetic epidemiology. *Am J Epidemiol* 2002;156:204-210.

41   Stewart LA, Clarke MJ. Practical methodology of meta-analyses (overviews) using updated individual patient data. Cochrane Working Group. *Stat Med* 1995;14:2057-2079.

42   Chan AW, Hrobjartsson A, Haahr MT, Gøtzsche PC, Altman DG. Empirical evidence for selective reporting of outcomes in randomized trials: Comparison of protocols to published articles. *JAMA* 2004;291:2457-2465.

43   Dwan K, Altman DG, Arnaiz JA, Bloom J, Chan AW, et al. Systematic review of the empirical evidence of study publication bias and outcome reporting bias. *PLoS ONE* 2008;3:e3081. doi:10.1371/journal.pone.0003081

44   Silagy CA, Middleton P, Hopewell S. Publishing protocols of systematic reviews: Comparing what was done to what was planned. *JAMA* 2002;287:2831-2834.

45   Centre for Reviews and Dissemination. Research projects. York: University of York, 2009. Available: http://www.crd.york.ac.uk/crdweb. Accessed 26 May 2009.

46   The Joanna Briggs Institute. Protocols & work in progress, 2009. Available: http://www.joannabriggs.edu.au/pubs/systematic_reviews_prot.php. Accessed 26 May 2009.

47   Bagshaw SM, McAlister FA, Manns BJ, Ghali WA. Acetylcysteine in the prevention of contrast-induced nephropathy: A case study of the pitfalls in the evolution of evidence. *Arch Intern Med* 2006;166:161-166.

48   Biondi-Zoccai GG, Lotrionte M, Abbate A, Testa L, Remigi E, et al. Compliance with QUOROM and quality of reporting of overlapping meta-analyses on the role of acetylcysteine in the prevention of contrast associated nephropathy: Case study. *BMJ* 2006;332:202-209.

49   Sacks HS, Berrier J, Reitman D, Ancona-Berk VA, Chalmers TC. Meta-analyses of randomized controlled trials. *N Engl J Med* 1987;316:450-455.

50   Schroth RJ, Hitchon CA, Uhanova J, Noreddin A, Taback SP, et al. Hepatitis B vaccination for patients with chronic renal failure. *Cochrane Database Syst Rev* 2004;(3):CD003775, doi:10.1002/14651858.CD003775.pub2

51   Egger M, Zellweger-Zahner T, Schneider M, Junker C, Lengeler C, et al. Language bias in randomised controlled trials published in English and German. *Lancet* 1997;350:326-329.

52   Gregoire G, Derderian F, Le Lorier J. Selecting the language of the publications included in a meta-analysis: Is there a Tower of Babel bias? *J Clin Epidemiol* 1995;48:159-163.

53   Jüni P, Holenstein F, Sterne J, Bartlett C, Egger M. Direction and impact of language bias in meta-analyses of controlled trials: Empirical study. *Int J Epidemiol* 2002;31:115-123.

54   Moher D, Pham B, Klassen TP, Schulz KF, Berlin JA, et al. What contributions do languages other than English make on the results of meta-analyses? *J Clin Epidemiol* 2000;53:964-972.

55   Pan Z, Trikalinos TA, Kavvoura FK, Lau J, Ioannidis JP. Local literature bias in genetic epidemiology: an empirical evaluation of the Chinese literature. *PLoS Med* 2005;2:e334. doi:10.1371/journal.pmed.0020334

56   Hopewell S, McDonald S, Clarke M, Egger M. Grey literature in meta-analyses of randomized trials of health care interventions. *Cochrane Database Syst Rev* 2007;(2):MR000010, doi:10.1002/14651858.MR000010.pub3.

57   Melander H, Ahlqvist-Rastad J, Meijer G, Beermann B. Evidence b(i)ased medicine—Selective reporting from studies sponsored by pharmaceutical industry: review of studies in new drug applications. *BMJ* 2003;326:1171-1173.

58   Sutton AJ, Duval SJ, Tweedie RL, Abrams KR, Jones DR. Empirical assessment of effect of publication bias on meta-analyses. *BMJ* 2000;320:1574-1577.

59   Gotzsche PC. Believability of relative risks and odds ratios in abstracts: Cross sectional study. *BMJ* 2006;333:231-234.

60   Bhandari M, Devereaux PJ, Guyatt GH, Cook DJ, Swiontkowski MF, et al. An observational study of orthopaedic abstracts and subsequent full-text publications. *J Bone Joint Surg Am* 2002;84-A:615-621.

61   Rosmarakis ES, Soteriades ES, Vergidis PI, Kasiakou SK, Falagas ME. From conference abstract to full paper: Differences between data presented in conferences and journals. *Faseb J* 2005;19:673-680.

62   Toma M, McAlister FA, Bialy L, Adams D, Vandermeer B, et al. Transition from meeting abstract to full-length journal article for randomized controlled trials. *JAMA* 2006;295:1281-1287.

63   Saunders Y, Ross JR, Broadley KE, Edmonds PM, Patel S. Systematic review of bisphosphonates for hypercalcaemia of malignancy. *Palliat Med* 2004;18:418-431.

64   Shojania KG, Sampson M, Ansari MT, Ji J, Doucette S, et al. How quickly do systematic reviews go out of date? A survival analysis. *Ann Intern Med* 2007;147:224-233.

65   Bergerhoff K, Ebrahim S, Paletta G. Do we need to consider 'in process citations' for search strategies? Ottawa, Ontario, Canada: 12th Cochrane Colloquium, 2-6 October 2004. Available: http://www.cochrane.org/colloquia/abstracts/ottawa/P-039.htm. Accessed 26 May 2009.

66   Zhang L, Sampson M, McGowan J. Reporting of the role of expert searcher in Cochrane reviews. *Evid Based Libr Info Pract* 2006;1:3-16.

67   Turner EH, Matthews AM, Linardatos E, Tell RA, Rosenthal R. Selective publication of antidepressant trials and its influence on apparent efficacy. *N Engl J Med* 2008;358:252-260.

68   Alejandria MM, Lansang MA, Dans LF, Mantaring JB. Intravenous immunoglobulin for treating sepsis and septic shock. *Cochrane Database Syst Rev* 2002;(1):CD001090, doi:10.1002/14651858.CD001090.

69   Golder S, McIntosh HM, Duffy S, Glanville J. Developing efficient search strategies to identify reports of adverse effects in MEDLINE and EMBASE. *Health Info Libr J* 2006;23:3-12.

70   Sampson M, McGowan J, Cogo E, Grimshaw J, Moher D, et al. An evidence-based practice guideline for the peer review of electronic search strategies. *J Clin Epidemiol* 2009; E-pub 2009 February 18.

71   Flores-Mir C, Major MP, Major PW. Search and selection methodology of systematic reviews in orthodontics (2000-2004). *Am J Orthod Dentofacial Orthop* 2006;130:214-217.

72   Major MP, Major PW, Flores-Mir C. An evaluation of search and selection methods used in dental systematic reviews published in English. *J Am Dent Assoc* 2006;137:1252-1257.

73   Major MP, Major PW, Flores-Mir C. Benchmarking of reported search and selection methods of systematic reviews by dental speciality. *Evid Based Dent* 2007;8:66-70.

74   Shah MR, Hasselblad V, Stevenson LW, Binanay C, O'Connor CM, et al. Impact of the pulmonary artery catheter in critically ill patients: Meta-analysis of randomized clinical trials. *JAMA* 2005;294:1664-1670.

75   Edwards P, Clarke M, DiGuiseppi C, Pratap S, Roberts I, et al. Identification of randomized controlled trials in systematic reviews: Accuracy and reliability of screening records. *Stat Med* 2002;21:1635-1640.

76   Cooper HM, Ribble RG. Influences on the outcome of literature searches for integrative research reviews. *Knowledge* 1989;10:179-201.

77   Mistiaen P, Poot E. Telephone follow-up, initiated by a hospital-based health professional, for postdischarge problems in patients discharged from hospital to home. *Cochrane Database Syst Rev* 2006;(4):CD004510, doi:10.1002/14651858.CD004510.pub3.

78   Jones AP, Remmington T, Williamson PR, Ashby D, Smyth RL. High prevalence but low impact of data extraction and reporting errors were found in Cochrane systematic reviews. *J Clin Epidemiol* 2005;58:741-742.

79   Clarke M, Hopewell S, Juszczak E, Eisinga A, Kjeldstrom M. Compression stockings for preventing deep vein thrombosis in airline passengers. *Cochrane Database Syst Rev* 2006;(2):CD004002, doi:10.1002/14651858.CD004002.pub2.

80   Tramer MR, Reynolds DJ, Moore RA, McQuay HJ. Impact of covert duplicate publication on meta-analysis: A case study. *BMJ* 1997;315:635-640.

81   von Elm E, Poglia G, Walder B, Tramer MR. Different patterns of duplicate publication: An analysis of articles used in systematic reviews. *JAMA* 2004;291:974-980.

82   Gotzsche PC. Multiple publication of reports of drug trials. *Eur J Clin Pharmacol* 1989;36:429-432.

83   Allen C, Hopewell S, Prentice A. Non-steroidal anti-inflammatory drugs for pain in women with endometriosis. *Cochrane Database Syst Rev* 2005;(4):CD004753, doi:10.1002/14651858.CD004753.pub2.

84   Glasziou P, Meats E, Heneghan C, Shepperd S. What is missing from descriptions of treatment in trials and reviews? *BMJ* 2008;336:1472-1474.

85   Tracz MJ, Sideras K, Bolona ER, Haddad RM, Kennedy CC, et al. Testosterone use in men and its effects on bone health. A systematic review and meta-analysis of randomized placebo-controlled trials. *J Clin Endocrinol Metab* 2006;91:2011-2016.

86   Bucher HC, Hengstler P, Schindler C, Guyatt GH. Percutaneous transluminal coronary angioplasty versus medical treatment for non-acute coronary heart disease: Meta-analysis of randomised controlled trials. *BMJ* 2000;321:73-77.

87   Gluud LL. Bias in clinical intervention research. *Am J Epidemiol* 2006;163:493-501.

88   Pildal J, Hróbjartsson A, Jorgensen KJ, Hilden J, Altman DG, et al. Impact of allocation concealment on conclusions drawn from meta-analyses of randomized trials. *Int J Epidemiol* 2007;36:847-857.

89   Moja LP, Telaro E, D'Amico R, Moschetti I, Coe L, et al. Assessment of methodological quality of primary studies by systematic reviews: Results of the metaquality cross sectional study. *BMJ* 2005;330:1053.

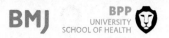

90 Moher D, Jadad AR, Tugwell P. Assessing the quality of randomized controlled trials. Current issues and future directions. *Int J Technol Assess Health Care* 1996;12:195-208.

91 Sanderson S, Tatt ID, Higgins JP. Tools for assessing quality and susceptibility to bias in observational studies in epidemiology: A systematic review and annotated bibliography. *Int J Epidemiol* 2007;36:666-676.

92 Greenland S. Invited commentary: A critical look at some popular meta-analytic methods. *Am J Epidemiol* 1994;140:290-296.

93 Jüni P, Altman DG, Egger M. Systematic reviews in health care: Assessing the quality of controlled clinical trials. *BMJ* 2001;323:42-46.

94 Kunz R, Oxman AD. The unpredictability paradox: Review of empirical comparisons of randomised and non-randomised clinical trials. *BMJ* 1998;317:1185-1190.

95 Balk EM, Bonis PA, Moskowitz H, Schmid CH, Ioannidis JP, et al. Correlation of quality measures with estimates of treatment effect in meta-analyses of randomized controlled trials. *JAMA* 2002;287:2973-2982.

96 Devereaux PJ, Beattie WS, Choi PT, Badner NH, Guyatt GH, et al. How strong is the evidence for the use of perioperative beta blockers in non-cardiac surgery? Systematic review and meta-analysis of randomised controlled trials. *BMJ* 2005;331:313-321.

97 Devereaux PJ, Bhandari M, Montori VM, Manns BJ, Ghali WA, et al. Double blind, you are the weakest link—Good-bye! *ACP J Club* 2002;136:A11.

98 van Nieuwenhoven CA, Buskens E, van Tiel FH, Bonten MJ. Relationship between methodological trial quality and the effects of selective digestive decontamination on pneumonia and mortality in critically ill patients. *JAMA* 2001;286:335-340.

99 Guyatt GH, Cook D, Devereaux PJ, Meade M, Straus S. Therapy. Users' guides to the medical literature. AMA Press, 2002:55-79.

100 Sackett DL, Gent M. Controversy in counting and attributing events in clinical trials. *N Engl J Med* 1979;301:1410-1412.

101 Montori VM, Devereaux PJ, Adhikari NK, Burns KE, Eggert CH, et al. Randomized trials stopped early for benefit: A systematic review. *JAMA* 2005;294:2203-2209.

102 Guyatt GH, Devereaux PJ. Therapy and validity: The principle of intention-to-treat. In: Guyatt GH, Rennie DR, eds. Users' guides to the medical literature. AMA Press, 2002:267-273.

103 Berlin JA. Does blinding of readers affect the results of meta-analyses? University of Pennsylvania Meta-analysis Blinding Study Group. *Lancet* 1997;350:185-186.

104 Jadad AR, Moore RA, Carroll D, Jenkinson C, Reynolds DJ, et al. Assessing the quality of reports of randomized clinical trials: Is blinding necessary? *Control Clin Trials* 1996;17:1-12.

105 Pittas AG, Siegel RD, Lau J. Insulin therapy for critically ill hospitalized patients: A meta-analysis of randomized controlled trials. *Arch Intern Med* 2004;164:2005-2011.

106 Lakhdar R, Al-Mallah MH, Lanfear DE. Safety and tolerability of angiotensin-converting enzyme inhibitor versus the combination of angiotensin-converting enzyme inhibitor and angiotensin receptor blocker in patients with left ventricular dysfunction: A systematic review and meta-analysis of randomized controlled trials. *J Card Fail* 2008;14:181-188.

107 Bobat R, Coovadia H, Stephen C, Naidoo KL, McKerrow N, et al. Safety and efficacy of zinc supplementation for children with HIV-1 infection in South Africa: A randomised double-blind placebo-controlled trial. *Lancet* 2005;366:1862-1867.

108 Deeks JJ, Altman DG. Effect measures for meta-analysis of trials with binary outcomes. In: Egger M, Smith GD, Altman DG, eds. Systematic reviews in healthcare: Meta-analysis in context. 2nd edn. London: BMJ Publishing Group, 2001.

109 Deeks JJ. Issues in the selection of a summary statistic for meta-analysis of clinical trials with binary outcomes. *Stat Med* 2002;21:1575-1600.

110 Engels EA, Schmid CH, Terrin N, Olkin I, Lau J. Heterogeneity and statistical significance in meta-analysis: An empirical study of 125 meta-analyses. *Stat Med* 2000;19:1707-1728.

111 Tierney JF, Stewart LA, Ghersi D, Burdett S, Sydes MR. Practical methods for incorporating summary time-to-event data into meta-analysis. *Trials* 2007;8:16.

112 Michiels S, Piedbois P, Burdett S, Syz N, Stewart L, et al. Meta-analysis when only the median survival times are known: A comparison with individual patient data results. *Int J Technol Assess Health Care* 2005;21:119-125.

113 Briel M, Studer M, Glass TR, Bucher HC. Effects of statins on stroke prevention in patients with and without coronary heart disease: A meta-analysis of randomized controlled trials. *Am J Med* 2004;117:596-606.

114 Jones M, Schenkel B, Just J, Fallowfield L. Epoetin alfa improves quality of life in patients with cancer: Results of metaanalysis. *Cancer* 2004;101:1720-1732.

115 Elbourne DR, Altman DG, Higgins JP, Curtin F, Worthington HV, et al. Meta-analyses involving cross-over trials: Methodological issues. *Int J Epidemiol* 2002;31:140-149.

116 Follmann D, Elliott P, Suh I, Cutler J. Variance imputation for overviews of clinical trials with continuous response. *J Clin Epidemiol* 1992;45:769-773.

117 Wiebe N, Vandermeer B, Platt RW, Klassen TP, Moher D, et al. A systematic review identifies a lack of standardization in methods for handling missing variance data. *J Clin Epidemiol* 2006;59:342-353.

118 Hrobjartsson A, Gotzsche PC. Placebo interventions for all clinical conditions. *Cochrane Database Syst Rev* 2004;(2):CD003974, doi:10.1002/14651858.CD003974.pub2.

119 Shekelle PG, Morton SC, Maglione M, Suttorp M, Tu W, et al. Pharmacological and surgical treatment of obesity. *Evid Rep Technol Assess (Summ)* 2004:1-6.

120 Chan AW, Altman DG. Identifying outcome reporting bias in randomised trials on PubMed: Review of publications and survey of authors. *BMJ* 2005;330:753.

121 Williamson PR, Gamble C. Identification and impact of outcome selection bias in meta-analysis. *Stat Med* 2005;24:1547-1561.

122 Williamson PR, Gamble C, Altman DG, Hutton JL. Outcome selection bias in meta-analysis. *Stat Methods Med Res* 2005;14:515-524.

123 Ioannidis JP, Trikalinos TA. The appropriateness of asymmetry tests for publication bias in meta-analyses: A large survey. *CMAJ* 2007;176:1091-1096.

124 Briel M, Schwartz GG, Thompson PL, de Lemos JA, Blazing MA, et al. Effects of early treatment with statins on short-term clinical outcomes in acute coronary syndromes: A meta-analysis of randomized controlled trials. *JAMA* 2006;295:2046-2056.

125 Song F, Eastwood AJ, Gilbody S, Duley L, Sutton AJ. Publication and related biases. *Health Technol Assess* 2000;4:1-115.

126 Schmid CH, Stark PC, Berlin JA, Landais P, Lau J. Meta-regression detected associations between heterogeneous treatment effects and study-level, but not patient-level, factors. *J Clin Epidemiol* 2004;57:683-697.

127 Higgins JP, Thompson SG. Controlling the risk of spurious findings from meta-regression. *Stat Med* 2004;23:1663-1682.

128 Thompson SG, Higgins JP. Treating individuals 4: Can meta-analysis help target interventions at individuals most likely to benefit? *Lancet* 2005;365:341-346.

129 Uitterhoeve RJ, Vernooy M, Litjens M, Potting K, Bensing J, et al. Psychosocial interventions for patients with advanced cancer—A systematic review of the literature. *Br J Cancer* 2004;91:1050-1062.

130 Fuccio L, Minardi ME, Zagari RM, Grilli D, Magrini N, et al. Meta-analysis: Duration of first-line proton-pump inhibitor based triple therapy for *Helicobacter pylori* eradication. *Ann Intern Med* 2007;147:553-562.

131 Egger M, Smith GD. Bias in location and selection of studies. *BMJ* 1998;316:61-66.

132 Ravnskov U. Cholesterol lowering trials in coronary heart disease: Frequency of citation and outcome. *BMJ* 1992;305:15-19.

133 Hind D, Booth A. Do health technology assessments comply with QUOROM diagram guidance? An empirical study. *BMC Med Res Methodol* 2007;7:49.

134 Curioni C, Andre C. Rimonabant for overweight or obesity. *Cochrane Database Syst Rev* 2006;(4):CD006162, doi:10.1002/14651858.CD006162.pub2.

135 DeCamp LR, Byerley JS, Doshi N, Steiner MJ. Use of antiemetic agents in acute gastroenteritis: A systematic review and meta-analysis. *Arch Pediatr Adolesc Med* 2008;162:858-865.

136 Pakos EE, Ioannidis JP. Radiotherapy vs. nonsteroidal anti-inflammatory drugs for the prevention of heterotopic ossification after major hip procedures: A meta-analysis of randomized trials. *Int J Radiat Oncol Biol Phys* 2004;60:888-895.

137 Skalsky K, Yahav D, Bishara J, Pitlik S, Leibovici L, et al. Treatment of human brucellosis: Systematic review and meta-analysis of randomised controlled trials. *BMJ* 2008;336:701-704.

138 Altman DG, Cates C. The need for individual trial results in reports of systematic reviews. *BMJ* 2001. Rapid response.

139 Gotzsche PC, Hrobjartsson A, Maric K, Tendal B. Data extraction errors in meta-analyses that use standardized mean differences. *JAMA* 2007;298:430-437.

140 Lewis S, Clarke M. Forest plots: Trying to see the wood and the trees. *BMJ* 2001;322:1479-1480.

141 Papanikolaou PN, Ioannidis JP. Availability of large-scale evidence on specific harms from systematic reviews of randomized trials. *Am J Med* 2004;117:582-589.

142 Duffett M, Choong K, Ng V, Randolph A, Cook DJ. Surfactant therapy for acute respiratory failure in children: A systematic review and meta-analysis. *Crit Care* 2007;11:R66.

143 Balk E, Raman G, Chung M, Ip S, Tatsioni A, et al. Effectiveness of management strategies for renal artery stenosis: A systematic review. *Ann Intern Med* 2006;145:901-912.

144 Palfreyman S, Nelson EA, Michaels JA. Dressings for venous leg ulcers: Systematic review and meta-analysis. *BMJ* 2007;335:244.

145 Ioannidis JP, Patsopoulos NA, Evangelou E. Uncertainty in heterogeneity estimates in meta-analyses. *BMJ* 2007;335:914-916.

146 Appleton KM, Hayward RC, Gunnell D, Peters TJ, Rogers PJ, et al. Effects of n-3 long-chain polyunsaturated fatty acids on depressed mood: systematic review of published trials. *Am J Clin Nutr* 2006;84:1308-1316.

147 Kirsch I, Deacon BJ, Huedo-Medina TB, Scoboria A, Moore TJ, et al. Initial severity and antidepressant benefits: A meta-analysis of data submitted to the Food and Drug Administration. *PLoS Med* 2008;5:e45. doi:10.1371/journal.pmed.0050045

148 Reichenbach S, Sterchi R, Scherer M, Trelle S, Burgi E, et al. Meta-analysis: Chondroitin for osteoarthritis of the knee or hip. *Ann Intern Med* 2007;146:580-590.

149 Hodson EM, Craig JC, Strippoli GF, Webster AC. Antiviral medications for preventing cytomegalovirus disease in solid organ transplant

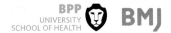

recipients. *Cochrane Database Syst Rev* 2008;(2):CD003774, doi:10.1002/14651858.CD003774.pub3.

150 Thompson SG, Higgins JP. How should meta-regression analyses be undertaken and interpreted? *Stat Med* 2002;21:1559-1573.

151 Chan AW, Krleza-Jeric K, Schmid I, Altman DG. Outcome reporting bias in randomized trials funded by the Canadian Institutes of Health Research. *CMAJ* 2004;171:735-740.

152 Hahn S, Williamson PR, Hutton JL, Garner P, Flynn EV. Assessing the potential for bias in meta-analysis due to selective reporting of subgroup analyses within studies. *Stat Med* 2000;19:3325-3336.

153 Green LW, Glasgow RE. Evaluating the relevance, generalization, and applicability of research: Issues in external validation and translation methodology. *Eval Health Prof* 2006;29:126-153.

154 Liberati A, D'Amico R, Pifferi, Torri V, Brazzi L. Antibiotic prophylaxis to reduce respiratory tract infections and mortality in adults receiving intensive care. *Cochrane Database Syst Rev* 2004;(1):CD000022, doi:10.1002/14651858.CD000022.pub2.

155 Gonzalez R, Zamora J, Gomez-Camarero J, Molinero LM, Banares R, et al. Meta-analysis: Combination endoscopic and drug therapy to prevent variceal rebleeding in cirrhosis. *Ann Intern Med* 2008;149:109-122.

156 D'Amico R, Pifferi S, Leonetti C, Torri V, Tinazzi A, et al. Effectiveness of antibiotic prophylaxis in critically ill adult patients: Systematic review of randomised controlled trials. *BMJ* 1998;316:1275-1285.

157 Olsen O, Middleton P, Ezzo J, Gotzsche PC, Hadhazy V, et al. Quality of Cochrane reviews: Assessment of sample from 1998. *BMJ* 2001;323:829-832.

158 Hopewell S, Wolfenden L, Clarke M. Reporting of adverse events in systematic reviews can be improved: Survey results. *J Clin Epidemiol* 2008;61:597-602.

159 Cook DJ, Reeve BK, Guyatt GH, Heyland DK, Griffith LE, et al. Stress ulcer prophylaxis in critically ill patients. Resolving discordant meta-analyses. *JAMA* 1996;275:308-314.

160 Jadad AR, Cook DJ, Browman GP. A guide to interpreting discordant systematic reviews. *CMAJ* 1997;156:1411-1416.

161 Clarke L, Clarke M, Clarke T. How useful are Cochrane reviews in identifying research needs? *J Health Serv Res Policy* 2007;12:101-103.

162 [No authors listed]. World Medical Association Declaration of Helsinki: Ethical principles for medical research involving human subjects. *JAMA* 2000;284:3043-3045.

163 Clarke M, Hopewell S, Chalmers I. Reports of clinical trials should begin and end with up-to-date systematic reviews of other relevant evidence: A status report. *J R Soc Med* 2007;100:187-190.

164 Dube C, Rostom A, Lewin G, Tsertsvadze A, Barrowman N, et al. The use of aspirin for primary prevention of colorectal cancer: A systematic review prepared for the U.S. Preventive Services Task Force. *Ann Intern Med* 2007;146:365-375.

165 Critchley J, Bates I. Haemoglobin colour scale for anaemia diagnosis where there is no laboratory: A systematic review. *Int J Epidemiol* 2005;34:1425-1434.

166 Lexchin J, Bero LA, Djulbegovic B, Clark O. Pharmaceutical industry sponsorship and research outcome and quality: Systematic review. *BMJ* 2003;326:1167-1170.

167 Als-Nielsen B, Chen W, Gluud C, Kjaergard LL. Association of funding and conclusions in randomized drug trials: A reflection of treatment effect or adverse events? *JAMA* 2003;290:921-928.

168 Peppercorn J, Blood E, Winer E, Partridge A. Association between pharmaceutical involvement and outcomes in breast cancer clinical trials. *Cancer* 2007;109:1239-1246.

169 Yank V, Rennie D, Bero LA. Financial ties and concordance between results and conclusions in meta-analyses: Retrospective cohort study. *BMJ* 2007;335:1202-1205.

170 Jorgensen AW, Hilden J, Gøtzsche PC. Cochrane reviews compared with industry supported meta-analyses and other meta-analyses of the same drugs: Systematic review. *BMJ* 2006;333:782.

171 Gotzsche PC, Hrobjartsson A, Johansen HK, Haahr MT, Altman DG, et al. Ghost authorship in industry-initiated randomised trials. *PLoS Med* 2007;4:e19. doi:10.1371/journal.pmed.0040019

172 Akbari A, Mayhew A, Al-Alawi M, Grimshaw J, Winkens R, et al. Interventions to improve outpatient referrals from primary care to secondary care. *Cochrane Database of Syst Rev* 2008;(2):CD005471, doi:10.1002/14651858.CD005471.pub2.

173 Davies P, Boruch R. The Campbell Collaboration. *BMJ* 2001;323:294-295.

174 Pawson R, Greenhalgh T, Harvey G, Walshe K. Realist review—A new method of systematic review designed for complex policy interventions. *J Health Serv Res Policy* 2005;10(Suppl 1):21-34.

175 Greenhalgh T, Robert G, Macfarlane F, Bate P, Kyriakidou O, et al. Storylines of research in diffusion of innovation: A meta-narrative approach to systematic review. *Soc Sci Med* 2005;61:417-430.

176 Lumley T. Network meta-analysis for indirect treatment comparisons. *Stat Med* 2002;21:2313-2324.

177 Salanti G, Higgins JP, Ades AE, Ioannidis JP. Evaluation of networks of randomized trials. *Stat Methods Med Res* 2008;17:279-301.

178 Altman DG, Moher D. [Developing guidelines for reporting healthcare research: scientific rationale and procedures.]. *Med Clin (Barc)* 2005;125(Suppl 1):8-13.

179 Delaney A, Bagshaw SM, Ferland A, Manns B, Laupland KB, et al. A systematic evaluation of the quality of meta-analyses in the critical care literature. *Crit Care* 2005;9:R575-582.

180 Altman DG, Simera I, Hoey J, Moher D, Schulz K. EQUATOR: Reporting guidelines for health research. *Lancet* 2008;371:1149-1150.

181 Plint AC, Moher D, Morrison A, Schulz K, Altman DG, et al. Does the CONSORT checklist improve the quality of reports of randomised controlled trials? A systematic review. *Med J Aust* 2006;185:263-267.

182 Simera I, Altman DG, Moher D, Schulz KF, Hoey J. Guidelines for reporting health research: The EQUATOR network's survey of guideline authors. *PLoS Med* 2008;5:e139. doi:10.1371/journal.pmed.0050139

183 Last JM. A dictionary of epidemiology. Oxford: Oxford University Press & International Epidemiological Association, 2001.

184 Antman EM, Lau J, Kupelnick B, Mosteller F, Chalmers TC. A comparison of results of meta-analyses of randomized control trials and recommendations of clinical experts. Treatments for myocardial infarction. *JAMA* 1992;268:240-248.

185 Oxman AD, Guyatt GH. The science of reviewing research. *Ann N Y Acad Sci* 1993;703:125-133; discussion 133-124.

186 O'Connor D, Green S, Higgins JPT. Chapter 5: Defining the review question and developing criteria for including studies. In: Higgins JPT, Green S, editors. Cochrane handbook for systematic reviews of interventions version 5.0.0 [updated February 2008]. The Cochrane Collaboration, 2008. Available: http://www.cochrane-handbook.org/. Accessed 26 May 2009.

187 McDonagh M, Whiting P, Bradley M, Cooper J, Sutton A, et al. A systematic review of public water fluoridation. Protocol changes (Appendix M). NHS Centre for Reviews and Dissemination. York: University of York, 2000. Available: http://www.york.ac.uk/inst/crd/pdf/appm.pdf.. Accessed 26 May 2009.

188 Moher D, Cook DJ, Jadad AR, Tugwell P, Moher M, et al. Assessing the quality of reports of randomised trials: Implications for the conduct of meta-analyses. *Health Technol Assess* 1999;3:i-iv, 1-98.

189 Devereaux PJ, Choi PT, El-Dika S, Bhandari M, Montori VM, et al. An observational study found that authors of randomized controlled trials frequently use concealment of randomization and blinding, despite the failure to report these methods. *J Clin Epidemiol* 2004;57:1232-1236.

190 Soares HP, Daniels S, Kumar A, Clarke M, Scott C, et al. Bad reporting does not mean bad methods for randomised trials: Observational study of randomised controlled trials performed by the Radiation Therapy Oncology Group. *BMJ* 2004;328:22-24.

191 Liberati A, Himel HN, Chalmers TC. A quality assessment of randomized control trials of primary treatment of breast cancer. *J Clin Oncol* 1986;4:942-951.

192 Moher D, Jadad AR, Nichol G, Penman M, Tugwell P, et al. Assessing the quality of randomized controlled trials: An annotated bibliography of scales and checklists. *Control Clin Trials* 1995;16:62-73.

193 Greenland S, O'Rourke K. On the bias produced by quality scores in meta-analysis, and a hierarchical view of proposed solutions. *Biostatistics* 2001;2:463-471.

194 Jüni P, Witschi A, Bloch R, Egger M. The hazards of scoring the quality of clinical trials for meta-analysis. *JAMA* 1999;282:1054-1060.

195 Fleiss JL. The statistical basis of meta-analysis. *Stat Methods Med Res* 1993;2:121-145.

196 Villar J, Mackey ME, Carroli G, Donner A. Meta-analyses in systematic reviews of randomized controlled trials in perinatal medicine: Comparison of fixed and random effects models. *Stat Med* 2001;20:3635-3647.

197 Lau J, Ioannidis JP, Schmid CH. Summing up evidence: One answer is not always enough. *Lancet* 1998;351:123-127.

198 DerSimonian R, Laird N. Meta-analysis in clinical trials. *Control Clin Trials* 1986;7:177-188.

199 Hunter JE, Schmidt FL. Fixed effects vs. random effects meta-analysis models: Implications for cumulative research knowledge. *Int J Sel Assess* 2000;8:275-292.

200 Deeks JJ, Altman DG, Bradburn MJ. Statistical methods for examining heterogeneity and combining results from several studies in meta-analysis. In: Egger M, Davey Smith G, Altman DG, eds. Systematic reviews in healthcare: Meta-analysis in context. London: BMJ Publishing Group, 2001:285-312.

201 Warn DE, Thompson SG, Spiegelhalter DJ. Bayesian random effects meta-analysis of trials with binary outcomes: Methods for the absolute risk difference and relative risk scales. *Stat Med* 2002;21:1601-1623.

202 Higgins JP, Thompson SG, Deeks JJ, Altman DG. Measuring inconsistency in meta-analyses. *BMJ* 2003;327:557-560.

203 Higgins JP, Thompson SG. Quantifying heterogeneity in a meta-analysis. *Stat Med* 2002;21:1539-1558.

204 Huedo-Medina TB, Sanchez-Meca J, Marin-Martinez F, Botella J. Assessing heterogeneity in meta-analysis: Q statistic or I2 index? *Psychol Methods* 2006;11:193-206.

205 Thompson SG, Turner RM, Warn DE. Multilevel models for meta-analysis, and their application to absolute risk differences. *Stat Methods Med Res* 2001;10:375-392.

206 Dickersin K. Publication bias: Recognising the problem, understanding its origin and scope, and preventing harm. In: Rothstein HR, Sutton AJ, Borenstein M, eds. Publication bias in meta-analysis—Prevention, assessment and adjustments. West Sussex: John Wiley & Sons, 2005:356.

207 Scherer RW, Langenberg P, von Elm E. Full publication of results initially presented in abstracts. *Cochrane Database Syst Rev* 2007;(2):MR000005, doi:10.1002/14651858.MR000005.pub3.

208 Krzyzanowska MK, Pintilie M, Tannock IF. Factors associated with failure to publish large randomized trials presented at an oncology meeting. *JAMA* 2003;290:495-501.

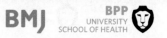

209 Hopewell S, Clarke M. Methodologists and their methods. Do methodologists write up their conference presentations or is it just 15 minutes of fame? *Int J Technol Assess Health Care* 2001;17:601-603.

210 Ghersi D. Issues in the design, conduct and reporting of clinical trials that impact on the quality of decision making. PhD thesis. Sydney: School of Public Health, Faculty of Medicine, University of Sydney, 2006.

211 von Elm E, Rollin A, Blumle A, Huwiler K, Witschi M, et al. Publication and non-publication of clinical trials: Longitudinal study of applications submitted to a research ethics committee. *Swiss Med Wkly* 2008;138:197-203.

212 Sterne JA, Egger M. Funnel plots for detecting bias in meta-analysis: guidelines on choice of axis. *J Clin Epidemiol* 2001;54:1046-1055.

213 Harbord RM, Egger M, Sterne JA. A modified test for small-study effects in meta-analyses of controlled trials with binary endpoints. *Stat Med* 2006;25:3443-3457.

214 Peters JL, Sutton AJ, Jones DR, Abrams KR, Rushton L. Comparison of two methods to detect publication bias in meta-analysis. *JAMA* 2006;295:676-680.

215 Rothstein HR, Sutton AJ, Borenstein M. Publication bias in meta-analysis: Prevention, assessment and adjustments. West Sussex: John Wiley & Sons, 2005.

216 Lau J, Ioannidis JP, Terrin N, Schmid CH, Olkin I. The case of the misleading funnel plot. *BMJ* 2006;333:597-600.

217 Terrin N, Schmid CH, Lau J. In an empirical evaluation of the funnel plot, researchers could not visually identify publication bias. *J Clin Epidemiol* 2005;58:894-901.

218 Egger M, Davey Smith G, Schneider M, Minder C. Bias in meta-analysis detected by a simple, graphical test. *BMJ* 1997;315:629-634.

219 Ioannidis JP, Trikalinos TA. An exploratory test for an excess of significant findings. *Clin Trials* 2007;4:245-253.

220 Sterne JAC, Egger M, Moher D. Chapter 10: Addressing reporting biases. In: Higgins JPT, Green S, eds. Cochrane handbook for systematic reviews of interventions version 5.0.0 [updated February 2008]. The Cochrane Collaboration, 2008. Available: http://www.cochrane-handbook.org/. Accessed 26 May 2009.

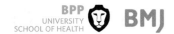

Consolidated Health Economic Evaluation Reporting Standards (CHEERS) statement

Don Husereau, senior associate; adjunct professor of medicine; senior scientist[1] [2] [3], Michael Drummond, co-editor-in-chief, Value in Health; professor of health economics[4], Stavros Petrou, professor of health economics[5], Chris Carswell, editor[6], David Moher, senior scientist[7], Dan Greenberg, associate professor and chairman; visiting assistant professor[8] [9], Federico Augustovski, director; professor of public health[10] [11], Andrew H Briggs, William R Lindsay chair of health economics, health economics and health technology assessment[12], Josephine Mauskopf, vice president of health economics[13], Elizabeth Loder, chief of division; clinical epidemiology editor, BMJ[14], on behalf of the CHEERS Task Force

[1]Institute of Health Economics, Edmonton, Canada

[2]Department of Epidemiology and Community Medicine. University of Ottawa, Ottawa, Canada

[3]University for Health Sciences, Medical Informatics and Technology, Hall in Tirol, Austria

[4]Centre for Health Economics, University of York, York, UK

[5]Warwick Medical School, University of Warwick, Coventry, UK

[6]Pharmacoeconomics, Adis International, Auckland, New Zealand

[7]Clinical Epidemiology Program, Ottawa Hospital Research Institute, Ottawa, Canada

[8]Department of Health Systems Management, Faculty of Health Sciences, Ben-Gurion University of the Negev, Beer-Sheva, Israel

[9]Center for the Evaluation of Value and Risk in Health, Tufts Medical Center, Boston MA, USA

[10]Health Economic Evaluation and Technology Assessment, Institute for Clinical Effectiveness and Health Policy (IECS), Buenos Aires, Argentina

[11]Universidad de Buenos Aires, Buenos Aires, Argentina

[12]Institute of Health and Wellbeing, University of Glasgow, Glasgow, Scotland

[13]RTI Health Solutions, Research Triangle Park NC, USA

[14]Division of Headache and Pain, Brigham and Women's/Faulkner Neurology, Faulkner Hospital, Boston MA, USA

Correspondence to: D Husereau, 879 Winnington Ave, Ottawa, ON K2B 5C4, Canada donh@donhusereau.com

Cite this as: BMJ 2013;346:f1049

http://www.bmj.com/content/346/bmj.f1049

ABSTRACT

Economic evaluations of health interventions pose a particular challenge for reporting. There is also a need to consolidate and update existing guidelines and promote their use in a user friendly manner. The Consolidated Health Economic Evaluation Reporting Standards (CHEERS) statement is an attempt to consolidate and update previous health economic evaluation guidelines efforts into one current, useful reporting guidance.

The primary audiences for the CHEERS statement are researchers reporting economic evaluations and the editors and peer reviewers assessing them for publication.

The need for new reporting guidance was identified by a survey of medical editors. A list of possible items based on a systematic review was created. A two round, modified Delphi panel consisting of representatives from academia, clinical practice, industry, government, and the editorial community was conducted. Out of 44 candidate items, 24 items and accompanying recommendations were developed. The recommendations are contained in a user friendly, 24 item checklist. A copy of the statement, accompanying checklist, and this report can be found on the ISPOR Health Economic Evaluations Publication Guidelines Task Force website (www.ispor.org/TaskForces/EconomicPubGuidelines.asp).

We hope CHEERS will lead to better reporting, and ultimately, better health decisions. To facilitate dissemination and uptake, the CHEERS statement is being co-published across 10 health economics and medical journals. We encourage other journals and groups, to endorse CHEERS. The author team plans to review the checklist for an update in five years.

Health economic evaluations are conducted to inform resource allocation decisions. Economic evaluation has been defined as "the comparative analysis of alternative courses of action in terms of both their costs and their consequences."[1] All economic evaluations assess costs, but approaches to measuring and valuing the consequences of health interventions may differ (see box).

Economic evaluations have been widely applied in health policy, including the assessment of prevention programmes (such as vaccination, screening, and health promotion), diagnostics, treatment interventions (such as drugs and surgical procedures), organisation of care, and rehabilitation. Economic evaluations are increasingly being used for decision making and are an important component of programmes for health technology assessment internationally.[2]

Reporting challenges and shortcomings in health economic evaluations

Compared with clinical studies, which report the consequences of an intervention only, economic evaluations require more reporting space for additional items, such as resource use, costs, preference related information, and cost effectiveness results. This creates challenges for editors, reviewers, and those who wish to scrutinise a study's findings.[3] There is evidence that the quality of reporting of economic evaluations varies widely and could potentially benefit from improved quality assurance mechanisms.[4] [5]

With the increasing number of publications available, and opportunity costs from decisions based on misleading study findings, transparency and clarity in reporting are important. In addition, outside of economic evaluations conducted alongside clinical trials, there are no widespread mechanisms for warehousing economic evaluation data to allow for independent interrogation, such as ethics review proceedings, regulator dossiers, or study registries. Instead, independent analysis may rely on the record keeping of individual investigators.

Even if measures to promote transparency exist, such as registries, biomedical journal editors have increasingly promoted and endorsed the use of reporting guidelines. Endorsement of guidelines by journals for randomised controlled trials has been shown to improve reporting.[6] The combination of the risk of making costly decisions due to poor reporting with the lack of mechanisms that promote accountability makes transparency in reporting economic evaluations especially important and a primary concern among journal editors and decision makers.[3] [7]

Aim and scope

The aim of the Consolidated Health Economic Evaluation Reporting Standards (CHEERS) statement is to provide recommendations, in the form of a checklist, to optimise reporting of health economic evaluations. The need for a contemporary reporting guidance for economic evaluations was recently identified by researchers and biomedical journal editors.[8] The CHEERS statement attempts to consolidate and update previous efforts [9] [10] [11] [12] [13] [14] [15] [16] [17] [18] [19] [20] into a single useful reporting guidance.

The primary audiences for the CHEERS statement are researchers reporting economic evaluations and the editors and peer reviewers evaluating their publication potential. We hope the statement (which consists of a 24 item checklist and accompanying recommendations on the minimum amount of information to be included when reporting economic evaluations) is a useful and practical tool for these audiences and will improve reporting and, in turn, health and healthcare decisions. To best understand and apply the recommendations contained within the statement, we encourage readers to access the Explanation and Elaboration Report.[21]

Development of the CHEERS statement

The statement was developed by a task force supported by the International Society for Pharmacoeconomics and Outcomes Research (ISPOR), as part of a broader initiative to facilitate and encourage the interchange of expert knowledge and develop best practices. The CHEERS Task Force members were chosen by the chair of the task force primarily based on their longstanding academic expertise and contribution to the multidisciplinary field of health economic evaluation. In addition to four members of the task force with doctorates in economics and its sub-discipline of health economics (AHB, MD, JM, SP), members included experts in health technology assessment and decision making (FA, AHB, DH, MD, JM) and in clinical epidemiology and biostatistics (AHB, EL, DM), those in active clinical practice (EL, FA), and those with previous experience in reporting guideline development (MD, DM). All members are researchers in applied health and health policy, with five members currently serving as editors for journals in the field (AHB, CC, MD, DG, EL).

The CHEERS Task Force followed current recommendations for developing reporting guidelines.[22] Briefly, the need for new guidance was first identified through a survey of members of the World Association of Medical Editors. Of the 6% (55/965) who responded, 91% (n=50) indicated they would use a standard if one were widely available.[8] Next, published checklists or guidance documents related to reporting economic evaluations were identified from a systematic review and survey of task force members.[23] Both of these activities were used to create a preliminary list of items to include when reporting economic evaluations. Recommendations of the minimum set of reporting items

were then developed through a modified Delphi panel process. Forty eight individuals identified by the task force with broad geographical representation and representing academia, biomedical journal editors, the pharmaceutical industry, government decision makers, and those in clinical practice were invited to participate. Thirty eight agreed to participate. Participants were asked to score importance on a Likert scale and the average scores, weighted by each individual's confidence in ability to score, were then used to rank items. A cut-off point was applied to the ranked list to determine the minimum number of items important for reporting.

The CHEERS statement recommendations have been independently reviewed and subsequently revised by task force members. The recommendations are entirely those of the task force—the sponsors of the study had no role in study design, data analysis, data interpretation, or writing of the final recommendations. A more complete description of the methods and findings of the Delphi panel are found in the larger explanation and elaboration document.[21]

Checklist items

The final recommendations are subdivided into six main categories: (1) title and abstract; (2) introduction; (3) methods; (4) results; (5) discussion; and (6) other. The recommendations are contained in a user friendly, 24 item checklist (table) to aid users who wish to follow them. A copy of the checklist can also be found on the CHEERS Task Force website. (www.ispor.org/TaskForces/EconomicPubGuidelines.asp). In order to encourage dissemination and use of a single international standard for reporting, the task force approached 14 journals identified as either the largest publishers of economic evaluations or widely read by the medical and research community. Thirteen journals responded, and 10 expressed their ability and interest in endorsing this guidance. The CHEERS statement is being simultaneously published in *BMC Medicine, BMJ, BJOG: An International Journal of Obstetrics and Gynaecology, Clinical Therapeutics, Cost Effectiveness and Resource Allocation, The European Journal of Health Economics, International Journal of Technology Assessment in Health Care, Journal of Medical Economics, Pharmacoeconomics,* and *Value in Health*. To facilitate wider dissemination and uptake of this reporting guidance, we encourage other journals and groups to consider endorsing CHEERS.

Concluding remarks

As the number of published health economic evaluations continues to grow, we believe more transparent and complete reporting of methods and findings will be increasingly important to facilitate interpretation and comparison of studies. We hope the CHEERS statement, consisting of recommendations in a 24 item checklist, will be viewed as an effective consolidation and update of previous efforts and serve as a starting point for standard reporting going forward.

We believe the CHEERS statement represents a considerable expansion over previous efforts. The strength of our approach is that it was developed in accordance with current recommendations for the development of reporting guidelines, using an international and multidisciplinary team of editors and content experts in economic evaluation and reporting.[22] Similar to the approach taken with other widely accepted guidelines, we have defined a minimum

---

BOX FORMS OF ECONOMIC EVALUATION[1]

Specific forms of analysis reflect different approaches to evaluating the consequences of health interventions. Health consequences may be estimated from a single analytical (experimental or non-experimental) study, a synthesis of studies, mathematical modelling, or a combination of modelling and study information.

- *Cost consequences analysis* examines costs and consequences without attempting to isolate a single consequence or aggregate consequences into a single measure
- *Cost minimisation analysis (CMA)*—The consequences of compared interventions are required to be equivalent, and only relative costs are compared
- *Cost effectiveness analysis (CEA)* measures consequences in natural units, such as life years gained, disability days avoided, or cases detected. In a variant of CEA, often called cost utility analysis, consequences are measured in terms of preference-based measures of health, such as quality adjusted life years or disability adjusted life years.
- *Cost benefit analysis*—Consequences are valued in monetary units.

Readers should be aware that an economic evaluation might be referred to as a "cost effectiveness analysis" or "cost benefit analysis" even if it does not strictly adhere to the definitions above. Multiple forms may also exist within a single evaluation. Different forms of analysis provide unique advantages or disadvantages for decision making. The Consolidated Health Economic Evaluation Reporting Standards (CHEERS) statement can be used with any form of economic evaluation.

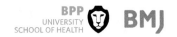

Table CHEERS checklist—Items to include when reporting economic evaluations of health interventions

Section/item	Item No	Recommendation	Reported on page No/ line No
Title and abstract			
Title	1	Identify the study as an economic evaluation or use more specific terms such as "cost-effectiveness analysis", and describe the interventions compared.	
Abstract	2	Provide a structured summary of objectives, perspective, setting, methods (including study design and inputs), results (including base case and uncertainty analyses), and conclusions.	
Introduction			
Background and objectives	3	Provide an explicit statement of the broader context for the study.	
		Present the study question and its relevance for health policy or practice decisions.	
Methods			
Target population and subgroups	4	Describe characteristics of the base case population and subgroups analysed, including why they were chosen.	
Setting and location	5	State relevant aspects of the system(s) in which the decision(s) need(s) to be made.	
Study perspective	6	Describe the perspective of the study and relate this to the costs being evaluated.	
Comparators	7	Describe the interventions or strategies being compared and state why they were chosen.	
Time horizon	8	State the time horizon(s) over which costs and consequences are being evaluated and say why appropriate.	
Discount rate	9	Report the choice of discount rate(s) used for costs and outcomes and say why appropriate.	
Choice of health outcomes	10	Describe what outcomes were used as the measure(s) of benefit in the evaluation and their relevance for the type of analysis performed.	
Measurement of effectiveness	11a	*Single study-based estimates:* Describe fully the design features of the single effectiveness study and why the single study was a sufficient source of clinical effectiveness data.	
	11b	*Synthesis-based estimates:* Describe fully the methods used for identification of included studies and synthesis of clinical effectiveness data.	
Measurement and valuation of preference based outcomes	12	If applicable, describe the population and methods used to elicit preferences for outcomes.	
Estimating resources and costs	13a	*Single study-based economic evaluation:* Describe approaches used to estimate resource use associated with the alternative interventions. Describe primary or secondary research methods for valuing each resource item in terms of its unit cost. Describe any adjustments made to approximate to opportunity costs.	
	13b	*Model-based economic evaluation:* Describe approaches and data sources used to estimate resource use associated with model health states. Describe primary or secondary research methods for valuing each resource item in terms of its unit cost. Describe any adjustments made to approximate to opportunity costs.	
Currency, price date, and conversion	14	Report the dates of the estimated resource quantities and unit costs. Describe methods for adjusting estimated unit costs to the year of reported costs if necessary. Describe methods for converting costs into a common currency base and the exchange rate.	
Choice of model	15	Describe and give reasons for the specific type of decision-analytical model used. Providing a figure to show model structure is strongly recommended.	
Assumptions	16	Describe all structural or other assumptions underpinning the decision-analytical model.	
Analytical methods	17	Describe all analytical methods supporting the evaluation. This could include methods for dealing with skewed, missing, or censored data; extrapolation methods; methods for pooling data; approaches to validate or make adjustments (such as half cycle corrections) to a model; and methods for handling population heterogeneity and uncertainty.	
Results			
Study parameters	18	Report the values, ranges, references, and, if used, probability distributions for all parameters. Report reasons or sources for distributions used to represent uncertainty where appropriate. Providing a table to show the input values is strongly recommended.	
Incremental costs and outcomes	19	For each intervention, report mean values for the main categories of estimated costs and outcomes of interest, as well as mean differences between the comparator groups. If applicable, report incremental cost-effectiveness ratios.	
Characterising uncertainty	20a	*Single study-based economic evaluation:* Describe the effects of sampling uncertainty for the estimated incremental cost and incremental effectiveness parameters, together with the impact of methodological assumptions (such as discount rate, study perspective).	
	20b	*Model-based economic evaluation:* Describe the effects on the results of uncertainty for all input parameters, and uncertainty related to the structure of the model and assumptions.	
Characterising heterogeneity	21	If applicable, report differences in costs, outcomes, or cost-effectiveness that can be explained by variations between subgroups of patients with different baseline characteristics or other observed variability in effects that are not reducible by more information.	
Discussion			
Study findings, limitations, generalisability, and current knowledge	22	Summarise key study findings and describe how they support the conclusions reached. Discuss limitations and the generalisability of the findings and how the findings fit with current knowledge.	
Other			
Source of funding	23	Describe how the study was funded and the role of the funder in the identification, design, conduct, and reporting of the analysis. Describe other non-monetary sources of support.	
Conflicts of interest	24	Describe any potential for conflict of interest of study contributors in accordance with journal policy. In the absence of a journal policy, we recommend authors comply with International Committee of Medical Journal Editors recommendations.	

For consistency, the CHEERS statement checklist format is based on the format of the CONSORT statement checklist

set of criteria though a modified Delphi technique and have translated these into recommendations, an explanatory document with explanations, and a checklist. Unlike some previous reporting guidance for economic evaluation, we have also made every effort to be neutral about the conduct of economic evaluation, allowing analysts the freedom to choose different methods.

There may be several limitations to our approach. A larger Delphi panel with a different composition could have led to a different final set of recommendations.[24] Some less common approaches and contexts (such as public health, developing countries, and system dynamic models) for conducting health economic evaluation may not be well represented by our sample of experts. Additionally, like many Delphi panel processes, we based decisions to reject or accept criteria on arbitrary levels of importance. However, we feel the group recruited to create the statement is sufficiently knowledgeable of the more common applications of economic evaluation, and the rules used to select criteria were created a priori and are consistent with previous efforts.

We believe it will be important to evaluate the effects of implementation of this statement and checklist on reporting in future economic evaluations. As methods for the conduct of economic evaluation continue to evolve, it will also be important to revisit or extend the guidance. The CHEERS Task Force feels that this statement should be reviewed for updating five years from its release.

Competing interests: All authors have completed the ICMJE uniform disclosure form at www.icmje.org/coi_disclosure.pdf and declare: FA served as board member for the study funder; FA, AHB, CC, MD, DG, DH, EL, JM, and SP were provided support for travel to a face-to-face meeting to discuss the contents of the report; FA and MD have received payment from the study sponsor for serving as co-editors for Value in Health; no other relationships or activities that could appear to have influenced the submitted work.

Elizabeth Loder—BMJ clinical epidemiology editor—played no part in the peer review or decision making of this paper at the editorial level, and contributed solely as an author.

The International Society for Pharmacoeconomics and Outcomes Research (ISPOR) Health Economic Evaluation Publication Guidelines—CHEERS Task Force acknowledge the support of Elizabeth Molsen; Donna Rindress, who provided the initial leadership for this effort; and the reviewers and Delphi panel participants, who are named in the larger explanation and elaboration document and on the CHEERS Task Force website.

Contributors: All authors provided a substantial contribution to the design and interpretation of the protocol and guidance, as well as writing sections of drafts, revising based on comments received, and approving the final version. DH conducted the analysis of Delphi panel responses, drafted and revised the protocol and the drafts of this paper, and is the guarantor for the study.

Funding: All CHEERS Task Force members are volunteers. Support for this initiative was provided by the International Society for Pharmacoeconomics and Outcomes Research.

1   Drummond MF, Sculpher MJ, Torrance G, O'Brien J, Stoddart GL. Methods for the economic evaluation of health care programmes . 3rd ed. Oxford University Press, 2005.

2   Drummond MF, Schwartz JS, Jönsson B, Luce BR, Neumann PJ, Siebert U, et al. Key principles for the improved conduct of health technology assessments for resource allocation decisions. Int J Technol Assess Health Care 2008;24:244-58.

3   Rennie D, Luft HS. Pharmacoeconomic analyses. JAMA 2000;283:2158-60.

4   Neumann PJ, Stone PW, Chapman RH, Sandberg EA, Bell CM. The quality of reporting in published cost-utility analyses, 1976-1997. Ann Intern Med 2000;132:964.

5   Rosen AB, Greenberg D, Stone PW, Olchanski NV, Neumann PJ. Quality of abstracts of papers reporting original cost-effectiveness analyses. Med Decis Making 2005;25:424-8.

6   Turner L, Shamseer L, Altman DG, Schulz KF, Moher D. Does use of the CONSORT Statement impact the completeness of reporting of randomised controlled trials published in medical journals? A Cochrane review. Syst Rev 2012;1:60.

7   Drummond MF. A reappraisal of economic evaluation of pharmaceuticals. Science or marketing? Pharmacoeconomics 1998;14:1-9.

8   McGhan WF, Al M, Doshi JA, Kamae I, Marx SE, Rindress D. The ISPOR Good Practices for Quality Improvement of Cost-Effectiveness Research Task Force report. Value Health 2009;12:1086-99.

9   Task Force on Principles for Economic Analysis of Health Care Technology. Economic analysis of health care technology. A report on principles. Ann Intern Med 1995;123:61-70.

10 Drummond MF, Jefferson TO. Guidelines for authors and peer reviewers of economic submissions to the BMJ. BMJ 1996;313:275-83.

11 Gold MR. Cost-effectiveness in health and medicine . Oxford University Press, 1996.

12 Siegel JE, Weinstein MC, Russell LB, Gold MR. Recommendations for reporting cost-effectiveness analyses. Panel on Cost-Effectiveness in Health and Medicine. JAMA 1996;276:1339-41.

13 Nuijten MJ, Pronk MH, Brorens MJ, Hekster YA, Lockefeer JH, de Smet PA, et al. Reporting format for economic evaluation: Part II: Focus on modelling studies. Pharmacoeconomics 1998;14:259-68.

14 Vintzileos AM, Beazoglou T. Design, execution, interpretation, and reporting of economic evaluation studies in obstetrics. Am J Obstet Gynecol 2004;191:1070-6.

15 Drummond M, Manca A, Sculpher M. Increasing the generalizability of economic evaluations: recommendations for the design, analysis, and reporting of studies. Int J Technol Assess Health Care 2005;21:165-71.

16 Ramsey S, Willke R, Briggs A, Brown R, Buxton M, Chawla A, et al. Good research practices for cost-effectiveness analysis alongside clinical trials: the ISPOR RCT-CEA Task Force report. Value Health 2005;8:521-33.

17 Goetghebeur MM, Wagner M, Khoury H, Levitt RJ, Erickson LJ, Rindress D. Evidence and value: impact on decisionmaking—the EVIDEM framework and potential applications. BMC Health Serv Rev 2008;8:270.

18 Davis JC, Robertson MC, Comans T, Scuffham PA. Guidelines for conducting and reporting economic evaluation of fall prevention strategies. Osteoporos Int 2010;22:2449-59.

19 Petrou S, Gray A. Economic evaluation using decision analytical modelling: design, conduct, analysis, and reporting. BMJ 2011;342:d1766.

20 Petrou S, Gray A. Economic evaluation alongside randomised controlled trials: design, conduct, analysis, and reporting. BMJ 2011;342:d1548.

21 Husereau D, Drummond M, Petrou S, Carswell C, Moher D, Greenberg D, et al. Consolidated Health Economic Evaluation Reporting Standards (CHEERS)—explanation and elaboration: a report of the ISPOR Health Economic Evaluations Publication Guidelines Task Force. Value in Health (forthcoming).

22 Moher D, Schulz KF, Simera I, Altman DG. Guidance for developers of health research reporting guidelines. PLoS Med 2010;7:e1000217.

23 Moher D, Simera I, Schulz K, Miller D, Grimshaw J, Hoey J, et al. Reporting guidelines for clinical research: a systematic review. Vancouver, BC, 2009. Available at: www.ama-assn.org/public/peer/abstracts-0912.pdf.

24 Campbell SM, Hann M, Roland MO, Quayle JA, Shekelle PG. The effect of panel membership and feedback on ratings in a two-round Delphi survey: results of a randomized controlled trial. Med Care 1999;37:964-8

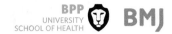

Economic evaluation alongside randomised controlled trials: design, conduct, analysis, and reporting

Stavros Petrou, professor[1], Alastair Gray, professor of health economics[2]

[1]Warwick Clinical Trials Unit, Warwick Medical School, University of Warwick, Coventry CV4 7AL, UK

[2]Health Economics Research Centre, Department of Public Health, University of Oxford, Oxford, UK

Cite this as: BMJ 2011;342:d1548

DOI: 10.1136/bmj.d1548

http://www.bmj.com/content/342/bmj.d1548

ABSTRACT

Collecting economic data at the same time as evidence of effectiveness maximises the information available for analysis but requires proper consideration at the design stage

Economic evaluation involves the comparative analysis of the costs and consequences of alternative programmes or interventions.[1] It has increasingly been used to inform decision making about healthcare in the United Kingdom and other industrialised nations.[2 3 4 5] Randomised controlled trials are commonly used as a vehicle for economic evaluations. Indeed, many funders, such as the UK National Institute for Health Research Health Technology Assessment Programme, routinely request that assessments of cost effectiveness are incorporated in the design of randomised trials. This article outlines some of the key issues concerning the design, conduct, analysis, and reporting of economic evaluations based on trials with individual patient data. Economic evaluations that synthesise data from disparate sources using decision analytical models (typically using summary rather than individual patient data) are discussed in an accompanying article.[6]

What are the objectives of economic evaluation?

Economic evaluations are typically concerned with two quantities: the additional cost of a new treatment compared with the existing alternative and the additional health benefits. If all the costs and outcomes relevant to this comparison can be measured, they can then be averaged across all patients in the treatment (t) or the control (c) group to obtain mean cost C and mean effect E for each group. It then becomes possible to calculate a third quantity: the cost effectiveness of the new treatment compared with the alternative. The incremental cost effectiveness ratio (ICER) will simply be the difference in costs divided by the difference in effects: $ICER = C_t - C_c / E_t - E_c = \Delta C / \Delta E$.

This can be shown neatly on the cost effectiveness plane (fig).[7] In the south east quadrant of the figure the new intervention is less costly and more effective and (assuming there is no uncertainty surrounding the cost effectiveness

ratio) should be adopted; equally, if the new intervention is less effective and more costly (the north west quadrant), it can readily be rejected. More controversially, new interventions may turn out to be more effective but also more costly (north east quadrant) or less effective but also less costly (south west quadrant): in either case, a trade-off then exists between effect and cost: additional health benefit can be obtained but at higher cost, or costs can be saved but only by giving up health benefit.

The question that then arises is whether the trade-off is acceptable: is the health gain (or cost saving) worth the additional cost (or health loss)? To address this question, we can imagine a diagonal line running through the figure depicting the maximum we are willing to pay for a unit of effect (sometimes represented by the Greek letter λ). All points to the right of this line involve a trade-off between costs and health benefits that a decision maker might consider acceptable; while all points to the left require an unacceptable trade-off. The steeper the slope of this diagonal line, the more decision makers are willing to pay for a unit of effect. There are various techniques for estimating the value of λ.[8] In many jurisdictions, however, it has tended to reflect externally determined decision rules that have evolved historically and with little scientific basis.[9] [10] The point to note is that economic evaluation involves two large uncertainties: where an intervention is located on the cost effectiveness plane, and how much a decision maker is willing to pay for health gains. Here we focus on the first question, and consider the use of trial based economic evaluations to obtain precise estimates of incremental cost effectiveness.

Design of trial based economic evaluations

Designing a rigorous trial based economic evaluation requires close collaboration between trialists and health economists. This collaboration should be reflected in the standard operating procedures of the coordinating clinical trials unit, including its data collection and informed consent procedures.[11] Where possible, the instruments and procedures used to collect economic data should be pilot tested for efficiency, clarity, and ease of use.[12] Pragmatic trials offer analysts an opportunity to evaluate the cost effectiveness of an intervention under real world conditions, with enrolled patients representative of typical clinical caseloads, a comparison of the intervention of interest with current practice, and follow-up under routine conditions.[1] With less naturalistic trial designs, such as explanatory trials designed primarily to answer questions about safety and efficacy, the generalisability of the economic evaluation may be impaired by stringent inclusion criteria and treatment protocols or by the absence of a "usual care" arm.[12] [13] These limitations are hard to overcome, although protocol driven costs can and should be factored out of cost effectiveness calculations.[14]

SUMMARY POINTS

- Economic evaluation is increasingly used to inform the regulatory and reimbursement decisions of government agencies
- Evaluations conducted alongside randomised controlled trials provide access to data on individual patients
- This enables a wide range of analytical techniques—for example, to examine the relation between events of interest and health related quality of life
- Designing a rigorous trial based economic evaluation requires close collaboration between trialists and health economists from the outset of the trial
- Key issues concerning the design, conduct, analysis, and reporting of economic evaluations based on randomised trial with individual patient data are outlined

Although several techniques have been proposed to estimate the appropriate sample size and statistical power for economic end points in randomised trials,[15][16][17] power calculations are almost invariably based on primary clinical outcomes. This is partly because of the complexity of trying to forecast the main outcome of interest to economists—the joint distribution of the difference in costs and benefits between treatment arms. Furthermore, large sample sizes may be needed to detect statistically significant differences because of the large variability in use of healthcare resources and cost measures,[18] and this may be neither financially nor ethically acceptable.[1] Economists therefore focus on estimating cost and effect differences and assessing the likelihood that an intervention is cost effective, rather than testing a particular hypothesis concerning cost effectiveness.[18]

Some people might wonder whether an economic evaluation should be included in a trial before we know whether the new treatment is more effective. However, if it is not included we risk losing the opportunity to collect information on use of resources and health related quality of life. Furthermore, as noted above, cost effectiveness is about the joint distribution of differences in cost and effect. This joint distribution could show clear cost effectiveness when neither cost nor effect differences are individually significant. Indeed, some economists have argued that reliance on traditional rules of statistical inference surrounding a single parameter, such as clinical effectiveness, is arbitrary and may result in inferior healthcare outcomes compared with decisions based on expected cost effectiveness.[1][19]

How are data measured and valued?

Use of resources

The resources used by patients, such as hospital admissions, consultations, and types and quantities of drugs administered, are normally recorded for each patient over the trial follow-up. The categories of resource use that are included in the study will be determined by the perspective of the analysis—whether it is confined to the healthcare system (sometimes referred to as the payer) or includes broader societal costs. The system perspective would typically include direct medical care, including the intervention itself, treatment of any side effects or complications, and follow-up care to the intervention or the underlying condition. It may also include medical care not directly associated with the underlying condition, although regression modelling may be required to disentangle background noise that often occurs when this is included.[20] In England and Wales, the National Institute for Health and Clinical Excellence (NICE) recommends including NHS and personal social services as a minimum.[2] The societal perspective also considers care provided by other sectors of the economy, costs incurred by patients, informal care provided by family and friends, and productivity losses from morbidity and premature death.

Use of many resources can normally be recorded on trial case report forms with little or no extra burden, but sometimes additional information will be required from medical records, patient questionnaires and diaries, and other sources.[21] A recent trial based economic evaluation of neonatal extracorporeal membrane oxygenation used observational research to estimate resource use associated with complications and parental questionnaires to document use of hospital and community health services after discharge.[22] Computerised record linkage may in future simplify the process of collecting these additional data.

When data are collected through patient or carer questionnaires, researchers have to balance recall bias against completeness of sampling information.[23] Shorter recall periods of a few days or weeks reduce the chance of a patient forgetting an episode or incorrectly recalling when it occurred, but if a study is trying to estimate resource use over a longer period, such as 12 months, sampling over a short recall period misses lots of data. It may be better to maximise completeness at the cost of some recall bias.[24]

Valuation of resource use

The total cost for an individual patient participating in a trial is the product of the quantity of each resource item they use and the unit cost of each item. Unit costs should theoretically be based on the economic notion of opportunity cost, which represents the value of the resource in its most highly valued alternative use.[1] In practice this is usually assumed to be approximated by nationally representative healthcare tariffs, such as the NHS payment by results tariffs[25] or the diagnosis related group payments in the US Medicare system.[26] However, unit costs are not always readily available from such sources and may have to be calculated using a combination of accounting data, time and motion studies, interviews with caregivers, and case note analysis.

Standard unit costs are often applied across all patients and trial centres, but non-standardised unit costs may be appropriate if the relative prices of factors such as labour and equipment vary between trial centres, especially in multinational trials.[27][28] All costs should be valued at the same price date, with adjustment using healthcare specific inflation indices when necessary.[29] Economic evaluations based on multinational trials should convert costs into a common currency by using purchasing power parity adjustments.[30]

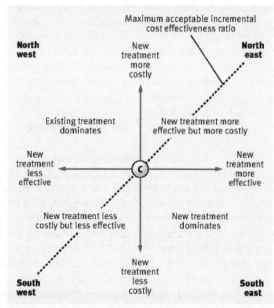

Fig The cost effectiveness plane. The x axis shows the difference in effectiveness between the new treatment and the comparator and the y axis shows the difference in cost. The slope of the line from any point on the figure to the origin is the incremental cost effectiveness ratio

Measurement and valuation of outcomes

Cost effectiveness may be reported in terms of many different outcome measures, ranging from biomedical markers to more final health outcomes.[12] The preferred outcome measure for many health economists, and many reimbursement agencies, remains the quality adjusted life year (QALY), a preference based measure of health outcome that combines length of life and health related quality of life.[31] For reimbursement agencies, the QALY has the advantage of allowing cost effectiveness comparisons between interventions for disparate health conditions. For economists, the QALY offers the additional advantage that it incorporates individual preferences for health outcomes, thereby moving beyond the narrow biomedical model for evaluative research.

To estimate QALYs patients typically complete at different time points a generic health related quality of life questionnaire with pre-existing preference weights that can be attached to each health state—for example EQ-5D,[32] the Health Utilities Index,[33] and the SF-6D.[34] The underpinning preference weights for these measures are generally drawn from surveys of the general population, and so descriptive data from patients are combined with health related quality of life weights (or utility scores) from the general population and survival data from the trial to generate QALY profiles. An alternative approach is to ask patients not only to describe their health status but also to value it using a complex scaling technique such as the standard gamble approach or time trade-off approach.[35] These techniques are more expensive and time consuming than using population weighting. For both approaches, the frequency and timing of assessments should be influenced by disease severity, speed of progression, and the questionnaire burden on patients.[36] When patients are too ill or do not have the cognitive competencies to complete a questionnaire, proxy measurements may be considered.[37]

If a trial has not included a quality of life assessment, mapping techniques can sometimes be used to predict preference based health related quality of life (or utility) scores based on responses to non-preference based measures.[38] This requires data from a separate study where both the preference based and non-preference based measures were completed. For example, Williamson and colleagues used data from a study that developed a utility algorithm for the OM8-30 otitis media with effusion questionnaire[39] to predict preference based health related quality of life scores, and consequently QALYs, for children participating in a randomised trial of topical intranasal corticosteroids for persistent bilateral otitis media with effusion.[40]

The QALY may be considered too restrictive or insensitive to the main outcomes of interest in some circumstances. Researchers are therefore developing instruments that try to measure broader outcomes such as attachment, security, enjoyment, role, and control that can still be used within an economic evaluation framework.[41]

Analysis and reporting of data
Discounting
Trial based economic evaluations often measure and value costs and outcomes over several years of patient follow-up. In this situation costs and outcomes that occur after the first year of follow-up are typically reduced by a discount factor so that they can be fairly compared. Some economists have argued for applying different discount rates to future costs and health outcomes,[42] but NICE recommends that economic evaluations conducted in England and Wales should discount both costs and outcomes at an annual rate of 3.5%.[2] Sensitivity analyses that test the effects of differential discount rates on costs and outcomes are recommended.[2]

Dealing with skewed, missing, and censored data
The costs and outcomes of the trial groups, and the respective differences between them, can be summarised in several ways. For costs, the crucial information is usually the arithmetic mean—that is, average cost—as this allows policy makers to estimate the total cost of implementing a programme or intervention.[43] Although cost data are often right skewed because a few patients use very high amounts of resource, producing a distribution that may violate the assumptions of standard statistical tests, it is not clear that the many alternative approaches suggested, such as bootstrapping, provide more reliable test results.[44] Indeed, simple approaches for analysing cost data that assume normal distributions may be preferable in large samples where the near-normality of sample means is assured, while relatively simple approaches, such as generalised linear models, may be sufficient in smaller samples to deal with problems such as skewness and excess zeros.[44] For clinical outcomes, it is generally most transparent to replicate the methods of the primary clinical analysis plan to summarise outcomes. Note, however, that economists will be interested in all events, whereas trialists may be more interested in time to the first event. For QALYs, it may be important to adjust for baseline differences in health status between the trial groups.[45]

Missing data are a particular problem for economic evaluations alongside trials, as the analysis may be drawing on information from case report forms, adverse event data, medication files, health related quality of life and resource use questionnaires, and other sources at all points across the study. The problem may be mitigated, in part, by approaches such as postal or telephone reminders to patients. Nevertheless, a complete case approach might require that most patients are dropped and is seldom a realistic option. Instead, analysts increasingly favour multiple imputation, where multivariate regression techniques are used to predict missing values on the basis of existing data.[46] The precise approach will depend on the nature of the missing data: (i) missing completely at random, with no relation to the value of any other factors in the study population; (ii) missing at random, but correlated in an observable way with the mechanism that generates the outcome; and (iii) not missing at random, but dependent on unobserved variables.[46] A particular form of missing data is censoring, where information on some patients is truncated and not available for the full duration of interest. In the past, analysts often ignored the effects of censoring on the estimation of costs and outcomes, but survival analysis methods are increasingly being used to deal with this problem.[8]

Handling uncertainty
As we noted when discussing the cost effectiveness plane, trial based economic evaluations result in different types of uncertainty. Sampling (or stochastic) uncertainty, usually reported as a confidence interval, depends on variation in both the numerator (incremental cost) and the denominator (incremental effectiveness) of the incremental cost effectiveness ratio. However, ratios are difficult statistics to work with: in cost effectiveness ratios the denominator (the effect difference) may be zero, producing an intractable result. Another problem is that the same negative value might represent improved outcomes and lower costs or worse outcomes and higher costs. This makes confidence intervals hard to compute and to interpret.

An alternative is to assume that the decision maker's willingness to pay for health gain is known and then rearrange the ratio on a linear scale to see whether the intervention produces any net benefit. For example, if the actual health benefits produced by the intervention are multiplied by the assumed willingness to pay for these benefits, and the net costs are subtracted, we produce a linear scale where a negative is unambiguously bad (the costs outweigh the value placed on the health benefits) and larger benefits are unambiguously better.[47] This net benefit approach makes it straightforward to examine decision uncertainty—that is, uncertainty over the value of the willingness to pay for health gain (λ)—by assessing the probability that the new intervention is cost effective across a range of values of λ. This is often displayed as a cost effectiveness acceptability curve.[48]

Heterogeneity in the trial population could also be explored by formulating a net benefit value for each patient from the observed costs and effects, and then constructing a regression model with a treatment variable and covariates such as age, sex, and disease severity. The magnitude and significance of the coefficients on the interaction between the covariates and the treatment variable might then provide an estimate of cost effectiveness by subgroup. Finally, methodological uncertainty, the uncertainty concerning issues such as the appropriate discount rate or cost perspective, can be explored by standard sensitivity analyses.

Longer term extrapolation

Cost effectiveness observed within a trial may be substantially different from what would have been observed with continued patient follow-up: for example, the benefits of reducing fatal outcomes typically continue well beyond the end of the trial. Consequently, extrapolation of cost effectiveness over an extended period, often a lifetime, is considered important.[36][49] Survival analysis models, such as the Cox proportional hazard model or Weibull model, are often used to estimate life expectancy with and without an intervention.[50] However, unbiased estimation of long term cost effectiveness may require more complex models of the disease process, accompanied by related information on the cost and utility of interventions and complications.

Trial based economic evaluations that use patient level data have important advantages in permitting the construction of such models and permitting them to be validated. A good example comes from the UK Prospective Diabetes Study.[51] The trial followed up patients for a median of 10 years. However, the wealth of individual patient data permitted the construction of a model consisting of a set of linked equations that predict the risks of major diabetes related complications, and this has been used to estimate the lifetime costs, utilities, and cost effectiveness of diabetes related interventions.[52] The interactions within the model between risk factors, individual characteristics, and disease history could not have been captured reliably without access to patient level data.

Advantages of trial based economic evaluations?

Economic evaluations conducted alongside randomised controlled trials provide an early opportunity to produce reliable estimates of cost effectiveness at low marginal cost. Access to individual patient data also permits a wide range of statistical and econometric techniques—for example, to examine the relation between events of interest and health

related quality of life or to explore subgroup differences. Although trial based evaluations have limitations—truncated time horizons, limited comparators, restricted generalisability to different settings or countries, and the failure to incorporate all relevant evidence[53]—they are likely to continue to have an important role in producing reliable estimates of cost effectiveness.

Competing interests: All authors have completed the unified competing interest form at www.icmje.org/coi_disclosure.pdf (available on request from the corresponding author) and declare no support from any organisation for the submitted work; The Warwick Clinical Trials Unit benefited from facilities funded through the Birmingham Science City Translational Medicine Clinical Research and Infrastructure Trials Platform, with support from Advantage West Midlands. The Health Economics Research Centre receives funding from the National Institute of Health Research. SP started working on this article while employed by the National Perinatal Epidemiology Unit, University of Oxford, and the Health Economics Research Centre, University of Oxford, and funded by a UK Medical Research Council senior non-clinical research fellowship. AG is an NIHR senior investigator. They have no other relationships or activities that could appear to have influenced the submitted work.

Provenance and peer review: Commissioned; externally peer reviewed.

1   Drummond MF, Sculpher MJ, Torrance GW, O'Brien BJ, Stoddart G. *Methods for the economic evaluation of health care programmes*, 3rd ed. Oxford University Press, 2005.
2   National Institute for Health and Clinical Excellence. *NICE guide to the methods of technology appraisal*. NICE, 2008.
3   Scottish Medicines Consortium. *Guidance to manufacturers for completion of new product assessment form (NPAF)*. SMC, 2007.
4   Pharmaceutical Benefits Advisory Committee. *Guidelines for the pharmaceutical industry on preparation of submissions to the Pharmaceutical Benefits Advisory Committee*. PBAC, 2002.
5   CDR Directorate at Canadian Coordinating Office for Health Technology Assessment. *Canada common drug review submission guidelines for manufacturers*. CCOHTA, 2003.
6   Petrou S, Gray A. Economic evaluation using decision analytical modelling: design, conduct, analysis and reporting. *BMJ* 2011;342:d1766.
7   Black WC. The CE plane: a graphic representation of cost-effectiveness. *Med Decis Making* 1990;10:212-4.
8   Gray A, Clarke P, Wolstenholme J, Wordsworth S. *Applied methods of cost-effectiveness analysis in health care*. Oxford University Press, 2010.
9   Devlin N, Parkin D. Does NICE have a cost-effectiveness threshold and what other factors influence its decisions? A binary choice analysis. *Health Econ* 2004;13:437-52.
10 Grosse S. Assessing cost-effectiveness in healthcare: history of the $50,000 per QALY threshold. *Expert Rev Pharmacoeconomics Outcomes Res* 2008;8:165-78.
11 Edwards RT, Hounsome B, Linck P, Russell IT. Economic evaluation alongside pragmatic randomised trials: developing a standard operating procedure for clinical trials units. *Trials* 2008;9:64.
12 Glick HA, Joshi JA, Sonnad SS, Polsky D. *Economic evaluation in clinical trials*. Oxford University Press, 2007.
13 O'Sullivan AK, Thompson D, Drummond MF. Collection of health-economic data alongside clinical trials: ils there a future for piggyback evaluations? *Value Health* 2005;8:67-79.
14 Coyle D, Lee LM. The problem of protocol driven costs in pharmacoeconomic analysis. *Pharmacoeconomics* 1998;14:357-63.
15 Briggs AH, Gray AM. Power and sample size calculations for stochastic cost-effectiveness analysis. *Med Decis Making* 1998;18:S81-92.
16 Gardiner JC, Sirbu CM, Rahbar MH. Updated on statistical power and sample size assessments for cost-effectiveness studies. *Expert Rev Pharmacoeconomics Outcomes Res* 2004;4:89-98.
17 Gafni A, Walter SD, Birch S, Sendi P. An opportunity cost approach to sample size calculation in cost-effectiveness analysis. *Health Econ* 2008;17:99-107.
18 Briggs A. Economic evaluation and clinical trials: size matters. *BMJ* 2000;321:1362.
19 Claxton K. The irrelevance of inference: a decision-making approach to the stochastic evaluation of health care technologies. *J Health Econ* 1999;18:341-64.
20 Simon J, Gray A, Duley L, Magpie Trial Collaborative Group. Cost-effectiveness of prophylactic magnesium sulphate for 9996 women with pre-eclampsia from 33 countries: economic evaluation of the Magpie Trial. *BJOG* 2006;113:144-51.
21 Drummond M, Manca A, Sculpher M. Increasing the generalizability of economic evaluations: recommendations for the design, analysis, and reporting of studies. *Int J Technol Assess* 2005;21:165-71.
22 Petrou S, Bischof M, Bennett C, Elbourne D, Field D, McNally H. Cost-effectiveness of neonatal ECMO based on seven year results from the UK Collaborative ECMO Trial. *Pediatrics* 2006;117:1640-9.
23 Ridyard CH, Hughes DA. Methods for the collection of resource use data within clinical trials: a systematic review of studies funded

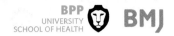

by the UK Health Technology Assessment program. *Value Health* 2010;13:867-72.

24   Clarke PM, Fiebig DG, Gerdtham UG. Optimal recall length in survey design. *J Health Econ* 2008;27:1275-84.

25   Department of Health, England. *Payment by results.* Department of Health, 2010. www.dh.gov.uk/en/Managingyourorganisation/ Financeandplanning/NHSFinancialReforms/DH_900.

26   Centers for Medicare and Medicaid Services. Acute inpatient PPS. www.cms.gov/InpatientPPS/.

27   Raikou M, Briggs A, Gray A, McGuire A. Centre-specific or average unit costs in multi-centre studies? Some theory and simulation. *Health Econ* 2000;9:191-8.

28   Torti FM, Reed SD, Schulman KA. Analytic considerations in economic evaluations of multinational cardiovascular clinical trials. *Value Health* 2006;9:281-91.

29   Curtis L. *Unit costs of health and social care 2009.* Personal Social Services Research Unit, University of Kent, 2009. www.pssru.ac.uk.

30   World Bank. *Global purchasing power parities and real expenditures 2005.* World Bank International Comparison Program, 2009. http:// siteresources.worldbank.org/ICPINT/Resources/icp-final.pdf.

31   Torrance GW, Feeny D. Utilities and quality-adjusted life years. *Int J Technol Assess Health Care* 1989;5:559-75.

32   Brooks R. EQ-5D, the current state of play. *Health Pol* 1996;37:53-72.

33   Torrance GW, Furlong W, Feeny D, Boyle M. Multi-attribute preference functions: Health Utilities Index. *PharmacoEcon* 1995;7:503-20.

34   Brazier J, Roberts J, Deverill M. The estimation of a preference-based measure of health from the SF-36. *J Health Econ* 2002;21:271-92.

35   Dolan P, Gudex C, Kind P, Williams A. Valuing health states: a comparison of methods. *J Health Econ* 1996;15:209-31.

36   Ramsey S, Willke R, Briggs A, Brown R, Buxton M, Chawla A, et al. Good research practices for cost-effectiveness analysis alongside clinical trials: the ISPOR RCT-CEA Task Force report. *Value Health* 2005;8:521-33.

37   Brazier J, Ratcliffe J, Salomon JA, Tsuchiya A. *Measuring and valuing health benefits for economic evaluation* . Oxford University Press, 2007.

38   Brazier J, Yang Y, Tsuchiya A, Rowen DL. A review of studies mapping (or cross walking) non-preference based measures of health to generic preference-based measures. *Eur J Health Econ* 2010;11:215-25.

39   Dakin H, Petrou S, Haggard M, Benge S, Williamson I. Mapping analyses to estimate health utilities based on responses to the OM8-30 otitis media questionnaire. *Qual Life Res* 2010:19:65-80.

40   Williamson I, Benge S, Barton S, Petrou S, Letley L, Fasey N, et al. A double-blind randomised placebo controlled trial of topical intra-nasal corticosteroids in 4-11 year old children with persistent bilateral otitis media with effusion in primary care. *Health Technol Assess* 2009;13:1-274.

41   Coast J, Flynn TN, Natarajan L, Sproston K, Lewis J, Louviere JJ, et al. Valuing the ICECAP capability index for older people. *Soc Sci Med* 2008;67:874-82.

42   Brouwer WBF, van Exel NJA. Discounting in decision making: the consistency argument revisited empirically. *Health Policy* 2004;67:187-94.

43   Thompson SG, Barber JA. How should cost data in pragmatic randomised trials be analysed? *BMJ* 2000;320:1197-200.

44   Mihaylova B, Briggs A, O'Hagan A, Thompson S. Review of statistical methods for analysing healthcare resources and costs. *Health Econ* 2010, doi:10.1002/hec.1653.

45   Manca A, Hawkins N, Sculpher MJ. Estimating mean QALYs in trial-based cost-effectiveness analysis: the importance of controlling for baseline utility. *Health Econ* 2005;14:487-96.

46   Sterne JAC, White IR, Carlin JB, Spratt M, Royston P, Kenward MG, et al. Multiple imputation for missing data in epidemiological and clinical research: potential and pitfalls. *BMJ* 2009;338:b2393.

47   Zethraeus N, Johannesson M, Jonsson B, Lothgren M, Tambour M. Advantages of using the net-benefit approach for analysing uncertainty in economic evaluation studies. *Pharmacoeconomics* 2003;21:39-48.

48   Fenwick E, O'Brien BJ, Briggs A. Cost-effectiveness acceptability curves: facts, fallacies and frequently asked questions. *Health Econ* 2004;13:405-15.

49   Hlatky MA, Owens DK, Sanders GD. Cost-effectiveness as an outcome in randomized clinical trials. *Clin Trials* 2006;3:543-51.

50   Mark DB, Hlatky MA, Califf RM, Naylor CD, Lee KL, Armstrong PW, et al. Cost-effectiveness of thrombolytic therapy with tissue plasminogen activator as compared with streptokinase for acute myocardial infarction. *N Engl J Med* 1995;332:1418-24.

51   UKPDS Group. Cost effectiveness analysis of improved blood pressure control in hypertensive patients with type 2 diabetes: UKPDS 40. *BMJ* 1998;317:720-6.

52   Clarke PM, Gray AM, Briggs A, Stevens R, Matthews DR, Holman RR. Cost-utility analyses of intensive blood glucose and tight blood pressure control in type 2 diabetes (UKPDS 72). *Diabetologia* 2005;48:868-77.

53   Sculpher MJ, Claxton K, Drummond M, McCabe C. Whither trial-based economic evaluation for health care decision making? *Health Econ* 2006;15:677-87.

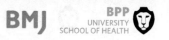

IDEAL framework for surgical innovation 3: randomised controlled trials in the assessment stage and evaluations in the long term study stage

Jonathan A Cook, methodologist[1], Peter McCulloch, clinical reader in surgery[2], Jane M Blazeby, professor of surgery[3], David J Beard, professor of musculoskeletal sciences[4][5], Danica Marinac-Dabic, director[6], Art Sedrakyan, associate professor of public health and cardiac surgery[7], On behalf of the IDEAL group

[1]Health Services Research Unit, University of Aberdeen, Aberdeen AB25 2ZD, UK

[2]Nuffield Department of Surgical Science, University of Oxford, Oxford, UK

[3]Centre for Surgical Research, School of Social and Community Medicine, University of Bristol, UK

[4]Nuffield Department of Orthopaedics, Rheumatology and Musculoskeletal Sciences, University of Oxford, UK

[5]National Institute for Health Research Oxford Musculoskeletal Biomedical Research Unit, Oxford, UK

[6]Division of Epidemiology, Office of Surveillance and Biometrics, Center for Devices and Radiological Health, Food and Drug Administration, MD, USA

[7]Weill Cornell Medical College of Cornell University and New York Presbyterian Hospital, New York, NY, USA

Correspondence to: J A Cook
j.a.cook@abdn.ac.uk

Cite this as: *BMJ* 2013;346:f2820

DOI: 10.1136/bmj.f2820

http://www.bmj.com/content/346/bmj.f2820

ABSTRACT

The complexity of surgical procedures often poses challenges for conducting a rigorous and comprehensive evaluation. This paper considers the final two IDEAL stages of surgical innovation. Surgical randomised controlled trials are often challenging to undertake and require careful consideration of the intervention definition, who should deliver it, and the impact of surgeon and patient preferences. In the long term study stage, better monitoring of surgical procedures is needed, along with improved surveillance of devices.

Introduction

The IDEAL framework describes the stages through which interventional therapy innovation normally passes: idea, development, exploration, assessment, and long term follow-up (also known as stages 1, 2a, 2b, 3, and 4, respectively). This paper focuses on the stages of assessment (specifically in relation to randomised trials) and long term follow-up. By the assessment stage, a new intervention will have shown early promise and be used increasingly by the surgical community; however, the intervention's relative benefit compared with alternative approaches will be uncertain. At the long term follow-up stage, a surgical intervention will need further assessment owing to technical refinements or to related devices or procedures being brought onto the market.

Surgical procedures are conducted with an almost infinite set of subtle variations: surgeon training, team expertise, personal practice, centre policy and infrastructure, anatomical features of the patient, and the use of a variety of medical devices. Beyond the procedure, other factors are implicitly part of the intervention: the type of anaesthesia used,[1] preoperative and postoperative management (including drug treatments such as aspirin),[2] physiotherapy,[3] and psychological interventions (including verbal guidance).[4] These linked and interdependent components produce a complex intervention.[5] At the assessment and long term stages, this complexity is most apparent and challenging for conducting a rigorous and comprehensive evaluation of a surgical intervention.

Another challenge is to measure outcomes comprehensively; surgical studies are also limited by their selection of outcomes, which are often short term, "operation" focussed, and inconsistently defined. Properly conducted randomised controlled trials and observational studies with agreed and defined core outcomes are needed at these critical stages.[6] The failure to conduct methodologically rigorous studies has resulted in some surgical interventions becoming and remaining standard practice without good evidence.[7][8] Similarly, new medical devices are widely used without due assessment.[9] In this paper, we consider in turn the roles of randomised controlled trials in the assessment stage and evaluations in the long term stage.

Randomised controlled trials in the assessment stage

The role of randomised controlled trials in evaluating surgical interventions has been debated over the past 30 years.[7][8][10][11] A consensus in favour of accepting properly conducted trials as the "gold standard" for comparisons of efficacy and effectiveness between surgical procedures has eventually emerged, although not without controversy.[8] While several surgical trials have been successful and influential,[10][12] others have been attempted and failed[13] or have not had the anticipated influence on the adoption of the intervention.[14] Even if a trial evaluation is undertaken successfully, factors out of the study investigators' control (for example, innovations and technological changes) can lead to uncertainty about the evaluation's applicability.[15]

The assessment stage provides a window of opportunity—albeit sometimes a brief one—to obtain definite randomised evidence about effectiveness. The IDEAL framework proposes that a large multicentre trial is most valuable and viable during the assessment stage, although small single centre trials might appear as early as IDEAL stage 2a. Randomised controlled trials have an array of potential problems in evaluating surgical techniques (box 1),[8][16][17] and most stem from three related issues: the intervention definition, who delivers the intervention, and the treatment preferences of surgeons and patients.

SUMMARY POINTS

- Rigorous evaluation of surgical innovations is needed in the assessment and long term study stages, which together meet the need for comprehensive outcome assessment
- Randomised trials of surgical interventions, along with observational studies in the long term study stage, should be designed which acknowledge the complexity of surgery
- Key issues for surgical trial design are specification of the interventions, who will deliver the interventions, and assessing the potential impact of patient and surgeon preferences
- Long term evaluations of the procedure and any related devices is needed, along with the development of data collection and methodology for surveillance

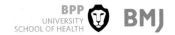

Intervention definition

How tightly the intervention should be defined will depend on the type of comparison (table). Trials investigating the auxiliary facets of the intervention are valuable, but studies evaluating the surgical core of an innovative procedure (whether a new procedure or a modification of an established procedure) are crucial. In a comparison of medical versus surgical trials, the definition of surgery can be broad. For example, in a trial of medical treatment versus hysterectomy, the type and route of the hysterectomy was left to the discretion of the gynaecologists, as was the medical treatment (although there was a suggested regimen).[18] In a trial comparing open versus laparoscopic repair of inguinal hernia, surgeons were allowed to choose the type of open and laparoscopic repair.[19]

If special equipment is needed, the medical device used does not typically need to be not restricted. In trials of medical devices, or where the related procedures being compared are similar, it may be necessary to define each intervention precisely and to introduce process control measures to check on compliance to preclude contamination and control the effect of ancillary care.[20] Small changes in technique or technology can have a substantial effect on outcomes, as shown by recent research relating to metal-on-metal hip devices.[9]

Measuring adherence regarding intervention delivery has been rare in surgical trials, but can help in interpreting the applicability (generalisability) of the results. Example measures include specimen margin examination or node counts in cancer procedures, or taking photographs after completion of key parts of the procedure.[21] [22] Deciding on restrictions requires careful consideration of the research question and the potential risk of bias and confounders (such as associated treatments), although as few restrictions as possible is preferable.

Who should deliver the intervention?

Every operation should be carried out or supervised closely by someone with appropriate level of expertise and training. Collectively, participating surgeons should have sufficient expertise in order for the surgical community to embrace the trial and its findings. The traditional approach—where each surgeon delivers both or all surgical interventions in the trial—has been criticised. A comparison could be deemed unfair if surgeons have more expertise in one intervention than another.

This problem can be managed in two ways. Firstly, trial participation can be restricted to surgeons with an acceptable level of expertise in both or all surgical interventions. Surgeon eligibility criteria have generally focussed on markers of training and previous experience of the intervention (for example, completing 10 laparoscopic hernia procedures). Professional grade, year of experience, and annual caseload can be used as markers, although a more rigorous standard of direct demonstration of surgical competency has also been proposed (for example, providing training and supervision before participation).[23] Under the second approach, participating surgeons deliver

---

BOX 1 POTENTIAL SOLUTIONS TO OVERCOME COMMON VARIATIONS IN SURGICAL RANDOMISED CONTROLLED TRIALS

Surgeon preferences
- Maximise flexibility in the delivery of surgical interventions, beyond the key distinctive elements, to allow for variation in surgeon and centre practices
- Implement recruitment of participants by a third party
- Use broad patient eligibility criteria
- Undertake preliminary work to establish consensus regarding community uncertainty
- Adopt an expertise based trial design

Patient preferences
- Undertake a qualitative evaluation of patients' perspectives and experiences

Quality control of the intervention
- Use criteria for surgeon eligibility (for example, training and previous number of cases)
- Record an objective measure of quality (for example, lymph node yield for gastric cancer surgery)
- Record indicators of surgical decision making (for example, conversion from partial to total knee replacement, or from laparoscopic to open surgery)

Table Surgical trials examples—standardisation of interventions and eligibility criteria of patients and surgeons

Research question	No of centres	Patient/surgeon eligibility	Standardisation of interventions Perioperative care	Preoperative and postoperative care
Stapler v hand sewn closure after distalpancreatectomy (DISPACT)[21]	21	Broad/training given to all participating surgeons (centre had to perform 10 pancreatic resections per year)	Resection and closure procedures standardised; stapler specified; type of incision not standardised; no additional intraoperative treatment or covering of the pancreatic remnant; splenectomy in addition to distal pancreatectomy at discretion of surgeon; standardised policy in relation to octreotide use at sites; pain management not standardised	Bowel preparation not standardised; standardised drain use; recovery not standardised (for example, location, feeding, and mobilisation)
Treatment of tibial fractures with reamed or non-reamed intrameduallary nails (SPRINT)[40]	29	Broad/no reported restrictions	Standardised reamed nailing and unreamed nailing procedures	Standardised antibiotic use in open and closed fractures; standardised mobilisation (both open and closed) and use of growth stimulation not allowed during first 12 months; wound closure (open); dynamisation of the nail (both) and reoperation (open) only allowed in specific circumstances
Treatment of abdominal aortic aneurysm (EVAR trial 1) with endovascular or open repair[15]	34	Broad/hospitals had to complete 20 endovascular repair procedures	Choice of EVAR device left to participating surgeons, otherwise no stated restrictions	No stated restrictions
Treatment of premenopausal women with abnormal uterine bleeding with surgical or medical treatment (Ms study)[18]	2	Broad/no stated restrictions	Type and route of hysterectomy at discretion of surgeon; prophylactic oophorectomies were discouraged	No stated restrictions
Treatment of osteoarthritis of the knee with arthroscopic débridement, arthroscopic lavage, or placebo surgery[41]	1	Broad/one surgeon performed all operations	Surgical interventions standardised	Standardised anaesthetic; mobilisation and pain management (analgesics)

only the interventions in which they have expertise (an expertise based trial).[24] There is limited evidence about how well this approach works to date, and such designs are not without statistical and practical disadvantages.[25] Whatever approach is adopted, other factors can lead to differences in outcome between surgeons (such as ancillary care and centre admission policies) although they are rarely, if ever, fully standardised.

Impact of treatment preferences

The preferences of both patients and surgeons are a key factor that affects the success of a randomised controlled trial, and can be the decisive influence upon recruitment.[26] If patients tend to prefer one of the treatments, they are unlikely to agree to be randomised in case they are assigned to another treatment. The merit of an otherwise well designed and conducted trial can be fatally undermined if too few surgeons are willing to be involved. There is, however, a strong relationship between the patient and the surgeon, who may have his or her own strong preferences and have traditionally acted as gatekeeper and facilitator.[27] Recent evidence[28] demonstrated that patients' preferences expressed during consultations could be influenced by surgeon recruiters, who seemed to unconsciously transmit their own preferences during the consent process. Properly informed patients could be more likely to consent to randomisation.

For multicentre trials, a pragmatic approach to patient eligibility that achieves general agreement and understanding is important. Surgeon preferences often depend on the patient's prognosis. The Spine Stabilisation Trial[29] explicitly adopted broad inclusion criteria, using an approach to recruitment based on the "uncertainty principle": surgeons could restrict randomisation to eligible patients which they personally were uncertain as to which intervention would be the best option (known as personal equipoise). However, this approach seems to have led to misunderstanding among participating surgeons about the pragmatic nature of the trial design and the explicit aim of seeking to recruit a wide spectrum of potential patients. A successful example is the first EVAR trial on endovascular aneurysm repair versus open repair in patients with abdominal aortic aneurysm, which had broad eligibility criteria and achieved its recruitment target.[12] Transmission of preference can be mitigated if consent is obtained by a trained and possibly neutral recruiter, who is not delivering any intervention (such as a research nurse). The merits of this approach will differ according to the research question.

Long term study stage

Although the benefit of a particular surgical intervention (for example, knee replacement) might be well established, the use of a particular variation in the approach (such as using a posterior approach) or device selection is often open to question long after widespread adoption. This provides an opportunity to obtain good evidence about safety and effectiveness of techniques or technologies from observational and surveillance studies. Current research on long term surveillance focuses mainly on medical devices and—in the case of surgery—implantable devices. One reason for this focus is the cost; the medical device market in 2008 was estimated to exceed £150bn (€177bn; $232bn) worldwide.[30] Surveillance of the long term effect of surgical innovation (both in terms of the procedure and devices) is imperative even if short term benefit has

been established (at IDEAL stages 1-3). The US Food and Drug Administration (FDA) recently developed a conceptual framework for medical devices specifically,[31] although it needs to be developed and refined in the context of long term surveillance. Box 2 provides an example of a long term surveillance study.

Long term evaluation of procedures

Well designed, large observational studies (for example, based on registries) can be used to evaluate procedures in the long term study stage; they can also provide data for outcomes in subgroups of interest as well as rare endpoints in safety and effectiveness.[32] From an assessment perspective, some national or nationally representative patient registries can be defined as observational studies collecting "uniform data, to evaluate specified outcomes for a population defined by a particular disease, condition, or exposure." Registries can be designed to capture data for specific conditions or exposures (such as surgery or devices), types of healthcare service delivered (such as surgical treatment or diagnostic procedure), or specific outcomes (such as an adverse event, disorder, or disease), to improve the delivery of care.

Practical factors often determine which data are collected, but in principle, disease based registries have the advantage of enabling consideration of selection for a procedure and potential for associated bias in an evaluation. Procedure registries can provide useful comparative evidence for different interventions and devices. Longstanding procedure registries include those developed by professional societies such as the United Kingdom's Society for Cardiothoracic Surgery's adult cardiac surgery database or the Society of Thoracic Surgeons' registry.[33] Other studies (including randomised controlled trials) can be nested in them. The Swedish national registry of gallstone surgery and endoscopic retrograde cholangiopancreatography (GallRiks) enabled a large cohort study to quantify survival and incidence of bile duct injuries and explore the relation between them.[34]

The choice of surgical procedure or medical device can often vary greatly, even for similar patients within and between centres. For example, the figure shows the proportion of operations using abdominal access (versus thoracic access) in hiatal hernia repair, in hospitals in the Nationwide Inpatient Sample.[35] The choice of access route was strongly influenced by surgeon practice and institutional culture, and was unlikely to be related to the hernia location for many hospitals.[35] In most hospitals, the majority of hernia repairs were conducted via abdominal access—that is, the hernia location did not dictate the approach and therefore any confounding by indication will probably be limited. Identifying such practice and surgeon patterns can, therefore, help clarify the extent to which selection of patients for receiving the procedure (or device) may have occurred. Exploration of variations in practice can improve the design of comparative studies, by providing insight regarding the likelihood of the main potential bias—confounding by indication.[36]

The modes of follow-up are critical,[32] as are completeness and accuracy of data collection, which can lead to loss of follow-up and various misclassification biases (for example, outcomes of difficult operative cases being attributed to revision surgery or a medical device). Standardisation of terminology, as in earlier stages,[36] would allow routine capture of information on surgical procedures such as the use of a laparoscopic approach, laterality (side of surgery), and device information. Similarly, standardised terminology for devices (such as from the Clinical Data Interchange Standards Consortium or product catalogues) will help to accurately describe the specific attributes and properly identify the technology used.

However, such studies have inherent and common limitations. Firstly, the concept of "intention to treat" does not readily map onto observation data, and only the first procedure or devices used is readily interpretable. If a patient subsequently receives another procedure that converts failure after the first procedure into success, this outcome could be misattributed to the first procedure. Observational studies (including registry based studies) should, whenever possible, construct intention to treat analyses that correspond to treatment decisions as they occur in the real world. However, key data are often not routinely collected. Reasoned inferences can be made from the clinical scenario using resource use data. For example, if routine data show that both partial and total knee devices were used in the same knee during an operation, it can be appropriately inferred that it was necessary to change a partial device to a total one, as it is impossible for the opposite to occur.

Secondly, the time between cohort entry (assignment to procedure) and date of first exposure (actual delivery of procedure) is often not recorded. This leads to "immortal time bias," a period of follow-up after assignment during which outcomes of treatment that determine the end of follow-up cannot occur, as the treatment has not

yet happened. This bias can confound results, because interventions that are delivered faster could look worse than those needing more time (for example, sicker patients might die before receiving the therapy and being accounted for). Finally, another difficult situation is when the originally assigned (intended) treatment switches before initiation. This switch can be due to patient refusal, financial factors, or other considerations. Again, such information is not typically collected by observational data sources but is often needed for meaningful interpretation.

Surveillance of devices
In the US and UK, manufacturers and importers are required to submit reports of device related deaths, serious injuries, and malfunctions to the regulatory bodies. US hospitals and nursing homes are required to submit reports of device related deaths and serious injuries to the manufacturer and only deaths to the FDA, but healthcare providers and consumers can submit reports voluntarily (through MedWatch).[37] Such passive reporting systems typically have important weaknesses, including:

- Incomplete or inaccurate data that are usually not independently verified
- Data reflecting reporting biases driven by event severity or uniqueness, publicity, or litigation
- Causality cannot be inferred from any individual report
- Events are generally under-reported and this, in combination with lack of denominator (exposure) data, precludes determination of event incidence or prevalence.

However, reports received through passive and enhanced systems are often useful and have resulted in important public health alerts related to:

- Transvaginal placement of surgical mesh
- Use of recombinant bone morphogenetic protein in cervical spine fusion
- Interactions induced by magnetic resonance imaging in patients with implanted neurological stimulators.[37]

In addition, the FDA has developed an enhanced surveillance system using several different modes of surveillance, including active surveillance. This system, known as the Medical Product Safety Network,[38] provides national surveillance of medical devices based on a representative subset of user facilities. Routine data collection and monitoring for devices need improvement. Finally, when resources are available, active surveillance based on registries can also help monitor high risk surgery and devices, such as a national registry of implanted ventricular assisted devices.[39]

Summary
A large, multicentre, randomised controlled trial in the assessment stage complements observational evaluation in the long term study stage. Large and preferably national patient registries are best suited for long term surveillance studies of surgical procedures. Surveillance of devices with improved data collection is needed. Owing to the inherent complexity of surgery and variation in practice, both randomised controlled trials and surveillance studies face particular challenges. However, solutions are often available, and such difficulties should not prevent rigorous and comprehensive evaluation of surgical innovations.

The Health Services Research Unit is core funded by the Chief Scientist Office of the Scottish Government Health Directorates. Views expressed are those of the authors and do not necessarily reflect the view of the Chief Scientist Office or the funders.

BOX 2 EXAMPLE OF OBSERVATIONAL STUDY AT THE LONG TERM STUDY STAGE[9]

Implanted devices for total hip replacement

Clinical background at time of conduct
- Total hip replacement is widely undertaken although revision is sometimes necessary, particularly in younger recipients
- Alternative devices with a larger head size and different bearing surface materials (such as metal-on-metal devices) have increasingly been used to reduce revisions

Design
- Long term, device surveillance study nested within a population based registry
- Primary stemmed operations of total hip replacement done between 2003 and 2011 (n=402051) were linked to revision operations
- Operations involving different types of devices (varying bearing surface and head size)

Findings
- Metal-on-metal devices had poorer survival than devices with alternative surfaces
- Lower device survival found in women, and for those devices with larger heads

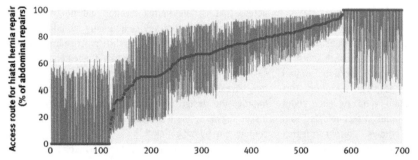

Fig Use of the abdominal route (versus thoracic route) as a proportion of operations in hiatal hernia repair, by hospital. Data taken from US hospitals in the Nationwide Inpatient Sample[35]; figure shows 708 hospitals (900 hospitals with 100% abdominal route use not shown). Blue=percentage of operations with abdominal route; black=95% exact (binomial) confidence intervals. Use of the abdominal route varied from 0% to 100% across hospitals

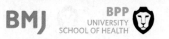

Contributors: JAC and PM formulated the IDEAL series to which this paper belongs. JAC and AS wrote the first draft of this paper; JMB, DJB, DM-D, and PM all commented on the draft. All authors approved the final version, and JAC and AS are the guarantors. The papers were informed by the IDEAL workshop in December 2010.

IDEAL workshop participants (December 2010): Doug Altman, Jeff Aronson, David Beard, Jane Blazeby, Bruce Campbell, Andrew Carr, Tammy Clifford, Jonathan Cook, Pierre Dagenais, Philipp Dahm, Peter Davidson, Hugh Davies, Markus Diener, Jonothan Earnshaw, Patrick Ergina, Shamiram Feinglass, Trish Groves, Sion Glyn-Jones, Muir Gray, Alison Halliday, Judith Hargreaves, Carl Heneghan, Jo Carol Hiatt, Sean Kehoe, Nicola Lennard, Georgios Lyratzopoulos, Guy Maddern, Danica Marinac-Dabic, Peter McCulloch, Jon Nicholl, Markus Ott, Art Sedrakyan, Dan Schaber, Frank Schuller, Bill Summerskill.

Funding: PM received funding from the National Institute for Health Research's Health Technology Assessment programme, Johnson & Johnson, Medtronic, and Zimmer (all unrestricted grants) for the IDEAL workshop in December 2010. JAC holds a Medical Research Council Methodology Fellowship (G1002292). JMB is supported in part by the Medical Research Council ConDuCT Hub for Trials Methodology Research. AS is supported in part by the US Food and Drug Administration contract for MDEpiNet Science and Infrastructure Centre (HHSF22321110172C).

Competing interests: All authors have completed the ICMJE uniform disclosure form at www.icmje.org/coi_disclosure.pdf and declare: PM received financial support from the National Institute for Health Research's Health Technology Assessment programme, Johnson & Johnson, Medtronic, and Zimmer for the IDEAL collaboration and for a workshop; DB has undertaken consultancy for ICNet and Stryker European Medicines Agency, and has received research grant funding from Genzyme; no other financial relationships with any organisations that might have an interest in the submitted work in the previous three years; no other relationships or activities that could appear to have influenced the submitted work.

Provenance and peer review: Not commissioned; externally peer reviewed.

1 Cuthbertson BH, Campbell MK, Stott SA, Vale L, Norrie J, Kinsella J, et al. A pragmatic multi-centre randomised controlled trial of fluid loading and level of dependency in high-risk surgical patients undergoing major elective surgery: trial protocol. Trials 2010;11:41.
2 Brown GA. Venous thromboembolism prophylaxis after major orthopaedic surgery: a pooled analysis of randomized controlled trials. J Arthroplasty 2009;24(6 suppl):77-83.
3 Hunter KF, Glazener CM, Moore KN. Conservative management for postprostatectomy urinary incontinence. Cochrane Database Syst Rev 2007;2:001843.
4 Powell R, McKee L, Bruce J. Information and behavioural instruction along the health-care pathway: the perspective of people undergoing hernia repair surgery and the role of formal and informal information sources. Health Expectations 2009;12:149-59.
5 Craig P, Dieppe P, Macintyre S, Michie S, Nazareth I, Petticrew M, et al. Developing and evaluating complex interventions: the new Medical Research Council guidance. BMJ 2008;337:a1655.
6 Comet Initiative. Home page. 2013. www.comet-initiative.org/.
7 McCulloch P, Taylor I, Sasako M, Lovett B, Griffin D. Randomised trials in surgery: problems and possible solutions. BMJ 2002;324:1448-51.
8 Cook JA. The challenges faced in the design, conduct and analysis of surgical randomised controlled trials. Trials 2009;10:9.
9 Smith AJ, Dieppe P, Vernon K, Porter M, Blom AW, National Joint Registry of England and Wales. Failure rates of stemmed metal-on-metal hip replacements: analysis of data from the National Joint Registry of England and Wales. Lancet 2012;379:1199-204.
10 Baum M. Reflections on randomised controlled trials in surgery. Lancet 1999;353(suppl 1):S6-8.
11 Pollock AV. Surgical evaluation at the crossroads. Br J Surg 1993;80:964-6.
12 EVAR trial participants. Endovascular aneurysm repair versus open repair in patients with abdominal aortic aneurysm (EVAR trial 1): randomised controlled trial. Lancet 2005;365:2179-86.
13 Challah S, Mays NB. The randomised controlled trial in the evaluation of new technology: a case study. Br Med J (Clin Res Ed) 1986;292:877-9.
14 Price AJ, Rees JL, Beard D, Juszczak E, Carter S, White S, et al. A mobile-bearing total knee prosthesis compared with a fixed-bearing prosthesis. J Bone Joint Surg Br 2003;85:62-7.
15 United Kingdom EVAR Trial I, Greenhalgh RM, Brown LC, Powell JT, Thompson SG, Epstein D, et al. Endovascular versus open repair of abdominal aortic aneurysm. N Engl J Med 2010;362:1863-71.
16 Ergina PL, Cook JA, Blazeby JM, Boutron I, Clavien PA, Reeves BC, et al. Challenges in evaluating surgical innovation. Lancet 2009;374:1097-104.
17 McCulloch P. Developing appropriate methodology for the study of surgical techniques. J R Soc Med 2009;102:51-5.
18 Kuppermann M, Varner RE, Summitt RL Jr, Learman LA, Ireland C, Vittinghoff E, et al. Effect of hysterectomy vs medical treatment on health-related quality of life and sexual functioning: the medicine or surgery (Ms) randomized trial. JAMA 2004;291:1447-55.

19 Ross S, Scott N, Grant AS, O'Dwyer P, Wright D, McIntosh E, et al. Laparoscopic versus open repair of groin hernia: a randomised comparison. Lancet 1999;354:185-90.
20 Bonenkamp JJ, Songun I, Hermans J, Sasako M, Welvaart K, Plukker JT, et al. Randomised comparison of morbidity after D1 and D2 dissection for gastric cancer in 996 Dutch patients. Lancet 1995;345:745-8.
21 Diener MK, Seiler CM, Rossion I, Kleeff J, Glanemann M, Butturini G, et al. Efficacy of stapler versus hand-sewn closure after distal pancreatectomy (DISPACT): a randomised, controlled multicentre trial. Lancet 2011;377:1514-22.
22 Fairbank J, Frost H, Wilson-MacDonald J, Yu LM, Barker K, Collins R; Spine Stabilisation Trial Group. Randomised controlled trial to compare surgical stabilisation of the lumbar spine with an intensive rehabilitation programme for patients with chronic low back pain: the MRC spine stabilisation trial. BMJ 2005;330:1233-9.
23 Cook JA, Ramsay CR, Fayers P. Statistical evaluation of learning effects in surgical trials. Clin Trials 2004;1:421-7.
24 Devereaux PJ, Bhandari M, Clarke M, Montori VM, Cook DJ, Yusuf S, et al. Need for expertise based randomised controlled trials. BMJ 2005;330:88-92.
25 Biau DJ, Porcher R. Letter to the editor re: Orthopaedic surgeons prefer to participate in expertise-based randomized trials. Clin Orthop Relat Res 2009;467:298-300.
26 Barkun JS, Aronson JK, Feldman LS, Maddern GJ, Strasberg SM, Balliol C, et al. Evaluation and stages of surgical innovations. Lancet 2009;374:1089-96.
27 Meakins JL. Innovation in surgery: the rules of evidence. Am J Surg 2002;183:399-405.
28 Mills N, Donovan JL, Wade J, Hamdy FC, Neal DE, Lane JA. Exploring treatment preferences facilitated recruitment to randomized controlled trials. J Clin Epidemiol 2011;64:1127-36.
29 Ziebland S, Featherstone K, Snowdon C, Barker K, Frost H, Fairbank J. Does it matter if clinicians recruiting for a trial don't understand what the trial is really about? Qualitative study of surgeons' experiences of participation in a pragmatic multi-centre RCT. Trials 2007;8:4.
30 Health Industries. Medical device industry assessment. 24 March 2010. www.ita.doc.gov/td/health/medical.html.
31 Sedrakyan A, Marinac-Dabic D, Normand ST, Mushlin AS, Gross T. A framework for evidence evaluation and methodological issues in implantable device studies. Med Care 2010;48(suppl 1):S121-8.
32 Dreyer NA, Garner S. Registries for robust evidence. JAMA 2009;302:790-1.
33 Peterson E, Kaul P, Kaczmarek R, Hammill B, Armstrong P, Bridges C, et al. From controlled trials to clinical practice: monitoring transmyocardial revascularization use and outcomes. J Am Coll Cardiol 2003;42:1611-6.
34 Tornqvist B, Stromberg C, Persson G, Nilsson M. Effect of intended intraoperative cholangiography and early detection of bile duct injury on survival after cholecystectomy: population based cohort study. BMJ 2012;345:e6457.
35 Healthcare Cost and Utilization Project. Overview of the National Inpatient Sample. 2013. www.hcup-us.ahrq.gov/nisoverview.jsp/.
36 Ergina PL, Barkun JS, McCulloch P, Cook JA, Altman DG, on behalf of the IDEAL group. IDEAL framework for surgical innovation 2: observational studies in the exploration and assessment stages. BMJ 2013;346:f3011.
37 US Food and Drug Administration. MedWatch: the FDA safety information and adverse event reporting program. 2013. www.fda.gov/Safety/MedWatch/.
38 US Food and Drug Administration. MedSun: medical product safety network. 2012. www.fda.gov/MedicalDevices/Safety/MedSunMedicalProductSafetyNetwork/default.htm.
39 University of Alabama at Birmingham School of Medicine. Interagency Registry for Mechanically Assisted Circulatory Support. 2013. www.intermacs.org.
40 Study to Prospectively Evaluate Reamed Intramedullary Nails in Patients with Tibial Fractures Investigators; Bhandari M, Guyatt G, Tornetta P 3rd, Schemitsch EH, Swiontkowski M, et al. Randomized trial of reamed and unreamed intramedullary nailing of tibial shaft fractures. J Bone Joint Surg Am 2008;90:2567-78.
41 Moseley JB, O'Malley K, Petersen NJ, Menke TJ, Brody BA, Kuykendall DH, et al. A controlled trial of arthroscopic surgery for osteoarthritis of the knee. N Engl J Med 2002;347:81-8.

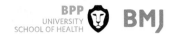

IDEAL framework for surgical innovation 2: observational studies in the exploration and assessment stages

Patrick L Ergina, assistant professor of surgery[1][2], Jeffrey S Barkun, professor of surgery[3],
Peter McCulloch, clinical reader in surgery[4], Jonathan A Cook, methodologist[5],
Douglas G Altman, director[6], On behalf of the IDEAL group

[1]Cardiothoracic Surgery Division, McGill University Health Centre, Royal Victoria Hospital, Montreal, Quebec, Canada H3A 1A1

[2]Oxford International Programme in Evidence-Based Health Care, University of Oxford, Oxford, UK

[3]Department of Surgery, McGill University, Montreal, Canada

[4]Nuffield Department of Surgical Science, University of Oxford, UK

[5]Health Services Research Unit, University of Aberdeen, Aberdeen, UK

[6]Centre for Statistics in Medicine, University of Oxford, UK

Correspondence to: P L Ergina
patrick.ergina@muhc.mcgill.ca

Cite this as: BMJ 2013;346:f3011

DOI: 10.1136/bmj.f3011

http://www.bmj.com/content/346/bmj.f3011

ABSTRACT

The IDEAL framework describes the stages of evaluation for surgical innovations. This paper considers the role of observational studies in the exploration and assessment stages. At the exploration stage, the surgical intervention is usually more widely used, and observational studies should collect prospective data from multiple surgeons, deal with factors such as case mix and learning, and prepare for a definitive evaluation at the next stage of assessment. Although a randomised controlled trial is preferable, a high quality observational study would be acceptable if a randomised trial is not feasible or, on rare occasions, deemed unnecessary.

Introduction

The evaluation of new innovations, from idea developed to accepted practice, has been less orderly in surgery and other interventional therapies than in clinical pharmacology. The IDEAL framework for surgical innovations and recommendations has been designed to describe the stages of evaluation for these interventional therapies (idea, development, exploration, assessment, and long term study), and to highlight the study designs and reporting standards that are likely to prove most useful at each stage.[1][2] The first two IDEAL stages are covered in the first paper in this series.[3] This second article focuses on the IDEAL recommendations for the use of observational studies in the exploration and assessment stages, and discusses the options for observational study designs and reporting protocols (box 1), using examples of surgical innovations. The final paper in the series covers the undertaking of a definitive randomised controlled trial, mainly in the assessment stage, as well as the long term stage.[4]

Reaching the exploration stage (IDEAL stage 2b)

By the exploration stage, the innovation is usually already practiced by many surgeons on an increasing number of less carefully selected patients. Promising evidence of safety and beneficial short term outcomes—without unacceptable complications—will have been generated, or further development would have been halted. Under the IDEAL framework, use of retrospective studies should be limited to hypothesis generation in the earliest stages. Typically, the early evaluation in the development stage (2a) will use small observational studies without contemporaneous comparison groups in highly selected cohorts of patients. The exploration stage (2b) offers the opportunity to obtain higher quality evidence in a more representative patient population and to deal with factors that could hinder the conduct of a proper methodological evaluation. Although developmental refinement of the intervention will probably not cease completely by this point, its adoption by multiple surgeons across different sites will increase variation in the patient case mix, driven by surgeons' practices and centre infrastructure and policies. One focus of studies in this stage should be to capture variation in practice. In addition, careful tabulation of patient characteristics could suggest potential covariates and confounders influencing outcomes.

Nature and challenges of the exploration stage: preparing for a definitive evaluation

In 1987, Martin Buxton observed that "It's always too early (to do a randomised trial) until, unfortunately, it's suddenly too late."[5] In observing past innovations, the exploration stage is often the "tipping point" of a surgical innovation (for example, laparoscopic procedures)—as described by Everett Rogers, where adopters' characteristics act as drivers or barriers (figs 1 and 2).[6] Factors such as whether the technique is too complex or too onerous to learn, and the strength of physician or patient preferences might critically affect its adoption.[7] This point could also be described as a time of "clinical equipoise," because further exponential adoption of this innovation by "early majority" and "late majority" adopters is consistent with a conviction of likely efficacy (for example, trends in diffusion of laparoscopic surgery[8]). It is at this stage when changes in regulatory structure might have the most profound effects in promoting randomised controlled trials in surgery (for example, approval requirements from the US Food and Drug Administration for drug trial phases for proof of safety and efficacy).

Several factors are needed to facilitate a definitive evaluation (preferably a randomised controlled trial). These include gathering practical information and fully evaluating the effect of the innovation (benefits and harms) that earlier evaluations would be ill equipped to represent. In the meantime, the new intervention still needs appropriate evaluation, and the highest possible methodological quality of evidence from observational studies should be

SUMMARY POINTS

- Observational studies at IDEAL exploration stage (2b) should collect data for consecutive patients from multiple surgeons, including key case mix characteristics that are likely to influence outcome. Where appropriate, adjustment or matching should be used to control for potential confounding in the statistical analysis

- Studies at the exploration stage should investigate the effect of technical parameters as well as skill and learning, assess the full range of outcomes, and prepare for a definitive (preferably randomised) evaluation at the assessment stage (3)

- A non-randomised controlled trial or interrupted time series could fulfil the role of a definitive evaluation at the assessment stage if a randomised controlled trial is not feasible, or on rare occasions, considered unnecessarily

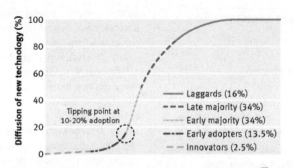

Fig 1 Theoretical adoption curve showing the different stages (according to adopter type) in the diffusion of a surgical innovation[6]

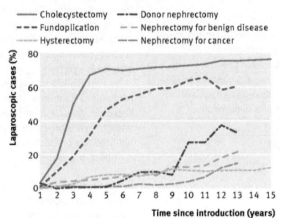

Fig 2 Example of surgical innovation: laparoscopic procedure adoption.[8] Reproduced from reference 8 with permission. Data are percentage of operations carried out using a laparoscopic approach in 1989-2003, from the Nationwide Inpatient Sample, a nationally representative annual sample of hospital admissions in the United States

sought at this stage. Prospective (and possibly controlled) observational studies are the most likely design at stage 2b—their value can be maximised, based on four recommendations.

Firstly, observational studies should collect data for consecutive patients from multiple surgeons (and preferably multiple centres) undertaking the new intervention.[9] Ideally, these studies would also be based on disease or diagnosis rather than solely on a new procedure, which would include patients irrespective of subsequent treatment. Such a prospective design is a substantial advance on the usual single surgeon (or single centre) retrospective case series of selected patients undergoing a novel intervention, which have predominated in the surgical literature. There is evidence that retrospective designs can be more susceptible to bias than prospective designs when comparing randomised studies with non-randomised (including both prospective and retrospective) studies.[10]

A well conducted, large prospective observational study can form the basis for identifying important patient characteristics (the case mix), technical intervention variables (including potential co-interventions), and clinical outcomes of interest. A recent example of this type of collaboration is the International Registry of Acute Aortic Dissection, which uses this design for evidence to guide surgical, endovascular, and medical practice in acute aortic dissection (box 2).[11] Data collection sponsored by professional organisations or the government can also help the conduct of later comparative observational studies (for example, the American College of Surgeons' national programme for surgical quality improvement).[12]

Secondly, studies at this stage should collect data for a range of outcomes using standardised definitions as well as key patient characteristics. Not only benefits but also harms should be assessed. Surgical research has focused considerably on the risks of short term harm (surgical complications), although with varying extensiveness and clarity. Standardised frameworks should be used—for example, the Dindo-Clavien system[14] for postoperative complications.

Thirdly, surgical skill differences and associated learning curves can affect outcomes,[15] and an evaluation of surgical variation and learning should be incorporated into study designs at this stage whenever possible.[16] We recommend identifying relevant variables that can measure the effect of skill and learning (for example, surgeon or centre "volume," operating times, quality measures, and appropriate outcomes), and analysing the data sequentially to assess learning, where possible.[17] In a sequential statistical analysis of cases (using a cumulative sum control chart) early in the use of robotic beating heart surgery, researchers detected several complications needing further investigation.[18]

Finally, studies should be conducted not necessarily to be definitive, but rather to prepare for a definitive evaluation study (preferably a randomised controlled trial). We suggest that professional or government bodies promote collaborative multicentre observational studies to evaluate important new interventions in their specialty, and incorporate their work as a strong foundation towards a definitive randomised controlled trial, as a secondary aim. Collected information can inform the timing of a trial (or another type of high quality, prospective study) with respect to equipoise, the key research question, and the appropriate study population. In addition, standardisation of the intervention, quality assurance techniques, and appropriate validated and measurable outcome measures can be assessed. Several successful examples of this approach to consensus development of a trial have been published.[19] In some circumstances, a feasibility or pilot trial could be a natural intermediate step between a prospective observational study and a definitive randomised controlled trial,[20] which can identify specific enablers and barriers.

Nature and challenges of assessment (IDEAL stage 3)

Use of observational studies as a definitive evaluation in lieu of a randomised controlled trial

Assessment is the stage in the IDEAL framework that requires a definitive evaluation, preferably a randomised controlled trial. On rare occasions, a randomised comparison might be considered unnecessary, owing to the magnitude of evidence from early evaluations (for example, the parachute scenario[21]). However, the risks of error due to bias are easily underestimated; therefore, as the magnitude of the treatment effect becomes smaller, one should be cautious about relying on such evidence. Criteria based on the signal to noise ratio suggesting that at least a 5-fold to 10-fold improvement in improvement or cure is needed for a randomised controlled trial to be considered unnecessary, have been proposed.[22] Few new interventions achieve such striking results, and most will need a randomised controlled trial to give confidence of their efficacy. More likely reasons for not using a randomised trial are that it is considered impractical; this can be due to anticipated recruitment difficulties, the low likelihood of a timely completion (for example, key technology becoming outdated by the end of the trial); or the study will be prohibitively expensive.

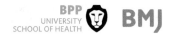

BOX 1 RECOMMENDATIONS FOR OBSERVATIONAL STUDIES AT STAGES 2B (EXPLORATION) AND 3 (ASSESSMENT)

Exploration

- Observational studies should generally be prospective and have a protocol
- A range of outcomes should be collected using standardised definitions
- Observational studies that are uncontrolled (for example, those based on registry and routine data collection) should be diagnosis based rather than procedure based whenever possible
- Important patient risk factors and variations in the interventions should be explored
- Studies should record and report surgeon experience (including any specific training received). Where possible, the effect of skill differences and learning should be assessed using appropriate data analysis
- Prospective, collaborative observational studies should be designed with a definite evaluation in mind (preferably a randomised controlled trial)

Assessment

- Definitive observational studies should use a quasi-experimental study design; protocol driven controlled studies with standardised eligibility and prospective data collection
- Possible designs include non-randomised controlled trials and interrupted time series
- Key patient and centre characteristics likely to confound analysis should be considered before conducting study and collecting appropriate data, which would facilitate assessment and adjustment of the case mix, and help matching to control for potential confounding

BOX 2 EXAMPLE OF OBSERVATIONAL STUDY AT EXPLORATION STAGE (2B)

International Registry of Acute Aortic Dissection study[13]

Clinical background at time of conduct

- Aortic dissection is defined as a tear in the aorta
- Acute aortic dissection (within 14 days of onset) needs urgent treatment because it is associated with increased mortality and morbidity
- There are two types of aortic dissection (A and B), according to location
- The effect of developments in surgical and medical management is uncertain

Design

- Observational study with registry data collection
- Eligibility was based on diagnosis—all patients with an acute aortic dissection in 12 large referral centres (six countries)
- Study included 464 patients between 1 January 1996 and 31 December 1998
- Data were collected at presentation and from routine hospital records until discharge

Findings

- Physical findings at presentation were diverse, classic findings were often absent
- For patients with a type A dissection, medical management was associated with a hospital mortality of 58%, compared with 26% mortality for surgical management
- For patients with a type B dissection, medical management was associated with a hospital mortality of 11%, compared with 31% for surgical management

BOX 3 EXAMPLE OF OBSERVATIONAL STUDY AT ASSESSMENT STAGE (3)

Minimally invasive, open radical prostatectomy with and without robotic assistance[28]

Clinical background at time of conduct

- Open retropubic radical prostatectomy (RRP) is commonly used to treat prostate cancer
- Use of minimally invasive radical prostatectomy (MIRP) with or without robotic assistance had been proposed as an alternative, and its use is increasing

Design

- Non-randomised controlled trial nested within data collection from a population based registry
- Men diagnosed with prostate cancer as their first and only cancer were eligible
- Men who underwent MIRP between 2002 and 2005 (n=1938) were compared with men who underwent RRP (n=6899) using a propensity score adjusted statistical analysis
- Registry data were linked with US Medicare administrative data

Findings

- Compared with RRP, MIRP resulted in a shorter length of stay, fewer strictures, and fewer 30 days respiratory and miscellaneous surgical complications—but a higher occurrence of incontinence, erectile dysfunction, and 30 day genitourinary complications
- Use of additional postoperative cancer treatments was similar for both approaches

In this scenario, careful consideration of how to obtain observational data of the greatest value and quality is particularly important.

Any observational study conducted as an alternative to a high quality, randomised controlled trial should have as many positive design features of such a trial as possible.[23] The study should have a prospective design with a detailed research protocol (ideally published at the outset) that clearly describes and defines a standardised intervention, the eligibility criteria and characteristics for patients being treated with the novel intervention, and the incorporation of quality control measures regarding delivery of the intervention. A unique circumstance when an observational study might be needed is if there is no viable alternative therapeutic option (for example, organ transplantation of the heart[24] or liver[25] for severe advanced stage disease). Many examples of prospective, uncontrolled observational studies have successfully provided evidence to guide practice in surgery.[26]

We consider in turn two quasi-experimental designs: non-randomised controlled trials and interrupted time series. These designs are methodologically stronger options than uncontrolled prospective observational studies,[27] and could fulfil the role of a definitive evaluation when a randomised controlled trial is infeasible (box 3 shows an example).

Non-randomised controlled trials

The preferred observational design is a non-randomised controlled trial; a study in which a cohort of patients undergoing a novel surgical intervention is compared with a concurrent control group undergoing standard treatment (standard surgical, medical, or no treatment). The study should incorporate the positive design features associated with a randomised controlled trial (for example, a prospective design and standardised data collection), with the exception of randomisation and blinding. Such studies provided the first convincing prospective evidence for benefits in coronary artery bypass surgery[29] and laparoscopic cholecystectomy.[30]

In a randomised controlled trial, random allocation will probably achieve balance for known and unknown risk factors and minimise bias. Selection bias in a non-randomised controlled trial can be addressed by controlling for known risk factors (case mix) in the analysis. Relevant risk factors, how they should be documented, and potential for bias should be considered before starting data collection. Patient characteristics at study entry should be thorough documented. Treatment group assignment can, however, have a different risk pattern at baseline, and this can lead to groups being less comparable after statistical adjustment (for example, regression) owing to the "constant risk fallacy" where the assumption of constant risk across different organisations (for example, hospitals) may be inappropriate.[31]

Nevertheless, adjustment or matching for known prognostic factors should generally be done where possible (for example, using propensity scoring and corresponding analysis, which is an increasingly popular approach[32]), while recognising the limitations of such analyses. The estimated treatment effects can be assumed to be unbiased only if matching stratified analyses or regression techniques are sufficient enough to fully deal with risk imbalance—that is, when treatment allocation is ignorable in terms of baseline risk.[33] A cautionary example of the importance of risk adjustment is the Veterans Affairs National Surgical Quality Improvement programme's study of long term outcomes after bariatric surgery. The survival advantage observed in the unmatched cohort disappeared when researchers used propensity scoring to analyse a matched cohort.[34] In some instances, results from randomised and observational studies have corresponded with respect to the magnitude of the effect size, although in general, observational studies have a greater risk of bias.[35] [36]

Interrupted time series

The interrupted time series is an alternative quasi-experimental design for an observational study that could potentially be used at the assessment stage.[37] The design uses a temporal rather than concurrent control group. A key outcome of interest (such as anastomotic leakage, graft failure, or death) is measured sequentially during a time period before the new intervention is introduced (that is, the interruption) and measured again during the same period afterwards.

Interrupted time series may be particularly suited to evaluating interventions that can be implemented at a centre with a long history of treating a particular disease (such as congenital heart disease). Although the design has been used to evaluate the effect of new interventions, it has not typically been used for evaluating clinical intervention efficacy. This design can be more susceptible to bias than non-randomised controlled trials, if not enough patient data are available to investigate and control risk factors. The design is particularly useful to assess secular trends in clinical care—that is, changes with time that could affect outcomes for all patients. The design should, whenever possible, be strengthened by adding a control group (that is, a parallel time series from a group where there the new intervention is not used).

An interrupted time series has been used to track the effect of new surgical interventions (such as laparoscopic cholecystectomy on rates of bile duct injury[38]), evaluate quality of care (for example, in relation to rates of cardiac surgery mortality[39]), and estimate associated healthcare costs.[40] Surgical studies are often complicated by the nature of complex interventions and potential co-intervention effects (for example, medical and anaesthesia treatment of surgical patients), and an interrupted time series could isolate these effects by tracking the onset of factors (that is, interruptions) other than the surgical intervention itself.

Summary

After the refinement and definition of the innovation in small studies with short endpoints for preliminary investigations at IDEAL development stage, the evaluation of a new surgical intervention enters the exploration stage. At this stage, researchers should obtain the highest possible quality of evidence from prospective observational studies and prepare for a definitive evaluation (preferably with a randomised trial design). Key factors for the evaluation to address include defining patient prognostic variables, characterising and standardising the surgical intervention, assessing learning, and identifying appropriate outcomes. Studies should use clear standardised definitions of key concepts, and be designed to promote a definitive evaluation at the assessment stage. Observational studies at the exploration stage should be based on a disease or indication, rather than just on the new procedure or technology of interest.

A randomised controlled trial is the preferred study design for definitive evidence and should be used wherever possible. But a high quality observational study may be acceptable if a trial is not feasible or, on rare occasions, deemed unnecessary. Observational studies should be carefully designed and conducted to maximally reduce the risk of bias. In such cases, quasi-experimental study designs should be considered (in particular non-randomised controlled trials or controlled interrupted series).

The Health Services Research Unit is core funded by the Chief Scientist Office of the Scottish Government Health and Social Care Directorates. Views expressed are those of the authors and do not necessarily reflect the view of the Chief Scientist Office or the funders.

Contributors: JAC and PM formulated the IDEAL series to which this paper belongs. PE and JB wrote the first draft of this paper, and JC, DA, and PM all commented on the draft. All authors approved the final version, and PE is guarantor. The papers were informed by the IDEAL workshop in December 2010.

IDEAL workshop participants (December 2010): Doug Altman, Jeff Aronson, David Beard, Jane Blazeby, Bruce Campbell, Andrew Carr, Tammy Clifford, Jonathan Cook, Pierre Dagenais, Philipp Dahm, Peter Davidson, Hugh Davies, Markus Diener, Jonothan Earnshaw, Patrick Ergina, Shamiram Feinglass, Trish Groves, Sion Glyn-Jones, Muir Gray, Alison Halliday, Judith Hargreaves, Carl Heneghan, Jo Carol Hiatt, Sean Kehoe, Nicola Lennard, Georgios Lyratzopoulos, Guy Maddern, Danica Marinac-Dabic, Peter McCulloch, Jon Nicholl, Markus Ott, Art Sedrakyan, Dan Schaber, Frank Schuller, Bill Summerskill.

Funding: The IDEAL group meeting in December 2010 was funded by the National Institute for Health Research's Health Technology Assessment programme, Johnson & Johnson, Medtronic and Zimmer (all unrestricted grants). JAC holds a Medical Research Council Methodology Fellowship (G1002292).

Competing interests: All authors have completed the ICMJE uniform disclosure form at www.icmje.org/coi_disclosure.pdf and declare: PM received financial support from the National Institute for Health Research's Health Technology Assessment programme, Johnson & Johnson, Medtronic, and Zimmer for the IDEAL collaboration and for a workshop; no other financial relationships with any organisations that might have an interest in the submitted work in the previous three years; no other relationships or activities that could appear to have influenced the submitted work.

Provenance and peer review: Not commissioned; externally peer reviewed.

1 Barkun JS, Aronson JK, Feldman LS, Maddern GJ, Strasberg SM, et al. Evaluation and stages of surgical innovations. Lancet 2009;374:1089-96.
2 McCulloch P, Altman DG, Campbell WB, Flum DR, Glasziou P, Marshall JC, et al. No surgical innovation without evaluation: the IDEAL recommendations. Lancet 2009;374:1105-12.
3 McCulloch P, Cook JA, Altman DG, Heneghan C, Diener MK. IDEAL framework for surgical innovation 1: the idea and development stages. BMJ 2013;346:f3012
4 Cook JA, McCulloch P, Blazeby JM, Beard DJ, Marinac-Dabic D, Sedrakyan A. IDEAL framework for surgical innovation 3: randomised controlled trials in the assessment stage and evaluations in the long term study stage. BMJ 2013;346:f2820.
5 Buxton MJ. Problems in the economic appraisal of new health technology: the evaluation of heart transplants in the UK. In: Drummond MF. Economic appraisal of health technology in the European Community. Oxford Medical Publications, 1987:103-18.
6 Wilson CB. Adoption of new surgical technology. BMJ 2006;332:112-4.
7 Ergina PL, Cook JA, Blazeby JM, Boutron I, Clavien PA, Reeves BC, et al. Challenges in evaluating surgical innovation. Lancet 2009;374:1097-104.
8 Miller DC, Wei JT, Dunn RL, Hollenbeck BK. Trends in the diffusion of laparoscopic nephrectomy. JAMA 2006;295:2480-2.
9 McCulloch P, Developing appropriate methodology for the study of surgical techniques. J R Soc Med 2009;102:51-5.
10 Ioannidis JP, Haidich AB, Pappa M, Pantazis N, Kokori SI, Tektonidou MG, et al. Comparison of evidence of treatment effects in randomized and nonrandomized studies. JAMA 2001;286:821-30.
11 Tsai TT, Trimarchi S, Nienaber CA. Acute aortic dissection: perspectives from the International Registry of Acute Aortic Dissection (IRAD). Eur J Vasc Endovasc Surg 2009;37:149-59.
12 Hall BL, Richards K, Ingraham A, Ko CY. New approaches to the National Surgical Quality Improvement Program: the American College of Surgeons experience. Am J Surg 2009;198(5 suppl):S56-62.
13 Hagan PG, Nienaber CA, Isselbacher EM, Bruckman D, Karavite DJ, Russman PL, et al. The International Registry of Acute Aortic Dissection (IRAD): new insights into an old disease. JAMA 2000;283:897-903.
14 Dindo D, Demartines N, Clavien PA. Classification of surgical complications: a new proposal with evaluation in a cohort of 6336 patients and results of a survey. Ann Surg 2004;240:205-13.
15 Vickers AJ, Savage CJ, Hruza M, Tuerk I, Koenig P, Martínez-Piñeiro L, et al. The surgical learning curve for laparoscopic radical prostatectomy: a retrospective cohort study. Lancet Oncol 2009;10:475-80.

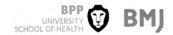

16   Lilford RJ, Braunholtz DA, Greenhalgh R, Edwards SJ. Trials and
     fast changing technologies: the case for tracker studies. *BMJ*
     2000;320:43-6.

17   Cook JA, Ramsay CR, Fayers P. Statistical evaluation of learning curve
     effects in surgical trials. *Clin Trials* 2004;1:421-7.

18   Novick RJ, Fox SA, Kiaii BB, Stitt LW, Rayman R, Kodera K, et al.
     Analysis of the learning curve in telerobotic, beating heart coronary
     artery bypass grafting: a 90 patient experience. *Ann Thorac Surg*
     2003;76:749-53.

19   Degiuli M, Sasako M, Ponti A, Calvo F. Survival results of a multicentre
     phase II study to evaluate D2 gastrectomy for gastric cancer. *Br J
     Cancer* 2004;90:1727-32.

20   Arnold DM, Burns KE, Adhikari NK, Kho ME, Meade MO, Cook DJ. The
     design and interpretation of pilot trials in clinical research in critical
     care. *Crit Care Med* 2009;37(1 suppl):S69-74.

21   Smith GC, Pell JP. Parachute use to prevent death and major trauma
     related to gravitational challenge: systematic review of randomised
     controlled trials. *BMJ* 2003;327:1459-61.

22   Glasziou P, Chalmers I, Rawlins M, McCulloch P. When are randomised
     trials unnecessary? Picking signal from noise. *BMJ* 2007;334:349-51.

23   Black N. Complementarity comes of age. *Transplantation*
     2008;86:28-29.

24   Robbins RC, Barlow CW, Oyer PE, Hunt SA, Miller JL, Reitz BA, et al.
     Thirty years of cardiac transplantation at Stanford University. *J Thorac
     Cardiovasc Surg* 1999;117:939-51.

25   Starzl TE, Klintmalm GB, Porter KA, Iwatsuki S, Schröter GP. Liver
     transplantation with use of cyclosporin A and prednisone. *N Engl J
     Med* 1981;305:266-9.

26   Rawlins M. De testimonio: on the evidence for decisions about the
     use of therapeutic interventions. *Lancet* 2008;372:2152-61.

27   Shadish WR, Cook TD, Campbell DT. Experimental and
     quasiexperimental designs for generalized causal inference. Houghton
     Mifflin, 2002.

28   Hu JC, Gu X, Lipsitz SR, Barry MJ, D'Amico AV, Weinberg AC, et al.
     Comparative effectiveness of minimally invasive vs open radical
     prostatectomy. *JAMA* 2009;302:1557-64.

29   Hultgren HN, Pfeifer JF, Angell W, Lipton MJ, Bilisoly J. Unstable angina:
     comparison of medical and surgical management. *Am J Cardiol*
     1977;39:734-40.

30   Attwood SE, Hill AD, Mealy K, Stephens RB. Prospective comparison
     of laparoscopic versus open cholecystectomy. *Ann R Coll Surg Engl*
     1992;74:397-400.

31   Nicholl J. Case-mix adjustment in nonrandomised observational
     evaluations: the constant risk fallacy. *J Epidemiol Community Health*
     2007;61:1010-3.

32   Heinze G, Jüni P. An overview of the objectives of and the approaches
     to propensity score analyses. *Eur Heart J* 2011;32:1704-8.

33   Johnson ML, Crown W, Martin BC, Dormuth CR, Siebert U. Good
     research practices for comparative effectiveness research: analytic
     methods to improve causal inference from nonrandomized studies
     of treatment effects using secondary data sources: the ISPOR good
     research practices for retrospective database analysis task force
     report—part III. *Value Health* 2009;12:1062-73.

34   Maciejewski ML, Livingston EH, Smith VA, et al. Survival among high-
     risk patients after bariatric surgery. *JAMA* 2011;305:2419-26.

35   Deeks JJ, Dinnes J, D'Amico R, Sowden AJ, Sakarovitch C, Song F, et
     al. Evaluating non-randomised intervention studies. *Health Technol
     Assess* 2003;7:iii-x, 1-173.

36   Shikata S, Nakayama T, Noguchi Y, et al. Comparison of effects in
     randomized controlled trials with observational studies in digestive
     surgery. *Ann Surg* 2006;244:668-76.

37   Matowe LK, Leister CA, Crivera C, Korth-Bradley JM. Interrupted time
     series analysis in clinical research. *Ann Pharmacother* 2003;37:1110-6.

38   Rutledge R, Fakhry SM, Baker CC, Meyer AA. The impact of
     laparoscopic cholecystectomy on the management and outcome of
     biliary tract disease in North Carolina: a statewide, population-based,
     time-series analysis. *J Am Coll Surg* 1996;183:31-45.

39   Marshall G, Shroyer AL, Grover FL, Hammermeister KE Time series
     monitors of outcomes. A new dimension for measuring quality of
     care. *Med Care* 1998;36:348-56.

40   Sun P, Chang J, Zhang J, Kahler KH. Evolutionary cost analysis of
     valsartan initiation among patients with hypertension: a time series
     approach. *J Med Econ* 2012;15:8-18.

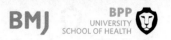

The Ottawa Statement on the ethical design and conduct of cluster randomised trials: précis for researchers and research ethics committees

Monica Taljaard, scientist, assistant professor[1] [2], Charles Weijer, professor[3] [4],
Jeremy M Grimshaw, senior scientist[5], professor[6],
Martin P Eccles, professor of clinical effectiveness[7], the Ottawa Ethics of Cluster Randomised Trials Consensus Group

[1]Ottawa Hospital Research Institute, Clinical Epidemiology Program, Ottawa Hospital, 1053 Carling Avenue, ASB2-004, Ottawa, ON, K1Y 4E9, Canada

[2]Department of Epidemiology and Community Medicine, University of Ottawa, Ottawa, ON, Canada

[3]Rotman Institute of Philosophy, Department of Philosophy, Western University, London, ON, Canada

[4]Departments of Medicine and of Epidemiology and Biostatistics, University of Western Ontario, London, ON, Canada

[5]Ottawa Hospital Research Institute, Clinical Epidemiology Program, Centre for Practice-Changing Research, The Ottawa Hospital, Ottawa, ON, Canada

[6]Department of Medicine, University of Ottawa, Ottawa, ON, Canada

[7]Institute of Health and Society, Newcastle University, Newcastle upon Tyne, UK

Correspondence to: M Taljaard
mtaljaard@ohri.ca

Cite this as: BMJ 2013;346:f2838

http://www.bmj.com/content/346/bmj.f2838

ABSTRACT

Cluster randomised trials have unique features that complicate the application of standard ethics guidelines for research. The Ottawa Statement on the ethical design and conduct of cluster randomised trials was developed to provide detailed guidance to researchers, research ethics committees, regulators, and sponsors as they seek to fulfil their respective roles. This article describes the development of the Ottawa Statement and outlines key implications for researchers and research ethics committees.

Introduction

An increasing number of studies in health system, public health, and knowledge translation research are using randomised controlled designs.[1] Examples are studies of changes in healthcare policies across a region, mass media health promotion campaigns, and training of health professionals with the view to improving the quality of patient care. For these types of interventions, which are naturally administered at the group level, cluster randomisation may be the only feasible choice. In a cluster randomised trial, the unit of allocation is an intact social unit or group (for example, a medical practice, community, worksite, or school), whereas the unit of outcome measurement is individuals within the group (for example, a patient, citizen, employee, or student).[2] [3] Even if the intervention is to be administered at the individual level, such as vitamin supplementation or patient leaflets, cluster randomisation may nevertheless be selected for either scientific reasons, such as avoidance of experimental contamination, or practical reasons.

Cluster randomised trials raise specific methodological and ethical issues. Although there is no shortage of guidance for handling the methodological issues,[4] [5] [6] little guidance exists for dealing with the ethical issues.[7] [8] [9] [10] Ethical issues arise because standard research ethics guidelines are not well attuned to the distinctive characteristics of cluster randomised trials. Most notably, cluster randomised trials may have differing units of allocation (for example, hospitals), intervention (for example, health professionals), and outcome measurement (for example, patients) within a single study. This complicates identification of those who ought to be considered as research participants and thus who are entitled to ethical and regulatory protections. Cluster level interventions and randomisation of clusters before identification of individual cluster members cause difficulties in seeking informed consent. Furthermore, cluster randomised trials often concern diverse social groups, communities, or organisations as the units of allocation, but the moral status of such groups, as well as the identification and authority of those who can morally speak on their behalf, are unclear. Because cluster randomised trials may have consequences for groups as well as for individuals, the assessments of benefits and harms are more challenging in such trials. In addition, protecting vulnerable participants in cluster randomised trials may require special consideration as their presence within clusters may go unnoticed, whereas risks to them may be amplified as a result of cluster membership.

The supplementary file presents a summary of the characteristics of cluster randomised trials and examples of the ethical challenges they raise. The absence of specific ethics guidelines for cluster randomised trials has led to considerable variability in the conduct and review of such trials[11] and to serious shortcomings in their reporting.[12] [13]

Aims

The Ottawa Statement[14] aims to provide guidance for researchers and research ethics committees primarily, and for policy makers, journal editors, and potential study participants, on the ethical design and conduct of cluster randomised trials in health research. It supplements national and international ethics guidelines to take into account the unique characteristics of cluster randomised trials. The statement should be interpreted in light of the laws and regulations of the country or countries in which the cluster randomised trial is conducted and other applicable international standards.

KEY POINTS

- Cluster randomised trials have many characteristics that complicate the application of standard research ethics guidelines; however, until recently there have been no comprehensive ethics guidelines specific to cluster randomised trials
- The Ottawa Statement aims to provide researchers and research ethics committees with detailed guidance on the ethical design, conduct, and review of cluster randomised trials
- The Ottawa Statement sets out 15 recommendations addressing the justification of the cluster randomised design, the need for ethics review, the identification of research participants, obtaining informed consent, the role of gatekeepers in protecting group interests, the assessment of benefits and harms, and the protection of vulnerable participants

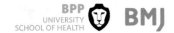

Development

The research team, comprising 15 investigators from Canada, the United Kingdom, and the United States (see supplementary file), was funded by the Canadian Institutes of Health Research in 2007. The goal of the project was to develop well grounded, international ethics guidelines for cluster randomised trials.[15] It was designed as a mixed methods project consisting of parallel empirical and ethical streams culminating in a consensus process. A series of empirical studies was designed to identify ethical problems arising in cluster randomised trials, elicit the views and experiences of investigators conducting these types of trials, and study the ethical review process of cluster randomised trials.[16 11] Based on the experience of the research team members and results of the empirical studies, the research team identified six ethical questions considered unique to cluster randomised trials.[17] The team conducted an in-depth ethical analysis of the identified issues and published the results as a series of articles in an open access journal.[18 19 20 21]

In year 5 of the project, the research team convened a multidisciplinary expert panel consisting of six members of the team and 13 external members (ethicists, experienced cluster trial investigators, consumer representatives, research ethics committee members, policy makers, representatives from funding agencies, and journal editors). A consensus conference was held in Ottawa, Canada, during November 2011 (video available at www.rotman. uwo.ca/resources/video-audio/cluster-randomized-trials-international-consensus-conference/). A detailed description of the consensus process is provided elsewhere.[12] A writing group produced a first draft of the guidelines, which the group circulated to the expert panel and then edited in response to their comments. In February 2012, the writing group posted the revised document on the project's website for public comment. It then edited the document in response to the received comments. The final draft was approved by all members of the expert panel in June 2012 and the full length Ottawa Statement was published in November 2012.[12]

Implications

The Ottawa Statement sets out 15 recommendations, each with a detailed commentary. Recommendations address the justification of the cluster randomised trial design, research ethics review, the identification of research participants, informed consent, the role and authority of gatekeepers, the evaluation of benefits and harms, and the protection of vulnerable participants. The table presents the recommendations for each of these ethical issues in the form of a checklist that may be used by researchers when designing their studies and when applying to research ethics committees. Equally, research ethics committees may consider the recommendations as a tool to help them judge the attributes of cluster randomised trials submitted to them. We recommend that researchers include discussion of each of the main ethical issues in their study protocols. The table may then be appended to their ethics application to direct the attention of the research ethics committee to the guidance and how the ethical issues have been dealt with in the study protocol.Here we outline key implications of the Ottawa Statement for researchers and research ethics committees.

Justifying the cluster randomised design

A cluster randomised trial is more complex to design and conduct and statistically inefficient than an individually randomised trial, and is vulnerable to multiple sources of biases. For these reasons, researchers should clearly justify their choice of cluster rather than individual randomisation (recommendation 1). Acceptable reasons include the evaluation of a cluster level intervention or group effects of an intervention; the need to avoid experimental contamination, reduce costs, enhance compliance, or secure cooperation of investigators; and administrative convenience. Researchers should not adopt this design in a veiled attempt to sidestep the requirements for informed consent.

Research ethics committee review

Research may be defined as a systematic investigation designed to produce generalisable knowledge.[22] Most cluster randomised trials in health research, including those evaluating knowledge translation, quality improvement, and public health interventions, meet this definition.[15] According to national and international research ethics guidelines, the trials must therefore be reviewed by a research ethics committee (recommendation 2). An expedited review may be appropriate if a cluster randomised trial poses a low risk to research participants and does not involve vulnerable participants.

Identifying research participants

Because cluster randomised trials may have differing units of allocation, intervention, and outcome measurement, determining which cluster members ought to be considered as research participants can be difficult. Yet appropriate identification of research participants is necessary for applying ethical and regulatory protections.[17] Recommendation 3 provides a definition and criteria for identifying research participants. Any cluster member who is the recipient or the direct target of a study intervention (including the control condition), with whom researchers interact for study purposes or about whom identifiable private information is collected, is a research participant. Figure 1 summarises the identification of research participants in cluster randomised trials.

The Ottawa Statement has three main implications for the identification of research participants. Firstly, researchers should clearly identify the research participants in the study protocol and other documents submitted for review by the research ethics committee. Secondly, in the case of a cluster level intervention, cluster members who are directly targeted by the intervention ought to be considered research participants. Thirdly, health professionals who are targeted by a knowledge translation intervention ought to be considered research participants; however, their patients are not research participants unless they are otherwise intervened upon or interacted with or their identifiable private information is collected for study purposes.

Obtaining informed consent

Informed consent procedures are complicated in cluster randomised trials for several reasons, including interventions administered at the cluster level, large cluster size, and randomisation of clusters before identification of individual research participants.[18] Figure 2 summarises the guidelines in the Ottawa Statement with respect to informed consent.

The Ottawa Statement has three main implications with respect to informed consent. Firstly, where possible, research participants (or their proxy decision makers) are required to provide informed consent, but not cluster members who are

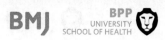

Table Ottawa Statement summary checklist for use in ethics applications, indicating page number in study protocol where an ethical issue is being addressed

	Ethical issue	Recommendation	Page No
1	Justifying the cluster randomised design	Researchers should provide a clear rationale for the use of the cluster randomised design and adopt statistical methods appropriate for this design	
2	Research ethics committee review	Researchers must submit a cluster randomised trial involving human research participants for approval by a research ethics committee before commencing	
3	Identifying research participants	Researchers should clearly identify the research participants in cluster randomised trials. A research participant can be identified as an individual whose interests may be affected as a result of study interventions or data collection procedures—that is, an individual who is the intended recipient of an experimental (or control) intervention; or who is the direct target of an experimental (or control) manipulation of his or her environment; or with whom an investigator interacts for the purpose of collecting data about that individual; or about whom an investigator obtains identifiable private information for the purpose of collecting data about that individual. Unless one or more of these criteria is met, an individual is not a research participant	
4	Obtaining informed consent	Researchers must obtain informed consent from human research participants in a cluster randomised trial, unless a waiver of consent is granted by a research ethics committee under specific circumstances	
5		When participants' informed consent is required, but recruitment of participants is not possible before randomisation of clusters, researchers must seek participants' consent for trial enrollment as soon as possible after cluster randomisation—that is, as soon as the potential participant has been identified, but before the participant has undergone any study interventions or data collection procedures	
6		A research ethics committee may approve a waiver or alteration of consent requirements when the research is not feasible without a waiver or alteration of consent, and the study interventions and data collection procedures pose no more than minimal risk	
7		Researchers must obtain informed consent from professionals or other service providers who are research participants unless conditions for a waiver or alteration of consent are met	
8	Gatekeepers	Gatekeepers should not provide proxy consent on behalf of individuals in their cluster	
9		When a cluster randomised trial may substantially affect cluster or organisational interests, and a gatekeeper possesses the legitimate authority to make decisions on the cluster or organisation's behalf, the researcher should obtain the gatekeeper's permission to enrol the cluster or organisation in the trial. Such permission does not replace the need for the informed consent of research participants	
10		When cluster randomised trial interventions may substantially affect cluster interests, researchers should seek to protect cluster interests through cluster consultation to inform study design, conduct, and reporting. Where relevant, gatekeepers can often facilitate such a consultation	
11	Assessing benefits and harms	The researcher must ensure that the study intervention is adequately justified. The benefits and harms of the study intervention must be consistent with competent practice in the field of study relevant to the cluster randomised trial	
12		Researchers must adequately justify the choice of the control condition. When the control arm is usual practice or no treatment, individuals in the control arm must not be deprived of effective care or programmes to which they would have access, were there no trial	
13		Researchers must ensure that data collection procedures are adequately justified. The risks of data collection procedures must be minimised consistent with sound design and stand in reasonable relation to the knowledge to be gained	
14	Protecting vulnerable participants	Clusters may contain vulnerable participants. In these circumstances, researchers and research ethics committees must consider whether additional protections are needed	
15		When individual informed consent is required, and there are individuals who may be less able to choose participation freely because of their position in a cluster or organisational hierarchy, research ethics committees should pay special attention to recruitment, privacy, and consent procedures for those participants	

Source: Weijer et al, 2012.[14]

not research participants (recommendation 4). Secondly, as far as possible researchers should identify participants and seek their consent before cluster randomisation. If consent is not feasible before randomisation, it should be sought as soon as possible after cluster randomisation and before any study interventions or data collection procedures (recommendation 5). Researchers should be aware that post-randomisation consent can introduce selection biases and should consider adopting design strategies that minimise the risk of bias.[23] Thirdly, because of the challenges in seeking informed consent in cluster randomised trials, waivers and alterations of consent procedures are especially important in this design. Waivers or alterations of consent can be justified only when the study would not otherwise be feasible and when the risks involved are minimal (recommendations 6 and 7). Minimal risk refers to the incremental risks associated with study participation and requires that such risks be consistent with the risks of daily life.[24] A waiver of consent means that the research ethics committee removes the requirement to obtain informed consent, whereas an alteration of consent means that the committee permits changes to or removal of some of the standard elements of disclosure in the informed consent—for example, to maintain blinding in the case of a behavioural intervention.

Gatekeepers

Gatekeepers are individuals or bodies (such as a school principal or municipal council) who may be called on to protect the interests of organisations or communities that are the setting for a cluster randomised trial. Researchers have historically relied on "cluster gatekeepers" to perform a variety of roles, including providing permission for clusters to participate in a cluster randomised trial and providing consent on behalf of individuals in a cluster—for example, for a cluster level intervention.[19]

The Ottawa Statement has three main implications with respect to gatekeepers. Firstly, gatekeepers may not legitimately provide proxy consent on behalf of individuals in a cluster (recommendation 8). Legitimate proxy consent requires that the potential participants be incapable of making their own decisions and that the decision makers be well acquainted with the potential participants' values and beliefs. Secondly, researchers should obtain permission from a gatekeeper to enrol a cluster or organisation in a cluster randomised trial when a trial poses important implications for group interests and a gatekeeper exists who has the legitimate authority to provide permission (recommendation 9). Thirdly, gatekeepers may help protect group interests in a cluster randomised trial by facilitating consultation between researchers and cluster members about the study (recommendation 10). Modes of consultation may include communication with communities through various media channels, open public forums, or meetings with opinion leaders.

Assessing benefits and harms

In individually randomised trials of clinical interventions, the analysis of benefits and harms usually focuses on the potential effects on individual patients, with the trial being justified on the basis of clinical equipoise. In a cluster randomised trial, however, study interventions may affect not only individuals but also clusters, organisations, and communities.[16] Moreover, cluster randomised trials may investigate the effectiveness of public health, health systems, and knowledge translation interventions. The justification of a cluster randomised trial must therefore take interests of a broader range of stakeholders into account.

The Ottawa Statement has three main implications when assessing benefits and harms in cluster randomised trials. Firstly, researchers must ensure that study interventions are consistent with competent practice in the specialty of study relevant to the cluster randomised trial, such as medical practice, public health, or health policy (recommendation 11). Random assignment is justified when the relevant community of experts (for example, public health practitioners, health policy researchers) is uncertain as to the better performing practice. Secondly, researchers must adequately justify the choice of the control condition; generally, at a minimum the control condition is usual care within the study context (recommendation 12). Researchers and research ethics committees may consider whether the control arm should receive a minimal level of intervention or "augmented" care, but they should be aware that this may bias the estimate of the intervention effect towards the null and may reduce generalisability. Thirdly, the risks associated with data collection procedures must be minimised and stand in reasonable relation to the knowledge to be gained (recommendation 13).

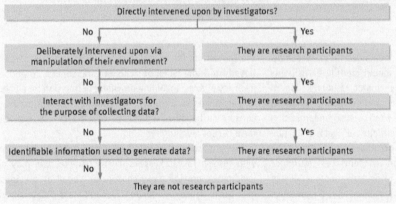

Fig 1 Identification of research participants in cluster randomised trials

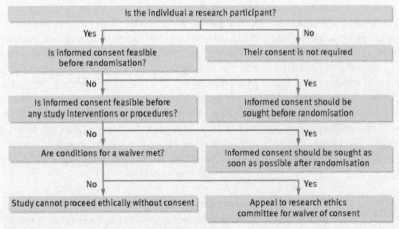

Fig 2 Informed consent procedures in cluster randomised trials

Protecting vulnerable participants

Vulnerable research participants include children, incapable adults (that is, those unable to provide informed consent), those at undue risk of harm as a result of study participation, and those in subordinate positions within social or organisational structures. Cluster randomised trials are commonly conducted in organisations, and research participants may include professionals, service staff, or employees whose position within the cluster makes them less able to express a free choice about trial participation.

The Ottawa Statement has two main implications with respect to vulnerable participants in cluster randomised trials. Firstly, special care must be taken to identify and protect vulnerable participants as their presence may not be apparent within clusters (recommendation 14). Secondly, discussions about informed consent with research participants in cluster randomised trials involving organisations should limit the potential for coercive influence from employers or cluster leaders, and such discussions should include career related risks, including risks from detection of negligence or incompetence (recommendation 15).

Discussion

The use of cluster randomisation in health research is increasing.[1] The substantial methodological differences between cluster randomised trials and conventional randomised trials pose serious challenges to the current conceptual framework for research ethics. Researchers need direction on these ethical challenges to guide the optimal design and conduct of cluster randomised trials. Research ethics committees may be unfamiliar with this increasingly important study methodology and, in the absence of formal guidelines for cluster randomised trials, they may fail to consider all the relevant ethical issues generated by a study protocol, resulting in inadequate protection of participants. Variable interpretation of ethical requirements for cluster randomised trials may lead to problems initiating multijurisdictional trials and to unequal treatment of participants in different jurisdictions.

Until the publication of The Ottawa Statement on the ethical design and conduct of cluster randomised trials,[12] there were no comprehensive ethics guidelines specific to this type of study design. The aim of the Ottawa Statement is to address this shortcoming by providing researchers and research ethics committees with recommendations for cluster randomised trials that meet international ethical standards in health research. Written by scientists and ethicists, the Ottawa Statement rests on a strong foundation of empirical study and detailed ethical analysis; it is the result of a transparent and robust consensus process. Applications of cluster randomised trials are found in a wide variety of sectors, including education, criminology, and welfare. Although the development of the Ottawa Statement has focused on applications in health research, it provides a starting point for future extension to these sectors.

The Ottawa Ethics of Cluster Randomised Trials Consensus Group includes: Fernando Althabe (Institute for Clinical Effectiveness and Health Policy, Buenos Aires, Argentina), Ariella Binik (Rotman Institute of Philosophy, London, Canada), Judith Belle Brown (Western University, London, Canada), Robert Boruch (University of Pennsylvania, Philadelphia, USA), Jamie C Brehaut (Ottawa Hospital Research Institute, Ottawa, Canada), Shazia Chaudhry (University of Ottawa, Ottawa, Canada), Allan Donner (Western University, London, Canada), Geneviève Dubois-Flynn (Canadian Institutes for Health Research Ethics Office, Ottawa, Canada), Martin P Eccles (Newcastle University, Newcastle upon Tyne, UK), Sarah Edwards (University

BMJ   BPP
UNIVERSITY
SCHOOL OF HEALTH

College London, London, UK), Diana Elbourne (London School of Hygiene and Tropical Medicine, London, UK), Sandra Eldridge (Queen Mary University of London, London, UK), David Forster (Western IRB, Olympia, USA), Antonio Gallo (Rotman Institute of Philosophy, London, Canada), Jeremy M Grimshaw (Ottawa Hospital Research Institute, Ottawa, Canada), Catarina Kiefe, University of Massachusetts Medical School, Worcester, USA), Jonathan Kimmelman (McGill University, Montreal, Canada), Melody Lin (Office for Human Research Protections, Rockville, USA), Elizabeth Loder (Harvard Medical School, Boston, USA), Kathleen Lohr (RTI International, Research Triangle Park, USA), Andrew D McRae (University of Calgary, Calgary, Canada), Eileen S Naughton (Rhode Island House of Representatives, Providence, USA), Rex J Polson (Solihull Hospital, Solihull, UK), Raphael Saginur (Ottawa Hospital, Civic Campus, Ottawa, CanadaAbha Saxena (World Health Organization, Geneva, Switzerland), Julie Spence (St Michael's Hospital, Toronto, Canada), Monica Taljaard (Ottawa Hospital Research Institute, Ottawa, Canada), Charles Weijer (Rotman Institute of Philosophy, London, Canada), Angela White (Rotman Institute of Philosophy, London, Canada), Gerald White (Health Council of Canada, Toronto, Canada), and Merrick Zwarenstein (Institute for Clinical Evaluative Studies, Toronto, Canada). Members of the Ottawa Ethics of Cluster Randomised Trials Consensus Group participated in this project as individuals and not as representatives of their employers. Authorship does not imply the approval of this document by the authors' employers or other organisations with which they are affiliated.

Contributors: MT, CW, and JMG are co-principal investigators of the project. MPE is a co-investigator of the project and chaired the consensus process. CW led the ethical analysis. MT drafted this article and is the guarantor. All authors commented on drafts of this article and revised the article critically for important intellectual content. All authors approved the final version.

Funding: This study was funded by the Canadian Institutes of Health Research (operating grants MOP85066 and MOP89790). The funding agency had no role in the study design, collection, analysis or interpretation of data, writing of the manuscript, or decision to submit the manuscript for publication. JMG and CW both hold Canada research chairs.

Competing interests: All authors have completed the ICMJE uniform disclosure form at www.icmje.org/coi_disclosure.pdf (available on request from the corresponding author) and declare: no support from any organisation for the submitted work; no financial relationships with any organisations which might have an interest in the submitted work in the previous three years; no other relationships or activities which could appear to have influenced the submitted work.

Ethical approval: This study was approved by the Ottawa Hospital research ethics board.

Provenance and peer review: Not commissioned; externally peer reviewed.

1   Bland MJ. Cluster randomised trials in the medical literature: two bibliometric surveys. *BMC Med Res Methodol* 2004;4:21. doi:10.1186/1471-2288-4-21.
2   Donner A, Klar N. Design and analysis of cluster randomization trials in health research. Arnold, 2000.
3   Eldridge S, Kerry S. A practical guide to cluster randomised trials in health services research. Chichester, Wiley, 2012.
4   Campbell MK, Mollison J, Steen N, Grimshaw JM, Eccles M. Analysis of cluster randomized trials in primary care: a practical approach. *Fam Pract* 2000;17:192-6.
5   Donner A, Klar N. Statistical considerations in the design and analysis of community intervention trials. *J Clin Epidemiol* 1996;49:435-9.
6   Hayes RJ, Bennett S. Simple sample size calculation for cluster-randomized trials. *Int J Epidemiol* 1999;28:319-26.
7   Edwards SJL, Braunholtz DA, Lilford RJ, Stevens AJ. Ethical issues in the design and conduct of cluster randomised controlled trials. *BMJ* 1999;318:1407-9.
8   Hutton JL. Are distinctive ethical principles required for cluster randomized controlled trials? *Stat Med* 2001;20:473-88.
9   Klar N, Donner A. Ethical challenges posed by cluster randomization. Wiley Encyclopedia of Clinical Trials. doi:10.1002/9780471462422. eoct050.
10 Hayes RJ, Moulton LH. Cluster randomised trials. Chapman and Hall/CRC, 2009.
11 Chaudhry SH, Brehaut JC, Grimshaw JM, Weijer C, Boruch R, Donner A, et al. Challenges in the research ethics review of cluster randomized trials: international survey of investigators. *Clin Trials* 2013;10:257-68.
12 Taljaard M, McRae A, Weijer C, Bennett C, Dixon S, Taleban J, et al. Inadequate reporting of research ethics review and informed consent in cluster randomized trials: review of a representative sample of published trials. *BMJ* 2011;342:d2496.
13 Campbell MK, Piaggio G, Elbourne DR, Altman DG, for the CONSORT Group. CONSORT 2010 statement: extension to cluster randomised trials. *BMJ* 2012;345:e5661.
14 Weijer C, Grimshaw JM, Eccles MP, McRae AD, White A, Brehaut JC, et al. The Ottawa Statement on the ethical design and conduct of cluster randomized trials. *PloS Med* 2012;9:e1001346.
15 Taljaard M, Weijer C, Grimshaw J, Belle Brown J, Binik A, Boruch R, et al. Study protocol: ethical and policy issues in cluster randomized trials: rationale and design of a mixed methods research study. *Trials* 2009;10:61.
16 McRae AD, Bennett C, Brown JB, Weijer C, Boruch R, Brehaut J, et al. Researchers' perceptions of ethical challenges in cluster randomized trials: a qualitative analysis. *Trials* 2013;14:1.
17 Weijer C, Grimshaw JM, Taljaard M, Binik A, Boruch R, Brehaut JC, et al. Ethical issues posed by cluster randomized trials in health research. *Trials* 2011;12:100.
18 Binik A, Weijer C, McRae AD, Grimshaw JM, Boruch R, Brehaut JC, et al. Does clinical equipoise apply to cluster randomized trials in health research? *Trials* 2011;12:118.
19 McRae AD, Weijer C, Binik A, White A, Grimshaw JM, Boruch R, et al. Who is the research subject in cluster randomized trials? *Trials* 2011;12:183.
20 McRae AD, Weijer C, Binik A, Grimshaw JM, Boruch R, Brehaut JC, et al. When is informed consent required in cluster randomized trials in health research? *Trials* 2011;12:202.
21 Gallo A, Weijer C, White A, Grimshaw JM, Boruch R, Brehaut JC, et al. What is the role and authority of gatekeepers in cluster randomized trials in health research? *Trials* 2012;13:116.
22 Levine RJ. Ethics and regulation of clinical research. Yale University Press, 1988.
23 Eldridge S, Kerry S, Torgerson DJ. Bias in identifying and recruiting participants in cluster randomised trials: what can be done? *BMJ* 2009;339:b4006.
24 Weijer C, Miller PB. When are research risks reasonable in relation to anticipated benefits? *Nat Med* 2004;10:570-3.

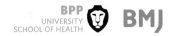

Preferred reporting items for systematic reviews and meta-analyses: the PRISMA statement

David Moher[1] [2], Alessandro Liberati[3] [4], Jennifer Tetzlaff[1], Douglas G Altman[5], for the PRISMA Group

[1]Ottawa Methods Centre, Ottawa Hospital Research Institute, Ottawa, Ontario, Canada

[2]Department of Epidemiology and Community Medicine, Faculty of Medicine, University of Ottawa, Ottawa, Ontario, Canada

[3]Università di Modena e Reggio Emilia, Modena, Italy

[4]Centro Cochrane Italiano, Istituto Ricerche Farmacologiche Mario Negri, Milan, Italy

[5]Centre for Statistics in Medicine, University of Oxford, Oxford, United Kingdom

Correspondence to: dmoher@ohri.ca

Cite this as:
BMJ 2009;338:b2535

DOI: 10.1136/bmj.b2535

http://www.bmj.com/content/339/bmj.b2535

ABSTRACT

David Moher and colleagues introduce PRISMA, an update of the QUOROM guidelines for reporting systematic reviews and meta-analyses

Systematic reviews and meta-analyses have become increasingly important in health care. Clinicians read them to keep up to date with their specialty,[1] [2] and they are often used as a starting point for developing clinical practice guidelines. Granting agencies may require a systematic review to ensure there is justification for further research,[3] and some medical journals are moving in this direction.[4] As with all research, the value of a systematic review depends on what was done, what was found, and the clarity of reporting. As with other publications, the reporting quality of systematic reviews varies, limiting readers' ability to assess the strengths and weaknesses of those reviews.

Several early studies evaluated the quality of review reports. In 1987 Mulrow examined 50 review articles published in four leading medical journals in 1985 and 1986 and found that none met all eight explicit scientific criteria, such as a quality assessment of included studies.[5] In 1987 Sacks and colleagues evaluated the adequacy of reporting of 83 meta-analyses on 23 characteristics in six domains.[6] Reporting was generally poor; between one and 14 characteristics were adequately reported (mean 7.7, standard deviation 2.7). A 1996 update of this study found little improvement.[7]

In 1996, to address the suboptimal reporting of meta-analyses, an international group developed a guidance called the QUOROM statement (QUality Of Reporting Of Meta-analyses), which focused on the reporting of meta-analyses of randomised controlled trials.[8] In this article, we summarise a revision of these guidelines, renamed PRISMA (Preferred Reporting Items for Systematic reviews and Meta-Analyses), which have been updated to address several conceptual and practical advances in the science of systematic reviews (see box).

Terminology

The terminology used to describe a systematic review and meta-analysis has evolved over time. One reason for changing the name from QUOROM to PRISMA was the desire to encompass both systematic reviews and meta-analyses. We have adopted the definitions used by the Cochrane Collaboration.[17] A systematic review is a review of a clearly formulated question that uses systematic and explicit methods to identify, select, and critically appraise relevant research, and to collect and analyse data from the studies that are included in the review. Statistical methods (meta-analysis) may or may not be used to analyse and summarise the results of the included studies. Meta-analysis refers to the use of statistical techniques in a systematic review to integrate the results of included studies.

Developing the PRISMA statement

A three-day meeting was held in Ottawa, Canada, in June 2005 with 29 participants, including review authors, methodologists, clinicians, medical editors, and a consumer. The objective of the Ottawa meeting was to revise and expand the QUOROM checklist and flow diagram as needed.

The executive committee completed the following tasks before the meeting: a systematic review of studies examining the quality of reporting of systematic reviews; a comprehensive literature search to identify methodological and other articles that might inform the meeting, especially in relation to modifying checklist items; and an international survey of review authors, consumers, and groups commissioning or using systematic reviews and meta-analyses (including the International Network of Agencies for Health Technology Assessment and the Guidelines International Network) to ascertain views of QUOROM, including the merits of the existing checklist items. The results of these activities were presented during the meeting and are summarised on the PRISMA website, www.prisma-statement.org/.

Only items deemed essential were retained or added to the checklist. Some additional items are nevertheless desirable, and review authors should include these, if relevant.[18] For example, it is useful to indicate whether the systematic review is an update of a previous review[19] and to describe any changes in procedures from those described in the original protocol.

Shortly after the meeting, a draft of the PRISMA checklist was circulated to the group, including those invited to the meeting but unable to attend. A disposition file was created containing comments and revisions from each respondent, and the checklist was subsequently revised 11 times. The group approved the checklist, flow diagram, and this summary paper.

Although no direct evidence was found to support retaining or adding some items, evidence from other domains was believed to be relevant. For example, item 5 asks authors to provide registration information about the systematic review, including a registration number if available. Although systematic review registration is not yet widely available,[20] [21] the participating journals of the International Committee of Medical Journal Editors[22] now require all clinical trials to be registered in an effort to increase transparency and accountability.[23] Those aspects are also likely to benefit systematic reviewers, possibly reducing the risk of an excessive number of reviews addressing the same question[24] [25] and providing greater transparency when updating systematic reviews.

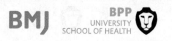

The PRISMA statement

The PRISMA statement consists of a 27 item checklist (table 1) and a four phase flow diagram (figure) (also available as extra items on bmj.com for researchers to download and re-use). The aim of the PRISMA statement is to help authors improve the reporting of systematic reviews and meta-analyses. We have focused on randomised trials, but PRISMA can also be used as a basis for reporting systematic reviews of other types of research, particularly evaluations of interventions. PRISMA may also be useful for critical appraisal of published systematic reviews. However, the

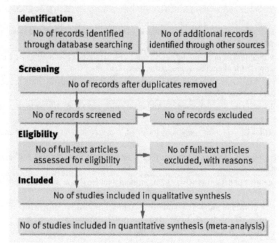

Fig Flow of information through the different phases of a systematic review.

PRISMA checklist is not a quality assessment instrument to gauge the quality of a systematic review.

From QUOROM to PRISMA

The new PRISMA checklist differs in several respects from the QUOROM checklist, and table 2 lists the substantive specific changes. Generally, the PRISMA checklist "decouples" several items present in the QUOROM checklist and, where applicable, several checklist items are linked to improve consistency across the systematic review report.

The flow diagram has also been modified. Before including studies and providing reasons for excluding others, the review team must first search the literature. This search results in records. Once these records have been screened and eligibility criteria applied, a smaller number of articles will remain. The number of included articles might be smaller (or larger) than the number of studies, because articles may report on multiple studies and results from a particular study may be published in several articles. To capture this information, the PRISMA flow diagram now requests information on these phases of the review process.

Endorsement

The PRISMA statement should replace the QUOROM statement for those journals that have endorsed QUOROM. We hope that other journals will support PRISMA; they can do so by registering on the PRISMA website. To emphasise to authors and others the importance of transparent reporting of systematic reviews, we encourage supporting journals to reference the PRISMA statement and include the PRISMA web address in their instructions to authors. We also invite editorial organisations to consider endorsing PRISMA and encourage authors to adhere to its principles.

The PRISMA explanation and elaboration paper

In addition to the PRISMA statement, a supporting explanation and elaboration document has been produced[26] following the style used for other reporting guidelines.[27] [28] [29] The process of completing this document included developing a large database of exemplars to highlight how best to report each checklist item, and identifying a comprehensive evidence base to support the inclusion of each checklist item. The explanation and elaboration document was completed after several face to face meetings and numerous iterations among several meeting participants, after which it was shared with the whole group for additional revisions and final approval. Finally, the group formed a dissemination subcommittee to help disseminate and implement PRISMA.

Discussion

The quality of reporting of systematic reviews is still not optimal.[9 30 31 32 33 34] In a recent review of 300 systematic reviews, few authors reported assessing possible publication bias,[9] even though there is overwhelming evidence for its existence[13] and its impact on the results of systematic reviews.[35] Even when the possibility of publication bias is assessed, there is no guarantee that systematic reviewers have assessed or interpreted it appropriately.[36] Although the absence of reporting such an assessment does not necessarily indicate that it was not done, reporting an assessment of possible publication bias is likely to be a marker of the thoroughness of the conduct of the systematic review.

BOX CONCEPTUAL ISSUES IN THE EVOLUTION FROM QUOROM TO PRISMA

Completing a systematic review is an iterative process

The conduct of a systematic review depends heavily on the scope and quality of included studies: thus systematic reviewers may need to modify their original review protocol during its conduct. Any systematic review reporting guideline should recommend that such changes can be reported and explained without suggesting that they are inappropriate. The PRISMA statement (items 5, 11, 16, and 23) acknowledges this iterative process. Aside from Cochrane reviews, all of which should have a protocol, only about 10% of systematic reviewers report working from a protocol.[9] Without a protocol that is publicly accessible, it is difficult to judge between appropriate and inappropriate modifications.

Conduct and reporting of research are distinct concepts

This distinction is, however, less straightforward for systematic reviews than for assessments of the reporting of an individual study, because the reporting and conduct of systematic reviews are, by nature, closely intertwined. For example, the failure of a systematic review to report the assessment of the risk of bias in included studies may be seen as a marker of poor conduct, given the importance of this activity in the systematic review process.[10]

Study-level versus outcome-level assessment of risk of bias

For studies included in a systematic review, a thorough assessment of the risk of bias requires both a study-level assessment (such as adequacy of allocation concealment) and, for some features, a newer approach called outcome-level assessment. An outcome-level assessment involves evaluating the reliability and validity of the data for each important outcome by determining the methods used to assess them in each individual study.[11] The quality of evidence may differ across outcomes, even within a study, such as between a primary efficacy outcome, which is likely to be carefully and systematically measured, and the assessment of serious harms,[12] which may rely on spontaneous reports by investigators. This information should be reported to allow an explicit assessment of the extent to which an estimate of effect is correct.[11]

Importance of reporting biases

Different types of reporting biases may hamper the conduct and interpretation of systematic reviews. Selective reporting of complete studies (such as publication bias),13 as well as the more recently empirically demonstrated "outcome reporting bias" within individual studies,14 15 should be considered by authors when conducting a systematic review and reporting its results. Although the implications of these biases on the conduct and reporting of systematic reviews themselves are unclear, some research has identified that selective outcome reporting may occur also in the context of systematic reviews.16

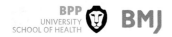

Table 1 Checklist of items to include when reporting a systematic review or meta-analysis

Section/topic	Item No	Checklist item	Reported on page No
Title			
Title	1	Identify the report as a systematic review, meta-analysis, or both	
Abstract			
Structured summary	2	Provide a structured summary including, as applicable, background, objectives, data sources, study eligibility criteria, participants, interventions, study appraisal and synthesis methods, results, limitations, conclusions and implications of key findings, systematic review registration number	
Introduction			
Rationale	3	Describe the rationale for the review in the context of what is already known	
Objectives	4	Provide an explicit statement of questions being addressed with reference to participants, interventions, comparisons, outcomes, and study design (PICOS)	
Methods			
Protocol and registration	5	Indicate if a review protocol exists, if and where it can be accessed (such as web address), and, if available, provide registration information including registration number	
Eligibility criteria	6	Specify study characteristics (such as PICOS, length of follow-up) and report characteristics (such as years considered, language, publication status) used as criteria for eligibility, giving rationale	
Information sources	7	Describe all information sources (such as databases with dates of coverage, contact with study authors to identify additional studies) in the search and date last searched	
Search	8	Present full electronic search strategy for at least one database, including any limits used, such that it could be repeated	
Study selection	9	State the process for selecting studies (that is, screening, eligibility, included in systematic review, and, if applicable, included in the meta-analysis)	
Data collection process	10	Describe method of data extraction from reports (such as piloted forms, independently, in duplicate) and any processes for obtaining and confirming data from investigators	
Data items	11	List and define all variables for which data were sought (such as PICOS, funding sources) and any assumptions and simplifications made	
Risk of bias in individual studies	12	Describe methods used for assessing risk of bias of individual studies (including specification of whether this was done at the study or outcome level), and how this information is to be used in any data synthesis	
Summary measures	13	State the principal summary measures (such as risk ratio, difference in means).	
Synthesis of results	14	Describe the methods of handling data and combining results of studies, if done, including measures of consistency (such as I^2 statistic) for each meta-analysis	
Risk of bias across studies	15	Specify any assessment of risk of bias that may affect the cumulative evidence (such as publication bias, selective reporting within studies)	
Additional analyses	16	Describe methods of additional analyses (such as sensitivity or subgroup analyses, meta-regression), if done, indicating which were pre-specified	
Results			
Study selection	17	Give numbers of studies screened, assessed for eligibility, and included in the review, with reasons for exclusions at each stage, ideally with a flow diagram	
Study characteristics	18	For each study, present characteristics for which data were extracted (such as study size, PICOS, follow-up period) and provide the citations	
Risk of bias within studies	19	Present data on risk of bias of each study and, if available, any outcome-level assessment (see item 12).	
Results of individual studies	20	For all outcomes considered (benefits or harms), present for each study (a) simple summary data for each intervention group and (b) effect estimates and confidence intervals, ideally with a forest plot	
Synthesis of results	21	Present results of each meta-analysis done, including confidence intervals and measures of consistency	
Risk of bias across studies	22	Present results of any assessment of risk of bias across studies (see item 15)	
Additional analysis	23	Give results of additional analyses, if done (such as sensitivity or subgroup analyses, meta-regression) (see item 16)	
Discussion			
Summary of evidence	24	Summarise the main findings including the strength of evidence for each main outcome; consider their relevance to key groups (such as health care providers, users, and policy makers)	
Limitations	25	Discuss limitations at study and outcome level (such as risk of bias), and at review level (such as incomplete retrieval of identified research, reporting bias)	
Conclusions	26	Provide a general interpretation of the results in the context of other evidence, and implications for future research	
Funding			
Funding	27	Describe sources of funding for the systematic review and other support (such as supply of data) and role of funders for the systematic review	

Several approaches have been developed to conduct systematic reviews on a broader array of questions. For example, systematic reviews are now conducted to investigate cost effectiveness,[37] diagnostic[38] or prognostic questions,[39] genetic associations,[40] and policy making.[41] The general concepts and topics covered by PRISMA are relevant to any systematic review, not just those summarising the benefits and harms of a healthcare intervention. However, some modifications of the checklist items or flow diagram will be necessary in particular circumstances. For example, assessing the risk of bias is a key concept, but the items used to assess this in a diagnostic review are likely to focus on issues such as the spectrum of patients and the verification of disease status, which differ from reviews of interventions. The flow diagram will also need adjustments when reporting meta-analysis of individual patient data.[42]

We have developed an explanatory document to increase the usefulness of PRISMA.[26] For each checklist item, this document contains an example of good reporting, a rationale for its inclusion, and supporting evidence, including references, whenever possible. We believe this document will also serve as a useful resource for those

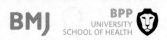

Table 2 Substantive specific changes between the QUOROM checklist and the PRISMA checklist (a tick indicates the presence of the topic in QUOROM or PRISMA)

Section/topic and item	QUOROM	PRISMA	Comment
Abstract	√	√	QUOROM and PRISMA ask authors to report an abstract. However, PRISMA is not specific about format
Introduction:			
Objective		√	This new item (4) addresses the explicit question the review addresses using the PICO reporting system (which describes the participants, interventions, comparisons, and outcome(s) of the systematic review), together with the specification of the type of study design (PICOS); the item is linked to items 6, 11, and 18 of the checklist
Methods:			
Protocol		√	This new item (5) asks authors to report whether the review has a protocol and if so how it can be accessed
Search	√	√	Although reporting the search is present in both QUOROM and PRISMA checklists, PRISMA asks authors to provide a full description of at least one electronic search strategy (item 8). Without such information it is impossible to repeat the authors' search
Assessment of risk of bias in included studies	√	√	Renamed from "quality assessment" in QUOROM. This item (12) is linked to reporting this information in the results (item 19). The new concept of "outcome level" assessment has been introduced
Assessment of risk of bias across studies		√	This new item (15) asks authors to describe any assessments of risk of bias in the review, such as selective reporting within the included studies. This item is linked to reporting this information in the results (item 22)
Discussion	√	√	Although both QUOROM and PRISMA checklists address the discussion section, PRISMA devotes three items (24-26) to the discussion. In PRISMA the main types of limitations are explicitly stated and their discussion required
Funding		√	This new item (27) asks authors to provide information on any sources of funding for the systematic review.

teaching systematic review methodology. We encourage journals to include reference to the explanatory document in their instructions to authors.

Like any evidence based endeavour, PRISMA is a living document. To this end we invite readers to comment on the revised version, particularly the new checklist and flow diagram, through the PRISMA website. We will use such information to inform PRISMA's continued development.

The following people contributed to the PRISMA statement: Doug Altman, Centre for Statistics in Medicine (Oxford); Gerd Antes, University Hospital Freiburg (Freiburg, Germany); David Atkins, Health Services Research and Development Service, Veterans Health Administration (Washington DC, USA); Virginia Barbour, *PLoS Medicine* (Cambridge, UK); Nick Barrowman, Children's Hospital of Eastern Ontario (Ottawa, Canada); Jesse A. Berlin, Johnson & Johnson Pharmaceutical Research and Development (Titusville NJ, USA); Jocalyn Clark, *PLoS Medicine* (at the time of writing, *BMJ*, London); Mike Clarke, UK Cochrane Centre (Oxford) and School of Nursing and Midwifery, Trinity College (Dublin, Ireland); Deborah Cook, Departments of Medicine, Clinical Epidemiology and Biostatistics, McMaster University (Hamilton, Canada); Roberto D'Amico, Università di Modena e Reggio Emilia (Modena, Italy) and Centro Cochrane Italiano, Istituto Ricerche Farmacologiche Mario Negri (Milan, Italy); Jonathan J Deeks, University of Birmingham (Birmingham); P J Devereaux, Departments of Medicine, Clinical Epidemiology and Biostatistics, McMaster University; Kay Dickersin, Johns Hopkins Bloomberg School of Public Health (Baltimore MD, USA); Matthias Egger, Department of Social and Preventive Medicine, University of Bern (Bern, Switzerland); Edzard Ernst, Peninsula Medical School (Exeter, UK); Peter C Gøtzsche, Nordic Cochrane Centre (Copenhagen, Denmark); Jeremy Grimshaw, Ottawa Hospital Research Institute (Ottawa, Canada); Gordon Guyatt, Departments of Medicine, Clinical Epidemiology and Biostatistics, McMaster University; Julian Higgins, MRC Biostatistics Unit (Cambridge, UK); John P A Ioannidis, University of Ioannina Campus (Ioannina, Greece); Jos Kleijnen, Kleijnen Systematic Reviews (York, UK) and School for Public Health and Primary Care (CAPHRI), University of Maastricht (Maastricht, Netherlands); Tom Lang, Tom Lang Communications and Training (Davis CA, USA); Alessandro Liberati, Università di Modena e Reggio Emilia, and Centro Cochrane Italiano, Istituto Ricerche Farmacologiche Mario Negri; Nicola Magrini, NHS Centre for the Evaluation of the Effectiveness of Health Care—CeVEAS (Modena, Italy); David McNamee, *Lancet* (London, UK); Lorenzo Moja, Centro Cochrane Italiano, Istituto Ricerche Farmacologiche Mario Negri; David Moher, Ottawa Methods Centre, Ottawa Hospital Research Institute (Ottawa, Canada); Cynthia Mulrow, *Annals of Internal Medicine* (Philadelphia PA, USA); Maryann Napoli, Center for Medical Consumers (New York, USA); Andy Oxman, Norwegian Health Services Research Centre (Oslo, Norway); Ba' Pham, Toronto Health Economics and Technology Assessment Collaborative (Toronto, Canada) (at the time of first meeting of the group, GlaxoSmithKline Canada, Mississauga, Ontario); Drummond Rennie, University of California San Francisco (San Francisco CA, USA); Margaret Sampson, Children's Hospital of Eastern Ontario (Ottawa, Canada); Kenneth F Schulz, Family Health International (Durham NC, USA); Paul G Shekelle, Southern California Evidence Based Practice Center (Santa Monica CA, USA); Jennifer Tetzlaff, Ottawa Methods Centre, Ottawa Hospital Research Institute; David Tovey, *Cochrane Library*, Cochrane Collaboration (Oxford, UK) (at the time of first meeting of the group, *BMJ*, London); Peter Tugwell, Institute of Population Health, University of Ottawa (Ottawa, Canada).

Author contributions: ICMJE criteria for authorship read and met—DM. Agree with the recommendations—DM, AL, JT, DGA. Wrote the first draft of the paper—DM, AL, DGA. Contributed to the writing of the paper—DM, AL, JT, DGA. Participated in regular conference calls, identified the participants, secured funds, planned the meeting, participated in the meeting, and drafted the manuscript—DM, AL, DGA. Participated in identifying the evidence base for PRISMA, refining the checklist, and drafting the manuscript—JT.

Funding: PRISMA was funded by the Canadian Institutes of Health Research; Università di Modena e Reggio Emilia, Italy; Cancer Research UK; Clinical Evidence BMJ Knowledge; the Cochrane Collaboration; and GlaxoSmithKline, Canada. AL is funded, in part, through grants of the Italian Ministry of University (COFIN-PRIN 2002 prot 2002061749 and COFIN-PRIN 2006 prot 2006062298). DGA is funded by Cancer Research UK. DM is funded by a University of Ottawa Research Chair. None of the sponsors had any involvement in the planning, execution, or writing of the PRISMA documents. No funder played a role in drafting this manuscript.

Competing interests: None declared.

Provenance and peer review: Not commissioned; externally peer reviewed.

In order to encourage dissemination of the PRISMA statement, this article is freely accessible on bmj.com and will also be published in *PLoS Medicine*, *Annals of Internal Medicine*, *Journal of Clinical Epidemiology*, and *Open Medicine*. The authors jointly hold the copyright of this article. For details on further use, see the PRISMA website (www.prisma-statement.org/).

1 Oxman AD, Cook DJ, Guyatt GH. Users' guides to the medical literature. VI. How to use an overview. Evidence-Based Medicine Working Group. *JAMA* 1994;272:1367-71.

2 Swingler GH, Volmink J, Ioannidis JP. Number of published systematic reviews and global burden of disease: database analysis. *BMJ* 2003;327:1083-4.

3 Canadian Institutes of Health Research. Randomized controlled trials registration/application checklist (12/2006). 2006. www.cihr-irsc.gc.ca/e/documents/rct_reg_e.pdf (accessed 19 May 2009).

4 Young C, Horton R. Putting clinical trials into context. *Lancet* 2005;366:107.

5 Mulrow CD. The medical review article: state of the science. *Ann Intern Med* 1987;106:485-8.

6 Sacks HS, Berrier J, Reitman D, Ancona-Berk VA, Chalmers TC. Meta-analysis of randomized controlled trials. *N Engl J Med* 1987;316:450-5.

7 Sacks HS, Reitman D, Pagano D, Kupelnick B. Meta-analysis: an update. *Mt Sinai J Med* 1996;63:216-24.

8 Moher D, Cook DJ, Eastwood S, Olkin I, Rennie D, Stroup DF, for the QUOROM group. Improving the quality of reporting of meta-analysis of randomized controlled trials: The QUOROM statement. *Lancet* 1999;354:1896-1900.

9 Moher D, Tetzlaff J, Tricco AC, Sampson M, Altman DG. Epidemiology and reporting characteristics of systematic reviews. *PLoS Med* 2007;4:e78, doi:10.1371/journal.pmed.0040078.

10 Moja LP, Telaro E, D'Amico R, Moschetti I, Coe L, Liberati A. Assessment of methodological quality of primary studies by systematic reviews: results of the metaquality cross sectional study. *BMJ* 2005;330:1053-5.

11 Guyatt GH, Oxman AD, Vist GE, Kunz R, Falck-Ytter Y, Alonso-Coello P, et al, for the GRADE Working Group. GRADE: an emerging consensus on rating quality of evidence and strength of recommendations. *BMJ* 2008;336:924-6.

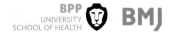

12   Schunemann HJ, Jaeschke R, Cook DJ, Bria WF, El-Solh AA, et al, for the ATS Documents Development and Implementation Committee. An official ATS statement: grading the quality of evidence and strength of recommendations in ATS guidelines and recommendations. *Am J Respir Crit Care Med* 2006;174:605-14.

13   Dickersin K. Publication bias: recognizing the problem, understanding its origins and scope, and preventing harm. In: Rothstein HR, Sutton AJ, Borenstein M, eds. *Publication bias in meta-analysis—prevention, assessment and adjustments* . Chichester: John Wiley, 2005:11-33.

14   Chan AW, Hrobjartsson A, Haahr MT, Gøtzsche PC, Altman DG. Empirical evidence for selective reporting of outcomes in randomized trials: comparison of protocols to published articles. *JAMA* 2004;291:2457-65.

15   Chan AW, Krleza-Jeric K, Schmid I, Altman DG. Outcome reporting bias in randomized trials funded by the Canadian Institutes of Health Research. *CMAJ* 2004;171:735-40.

16   Silagy CA, Middleton P, Hopewell S. Publishing protocols of systematic reviews: comparing what was done to what was planned. *JAMA* 2002;287:2831-4.

17   Green S, Higgins J, eds. Glossary. *Cochrane Handbook for Systematic Reviews of Interventions 4.2.5* [updated May 2005]. www.cochrane. org/resources/glossary.htm (accessed 19 May 2009).

18   Strech D, Tilburt J. Value judgments in the analysis and synthesis of evidence. *J Clin Epidemiol* 2008;61:521-4.

19   Moher D, Tsertsvadze A. Systematic reviews: when is an update an update? *Lancet* 2006;367:881-3.

20   University of York. Centre for Reviews and Dissemination, 2009. www. york.ac.uk/inst/crd/ (accessed 19 May 2009).

21   Joanna Briggs Institute. Protocols & work in progress, 2008. www. joannabriggs.edu.au/pubs/systematic_reviews_prot.php (accessed 19 May 2009).

22   De Angelis C, Drazan JM, Frizelle FA, Haug C, Hoey J, et al, for the International Committee Medical Journal Editors. Clinical trial registration: a statement from the International Committee of Medical Journal Editors. *CMAJ* 2004;171:606-7.

23   Whittington CJ, Kendall T, Fonagy P, Cottrell D, Cotgrove A, et al. Selective serotonin reuptake inhibitors in childhood depression: systematic review of published versus unpublished data. *Lancet* 2004;363:1341-5.

24   Bagshaw SM, McAlister FA, Manns BJ, Ghali WA. Acetylcysteine in the prevention of contrast-induced nephropathy: a case study of the pitfalls in the evolution of evidence. *Arch Intern Med* 2006;166:161-6.

25   Biondi-Zoccai GG, Lotrionte M, Abbate A, Testa L, Remigi E, et al. Compliance with QUOROM and quality of reporting of overlapping meta-analyses on the role of acetylcysteine in the prevention of contrast associated nephropathy: case study. *BMJ* 2006;332:202-9.

26   Liberati A, Altman DG, Tetzlaff J, Mulrow C, Gøtzsche PC, Ioannidis JPA, et al, for the PRISMA Group. The PRISMA statement for reporting systematic reviews and meta-analyses of studies that evaluate healthcare interventions: explanation and elaboration. *BMJ* 2009;339:b2700.

27   Altman DG, Schulz KR, Moher D, Egger M, Davidoff F, et al, for the CONSORT group. The revised CONSORT statement for reporting randomized trials: explanation and elaboration. *Ann Intern Med* 2001;134:663-94.

28   Bossuyt PM, Reitsma JB, Bruns DE, Gatsonis CA, Glasziou PP, et al, for the STARD group. Towards complete and accurate reporting of studies of diagnostic accuracy: the STARD explanation and elaboration. *Ann Intern Med* 2003;138:W1-12.

29   Vandenbroucke JP, von Elm E, Altman DG, Gøtzsche PC, Mulrow CD, et al, for the STROBE initiative. Strengthening the reporting of observational studies in epidemiology (STROBE): explanation and elaboration. *Ann Intern Med* 2007;147:W163-94.

30   Bhandari M, Morrow F, Kulkarni AV, Tornetta P. Meta-analyses in orthopaedic surgery: a systematic review of their methodologies. *J Bone Joint Surg Am* 2001;83-A:15-24.

31   Kelly KD, Travers A, Dorgan M, Slater L, Rowe BH. Evaluating the quality of systematic reviews in the emergency medicine literature. *Ann Emerg Med* 2001;38:518-26.

32   Richards D. The quality of systematic reviews in dentistry. *Evid Based Dent* 2004;5:17.

33   Choi PT, Halpern SH, Malik N, Jadad AR, Tramer MR, et al. Examining the evidence in anesthesia literature: a critical appraisal of systematic reviews. *Anesth Analg* 2001;92:700-9.

34   Delaney A, Bagshaw SM, Ferland A, Manns B, Laupland KB. A systematic evaluation of the quality of meta-analyses in the critical care literature. *Crit Care* 2005;9:R575-82.

35   Sutton AJ. Evidence concerning the consequences of publication and related biases. In: Rothstein HR, Sutton AJ, Borenstein M, eds. *Publication bias in meta-analysis—prevention, assessment and adjustments*. Chichester: John Wiley, 2005:175-92.

36   Lau J, Ioannidis JP, Terrin N, Schmid CH, Olkin I. The case of the misleading funnel plot. *BMJ* 2006;333:597-600.

37   Ladabaum U, Chopra CL, Huang G, Scheiman JM, Chernew ME, et al. Aspirin as an adjunct to screening for prevention of sporadic colorectal cancer: a cost-effectiveness analysis. *Ann Intern Med* 2001;135:769-81.

38   Deeks JJ. Systematic reviews in health care: systematic reviews of evaluations of diagnostic and screening tests. *BMJ* 2001;323:157-62.

39   Altman DG. Systematic reviews of evaluations of prognostic variables. *BMJ* 2001;323:224-8.

40   Ioannidis JP, Ntzani EE, Trikalinos TA, Contopoulos-Ioannidis DG. Replication validity of genetic association studies. *Nat Genet* 2001;29:306-9.

41   Lavis J, Davies H, Oxman A, Denis J, Golden-Biddle K, et al. Towards systematic reviews that inform health care management and policy-making. *J Health Serv Res Policy* 2005;10:35-48.

42   Stewart LA, Clarke MJ. Practical methodology of meta-analyses (overviews) using updated individual patient data. Cochrane Working Group. *Stat Med* 1995;14:2057-79.

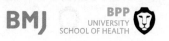

Evaluating policy and service interventions: framework to guide selection and interpretation of study end points

Richard J Lilford, professor of clinical epidemiology[1], Peter J Chilton, research associate[1], Karla Hemming, senior research fellow[1], Alan J Girling, senior research fellow[1], Celia A Taylor, senior lecturer[2], Paul Barach, visiting professor[3]

[1]Public Health, Epidemiology and Biostatistics, University of Birmingham, Edgbaston, West Midlands B15 2TT

[2]Department of Clinical and Experimental Medicine, University of Birmingham

[3]Patient Safety Centre, University Medical Centre Utrecht, PO Box 85500, 3508 GA Utrecht, Netherlands

Correspondence to: R J Lilford
r.j.lilford@bham.ac.uk

Cite this as:
BMJ 2010;341:c4413

DOI: 10.1136/bmj.c4413

http://www.bmj.com/content/341/bmj.c4413

ABSTRACT

The effect of many cost effective policy and service interventions cannot be detected at the level of the patient. This new framework could help improve the design (especially choice of primary end point) and interpretation of evaluative studies

There is broad consensus that clinical interventions should be compared in randomised trials measuring patient outcomes. However, methods for evaluation of policy and service interventions remain contested. This article considers one aspect of this complex issue—the selection of the primary end point (the end point used to determine sample size and given most weight in the interpretation of results). Other methodological issues affecting the design and interpretation of evaluations of policy and service interventions (including attributing effect to cause) have been discussed elsewhere,[1] and we will consider them only in so far as they may affect selection of the primary end point. Our analysis begins with a classification of policy and service interventions based on an extended version of Donabedian's causal chain.

Avedis Donabedian conceptualised a chain linking structure, process, and outcome.[2] The classification we propose is based on a model in which the process level is divided into three further categories or sublevels as shown in fig 1.[3] [4] [5] Starting closest to the patient these are: clinical processes (encompassing treatments such as drugs, devices, procedures, "talking" therapy, complementary therapy, and so on); targeted processes (those aimed at improving particular clinical processes, such as training in the use of a device, or a decision rule built into a computer system); and generic processes (for example, the human resource policy adopted by an organisation).

When an intervention is designed, the level at which it first affects this chain should be clarified along with its plausible effects.[6] There are four levels in the extended Donabedian chain at which it is possible to intervene. Starting closest to the patient these levels are:

- Clinical interventions—for example, use of clot busting drugs for thrombotic stroke
- Targeted (near patient) service interventions—for example, establishing a service to expedite administration of clot busting drugs for thrombotic stroke
- Generic (far patient) service interventions—for example, providing yearly appraisal for all staff)
- Structural (policy) interventions—for example, improving the nurse to patient ratio.

Evaluation of targeted and generic service interventions tends to be lumped together under portmanteau terms such as management research, service delivery and organisational research, or health services research. We shall show that, from a methodological point of view, generic service interventions have more in common with policy interventions than with targeted service interventions.

Assessing targeted service interventions

Clinical interventions have only one downstream level at which evidence of effectiveness may be observed—patient outcomes. However, the effect of targeted service interventions can be assessed by using either clinical processes (for example, the proportion of eligible patients who receive timely thrombolysis) or outcomes (proportion of patients who recover from stroke). Selecting a sample of sufficient size to measure changes in end points at both levels risks wasteful redundancy. If there is an established link between a clinical process and its corresponding outcome, then the least expensive option should be chosen. Costs are a function of sample size (number of participating centres and the number of patients sampled in each centre) and the cost of making each observation.

Changes in clinical outcome (such as mortality or infection rates) can never be bigger than changes in the clinical error rates on which they depend and are usually much smaller; it is rare for the risk of an adverse outcome to be wholly attributable to clinical error. Thus detection of changes in outcome requires larger, often much larger, samples than those needed to detect changes in the corresponding clinical process. Figure 2 compares the sample sizes for a standard simple before and after study designed to measure the effect of an intervention on compliance with a clinical standard (process study) and the risk of an associated adverse clinical outcome (outcome study). The sample size for the outcome study is about four times that of the corresponding process study even when the adverse outcome is 100% attributable to clinical error (that is, can arise only if the corresponding error has occurred, as in reaction to incompatible blood transfusion). The outcome study must be more than 200 times larger than the process study if the attributable risk is 25% (as in failure to carry out timely thrombolysis therapy after thrombotic stroke).

The actual numbers will depend on baseline rates of compliance and adverse outcome and the study design—cluster studies with contemporaneous controls will require even larger samples than simple randomised controlled trials.[7] [8] [9] However, study costs are a function not only of the number of observations, but also of the costs of making each observation. Although outcomes such as mortality and rates of infection are often collected routinely, health service systems seldom carry the numerator (process failure) and denominator (opportunity for failure) data required to calculate the rates of process failure.[10] This information usually has to be obtained from case notes, bespoke data collection forms, or direct observation.[11] The cost of reliably measuring failures in clinical process may therefore be considerable, depending on the process concerned.[12]

There are thus competing forces at work when evaluating a targeted service   tension with the greater number of cases that must be sampled to measure outcomes with commensurate precision. The greater the size (in absolute terms) of the hypothesised effect on outcome and the more expensive the collection of data, the stronger the argument to rely on outcome measures. For example, an

influential study to assess the effect of targeted processes to reduce infection associated with central venous lines used bloodstream infections as the outcome measure.[13] Real time observations to assess the clinical processes that reduce infection risk would have been very expensive and substantial effects on the outcome (infection rates) were expected (and observed).[13] However, as the signal (change in outcome due to intervention) diminishes in relation to the noise (changes in outcome due to uncontrolled sources of variation), a study based on process measurement will become more cost effective. Such was the case in Landrigan's study of the effects of fatigue on the quality of care delivered by medical interns in the intensive care unit, which used direct observation of clinical processes.[14]

The above argument is predicated on circumstances where the clinical process of interest is a valid surrogate (proxy) for the relevant patient outcome. If this is not the case, the link between clinical process and patient outcome should first be confirmed—for example, with a double masked randomised controlled trial. However, the link between process and outcome cannot always be established robustly, particularly when the outcome in question is the egregious consequences of a rare clinical process failure—for example, transfusion of incompatible blood, oesophageal intubation, or intrathecal injection of vincristine.

Policy and generic service interventions

Generic service interventions have the potential to affect targeted processes, clinical processes, and outcomes. They may affect clinical processes directly through targeted processes or indirectly through intervening variables (such as morale, sickness absence, culture, knowledge, time spent with each patient).[15] Figure 1 shows that there are four downstream levels at which effects may be observed. Policy interventions (such as building a new hospital, increasing reimbursement rates, or conferring 'teaching' status) can exert effects through five levels.

Narrow versus diffuse effects

The further to the left an intervention is applied in the causal chain, the greater the number of downstream processes that may be affected. For example, a targeted service intervention to prevent misconnection of oxygen delivery pipes in the operating theatre would affect only one clinical process—gas delivery. This is a narrow or tightly coupled effect. However, a generic service intervention (such as applying a system of appraisal for all staff) or a policy level intervention (such as increasing resources to improve the nurse to patient ratio) has the potential to affect myriad clinical processes across an institution—a diffuse effect. Nevertheless, these clinical processes converge on outcomes that can be placed in a limited number of discrete, identifiable groups (fig 3). For example, mortality, quality of life scores, patient satisfaction, and numbers treated are the final common pathway for hundreds, if not thousands, of individual clinical processes.

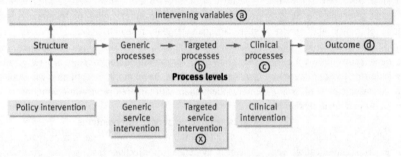

Fig 1 Modified Donabedian causal chain. Interventions at structural (policy) and generic service level can achieve effects through intervening variables (such as motivation and staff-patient contact time) further down the chain. For example, an intervention at (x) produces effects (good or bad) downstream at (a), (b), (c), and (d)

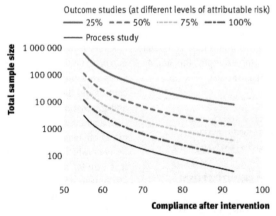

Fig 2 Specimen sample sizes for a simple before and after study or randomised controlled trial to detect an improvement in process compliance using process and outcome measures with conventional 80% power and 5% significance levels. At baseline, compliance with the targeted clinical process is 50% and the rate of adverse outcomes is 20%. The numbers needed for the outcome study increase as the percentage of outcome risk attributable to non-compliance with the process (attributable risk) decreases

Selecting end points

It may be impractical to measure the effectiveness of an intervention with diffuse effects by observing hundreds or thousands of downstream clinical processes. For example, Donchin and colleagues estimated that patients in intensive care units experience a mean of 178 clinical processes every day.[16] The hospital as a whole would provide many thousands of actions that could be affected by a change such as the ratio of doctors to patients. The effect on each clinical process might be so small that impracticably large

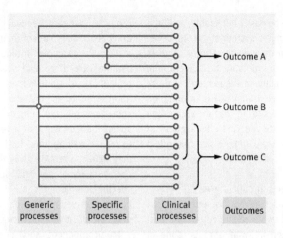

Fig 3 Interventions applied towards the far left of an extended causal chain can have diffuse effects on clinical processes but show convergence on outcomes

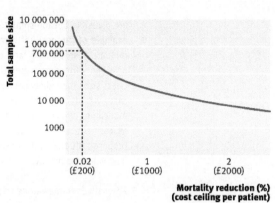

Fig 4 Sample size needed in a simple before and after study to detect reductions in mortality from a baseline of 10% using conventional 80% power and 5% significance levels. Each death avoided is assumed to result in a patient benefit of five years of healthy life, which is used to generate the cost ceiling for the intervention using a threshold of £20 000 per quality adjusted life year

samples would be required to avoid high probabilities (or the near certainty) of false null results. It would be logistically taxing to enumerate compliance with all (or even a meaningful proportion) of the clinical processes that might be affected downstream.

Given limited resources, it makes more sense to study the effects of such interventions by using outcomes on which large numbers of processes converge and which often can be measured at low cost. Patient outcomes also encapsulate the net effect of generic interventions on many individual processes, some of which may be negatively affected; various positive and negative effects are consolidated among a limited number of outcomes. However, this still leaves the question of the sample size required to investigate such outcomes.

Cost effectiveness of studies using patient level end points

Rare problems and small effect sizes

Sometimes it is not cost effective, or logistically possible, to measure the effectiveness of policy or service delivery interventions at either the clinical process or patient outcome level. In the case of targeted service delivery this situation arises in the context of rare incidents, such as transfusion of incompatible blood. For policy and generic service interventions the problem arises when the cost of the intervention is small relative to the magnitude of the plausible effect size.

In England and Wales, the National Institute for Health and Clinical Excellence (NICE), uses a heuristic maximum of between £20 000 (€24 000; $31 000) and £30 000 for a healthy life year.[17] An intervention, such as a clinical computing system costing £10m a year might sound expensive, but would average £200 per patient in a hospital with 50 000 admissions a year. It would have to save only around two lives (of five years mean duration in good health) per 1000 patients admitted to be cost effective. In such a case the cost per life year saved is calculated as:

$$\text{Cost per life year saved} = \frac{\text{Cost per patient} \times \text{No of patients}}{\text{No of lives saved} \times \text{Mean duration of a saved life}}$$

$$= \frac{£200 \times 1000}{2 \times 5} = £20\,000$$

(Discounting at 3.5% a year increases the cost slightly to £21 500, which is still below the NICE threshold.)

If we assume a baseline mortality of 10%, as in fig 4, 700 000 patients would be required to detect a change of two lives per 1000 patients in a simple before and after study. Furthermore it would be risky to make a causal inference on so small a difference (0.2 percentage points) from a study with no contemporaneous controls—moderate biases are more important when measured differences are small. Even more patients would be needed to conduct a more valid cluster study incorporating a sample of control hospitals that were not exposed to the intervention.

The above estimate of effect (two lives saved per 1000 admissions) is not unduly pessimistic. Many people were shocked to hear that one in 400 inpatients died as a result of deficiencies in their care in the famous Harvard malpractice study.[18] If this could be halved (arguably an ambitious target), hospital mortality would decline by 0.125 percentage points (that is, by less than 2 in 1000). Figure 4 shows that the rate at which sample size increases as a function of diminishing effect size is such that detecting plausible effects of an intervention on death rates may be not only expensive but logistically impossible.[19]

Modelling cost effectiveness

Sometimes it is difficult to decide whether it would be cost effective to carry out a study that is powered on the basis of patient level outcomes (clinical processes or patient outcomes). In many cases, the decision can be informed by modelling effectiveness and cost effectiveness.

Effectiveness is modelled by mapping the pathway through which the intervention is hypothesised to work. For instance, the plausible effectiveness of a programme of rotating ward closures was based on observed rates of bacterial recontamination of cleaned surfaces and expert opinion on plausible consequences for hospital acquired infection.[20]

Cost effectiveness can then be modelled by offsetting putative benefits against costs. A simple "back of the envelope" calculation may be informative.[21] In the above example, it turned out that the costs (particularly opportunity costs of ward closure) were not commensurate with even the most optimistic expert estimates of benefit.[20] More often simple models will reveal an "inconvenient truth" that cost effective effects on patient level outcomes are plausible but too small to be easily detectable, as in the example of the hospital computer system above. However, in some cases, particularly in developing country contexts or when outcomes other than mortality are salient, the effect sizes may allow cost effective measurement. In these cases we advocate the use of bayesian value of information modelling, which has been used in health technology assessment,[22] [23] [24] to investigate the cost effectiveness of proposed studies and to select the sample size that offers best value for money.

Alternatives to measuring effects at patient level

Situations where interventions may be cost effective, but are unlikely to produce measurable effects on patient level end points, raise the question of what is to be done in such cases. We take our cue from Walter Charleton, who in the 17th century, said that, "The 'reasonable man' will not require demonstrations or proofs that 'exclude all dubiosity, and compel assent,' but will accept moral and physical proofs that are the best that may be gained."[25] When end points at the patient level are unlikely to be sensitive to the intervention, evaluations must turn on theory and on other types of observation. These observations will be components of a general framework for all evaluations[1] [3] [4] [6] [15] and include outcome of previous studies of similar interventions, results of preimplementation evaluations (alpha testing),[3] and observations upstream in the extended Donabedian chain. These upstream observations include the fidelity of uptake of the intervention[15] and effects on intervening variables,[15] and could require the synthesis of quantitative and qualitative data.[4]

Clinical processes and outcome can still be measured even though they are not the primary end point. This will determine whether the observed effect is larger than expected and make data available for possible future systematic reviews. However, these patient level end points will not be used to determine sample size. Care must also be taken not to misinterpret a null result (no evidence of effect) as evidence of no effect since studies that examine upstream effects are not powered to detect changes in patient level end points.

Consider for example, the effect of an online intervention package to improve the general knowledge and attitudes of all clinical staff towards patient safety. Here it might be asking too much to expect to observe improvements in clinical processes or outcomes. The finding that staff attended the educational events, reported positively on the experience, and had improved scores on a reliable patient safety culture tool, may provide sufficient encouragement to continue the intervention, especially against a theoretical backdrop linking culture to safety built up from studies in many healthcare and non-healthcare settings.[26]

Discussion

The classification we propose is based on a deconstructed version of Donabedian's process level and does not readily map on to other classifications such as safety versus quality. The insight derived from the distinction between targeted and generic service interventions relates to the downstream effects of the intervention—targeted interventions with narrow effects versus policy and generic service interventions with diffuse effects.

We have described the causal chain as operating from left to right. However, bidirectional flow is plausible in some circumstances—a specific targeted intervention may produce upstream (feedback) effects. These in turn could bring about downstream changes (feed-forward) in a related activity. For example, introduction of clinical guidelines for asthma care in general practice may sensitise clinicians to the use of guidelines in general and thereby produce improvements in diabetes care.[27] This phenomenon is sometimes referred to as the "halo effect,"[28] although such spillover effects can also be harmful—for example, incentives to reduce waiting times for investigation of possible cancer may deflect attention away from other important diseases. The corollary of potential spillover effects when targeted specific interventions are implemented is that the end points observed may need to be widened to take account of plausible positive and negative effects in related practices.

Multicomponent service interventions may comprise both generic and targeted elements, such as the Health Foundation's Safer Patients Initiative, which seeks to promote leadership and safety culture while strengthening specific practices by, for instance, promulgating evidence based guidelines.[29] An evaluation in this case should consist of observations relevant to both generic elements (such as measurements of effects on intervening variables and perhaps outcomes) and the specific components (where targeted clinical processes are relevant).

Surrogate outcomes and publication bias

The observation that it may not be possible to detect worthwhile effects at the patient level inevitably places greater weight on upstream end points, which become surrogates for patient outcomes. It is therefore important to increase our knowledge of the construct validity of intervening variables such as culture, leadership, and morale. The literature correlating these upstream variables with patient outcomes is likely to be distorted by publication bias—an endemic problem in clinical epidemiology.[30] Thus authors should consider using statistical methods that provide evidence of publication bias, as in a recent study of service interventions to improve acute paediatric care in developing countries.[31] Readers should be aware that when they encounter strongly positive results, they may be sampling the most optimistic tail of a distribution of results, most of which is hidden from view. Suspicion that one may be dealing with an example of publication bias must be heightened if the results exceed the most optimistic of prior expectations.

Bayesian methods and decision analysis

Our analysis has been couched, for the most part, in terms of primary end points and statistical methods for hypothesis testing. This is partly because these conform to contemporary methodological models in quantitative research and partly because they provide convenient "handles" to help describe the underlying ideas. These ideas would still be relevant under alternative models where, for example, multiple end points were weighted on a sliding scale according to their contribution to a decision analysis model.[32] Likewise, the relation between interventions and effect size would be relevant when considering cost effective sample sizes in a bayesian model.[24] Here changes in credible limits and the centre of updated probability distributions would be the relevant considerations, but it would still be necessary to think carefully about sample size, cost effectiveness, and the distinction between interventions with diffuse and narrow effects. Bayesian methods can also be used to integrate multiple observations (including qualitative data).[33]

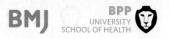

Representational nature of the model

The model we present is more fine grained than Donabedian's original framework, but even so the process level could have been divided into more than three sublevels; the underlying construct is, in all likelihood, a continuum. The nub of the argument is that the further to the left an intervention is applied, the greater the number of downstream end points that might be affected until a point is reached where there are too many to capture at the clinical processes level. However, the effect on patient outcomes might be too small to detect, yet worth while, given an intervention that is inexpensive on a per patient basis. Our framework, like all representational models, is a "simplified view of the world to help us think about complex issues, but is not a true representation of the complexity itself."[34] Just as the map of the London underground does not need to represent the geography of track and stations literally to be helpful, so we hope that our model will be useful for those who navigate the complex intellectual terrain of policy and service evaluation.

We thank Peter Lilford, Tim Hofer, Mary Dixon-Woods, Mohammed Mohammed, Cor Kalkman, Jon Nicholl, William Runciman, and Tim Cole for helpful comments.

Contributors RJL conceived the idea for the paper and drafted the initial core manuscript; KH, CAT, and AJG performed statistical analysis; PJC, KH, CAT, AJG, and PB contributed sections and critically reviewed and commented on the document. RJL is the guarantor.

Funding: National Institute for Health Research Collaborations for Leadership in Applied Health Research and Care for Birmingham and Black Country; European Union FP7 handover project: improving the continuity of patient care through identification and implementation of novel patient handoff processes in Europe; and the MATCH programme (EPSRC Grant GR/S29874/01). The views expressed in this work do not necessarily reflect those of the funders.

Competing interest: All authors have completed the unified competing interest form at www.icmje.org/coi_disclosure.pdf (available on request from the corresponding author) and declare financial support for the submitted work from the National Institute for Health Research Collaborations for Leadership in Applied Health Research and Care for Birmingham and Black Country, European Union FP7 handover project: improving the continuity of patient care through identification and implementation of novel patient handoff processes in Europe, and the MATCH programme; no financial relationships with commercial entities that might have an interest in the submitted work; no spouses, partners, or children with relationships with commercial entities that might have an interest in the submitted work; and no non-financial interests that may be relevant to the submitted work.

Provenance and peer review: Not commissioned; externally peer reviewed.

1   Brown C, Hofer T, Johal A, Thomson R, Nicholl J, Franklin BD, et al. An epistemology of patient safety research: a framework for study design and interpretation. Part 2. Study design. *Qual Saf Health Care* 2008;17:163-9.
2   Donabedian A. Explorations in quality assessment and monitoring. Health Administration Press, 1980.
3   Brown C, Hofer T, Johal A, Thomson R, Nicholl J, Franklin BD, et al. An epistemology of patient safety research: a framework for study design and interpretation. Part 1. Conceptualising and developing interventions. *Qual Saf Health Care* 2008;17:158-62.
4   Brown C, Lilford R. Evaluating service delivery interventions to enhance patient safety. *BMJ* 2008;337:a2764.
5   Cornford T, Doukidis GI, Forster D. Experience with a structure, process and outcome framework for evaluating an information system. *Omega-Int J Manage S* 1994;22:491-504.
6   Craig P, Dieppe P, Macintyre S, Mitchie S, Nazareth I, Petticrew M. Developing and evaluating complex interventions: the new Medical Research Council guidance. *BMJ* 2008;337:a1655.
7   Edwards SJ, Braunholtz DA, Lilford RJ, Stevens AJ. Ethical issues in the design and conduct of cluster randomised controlled trials. *BMJ* 1999;318:1407-9.
8   Murray DM, Blitstein JL. Methods to reduce the impact of intraclass correlation in group-randomized trials. *Eval Rev* 2003;27:79-103.
9   Campbell MK, Fayers PM, Grimshaw JM. Determinants of the intracluster correlation coefficient in cluster randomized trials: the case of implementation research. *Clin Trials* 2005;2:99-107.
10 Lilford RJ, Mohammed MA, Braunholtz D, Hofer TP. The measurement of active errors: methodological issues. *Qual Saf Health Care* 2003;12(suppl 2):ii8-12S.
11 Barach P, Johnson JK, Ahmad A, Galvan C, Bognar A, Duncan R, et al. A prospective observational study of human factors, adverse events, and patient outcomes in surgery for pediatric cardiac disease. *J Thorac Cardiovasc Surg* 2008;136:1422-8.
12 Lilford R, Edwards A, Girling A, Hofer T, Di Tanna GL, Petty J, et al. Inter-rater reliability of case-note audit: a systematic review. *J Health Serv Res Policy* 2007;12:173-80.
13 Pronovost P, Needham D, Berenholtz S, Sinopoli D, Chu H, Cosgrove S, et al. An intervention to decrease catheter-related bloodstream infections in the ICU. *N Engl J Med* 2006;355:2725-32.
14 Landrigan CP, Rothschild JM, Cronin JW, Kaushal R, Burdick E, Katz JT, et al. Effect of reducing interns' work hours on serious medical errors in intensive care units. *N Engl J Med* 2004;351:1838-48.
15 Brown C, Hofer T, Johal A, Thomson R, Nicholl J, Franklin BD, et al. An epistemology of patient safety research: a framework for study design and interpretation. Part 3. End points and measurement. *Qual Saf Health Care* 2008;17:170-7.
16 Donchin Y, Gopher D, Olin M, Badihi Y, Biesky M, Sprung CL, et al. A look into the nature and causes of human errors in the intensive care unit. *Crit Care Med* 1995;23:294-300.
17 National Institute for Health and Clinical Excellence. Guide to the methods of technology appraisal. Reference No515. NICE, 2008.
18 Brennan TA, Leape LL, Laird NM, Hebert L, Localio AR, Lawthers AG, et al. Incidence of adverse events and negligence in hospitalized patients. Results of the Harvard Medical Practice Study I. *N Engl J Med* 1991;324:370-6.
19 Runciman WB. Qualitative versus quantitative research—balancing cost, yield and feasibility. *Anaesth Intens Care* 1993;21:502-5.
20 Brown CA, Lilford RJ. Should the UK government's deep cleaning of hospitals programme have been evaluated? *J Infect Prevent* 2009;10:143-7.
21 Cosh E, Girling A, Lilford R, McAteer H, Young T. Investing in new medical technologies: a decision framework. *J Commerc Biotechnol* 2007;13:263-7.
22 Conti S, Claxton K. Dimensions of design space: a decision-theoretic approach to optimal research design. *Med Decis Making* 2009;29:643-60.
23 Girling AJ, Freeman G, Gordon JP, Poole-Wilson P, Scott DA, Lilford RJ. Modeling payback from research into the efficacy of left-ventricular assist devices as destination therapy. *Int J Technol Assess Health Care* 2007;23:269-77.
24 Girling AJ, Lilford RJ, Braunholtz DA, Gillett WR. Sample-size calculations for trials that inform individual treatment decisions: a 'true-choice' approach. *Clin Trials* 2007;4:15-24.
25 Charleton W. The immortality of the human soul, demonstrated by the light of nature: In two dialogues. Printed by W Wilson for H Herringman, 1657.
26 Vohra PD, Johnson JK, Daugherty CK, Wen M, Barach P. Housestaff and medical student attitudes toward medical errors and adverse events. *Jt Comm J Qual Patient Saf* 2007;33:493-501.
27 Eccles M, Clapp Z, Grimshaw J, Adams PC, Higgins B, Purves I, et al. North of England evidence based guidelines development project: methods of guideline development. *BMJ* 1996;312:760-2.
28 Francis J, Perlin JB. Improving performance through knowledge translation in the Veterans Health Administration. *J Contin Educ Health Prof* 2006;26:63-71.
29 Shirley PJ. The Safer Patients Initiative: the UK experience of attempting to improve safe clinical care. *Med J Aust* 2008;189:414.
30 Dickersin K, Min YI. Publication bias: the problem that won't go away. *Ann N Y Acad Sci* 1993;703:135-46.
31 Sazawal S, Black RE, Pneumonia Case Management Trials Group. Effect of pneumonia case management on mortality in neonates, infants, and preschool children: a meta-analysis of community-based trials. *Lancet Infect Dis* 2003;3:547-56.
32 Thornton JG, Lilford RJ. Decision analysis for medical managers. *BMJ* 1995;310:791-4.
33 Lilford RJ, Braunholtz D. Reconciling the quantitative and qualitative traditions: the Bayesian approach. *Public Money and Management* 2003;23:203-8
34 Demeulemeester J, Diebolt C. Letters: economic reasoning. *Economist* 2009;392:15.

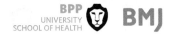

Publication guidelines for quality improvement studies in health care: evolution of the SQUIRE project

Frank Davidoff, executive editor[1], Paul Batalden, director[2], David Stevens, director of the quality literature programme[2], Greg Ogrinc, associate director of the quality literature programme[2 3], Susan E Mooney, medical director for quality improvement[2 4], for the SQUIRE development group

[1]Institute for Healthcare Improvement, 143 Garden Street, Wethersfield, CT 06109, USA

[2]Center for Leadership and Improvement, Dartmouth Institute for Health Policy and Clinical Practice Lebanon, NH 03766, USA

[3]White River Junction VA Hospital, White River Junction, VT 05009-0001, USA

[4]Alice Peck Day Memorial Hospital, Lebanon, NH 03766, USA

Correspondence to: F Davidoff
fdavidoff@cox.net

Cite this as:
BMJ 2009;338:a3152

DOI: 10.113/bmj.f3012

http://www.bmj.com/content/338/bmj.a3152

ABSTRACT

In 2005 we published draft guidelines for reporting studies of quality improvement, as the initial step in a consensus process for development of a more definitive version. The current article contains the revised version, which we refer to as standards for quality improvement reporting excellence (SQUIRE). This narrative progress report summarises the special features of improvement that are reflected in SQUIRE, and describes major differences between SQUIRE and the initial draft guidelines. It also briefly describes the guideline development process; considers the limitations of and unresolved questions about SQUIRE; describes ancillary supporting documents and alternative versions under development; and discusses plans for dissemination, testing, and further development of SQUIRE.

Introduction

A great deal of meaningful and effective work is now done in clinical settings to improve the quality and safety of care. Unfortunately, relatively little of that work is reported in the biomedical literature, and much of what is published could be described more effectively. Failure to publish is potentially a serious barrier to the development of improvement science, because public sharing of concepts, methods, and findings is essential to the progress of all scientific work, both theoretical and applied. To help strengthen the evidence base for improvement in health care, we proposed draft guidelines for reporting planned original studies of improvement interventions in 2005.[1] Our aims were to stimulate the publication of high calibre improvement studies and to increase the completeness, accuracy, and transparency of published reports of that work.

Our initial draft guidelines were based largely on personal experience with improvement work, and were intended only as an initial step toward creation of recognised publication standards. We have now refined and extended that draft, and present here the resulting revised version, which we refer to as the standards for quality improvement reporting excellence or SQUIRE (table). In this narrative progress report, we describe the special features of quality improvement that are reflected in SQUIRE and examine the major differences between SQUIRE and the initial draft guidelines. We also briefly outline the consensus process used to develop SQUIRE, including our responses to critical feedback obtained during that process. Finally, we consider the limitations of and questions about the SQUIRE guidelines, describe ancillary supporting documents and various versions currently under development, and explain plans for their dissemination, testing, and further development.

Special features of quality improvement

Unlike conceptually neat and procedurally unambiguous interventions such as drugs, tests, and procedures that directly affect the biology of disease, and are the objects of study in most clinical research, improvement is essentially a social process. Improvement is an applied science rather than an academic discipline[2]; its immediate purpose is to change human performance, rather than generate new, generalisable knowledge,[3] and it is driven primarily by experiential learning.[4 5] Like other social processes, improvement is inherently context dependent; it is reflexive, meaning that improvement interventions are repeatedly modified in response to outcome feedback, with the result that both its interventions and outcomes are relatively unstable; and it generally involves complex, multicomponent interventions. Although traditional experimental and quasi-experimental methods are important for learning whether improvement interventions change behaviour, they do not provide appropriate and effective methods for addressing the crucial pragmatic (or "realist") questions about improvement that are derived from its complex social nature: what is it about the mechanism of a particular intervention that works, for whom, and under what circumstances?[2 3 6]

Using combinations of methods that answer both the experimental and pragmatic questions is not an easy task, because those two contrasting methodologies can sometimes work at cross purposes. For example, true experimental studies are designed to minimise the confounding effects of context, such as the impact of the heterogeneity of local settings, staff and other study participants, resources, and culture, on measured outcomes. But trying to control context out of improvement interventions is both inappropriate and counterproductive because improvement interventions are inherently and strongly context dependent.[2 3] Similarly, true experimental studies require strict adherence to study protocols because it reduces the impact of many potential confounders. But rigid adherence to initial improvement plans is incompatible with an essential element of improvement, which is continued modification of those plans in response to outcome feedback (reflexiveness). We have attempted to maintain a balance between experimental and pragmatic (or realist) methodologies in the SQUIRE guidelines; both are important and necessary, and they are mutually complementary.

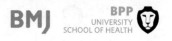

Table SQUIRE guidelines (Standards for QUality Improvement Reporting Excellence)

Title and abstract
Did you provide clear and accurate information for finding, indexing, and scanning your paper?
1. Title
(a) Indicates the article concerns the improvement of quality (broadly defined to include the safety, effectiveness, patient centeredness, timeliness, efficiency, and equity of care)
(b) States the specific aim of the intervention
(c) Specifies the study method used—for example, qualitative study or randomised cluster trial
2. Abstract
Summarises precisely all key information from various sections of the text using the abstract format of the intended publication
Introduction
Why did you start?
3. Background knowledge
Provides a brief, non-selective summary of current knowledge of the care problem being investigated and characteristics of organisations in which it occurs
4. Local problem
Describes the nature and severity of the specific local problem or system dysfunction that was investigated
5. Intended improvement
(a) Describes the specific aim (changes/improvements in care processes and patient outcomes) of the proposed intervention
(b) Specifies who (champions, supporters) and what (events, observations) triggered the decision to make changes and why now (timing)
6. Study question
States precisely the primary improvement related question and any secondary questions that the study of the intervention was designed to answer
Methods
What did you do?
7. Ethical issues
Describes ethical aspects of implementing and studying the improvement, such as privacy concerns, protection of participants' physical wellbeing, and potential author conflicts of interest, and how ethical concerns were addressed
8. Setting
Specifies how elements of the local care environment considered most likely to influence change/improvement in the involved site or sites were identified and characterised
9. Planning theintervention
(a) Describes the intervention and its component parts in sufficient detail that others could reproduce it
(b) Indicates main factors that contributed to choice of the specific intervention—eg, analysis of causes of dysfunction, matching relevant improvement experience of others with the local situation
(c) Outlines initial plans for how the intervention was to be implemented—eg, what was to be done (initial steps, functions to be accomplished by those steps, how tests of change would be used to modify intervention) and by whom (intended roles, qualifications, and training of staff)
10. Planning the study of the intervention
(a) Outlines plans for assessing how well the intervention was implemented (dose or intensity of exposure)
(b) Describes mechanisms by which intervention components were expected to cause changes and plans for testing whether those mechanisms were effective
(c) Identifies the study design (eg, observational, quasi-experimental, experimental) chosen for measuring impact of the intervention on primary and secondary outcomes, if applicable
(d) Explains plans for implementing essential aspects of the chosen study design, as described in publication guidelines for specific designs, if applicable (see for example www.equator-network.org)
(e) Describes aspects of the study design that specifically concerned internal validity (integrity of the data) and external validity (generalisability)
11. Methods of evaluation
(a) Describes instruments and procedures (qualitative, quantitative, or mixed) used to assess the effectiveness of implementation; the contributions of intervention components and context factors to effectiveness of the intervention; and primary and secondary outcomes
(b) Reports efforts to validate and test reliability of assessment instruments
(c) Explains methods used to assure data quality and adequacy—eg, blinding, repeating measurements and data extraction, training in data collection, collection of sufficient baseline measurements
12. Analysis
(a) Provides details of qualitative and quantitative (statistical) methods used to draw inferences from the data
(b) Aligns unit of analysis with level at which the intervention was implemented, if applicable
(c) Specifies degree of variability expected in implementation, change expected in primary outcome (effect size), and ability of study design (including size) to detect such effects
(d) Describes analytical methods used to show effects of time as a variable (eg, statistical process control)
Results
What did you find?
13. Outcomes
(a) Nature of setting and improvement intervention:
i) Characterises relevant elements of setting or settings (eg, geography, physical resources, organisational culture, history of change efforts) and structures and patterns of care (eg, staffing, leadership) that provided context for the intervention
ii) Explains the actual course of the intervention (eg, sequence of steps, events, or phases; type and number of participants at key points), preferably using a timeline diagram or flow chart
iii) Documents degree of success in implementing intervention components
iv) Describes how and why the initial plan evolved, and the most important lessons learnt from that evolution, particularly the effects of internal feedback from tests of change (reflexiveness)
(b) Changes in processes of care and patient outcomes associated with the intervention:
i) Presents data on changes observed in the care delivery process
ii) Presents data on changes observed in measures of patient outcome (eg, morbidity, mortality, function, patient/staff satisfaction, service utilisation, cost, care disparities)
iii) Considers benefits, harms, unexpected results, problems, failures
iv) Presents evidence regarding the strength of association between observed changes or improvements and intervention components or context factors
v) Includes summary of missing data for intervention and outcomes
Discussion

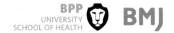

What do the findings mean?
14. Summary
(a) Summarises the most important successes and difficulties in implementing intervention components, and main changes observed in care delivery and clinical outcomes
(b) Highlights the study's particular strengths
15. Relation toother evidence
Compares and contrasts study results with relevant findings of others, drawing on broad review of the literature; use of a summary may be helpful in building on existing evidence
16. Limitations
(a) Considers possible sources of confounding, bias, or imprecision in design, measurement, and analysis that might have affected study outcomes (internal validity)
(b) Explores factors that could affect generalisability (external validity)—eg, representativeness of participants, effectiveness of implementation, dose-response effects, features of local care setting
(c) Considers likelihood that observed gains may weaken over time and describes plans, if any, for monitoring and maintaining improvement; explicitly states if such planning was not done
(d) Reviews efforts made to minimise and adjust for study limitations
(e) Assesses the effect of study limitations on interpretation and application of results
17. Interpretation
(a) Explores possible reasons for differences between observed and expected outcomes
(b) Draws inferences consistent with the strength of the data about causal mechanisms and size of observed changes, paying particular attention to components of the intervention and context factors that helped determine the intervention's effectiveness (or lack thereof), and types of settings in which this intervention is most likely to be effective
(c) Suggests steps that might be modified to improve future performance
(d) Reviews issues of opportunity cost and actual financial cost of the intervention
18. Conclusions
(a) Considers overall practical usefulness of the intervention
(b) Suggests implications of this report for further studies of improvement interventions
Other information
Were there other factors relevant to the conduct and interpretation of the study?
19. Funding
Describes funding sources, if any, and role of funding organisation in design, implementation, interpretation, and publication of study

These guidelines provide a framework for reporting formal, planned studies designed to assess the nature and effectiveness of interventions to improve the quality and safety of care. It may not always be appropriate, or even possible, to include information about every numbered guideline item in reports of original studies, but authors should at least consider every item in writing their reports.

Although each major section (introduction, methods, results, and discussion) of a published original study generally contains some information about the numbered items within that section, information about items from one section (for example, the introduction) is also often needed in other sections (for example, the discussion).

Differences between SQUIRE and draft guidelines

The SQUIRE guidelines differ in several important ways from the initial draft guidelines. Firstly, as noted, SQUIRE highlights more explicitly the essential and unique properties of improvement interventions, particularly their social nature, focus on changing performance, context dependence, complexity, nonlinearity, adaptation, and iterative modification based on outcome feedback (reflexiveness). Secondly, SQUIRE distinguishes more clearly between improvement practice (planning and implementing improvement interventions) and the evaluation of improvement projects (designing and carrying out studies to assess whether those interventions work and why they do or do not work). Thirdly, SQUIRE now explicitly specifies elements of study design that make it possible to assess both whether improvement interventions work (by minimising bias and confounding) and why interventions are or are not effective (by identifying the effects of context and identifying mechanisms of change). And finally, SQUIRE explicitly addresses the often confusing ethical dimensions of improvement projects and improvement studies.[7] [8] Other differences between SQUIRE and the draft guidelines are available on the SQUIRE website (www.squire-statement.org).

The development process

The SQUIRE development process was designed to produce consensus among a broad constituency of experts and users on both the content and format of guideline items. It proceeded along the following six lines. We first obtained informal feedback on the utility, strengths, and limitations of the draft guidelines from potential authors in a series of seminars at national and international meetings, as well as from experienced publication guideline developers at the organisational meeting of the EQUATOR network.[9] Authors, peer reviewers, and journal editors then "road tested" the draft guidelines as a working tool for editing and revising submitted manuscripts.[10] [11] Next, we solicited and published written commentaries on the initial version of the guidelines.[12] [13] [14] [15] [16] We also did a literature review on epistemology, methodology, and the evaluation of complex interventions, particularly in social sciences. In April 2007, we subjected the draft guidelines to intensive analysis, comment, and recommendations for change at a two day meeting of 30 stakeholders. After that meeting, we obtained further critical appraisal of the guidelines through three cycles of a Delphi process with an international group of more than 50 consultants.

Informal feedback

Informal input about the draft guidelines from authors and peer reviewers raised four particularly relevant issues: uncertainty as to which studies the guidelines apply; the possibility that their use might force quality improvement reports into a rigid, narrow format; the concern that their slavish application might result in lengthy and unreadable reports that are indiscriminately laden with detail; and difficulty knowing if, when, and how other publication guidelines should be used in conjunction with guidelines for reporting quality improvement studies.

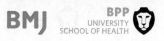

Deciding when to use the guidelines

Publications on improvement in health care are emerging in four general categories: empirical studies on the effectiveness of quality improvement interventions; stories, theories, and frameworks; literature reviews and syntheses; and the development and testing of improvement related tools and methods (L Rubenstein et al, unpublished data). Our guideline development process has made it clear that the SQUIRE guidelines can and should apply to reports in the first category: original, planned studies of interventions that are designed to improve clinical outcomes by delivering clinically proved care measures more appropriately, effectively, and efficiently.

Forcing articles into a rigid format

Publication guidelines are often referred to as checklists because, like other such documents, they serve as aide-mémoires, which have proved increasingly valuable in managing information in complex systems.[17] Rigid or mechanical application of checklists can prevent users from making sense of complex information.[18][19] At the same time, however (and paradoxically), checklists, like all constraints and reminders, can serve as important drivers for creativity. The SQUIRE guidelines must therefore always be understood and used as signposts, not shackles.[20]

Creating longer articles

Improvement is a complex undertaking, and its evaluation can produce substantial amounts of qualitative and quantitative information. Adding irrelevant information simply to "cover" guideline items would be counterproductive; on the other hand, added length that makes reports of improvement studies more complete, coherent, usable, and systematic helps the guidelines meet a principal aim of SQUIRE. Publishing portions of improvement studies only in electronic form can make the content of long articles publicly available while conserving space in print publication.

Conjoint use with other publication guidelines

Most other biomedical publication guidelines are designed to improve the reporting of studies that use specific experimental designs. The SQUIRE guidelines, in contrast, are concerned with the reporting of studies in a defined content area—improvement and safety. These two guideline types are therefore complementary, rather than redundant or conflicting. When appropriate, other specific design related guidelines can and should be used in conjunction with SQUIRE.

Formal commentaries

The written commentaries provided both supportive and critical input on the draft guidelines.[12][13][14][15][16] One suggested that the guidelines' "pragmatic" focus was an important complement to guidelines for reporting traditional experimental clinical science.[12] The guidelines were also seen as a potentially valuable instrument for strengthening the design and conduct of improvement research, resulting in greater synergy with improvement practice[15] and increasing the feasibility of combining improvement studies in systematic reviews. However, other commentaries on the draft guidelines raised concerns: that they were inattentive to racial and ethnic disparities in care[14]; that their proposed introduction, methods, results, and discussion (IMRaD) structure might be incompatible with the reality that

improvement interventions are designed to change over time[13]; and that their use could result in a "dumbing down" of improvement science.[16] Our responses to these concerns are as follows.

Health disparities

We do not believe it would be useful, even if it were possible, to address every relevant content issue in a concise set of quality improvement reporting guidelines. We do agree, however, that disparities in care are not considered often enough in improvement work, and that improvement initiatives should address this important issue whenever possible. We have therefore highlighted this issue in the SQUIRE guidelines (table, item 13.b.1).

IMRaD structure

The study protocols traditionally described in the methods section of clinical trials are rigidly fixed, as required by the dictates of experimental design.[21] In contrast, improvement is a reflexive learning process—that is, improvement interventions are most effective when they are modified in response to outcome feedback. On these grounds, it has been suggested that reporting improvement interventions in the IMRaD format logically requires multiple, sequential pairs of methods and results sections, one pair for each iteration of the evolving intervention.[13] We maintain, however, that the changing, reflexive nature of improvement does not exempt improvement studies from answering the four fundamental questions required in all scholarly inquiry: Why did you start? What did you do? What did you find? What does it mean? These same questions define the four elements of the IMRaD framework.[22][23]

Although some authors and editors might understandably choose to use a modified IMRaD format that involves a series of small sequential methods and results sections, we believe that approach is often both unnecessary and confusing. We therefore continue to support describing the initial improvement plan, and the theory (mechanism) on which it is based, in a single methods section. Because the changes in interventions over time and the learning that comes from making those changes are themselves important outcomes in improvement projects, in our view they belong collectively in a single results section.[1]

Dumbing down improvement reports

The declared purpose of all publication guidelines is to improve the completeness and transparency of reporting. Because it is precisely these characteristics of reporting that make it possible to detect weak, sloppy, or poorly designed studies, it is difficult to understand how use of the draft guidelines might lead to a dumbing down of improvement science. The underlying concern here therefore seems to have less to do with transparency than with the inference that the draft guidelines failed to require sufficiently rigorous standards of evidence.[16][21] We recognise that those traditional experimental standards are powerful instruments for protecting the integrity of outcome measurements, largely by minimising selection bias.[21][24] Although those standards are necessary in improvement studies, they are not sufficient because they fail to take into account the particular epistemology of improvement that derives from its applied purpose and social nature. As noted, the SQUIRE guidelines specify methodologies that are appropriate for both experimental and pragmatic (or realist) evaluation of improvement programmes.

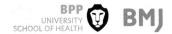

Consensus meeting of editors and research scholars

With support from the Robert Wood Johnson Foundation, we undertook an intensive critical appraisal of the draft guidelines at a two day meeting in April 2007. Thirty participants attended, including clinicians, improvement professionals, epidemiologists, clinical researchers, and journal editors, several from outside the United States. Before the meeting, we sent participants a reading list and a concept paper on the epistemology of improvement. In plenary and small group sessions, participants critically discussed and debated the content and wording of every item in the draft guidelines and recommended changes. They also provided input on plans for dissemination, adoption, and future uses of the guidelines. Working from transcribed audiorecordings of all meeting sessions and flip charts listing the key discussion points, a coordinating group (the authors of this paper) then revised, refined, and expanded the draft guidelines.

Delphi process

Following the consensus meeting, we circulated sequential revisions of the guidelines for further comment and suggestions in three cycles of a Delphi process. The group involved in that process included the meeting participants and roughly 20 additional expert consultants. We then surveyed all participants as to their willingness to endorse the final consensus version (SQUIRE).

Limitations and questions

The SQUIRE guidelines have been characterised as providing both too little and too much information: too little, because they fail to represent adequately the many unique and nuanced issues in the practice and evaluation of improvement[2 3 4 12 13 14 15 16 21 24 25]; too much, because the detail and density of the item descriptions might seem intimidating to authors. We recognise that the SQUIRE item descriptions are much more detailed than those of some other publication guidelines. In our view, however, the complexity of the improvement process, plus the relative unfamiliarity of improvement interventions and of the methods for evaluating them, justify that level of detail, particularly in light of the diverse backgrounds of people working to improve health care. Moreover, the level of detail in the SQUIRE guidelines is quite similar to that of recently published guidelines for reporting observational studies, which also involve considerable complexities of study design.[26] To increase the usability of SQUIRE, we are making available a shortened electronic version on the SQUIRE website, accompanied by a glossary of terms used in the item descriptions that may be unfamiliar to users.

Applying SQUIRE

Authors' interest in using publication guidelines increases when journals make them part of the peer review and editorial process. We therefore encourage the widest possible use of the SQUIRE guidelines by editors. Unfortunately, little is known about the most effective ways to apply publication guidelines in practice. Therefore, editors have been forced to learn from experience how to use other publication guidelines, and the specifics of their use vary widely from journal to journal. We also lack systematic knowledge of how authors can use publication guidelines most productively. Our experience suggests, however, that SQUIRE is most helpful if authors simply keep the general content of the guideline items in mind as they write their initial drafts, then refer to the details of individual items as they critically appraise what they have written during the revision process. The most effective way to use publication guidelines in practice seems to us to be an empirical question; we therefore strongly encourage editors and authors to collect, analyse, and report their experiences in using SQUIRE and other publication guidelines.

Current and future directions

A SQUIRE explanation and elaboration document has been published elsewhere.[27] Like other such documents,[28 29 30 31] this document provides much of the necessary depth and detail that cannot be included in a set of concise guideline items. It presents the rationale for including each guideline item in SQUIRE, along with published examples of reporting for each item, and commentary on the strengths and weaknesses of those examples.

The SQUIRE website (www.squire-statement.org) will provide an authentic electronic home for the guidelines and a medium for their progressive refinement. We also intend the site to serve as an interactive electronic community for authors, students, teachers, reviewers, and editors who are interested in the emerging body of scholarly and practical knowledge on improvement.

Although the primary purpose of SQUIRE is to enhance the reporting of improvement studies, we believe the guidelines can also be useful for educational purposes, particularly for understanding and exploring further the epistemology of improvement and the methods for evaluating improvement work. We believe, similarly, that SQUIRE can help in planning and executing improvement interventions, carrying out studies of those interventions, and developing skill in writing about improvement. We encourage these uses, as well as efforts to assess SQUIRE's impact on the completeness and transparency of published improvement studies[32 33] and to obtain empirical evidence that individual guideline items contribute materially to the value of published information in improvement science.

We thank Rosemary Gibson and Laura Leviton for support of this project; the Institute for Healthcare Improvement for help in hosting the review meeting in Cambridge; and Joy McAvoy for administrative work in coordinating the entire development process.

The following people contributed critical input to the guidelines during their development: Kay Dickersin, Donald Goldmann, Peter Goetzsche, Gordon Guyatt, Hal Luft, Kathryn McPherson, Victor Montori, Dale Needham, Duncan Neuhauser, Kaveh Shojania, Vincenza Snow, Ed Wagner, Val Weber. The following participants in the consensus process also provided critical input on the guidelines, and endorsed the final version. Their endorsements are personal and do not imply endorsement by any group, organisation, or agency: David Aron, Virginia Barbour, Jesse Berlin, Steven Berman, Donald Berwick, Maureen Bisognano, Andrew Booth, Isabelle Boutron, Peter Buerhaus, Marshall Chin, Benjamin Crabtree, Linda Cronenwett, Mary Dixon-Woods, Brad Doebbling, Denise Dougherty, Martin Eccles, Susan Ellenberg, William Garrity, Lawrence Green, Trisha Greenhalgh, Linda Headrick, Susan Horn, Julie Johnson, Kate Koplan, David Korn, Uma Kotegal, Seth Landefield, Elizabeth Loder, Joanne Lynn, Susan Mallett, Peter Margolis, Diana Mason, Don Minckler, Brian Mittman, Cynthia Mulrow, Eugene Nelson, Paul Plsek, Peter Pronovost, Lloyd Provost, Philippe Ravaud, Roger Resar, Jane Roessner, John-Arne Røttingen, Lisa Rubenstein, Harold Sox, Ted Speroff, Richard Thomson, Erik von Elm, Elizabeth Wager, Doug Wakefield, Bill Weeks, Hywel Williams, Sankey Williams. All authors contributed substantively to the ideas developed in the SQUIRE project, and provided critical input on the guidelines. All authors reviewed, commented on, and approved the final version of the paper. FD drafted the paper and is the guarantor.

Funding: The SQUIRE project was supported in part by a grant from the Robert Wood Johnson Foundation (RWJF grant number 58073).

Competing interests: None declared.

Provenance and peer review: Not commissioned; externally peer reviewed.

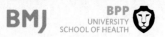

1   Davidoff F, Batalden P. Toward stronger evidence on quality improvement. Draft publication guidelines: the beginning of a consensus project. *Qual Saf Health Care* 2005;14:319-25.

2   Walshe K, Freeman T. Effectiveness of quality improvement: learning from evaluations. *Qual Saf Health Care* 2002;11:85-7.

3   Pawson R, Greenhalgh T, Harvey G, Walshe K. Realist review—a new method of systematic review designed for complex policy interventions. *J Health Serv Res Policy* 2005;10(suppl 1):21-34.

4   Batalden P, Davidoff F. Teaching quality improvement: the devil is in the details [Editorial]. *JAMA* 2007;298:1059-61.

5   Kolb DA. *Experiential learning. experience as the source of learning and development.* Englewood Cliffs, NJ: Prentice-Hall, 1984.

6   Pawson R, Tilley N. *Realistic evaluation.* Thousand Oaks, CA: SAGE, 1997.

7   Jennings B, Baily MA, Bottrell M, Lynn J, eds. *Health care quality improvement: ethical and regulatory issues.* Garrison, NY: Hastings Center, 2007.

8   Lynn J, Baily MA, Bottrell M, Jennings B, Levine RJ, Davidoff F, et al. The ethics of using quality improvement methods in health care. *Ann Intern Med* 2007;146:666-73.

9   EQUATOR Network. Enhancing the QUality And Transparency Of health Research. www.equator-network.org.

10 Janisse T. A next step: reviewer feedback on quality improvement publication guidelines. *Permanente J* 2007;11:1.

11 Quality and Safety in Health Care. *Guidelines for authors: guidelines for submitting more extensive quality research.* http://qshc.bmj.com/ifora/article_type.dtl#extensive.

12 Berwick DM. Broadening the view of evidence-based medicine. *Qual Saf Health Care* 2005;14:315-6.

13 Thomson RG. Consensus publication guidelines: the next step in the science of quality improvement? *Qual Saf Health Care* 2005;14:317-8.

14 Chin MH, Chien AT. Reducing racial and ethnic disparities in health care: an integral part of quality improvement scholarship. *Qual Saf Health Care* 2006;15:79-80.

15 Baker GR. Strengthening the contribution of quality improvement research to evidence based health care. *Qual Saf Health Care* 2006;15:150-1.

16 Pronovost P, Wachter R. Proposed standards for quality improvement research and publication: one step forward and two steps back. *Qual Saf Health Care* 2006;15:152-3.

17 Gawande A. The checklist: if something so simple can transform intensive care, what else can it do? *New Yorker* 2007:86-101.

18 Rennie D. Reporting randomized controlled trials. An experiment and a call for responses from readers [Editorial] *JAMA* 1995;273:1054-5.

19 Williams JW Jr, Holleman DR Jr, Samsa GP, Simel DL. Randomized controlled trial of 3 vs 10 days of trimethoprim/sulfamethoxazole for acute maxillary sinusitis. *JAMA* 1995;273:1015-21.

20 Rutledge A. *On creativity.* www.alistapart/articles/oncreativity.

21 Shadish WR, Cook TD, Campbell DT. *Experimental and quasi-experimental designs for generalized causal inference.* New York: Houghton-Mifflin, 2002.

22 Day RA. The origins of the scientific paper: the IMRaD format. *J Am Med Writers Ass* 1989;4:16-8.

23 Huth EJ. The research paper: general principles for structure and content. In: *Writing and publishing in medicine.* 3rd ed. Philadelphia: Williams and Wilkins, 1999:63-73.

24 Jadad AR, Enkin MW. *Randomized controlled trials. Questions, answers, and musings* . 2nd ed. London: Blackwell/BMJ Books, 2007.

25 Glouberman S, Zimmerman B. *Complicated and complex systems: what would successful reform of medicine look like? Discussion paper No 8* . Commission on the Future of Health Care in Canada, 2002. www.change-ability.ca/Health_Care_Commission_DP8.pdf.

26 STROBE Initiative. The strengthening the reporting of observational studies in epidemiology (STROBE) statement: guidelines for reporting observational studies. *Ann Intern Med* 2007;147:573-7.

27 Ogrinc G, Mooney SE, Estrada C, Foster T, Hall LW, Huizinga MM, et al. The SQUIRE (Standards for Quality Improvement Reporting Excellence) guidelines for quality improvement reporting: explanation and elaboration. *Qual Saf Health Care* 2008;17(suppl 1):i13-32

28 CONSORT Group (Consolidated Standards of Reporting Trials). The revised CONSORT statement for reporting randomized trials: explanation and elaboration. *Ann Intern Med* 2001;134:663-94.

29 Standards for Reporting of Diagnostic Accuracy. The STARD statement for reporting studies of diagnostic accuracy: explanation and elaboration. *Clin Chem* 2003;49:7-18.

30 STROBE Initiative. Strengthening the reporting of observational studies in epidemiology (STROBE): explanation and elaboration. *Ann Intern Med* 2007;147:w163-94.

31 Keech A, Gebski V, Pike R. *Interpreting and reporting clinical trials. A guide to the CONSORT statement and the principles of randomized trials* . Sydney: Australian Medical Publishing Company, 2007.

32 Plint AC, Moher D, Morrison A, Schulz K, Altman DG, Hill C, et al. Does the CONSORT checklist improve the quality of reports of randomised controlled trials? A systematic review. *Med J Aust* 2006;185:263-7.

33 CONSORT Group. Value of flow diagrams in reports of randomized controlled trials. *JAMA* 2001;285:1996-9.

More titles in
The BMJ Series

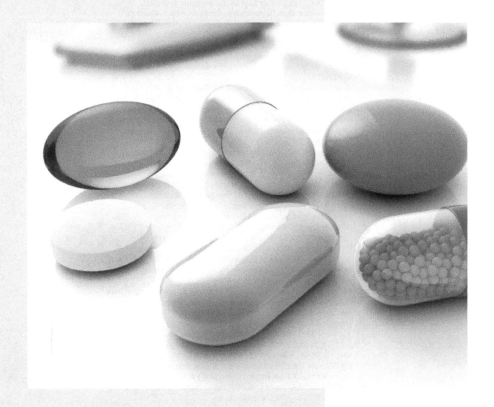

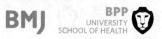
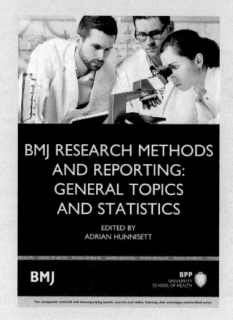
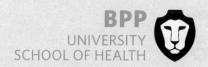

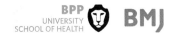

More titles in The BMJ Easily Missed? Series

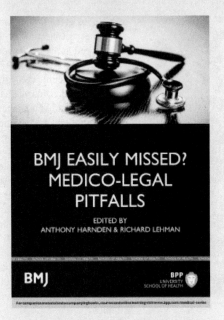

BMJ EASILY MISSED? MEDICO-LEGAL PITFALLS

EDITED BY
ANTHONY HARNDEN & RICHARD LEHMAN

£29.99
January 2016
Paperback
978-1-472738-95-0

This book groups together a series of useful articles on cancer diagnoses that may be easily missed at first presentation in primary care together with other articles on the early diagnosis of important infections and inflammatory conditions. The spectrum of conditions ranges from colorectal, lung, ovarian and pancreatic cancers to primary HIV infection, infective endocarditis, giant cell arteritis and appendicitis. All articles describe data to support the assertion that the conditions are often overlooked in primary care and that failure to recognise the diagnosis may have serious implications for the patient. Subjects dealt with include:

- Diagnoses that are important not to miss in primary care
- Evidence that the diagnoses are easily missed in primary care
- Succinct articles with specific learning points and take home messages
- Spectrum of important cancer, infective and inflammatory conditions

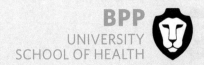

BPP UNIVERSITY SCHOOL OF HEALTH

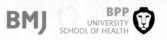
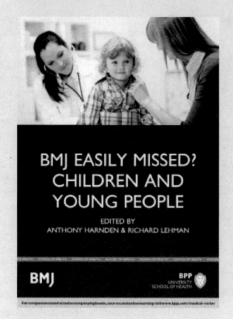
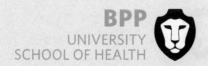

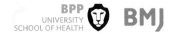
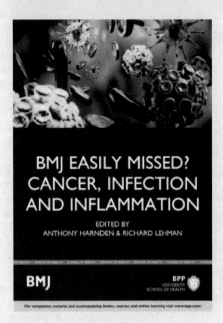
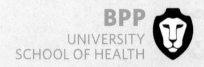

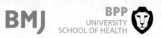
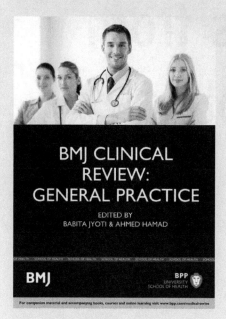
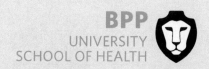

More titles from BPP School of Health

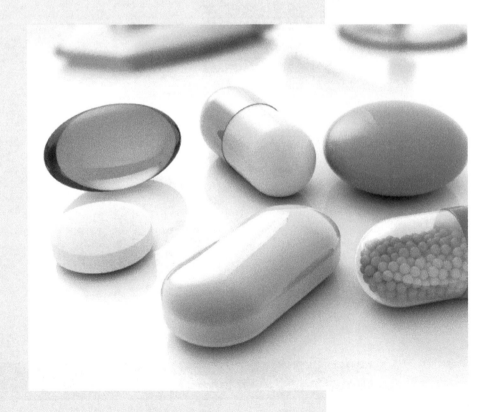

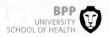

More titles in The Progressing your Medical Career Series

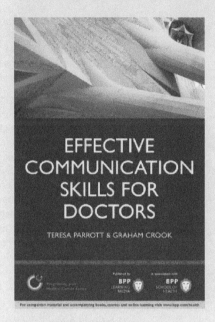

£19.99

September 2011

Paperback

978-1-445379-56-2

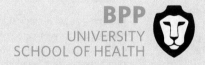

Would you like to know how to improve your communication skills? Are you looking for a clearly written book which explores all aspects of effective medical communication?

There is an urgent need to improve doctors' communication skills. Research has shown that poor communication can contribute to patient dissatisfaction, lack of compliance and increased medico-legal problems. Improved communication skills will impact positively on all of these areas.

The last fifteen years have seen unprecedented changes in medicine and the role of doctors. Effective communication skills are vital to these new roles. But communication is not just related to personality. Skills can be learned which can make your communication more effective, and help you to improve your relationships with patients, their families and fellow doctors.

This book shows how to learn those skills and outlines why we all need to communicate more effectively. Healthcare is increasingly a partnership. Change is happening at all levels, from government directives to patient expectations. Communication is a bridge between the wisdom of the past and the vision of the future.

Readers of this book can also gain free access to an online module which upon successful completion can download a certificate for their portfolio of learning/ Revalidation/CPD records.

This easy-to-read guide will help medical students and doctors at all stages of their careers improve their communication within a hospital environment.

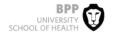
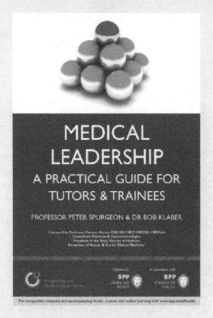
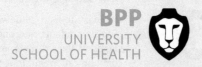

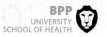

More Titles in The Progressing Your Medical Career Series

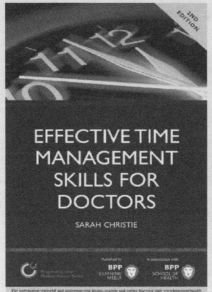

£19.99

February 2012

Paperback

978-1-445390-15-4

Do you find it difficult to achieve a work-life balance? Would you like to know how you can become more effective with the time you have?

With the introduction of the European Working Time Directive, which will severely limit the hours in the working week, it is more important than ever that doctors improve their personal effectiveness and time management skills. This interactive book will enable you to focus on what activities are needlessly taking up your time and what steps you can take to manage your time better.

By taking the time to read through, complete the exercises and follow the advice contained within this book you will begin to:

- Understand where your time is being needlessly wasted
- Discover how to be more assertive and learn how to say 'No'
- Set yourself priorities and stick to them
- Learn how to complete tasks more efficiently
- Plan better so you can spend more time doing the things you enjoy

In recent years, with the introduction of the NHS Plan and Lord Darzi's commitment to improve the quality of healthcare provision, there is a need for doctors to become more effective within their working environment. This book will offer you the chance to regain some clarity on how you actually spend your time and give you the impetus to ensure you achieve the tasks and goals which are important to you.

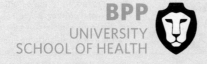

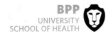
More titles in The Essential Clinical Handbook Series

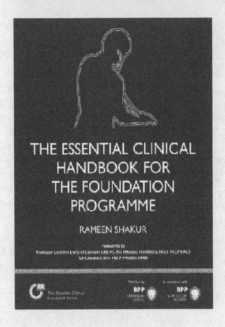

THE ESSENTIAL CLINICAL
HANDBOOK FOR
THE FOUNDATION
PROGRAMME

RAMEEN SHAKUR

£24.99

October 2011

Paperback

978-1-445381-63-3

Unsure of what clinical competencies you must gain to successfully complete the Foundation Programme? Unclear on how to ensure your ePortfolio is complete to enable your progression to ST training?

This up-to-date clinical handbook is aimed at current foundation doctors and clinical medical students and provides a comprehensive companion to help you in the day-to-day management of patients on the ward. Together with this it is the first handbook to also outline clearly how to gain the core clinical competencies required for successful completion of the Foundation Programme. Written by doctors for doctors this comprehensive handbook explains how to successfully manage all of the common cases you will face during the Foundation Programme and:

- Introduces the Foundation Programme and what is expected of a new doctor especially with the introduction of Modernising Medical Careers
- Illustrates clearly the best way to manage, step-by-step, over 150 commonly encountered clinical diseases, including NICE guidelines to ensure a gold standard of clinical care is achieved.
- Describes how to successfully gain the core clinical competencies within Medicine and Surgery including an extensive list of differentials and conditions explained
- Explores the various radiology images you will encounter and how to interpret them
- Tells you how to succeed in the assessment methods used including DOP's, Mini-CEX's and CBD's
- Has step by step diagrammatic guide to doing common clinical procedures competently and safely.
- Outlines how to ensure your ePortfolio is maintained properly to ensure successful completion of the Foundation Programme.
- Provides tips and advice on how to start preparing now to ensure you are fully prepared and have the competitive edge for your CMT/ST application.

The introduction of the e-Portfolio as part of the Foundation Programme has paved the way for foundation doctors to take charge of their own learning and portfolio. Through following the expert guidance laid down in this handbook you will give yourself the best possible chance of progressing successfully through to CMT/ST training.

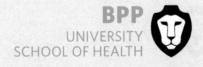

BPP
UNIVERSITY
SCHOOL OF HEALTH

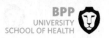

More titles in The Essential Clinical Handbook Series

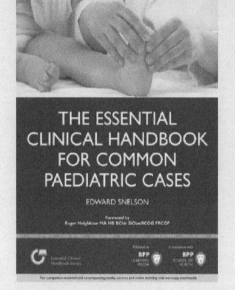

THE ESSENTIAL CLINICAL HANDBOOK FOR COMMON PAEDIATRIC CASES

EDWARD SNELSON

Foreword by
Roger Neighbour MA MB BChir DObstRCOG FRCGP

£24.99
September 2011
Paperback
978-1-445379-60-9

Not sure what to do when faced with a crying baby and demanding parent on the ward? Would you like a definitive guide on how to manage commonly encountered paediatric cases?

This clear and concise clinical handbook has been written to help healthcare professionals approach the initial assessment and management of paediatric cases commonly encountered by Junior Doctors, GPs, GP Specialty Trainees and allied healthcare professionals. The children who make paediatrics so fun, can also make it more than a little daunting for even the most confident person. This insightful guide has been written based on the author's extensive experience within both a General Practice and hospital setting.

Intended as a practical guide to common paediatric problems it will increase confidence and satisfaction in managing these conditions. Each chapter provides a clear structure for investigating potential paediatric illnesses including clinical and non-clinical advice covering: background, how to assess, pitfalls to avoid, FAQs and what to tell parents. This helpful guide provides:

- A problem/symptom based approach to common paediatric conditions
- An essential guide for any doctor assessing children on the front line
- Provides easy-to-follow and step-by-step guidance on how to approach different paediatric conditions
- Useful both as a textbook and a quick reference guide when needed on the ward

This engaging and easy to use guide will provide you with the knowledge, skills and confidence required to effectively diagnose and manage commonly encountered paediatric cases both within a primary and secondary care setting.

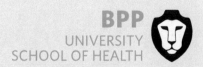

BPP
UNIVERSITY
SCHOOL OF HEALTH

www.bpp.com/medical-series

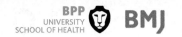